The Obstetric Hematology
Manual

The Obstetric Hematology Manual

Second Edition

Edited by

Sue Pavord
Oxford University Hospitals NHS Foundation Trust

Beverley Hunt
Guy's and St. Thomas' NHS Foundation Trust and King's College, London

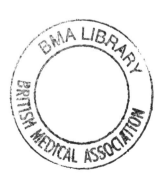

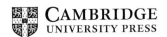
CAMBRIDGE
UNIVERSITY PRESS

CAMBRIDGE
UNIVERSITY PRESS

University Printing House, Cambridge CB2 8BS, United Kingdom

One Liberty Plaza, 20th Floor, New York, NY 10006, USA

477 Williamstown Road, Port Melbourne, VIC 3207, Australia

314–321, 3rd Floor, Plot 3, Splendor Forum, Jasola District Centre, New Delhi – 110025, India

79 Anson Road, #06–04/06, Singapore 079906

Cambridge University Press is part of the University of Cambridge.

It furthers the University's mission by disseminating knowledge in the pursuit of education, learning, and research at the highest international levels of excellence.

www.cambridge.org
Information on this title: www.cambridge.org/9781107125605
DOI: 10.1017/9781316410837

© Cambridge University Press 2018

First published 2010
Second edition 2018

Printed in the United Kingdom by Clays, St Ives plc

A catalog record for this publication is available from the British Library.

Library of Congress Cataloging-in-Publication Data
Names: Pavord, Sue, editor. | Hunt, Beverley J., editor.
Title: The obstetric hematology manual / edited by Sue Pavord, Beverley J. Hunt.
Description: Second edition. | Cambridge, United Kingdom ; New York, NY : Cambridge University Press, 2017. | Includes bibliographical references and index.
Identifiers: LCCN 2017057520 | ISBN 9781107125605 (hardback : alk. paper)
Subjects: | MESH: Pregnancy Complications, Hematologic | Postpartum Hemorrhage | Hemostatic Techniques
Classification: LCC RG580.H47 | NLM WQ 252 | DDC 618.3/261–dc23
LC record available at https://lccn.loc.gov/2017057520

ISBN 978-1-107-12560-5 Hardback

....

To our families

Contents

vii

Contributors

Sahra Ali
Department of Haematology, Queen's Center, Castle Hill Hospital Hull and East Yorkshine Hospitals NHS Trust, Hull, UK

Susan Bewley
Women's Services, Guy's and St Thomas' NHS Foundation Trust, London, UK

Annette Briley
Maternal and Fetal Research, Guy's and St Thomas' NHS Foundation Trust, London, UK

Peter Collins
Institute of Infection and Immunity, School of Medicine, Cardiff University, Cardiff, UK

Catherine Collinson
Department of Anaesthesia, Royal Infirmary of Edinburgh, Edinburgh, UK

Rachel Collis
Department of Anaesthetics, Cardiff and Vale University Health Board, Cardiff, UK

Nicola Curry
Oxford Haemophilia and Thrombosis Center, Oxford University Hospitals NHS Foundation Trust, Oxford, UK

Athanasios Diamantopoulos
Department of Radiology, Guy's and St Thomas' NHS Foundation Trust, London, UK

Ian Greer
School of Medicine, The University of Manchester, Manchester, UK

Claire Harrison
Department of Haematology, Guy's and St Thomas' NHS Foundation Trust, London, UK

Shirley Henderson
Department of Haematology, Oxford University Hospitals NHS Foundation Trust, Oxford, UK

Jo Howard
Department of Haematology, Guy's and St Thomas' NHS Foundation Trust, London, UK

Beverley Hunt
Department of Haematology, Guy's and St Thomas' NHS Foundation Trust, London, UK

Narayan Karunanithy
Department of Radiology, Guy's and St Thomas' NHS Foundation Trust, London, UK

Alesia Khan
Department of Haematology, Guy's and St Thomas' NHS Foundation Trust, London, UK

Amma Kyei-Mensah
Department of Obstetrics & Gynaecology, Whittington Health NHS Trust, London, UK

Anna Lawin-O'Brien
Department of Obstetrics, Imperial College Healthcare NHS Trust, London, UK

Eleftheria Lefkou
Department of Haematology, Hippokrateion University Hospital of Thessaloniki, Greece

Andrew Ling
Department of Anaesthesia, University Hospitals of Leicester NHS Trust, Leicester, UK

Karyn Longmuir
Department of Haematology, Kettering General Hospital, Kettering, UK

Hamish Lyall
Department of Haematology, Norfolk and Norwich University Hospitals NHS Foundation Trust, Norwich, UK

Alec McEwan
Department of Obstetrics and Gynaecology, Nottingham University Hospitals NHS Trust, Nottingham, UK

Claire McLintock
National Women's Health Auckland City Hospital, Auckland, New Zealand

Saskia Middeldorp
Department of Vascular Medicine, Academic Medical Centre, University of Amsterdam, The Netherlands

Carolyn Millar
Department of Haematology, Imperial Hospital, London, UK

Andrew Mumford
Bristol Haemophilia Centre, Bristol Haematology and Oncology Center, Bristol, UK

Michael Murphy
NHS Blood & Transplant, Oxford University Hospitals NHS Foundation Trust and University of Oxford, Oxford, UK

Bethan Myers
Department of Haematology, University Hospitals of Leicester NHS Trust and Lincoln Country Hospital, Leicester, UK

Catherine Nelson-Piercy
Department of Obstetrics, Guy's and St Thomas' NHS Foundation Trust, London, UK

Pat O'Brien
Department of Obstetrics, University College London Hospitals NHS Foundation Trust, London, UK

Christina Oppenheimer
Department of Obstetrics and Gynaecology, University of Leicester, Leicester, UK

Sue Pavord
Department of Haematology, Oxford University Hospitals NHS Foundation Trust, Oxford, UK

Emma Prescott
Whittington Health NHS Trust, London, UK

Seonaid Pye
Department of Haematology, Charing Cross Hospital, London, UK

Margaret Ramsay
Department of Obstetrics and Gynaecology, Nottingham University Hospitals NHS Trust, Nottingham, UK

Rachel Rayment
Department of Haematology, Cardiff and Vale University Health Board, Wales, UK

Susan Robinson
Department of Haematology, Guy's and St Thomas' NHS Foundation Trust, London, UK

Noemi Roy
Department of Haematology, Oxford University Hospitals NHS Foundation Trust, Oxford, UK

Nina Salooja
Faculty of Medicine, Imperial College, London, UK

Luuk Scheres
Department of Vascular Medicine, Academic Medical Centre, University of Amsterdam, The Netherlands

Savino Sciascia
Department of Haematology, Guy's and St Thomas' NHS Foundation Trust, London, UK

Marie Scully
Department of Haematology, University College London Hospitals NHS Foundation Trust, London, UK

Farrukh Shah
Department of Haematology, University College London Hospitals NHS Foundation Trust, London, UK

Paul Sharpe
Department of Anaesthesia, University Hospitals of Leicester NHS Trust, Leicester, UK

Gill Swallow
Department of Haematology, Nottingham University Hospitals NHS Trust, Nottingham, UK

Andrew Thomson
Department of Obstetrics and Gynaecology, Royal Alexandra Hospital, Paisley, UK

Isobel Walker
Department of Haematology, Glasgow Royal Infirmary, NHS Greater Glasgow and Clyde, Glasgow, UK

Arlene Wise
Department of Anaesthesia, Royal Infirmary of Edinburgh, Edinburgh, UK

Josh Wright
Department of Haematology, Royal Hallamshire Hospital, Sheffield, UK

Xiao-Yin Zhang
Department of Haematology, Oxford University Hospitals NHS Foundation Trust, Oxford, UK

Preface to the Second Edition

We are delighted to have been asked to produce a second edition of *The Obstetric Hematology Manual*. Since the publication of the first edition, this high-stakes area of medicine has continued to thrive as a specialty, with designated hematologists and multidisciplinary clinics established in many UK Trusts and with an expanding international network. Additionally, obstetric hematological problems increasingly frequent the membership examinations for the Royal College of Pathologists and the Royal College of Obstetricians and Gynaecologists. This book is aimed at clinicians at all levels; it is intended to be highly practical, pulling together research, insights, and guidelines. It is larger than the first edition, reflecting the growth in knowledge and important advances in the field over the last 5 years; each chapter has been revised and new chapters have been added. We have chosen authors who are leaders in their field and represent practice across the globe.

The mutual impact of hematological disease on pregnancy continues to challenge and stimulate us in our pursuit of best care for our patients. The physiological changes that occur during pregnancy, to meet the needs of the developing fetus and to ensure safe delivery, may lead to complications in vulnerable patients. For example, close proximity of fetal and maternal circulations enables effective transfer of nutrients and oxygen, but the increased demand for iron and other hematinics by the growing fetus can cause significant maternal deficiencies. Furthermore, transfer of certain maternal substances and drugs can have disastrous consequences for the baby, thus limiting treatment options for many hematological diseases. Similarly, passage of fetal antigenic material into the maternal circulation may cause alloimmune sensitization, with potential destruction of fetal red cells or platelets. Exciting new management strategies for these conditions are discussed in this book.

The considerable increase in uterine blood flow and vascular compliance needed to maintain the blood supply to the developing fetus can cause significant hemorrhage at the time of placental separation. Conversely, the alteration of coagulation factors necessary to combat this risk inadvertently increases the potential for systemic thromboembolic events. These two catastrophes remain the leading causes of direct maternal death, although with improved knowledge and awareness, the incidence is slowly declining. In these, like all other areas of obstetric hematology, we continue to strive for good outcomes.

We hope this edition will be helpful to those experienced in obstetric hematology and will enthuse those who are new to the area. We aim to encourage and inspire clinicians to immerse themselves in this hugely rewarding specialty.

Sue Pavord
Beverley Hunt

Normal Cellular Changes during Pregnancy and the Puerperium

Margaret Ramsay

Introduction

There are both subtle and substantial changes in hematological parameters during pregnancy and the puerperium, orchestrated by changes in the hormonal milieu. A thorough understanding of these is important to avoid both over- and under-diagnosing abnormalities. Some of the quoted reference ranges may differ among centers, depending on laboratory techniques. However, the principles of recognizing physiological changes can still be applied.

Red Cells

During pregnancy, the total blood volume increases by 1.5 L, mainly to supply the needs of the new vascular bed. Almost 1 L of blood is contained within the uterus and maternal blood spaces of the placenta. Expansion of plasma volume by 25–80% is one of the most marked changes, reaching its maximum by mid-pregnancy. Red cell mass also increases by 10–20%, but the net result is that hemoglobin (Hb) concentration falls[1]. Typically, this is by 10–20 g/L by the late second trimester and stabilizes thereafter. Women who take iron supplements have less pronounced Hb changes, as they increase their red cell mass proportionately more than those without dietary supplements; typically, the increase is 30% over pre-pregnancy values[1].

It is hard to define a normal reference range for Hb during pregnancy and the limit for diagnosing anemia. The World Health Organization has suggested that anemia is present in pregnancy when Hb concentration is <110 g/L. However, large studies in healthy Caucasian women taking iron supplements from midpregnancy found Hb values in the early third trimester to be 104–135 g/L (2.5th–97.5th centiles)[2]. A randomized, placebo-controlled trial of iron supplementation in pregnancy found that Hb levels in those who had received 66 mg ferrous iron per day from 9 to 18 weeks' gestation were significantly higher from the beginning of the second trimester to 8 weeks postpartum[3].

Studies from other ethnic populations have documented lower third trimester Hb concentrations, which may be attributable to the women entering pregnancy with poor iron stores or with dietary deficiencies of iron and folic acid. However, a study of healthy women in China who were all given iron, folate, and vitamin B_{12} supplements during pregnancy found Hb levels of 95–130 g/L in the second trimester and 96–135 g/L in the third trimester (5th–95th centiles), so there may be genuine racial differences[4].

Women living at an altitude of 2240 m above sea level in Mexico City were found to have a progressive drop in Hb levels during pregnancy, from 122 to 152 g/L in the first trimester to 111–138 g/L in the early third trimester and 108–142 g/L by term (5th–95th centiles)[5]. All these women took iron, folate, and vitamin B_{12} supplements. The progressive drop in Hb was similar to what has been observed in other studies on women not given iron supplements during pregnancy[3]. Although altitude hypoxia stimulates erythropoiesis, it is not known what effect altitude has on plasma volume expansion in pregnancy. Other studies from even higher altitudes, up to 4340 m above sea level, have confirmed that Hb levels progressively drop as gestation advances, rather than stabilizing after the second trimester[5].

Red cell count and hematocrit (Hct) values are likewise lower in pregnancy, but the other red cell indices change little (Table 1.1), although red cells show more variation in size and shape than in the non-pregnant state. There is a small increase in mean cell volume (MCV), on average 4 fL for iron-replete women, which reaches a maximum at 30–35 weeks' gestation and occurs independently of any deficiency of B_{12} and folate[2]. Hemoglobin and hematocrit increase after delivery. Significant increases have been documented between measurements taken at 6–8 weeks postpartum and those at 4–6 months postpartum, demonstrating that this length of time is needed to restore them to non-pregnant values[1].

Table 1.1 Red cell indices during pregnancy and the puerperium

Red cell indices	Gestation			
	18 weeks	32 weeks	39 weeks	8 weeks postpartum
Hemoglobin (Hb) g/L	119 (106–133)	119 (104–135)	125 (109–142)	133 (119–148)
Red cell count × 10^{12}/L	3.93 (3.43–4.49)	3.86 (3.38–4.43)	4.05 (3.54–4.64)	4.44 (3.93–5.00)
Mean cell volume (MCV) fL	89 (83–96)	91 (85–97)	91 (84–98)	88 (82–94)
Mean cell hemoglobin (MCH) pg	30 (27–33)	30 (28–33)	30 (28–33)	30 (27–32)
Mean cell hemoglobin concentration (MCHC) g/dL	34 (33–36)	34 (33–36)	34 (33–36)	34 (33–36)
Hematocrit	0.35 (0.31–0.39)	0.35 (0.31–0.40)	0.37 (0.32–0.42)	0.39 (0.35–0.44)

Mean and reference ranges (2.5th–97.5th centiles). Samples were collected longitudinally from 434 women. Adapted from Ref. [2].

Table 1.2 Hematinic factors during pregnancy and the puerperium

Hematinic factors	Gestation			
	18 weeks	32 weeks	39 weeks	8 weeks postpartum
Serum ferritin (μg/L)	32 (8–123)	18 (6–48)	21 (7–64)	46 (15–144)
Plasma folate (nmol/L)	15 (6–34)	10 (5–22)	10 (4–22)	9 (4–22)
Erythrocyte folate (μmol/L)	0.85 (0.46–1.59)	0.76 (0.41–1.40)	0.66 (0.33–1.33)	0.55 (0.29–1.01)
Plasma B_{12} (pmol/L)	216 (96–484)	169 (73–388)	154 (71–333)	315 (148–672)

Mean and reference ranges (2.5th–97.5th centiles). Samples were collected longitudinally from 434 women. Adapted from Ref. [2].

Changes in hematinic factors are shown in Table 1.2. Red cell folate levels have been shown in some studies to decrease during pregnancy, but in others to increase; plasma or serum folate levels always decrease during pregnancy[2,6]. These differences probably relate to dietary intake of folic acid or use of supplements. Folate levels may be low in the puerperium, especially in those who breast-feed. Vitamin B_{12} levels decrease during pregnancy, but recover by 6–8 weeks postpartum[2,6]. Iron stores, as judged by serum ferritin levels, become depleted in pregnancy, even when iron supplements are given, but are restored to early pregnancy levels by 5–8 weeks after delivery[2,7].

Summary Points

- Hb concentrations decrease in pregnancy.
- Hb <104 g/L suggests anemia.
- Hb >135–g/L is unusual and suggests inadequate plasma volume expansion (which can be associated with pregnancy problems including pre-eclampsia and poor fetal growth) or rarely a myeloproliferative disorder.
- MCV is normally slightly increased.
- MCH and MCHC are normally unchanged in pregnancy and do not change with gestation.

- Iron stores become depleted during pregnancy.
- B_{12} levels may be very low during pregnancy.
- Folate levels may decrease during pregnancy, depending on dietary intake.

White Cells

The white cell count (WBC) is increased in pregnancy [2], with a typical reference range of 6–16 × 10^9/L (Figure 1.1). Supplementation with iron and folate does not affect the total white cell count during or after pregnancy. In the hours after delivery[8], healthy women have been documented as having a WBC of 9–25 × 10^9/L. These naturally high WBCs have implications for the diagnosis of sepsis, especially during labor or soon after delivery[9]. White cell counts may also be transiently elevated after administration of corticosteroids in pregnancy, such as those given to promote fetal lung maturity when premature delivery is anticipated. By 4–8 weeks post-delivery, typical WBC ranges are similar to those in healthy non-pregnant women (4–10 × 10^9/L).

There has been much discussion about the normal ranges for the different types of white cells (Table 1.3) [8,10,11]. Neutrophils contribute most to the overall higher WBC. There is an increase in immature forms

Table 1.3 Total and differential white cell count in late pregnancy and the early puerperium

	Total and differential white cell count			
	Week 33 (n=151)	Week 36 (n=146)	Week 39 (n=130)	1–3 hours post-delivery (n=91)
Total white cell count × 10^9/L	9.1 (5.7–14)	8.9 (6.1–15)	9.0 (6.0–16)	16 (9.4–25)
Neutrophils × 10^9/L	6.5 (3.5–11)	6.4 (4.1–11)	6.5 (3.7–13)	14 (6.6–23)
Lymphocytes × 10^9/L	1.7 (0.9–2.8)	1.8 (1.1–2.8)	1.8 (1.1–2.9)	1.1 (0.5–2.4)
Monocytes × 10^9/L	0.50 (0.2–1.0)	0.50 (0.3–1.0)	0.50 (0.28–0.90)	0.53 (0.3–1.2)
Eosinophils × 10^9/L	0.10 (0.0–0.40)	0.10 (0.0–0.30)	0.10 (0.0–0.40)	0.0 (0.0–0.50)
Basophils × 10^9/L	0.0 (0.0–0.10)	0.03 (0.0–0.10)	0.04 (0.0–0.10)	0.08 (0.0–0.20)

Median and reference ranges (2.5th–97.5th centiles). From a longitudinal study of 154 women who were taking iron supplements during pregnancy and had undergone at least one previous normal pregnancy. Post-delivery samples were excluded for cases delivered by cesarean section. Adapted from Ref. [8].

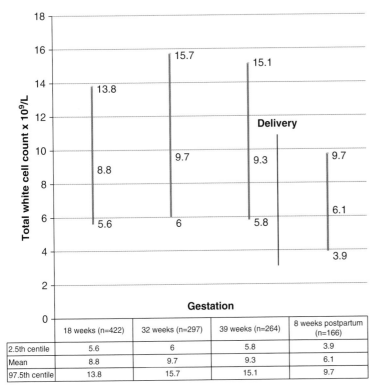

Figure 1.1 Normal values for white cell counts during pregnancy. Mean and reference ranges (2.5th –97.5th centiles). Samples were collected longitudinally from 434 women. Adapted from ref [2].

	18 weeks (n=422)	32 weeks (n=297)	39 weeks (n=264)	8 weeks postpartum (n=166)
2.5th centile	5.6	6	5.8	3.9
Mean	8.8	9.7	9.3	6.1
97.5th centile	13.8	15.7	15.1	9.7

and the cytoplasm shows toxic granulation. The count is relatively constant throughout gestation (3– 10 × 10^9/ L), markedly elevated in the hours after delivery (up to 23 × 10^9/L) and back to non-pregnant values by 4–8 weeks postpartum (1.5–6 × 10^9/L). Neutrophil chemotaxis and phagocytic activity are depressed, the latter being inhibited by factors present in pregnancy serum. There is also evidence of increased oxidative metabolism in neutrophils during pregnancy.

The lymphocyte count decreases during pregnancy through the first and second trimesters, increases during the third trimester, but remains low in the early puerperium as compared to normal non-pregnant values[8,10,11]. The typical pregnancy range for lymphocyte count is from 1.1 × 10^9/L to 2.8 × 10^9/L, compared with the non-pregnant reference range of from 0.8 × 10^9/L to 4.0 × 10^9/L. The lymphocyte count is restored to normal range by 4–8 weeks after delivery.

Detailed studies of T- and B-lymphocyte subsets in peripheral blood and the proliferative responses of these cells to mitogens found more helper and suppressor cells and less killer cells during pregnancy. Lymphocyte proliferation in response to a variety of agents was found to be impaired in pregnancy, suggesting that there is an immunosuppressant factor present.

The monocyte count is higher in pregnancy, especially in the first trimester[8,10,11]. Typical values in the third trimester are $0.2-1.0 \times 10^9$/L, as compared to non-pregnant values of $0.1-0.9 \times 10^9$/L. The monocyte to lymphocyte ratio is markedly increased in pregnancy. The eosinophil count does not change significantly during pregnancy ($0.03-0.5 \times 10^9$/L) [8,11]. The basophil count has been found in one study to be low in the second trimester[11], but in a detailed study during the third trimester and early puerperium[8], levels were similar to those found in non-pregnant subjects (up to 0.1×10^9/L). Myelocytes and metamyelocytes may be found in the peripheral blood film of healthy women during pregnancy and do not have pathological significance.

Summary Points

- WBC is elevated in pregnancy, mostly due to neutrophilia.
- Lymphocyte count is lower and monocyte count higher.
- During pregnancy, only WBC $>16 \times 10^9$/L is considered abnormal.
- Soon after delivery, only WBC $>25 \times 10^9$/L is considered abnormal.
- Eosinophil and basophil counts do not change significantly in pregnancy.

Platelets

Like the red cell mass, the platelet mass increases in pregnancy but not to the same extent as the plasma volume, so that the platelet count appears to fall in a full blood count. Large cross-sectional studies in pregnancy of healthy women (specifically excluding any with hypertension) have shown that there is also a left-shift of the platelet count distribution histogram. Thus, platelet counts are lower during pregnancy (Table 1.4), particularly in the third trimester[12,13]. This is termed "gestational thrombocytopenia." Almost 12% of women in one study[13] were found

Table 1.4 Platelet count in pregnant and non-pregnant women

Platelet count $\times 10^9$/L	Pregnant women (n=6770)	Non-pregnant women (n=287)
Mean	213	248
Median	206	242
2.5th centile	116	164
97.5th centile	346	362
Count $<150 \times 10^9$/L	11.6%	1.0%

Cross-sectional study of women in pregnancy, all 36 or more weeks' gestation; compared to healthy women of similar age. Adapted from Ref. [13].

to have a platelet count of $<150 \times 10^9$/L late in pregnancy. Of these women, 79% had platelet counts of $116-149 \times 10^9$/L; none had complications related to thrombocytopenia and none of their babies had severe thrombocytopenia (platelet count $<20 \times 10^9$/L). Thus, it has been recommended that the lower limit of platelet count in late pregnancy should be considered as 115×10^9/L. Less than 1% of healthy women in pregnancy have platelet counts of $<100 \times 10^9$/L [12,13]. Platelet counts increase within 2–3 days of delivery in women with gestational thrombocytopenia[12].

Platelet size is an indicator of the age of the platelets; young ones are large and they become progressively smaller with age. Platelet volume has a skewed distribution, tailing off at larger volumes. The platelet volume distribution width increases significantly and continuously as gestation advances and the mean platelet volume becomes an insensitive measure of platelet size. Studies suggest that platelet lifespan is shorter in pregnancy. The decrease in platelet count and increase in platelet size in pregnancy suggests that there is hyper-destruction of platelets[14].

Platelet function, as assessed by the time required for whole blood to occlude a membrane impregnated with either epinephrine or adenosine 5′ diphosphate (ADP), has been studied in late pregnancy[15,16]. No correlation was found between platelet count and the "closure times" over a range of platelet counts of $44-471 \times 10^9$/L in healthy women[16]. Another study found that the closure times were increased in women with severe pre-eclampsia, although they did not correlate with clinical bleeding problems in these women [17]. In women with gestational thrombocytopenia, platelet closure times are influenced by hemoglobin level, being prolonged when there is both thrombocytopenia and anemia[15]. This is perhaps not surprising, given the contribution of red cells to the hemostatic process, in part due to ADP donation. The increase in fibrinogen during pregnancy maintains platelet function, as fibrinogen is the ligand for platelet to platelet aggregation.

Summary Points

- Platelet count decreases during pregnancy in some patients.
- The lower limit of normal platelet count at term is 115×10^9/L.
- There is evidence of increased platelet destruction in pregnancy.
- Platelet closure times are not affected by absolute platelet count in healthy women during pregnancy.
- Platelet closure times are prolonged when there is anemia in addition to a low platelet count.
- The increase in fibrinogen during pregnancy more than compensates for the fall in platelet count.

Case Studies

Case Study 1

A woman was admitted for an elective cesarean section at 39 weeks. Her full blood count showed a platelet count of 90×10^9/L. She was not hypertensive, had no history of medical disorders and was not taking any medication other than pregnancy vitamin supplements. A repeat platelet count was requested (84×10^9/L) and a coagulation screen performed, which was normal. She had never been previously told that her platelet count was low and had never experienced unexplained bruising or significant bleeding complications, during childhood and early adulthood, nor at the time of her previous cesarean delivery, 3 years earlier. The laboratory records revealed a platelet count of 158×10^9/L in early pregnancy and 110×10^9/L at 28 weeks' gestation, but there were no records prior to confirmed pregnancy. Gestational thrombocytopenia with a low–normal platelet count at the start of pregnancy was diagnosed. The cesarean section went ahead under a spinal anesthetic. There were no anesthetic or surgical complications. After 48 hours, the platelet count was 110×10^9/L and 4 weeks later it was 194×10^9/L. This case illustrates how a falling platelet count during pregnancy became "noticed" because the absolute count was low enough to attract attention and surgical delivery was planned. The prompt rise in platelet count after delivery and subsequent normal-range value makes gestational thrombocytopenia the most likely diagnosis, rather than immune thrombocytopenia.

Case Study 2

A woman who had delivered with the assistance of obstetric forceps was reviewed on the postnatal ward the following morning. The midwife had taken a full blood count and was concerned about the results: hemoglobin 96 g/L, white cell count 22×10^9/L, platelet count 176×10^9/L. The bedside Modified Obstetric Early Warning Score chart was reviewed. In the 24 hours since delivery, temperature had been 36.9–37.4°C, pulse rate 80–95 beats per minute, respiratory rate 18–22 breaths per minute, blood pressure between 102/63 mmHg and 113/66 mmHg. Lochia were normal in amount and non-offensive. The uterus felt well contracted and was not tender. The woman complained of dysuria. A urine sample had shown 2+ blood, 1+ white cells, 1+ protein but was negative for nitrites and a sample had been sent to the laboratory for culture. The midwife questioned whether the high white cell count and complaints of dysuria indicated urinary tract infection, suggesting that antibiotics could be prescribed. However, none of the observations, bedside tests, or the full blood count were actually abnormal for a woman recently delivered and she seemed well. It was explained that the white cell count on its own did not indicate sepsis and a high white cell count was typical during labor and in the early puerperium. It was agreed that the result of the urinary culture would be awaited and that antibiotics would only be prescribed if this confirmed infection, or if continued observations of temperature, pulse, respiratory rate, or blood pressure became abnormal.

References

1. Taylor DJ, Lind T. Red cell mass during and after normal pregnancy. *British Journal of Obstetrics and Gynecology* 1979; **86**: 364–370.

2. Milman N, Bergholt T, Byg K-E *et al.* Reference intervals for hematological variables during normal pregnancy and postpartum in 434 healthy Danish women. *European Journal of Hematology* 2007; **79**: 39–46.

3. Milman N, Byg K-E, Agger AO. Hemoglobin and erythrocyte indices during normal pregnancy and postpartum in 206 women with and without iron supplementation. *Acta Obstetricia et Gynecologica Scandinavica* 2000; **79**: 89–98.

4. Shen C, Jiang YM, Shi H *et al.* A prospective, sequential and longitudinal study of hematological profile during normal pregnancy in Chinese women. *Journal of Obstetrics and Gynecology* 2010; **30**: 357–361.

5. Gaitán-González MJ, Echeverría-Arjonilla JC, Vargas-García C *et al.* Valores de hemoglobina en mujeres embarazadas residentes en zonas de altitud media. *Salud Pública Méx* [online series] 2013; **55**(4): 379–386. Available from: http://www.scielosp.org/scielo.php?script=sci_arttext&pid=S0036-36342013000500003&lng=en (accessed March 28 2015).

6. Cikot RJLM, Steegers-Theunissen RPM, Thomas CMG *et al.* Longitudinal vitamin and homocysteine levels in normal pregnancy. *British Journal of Nutrition* 2001; **85**: 49–58.

7. Fenton V, Cavill I, Fisher J. Iron stores in pregnancy. *British Journal of Hematology* 1977; **37**: 145–149.

8. Edlestam G, Lowbeer C, Kral G *et al.* New reference values for routine blood samples and human neutrophilic lipocalin during third trimester pregnancy. *Scandinavian Journal of Clinical Laboratory Investigation* 2001; **61**: 583–592.

9. Bauer ME, Bauer ST, Rajala B *et al.* Maternal physiological parameters in relationship to systemic inflammatory response syndrome criteria. *Obstetrics and Gynecology* 2014; **124**: 535–541.

10. Valdimarsson H, Mulholland C, Fridriksdottir V *et al.* A longitudinal study of leucocyte blood counts and lymphocyte responses in pregnancy: a marked early increase of monocyte-lymphocyte ratio. *Clinical and Experimental Immunology* 1983; **53**: 437–443.

11. Lurie S, Rahamin E, Piper I *et al.* Total and differential leukocyte counts percentiles in normal pregnancy. *European Journal of Obstetrics & Gynecology and Reproductive Biology* 2008; **136**: 16–19.

12. Sainio S, Kekomaki R, Riikonen S, Teramo K. Maternal thrombocytopenia at term: a population-based study. *Acta Obstetricia et Gynecologica Scandinavica* 2000; **79**: 744–749.

13. Boehlen F, Hohfeld P, Extermann P *et al.* Platelet count at term pregnancy: a reappraisal of the threshold. *Obstetrics and Gynecology* 2000; **95**: 29–33.

14. Fay RA, Hughes AO, Farron NT. Platelets in pregnancy: hyperdestruction in pregnancy. *Obstetrics and Gynecology* 1983; **61**: 238–240.

15. Vincelot A, Nathan N, Collert D *et al.* Platelet function during pregnancy: an evaluation using the PFA-100 analyser. *British Journal of Anesthesia* 2001; **87**: 890–893.

16. Beilin Y, Arnold I, Hossain S. Evaluation of the platelet function analyzer (PFA-100®) vs. the thromboelastogram (TEG) in the parturient. *International Journal of Obstetric Anesthesia* 2006; **15**: 7–12.

17. Davies JR, Roshan F, Hallworth SP. Hemostatic function in healthy pregnant and preeclamptic women: an assessment using the platelet function analyzer (PFA-100®) and Thromboelastograph®. *Anesthesia and Analgesia* 2007; **104**: 416–420.

Chapter 2

Normal Coagulation Changes during Pregnancy

Rachel Rayment

Introduction

During pregnancy, the hemostatic system alters in preparation for delivery of the fetus. In an uncomplicated vaginal delivery, bleeding is largely prevented by the mechanical events of uterine contraction and retraction of the interlacing myometrial fibers surrounding maternal spiral arteries of the placental bed. Myometrial contraction compresses the spiral arteries and veins, thereby obliterating their lumina[1]. As a result of myometrial contraction, the uterine walls are firmly opposed, providing further support for hemostasis. However, on occasion this process fails, e.g. uterine atony, placental abruption, placental retention, and bleeding occurs. The maternal blood supply to the placenta at term is 600–700 mL/min[2], and failure to occlude the blood supply at delivery results in catastrophic hemorrhage and consumption of coagulation factors. In preparation for this possibility, the normal balance of hemostasis alters, becoming prothrombotic and hypofibrinolytic. An unfortunate consequence of this is an increased incidence of venous thrombotic events during pregnancy and the puerperium. This chapter will discuss the changes in hemostasis seen during normal pregnancy, and the role of coagulation tests in its assessment.

Primary Hemostasis

Primary hemostasis is the initial response of the body to a breach in the integrity of the endothelium and is dependent on the interaction between von Willebrand factor and platelets. von Willebrand factor is anchored to the subendothelial matrix through collagen binding. It then binds circulating platelets which are recruited to the site of injury and ultimately form a temporary plug which both stops bleeding and serves to provide a phospholipid surface on which coagulation factors can function in order to form a more durable fibrin clot (Figure 2.1).

Defects in primary hemostasis result in a tendency toward mucocutaneous bleeding, in particular menorrhagia, and women with von Willebrand disease are at risk of postpartum hemorrhage. It is therefore perhaps unsurprising that von Willebrand factor rises during normal pregnancy. Estrogen directly stimulates endothelial cells to increase their rate of production of VWF[3], and this is thought to be the mechanism for the increase in pregnancy, where a doubling of levels may occur. Since von Willebrand factor is the carrier molecule for factor VIII, there is an equivalent increase in factor VIII levels by the third trimester of pregnancy. Levels of von Willebrand factor begin to fall around 3 days postpartum[4], returning to preconception levels in the subsequent 2–3 weeks. This may be associated with delayed postpartum hemorrhage in women with von Willebrand disease.

As discussed in Chapter 1, the platelet count is lower during pregnancy. In approximately 5% of pregnancies, the platelet concentration is reduced in the absence of any detectable pathology. This is thought to be due to consumption of platelets in the uteroplacental bed and is of no clinical consequence to either the mother or fetus. In this so-called gestational thrombocytopenia, the platelet count starts in general to fall in the second trimester and to plateau when the pregnancy reaches 36–37 weeks. The platelet count nadir is often above 100×10^9/L, but can be lower. In general, a platelet count below 80×10^9/L should be investigated for alternative causes, such as immune thrombocytopenia or a microangiopathic hemolysis. It is unlikely that a platelet count below 50×10^9/L is due to gestational thrombocytopenia alone[5]. Gestational thrombocytopenia does tend to recur with subsequent pregnancies and, where there has been some doubt about the etiology of the thrombocytopenia, this can be removed by simply checking the platelet count outside of pregnancy since complete recovery is

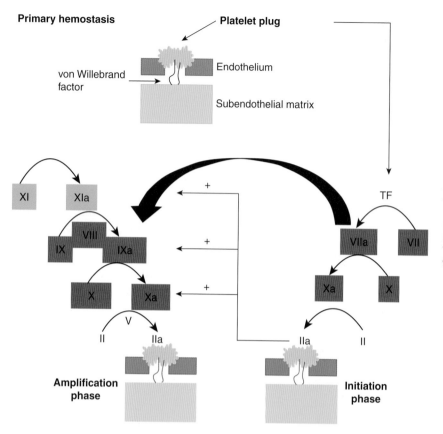

Primary hemostasis

Platelet plug

Endothelium

von Willebrand factor

Subendothelial matrix

XI → XIa

VIII

IX   IXa

X   Xa

V

II   IIa

Amplification phase

TF

VIIa   VII

Xa   X

IIa   II

Initiation phase

Figure 2.1 Thrombin generation and normal changes in coagulation in pregnancy. Following formation of a primary hemostatic plug tissue factor activates factor VII on the phospholipid surface created by activated platelets. Factor VII then activates factor X which cleaves prothrombin to thrombin. This sets off the amplification phase of coagulation, generating a "burst" of thrombin generation. Subsequent formation of fibrin glues the primary hemostatic plug through its interaction with platelets. Clotting factors which rise during pregnancy are highlighted in red, and those which may increase or decrease, in green.

to be expected, usually within days of delivery, but always within weeks.

Thrombin Generation

A primary platelet plug will disaggregate over time, since it is held together by non-covalent bonds. Tissue factor activates factors IX and X to enable production of thrombin and ultimately a fibrin clot at the site of a primary platelet plug. The process is largely controlled by thrombin, which not only cleaves fibrinogen to its fibrin monomer, but also activates coagulation factors, V, VIII, and XI, allowing the generation of a large "burst" of thrombin. Thrombin activity is limited to the site of need by the natural anticoagulants, protein C and antithrombin.

Thrombin generation is increased during pregnancy[6]. Many of the procoagulant factors increase during pregnancy, predominantly during the second trimester (Figure 2.1), although interestingly levels of prothrombin itself are unchanged during pregnancy [7]. This increased thrombin generation is evidenced by an increase in prothrombin fragments 1 and 2

(which result from the cleavage of prothrombin)[8] and thrombin–antithrombin complexes[9] (which are formed in the presence of free thrombin).

Coagulation factors have usually returned to prepregnancy levels by 4–6 weeks postpartum[10].

Fibrinogen

Fibrinogen is cleaved to fibrin monomer by thrombin. This "glue" binds the primary hemostatic plug, through its interactions with platelets. The fibrin clot is further stabilized through cross-linking by factor XIII. Fibrinogen concentration increases during pregnancy, the normal range rising from 2–4 g/L to 4–6 g/L. Fibrinogen is essential for hemostasis and in the event of bleeding is often the first coagulation factor to fall to critical levels[11]. At the time of delivery, the raised fibrinogen levels protect against bleeding, in an otherwise uncomplicated delivery. Fibrinogen levels have been shown to correlate with the likelihood of ongoing bleeding in the event of a postpartum hemorrhage[12] and a fibrinogen level >4 g/L is rarely associated with continued bleeding.

Factor XIII levels fall early in pregnancy, then gradually rise, such that levels are about 50% of baseline toward the end of pregnancy[13].

Fibrinolysis

Once fibrinogen has been cross-linked by factor XIII the clot is stable (allowing repair of the underlying endothelium) until it is broken down by an enzymatic process called fibrinolysis (Figure 2.2). In the presence of a fibrin clot, tissue plasminogen activator (tPA) cleaves plasminogen, generating plasmin, which in turn digests fibrin at exposed lysine residues, resulting in the formation of fibrin degradation products.

tPA is inhibited by plasminogen activator inhibitor (PAI). Outside of pregnancy the only detectable plasminogen inhibitor is PAI-1, which is produced by endothelial cells. However, during pregnancy the placenta produces PAI-2. Both PAI-1 and PAI-2 rise in pregnancy, thus creating a hypofibrinolytic state. Since PAI-2 is produced by the placental villous cells, placental and fetal wellbeing can affect levels of PAI-2 in pregnancy[14]. Levels fall following delivery and are back to pre-pregnancy levels by about 5 weeks postpartum[15,16]. Interestingly, although PAI is increased during pregnancy, one of the markers of fibrinolysis, the D-dimer, is often raised throughout pregnancy, reflecting the overall increase in fibrin production through pregnancy [7]. This causes difficulty in the clinical assessment of suspected venous thromboembolism, and there is currently an ongoing study ascertaining a normal range for D-dimers during pregnancy[17].

Fibrinolysis is also inhibited by thrombin-activatable inhibitor of fibrinolysis (TAFI). Plasmin binds to and digests fibrin on exposed lysine residues. TAFI removes the exposed binding sites, thus limiting the action of plasmin[18]. TAFI concentrations are unaffected by pregnancy[19]. Tranexamic acid is a lysine analog that binds to the lysine binding site on plasminogen and inhibits plasmin formation. It is used clinically to inhibit fibrinolysis and reduce bleeding.

Plasmin is also inhibited by the antifibrinolytics α2-antiplasmin and α2-macroglobulin. α2-antiplasmin levels are not affected in pregnancy in general, although they may sometimes increase[19]. A pregnancy-associated form of α2-macroglobulin has been reported, the levels of which rise significantly during the first trimester, persist throughout pregnancy, and fall 8 weeks postpartum[20].

Physiological Anticoagulants

The physiological anticoagulants include protein C, protein S, and antithrombin. These serine proteases serve to limit thrombin generation (Figure 2.3).

Thrombin generation is limited by the action of the natural anticoagulants, antithrombin, protein C, and its cofactor, protein S. Antithrombin binds free thrombin but also inactivates factors IXa, Xa, and XIa. Activated protein C inhibits factors Va and VIIIa.

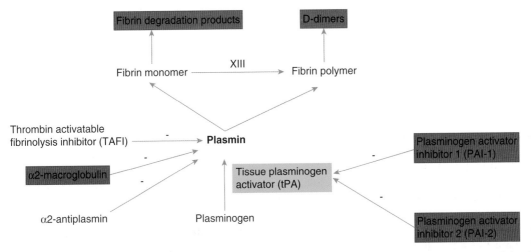

Figure 2.2 Fibrinolysis and the normal changes during pregnancy. Breakdown of fibrin is through the enzymatic action of plasmin and results in the formation of fibrin degradation products. Pregnancy is considered an altered fibrinolytic state, due to the increase in plasminogen activator inhibitors 1 and 2. Factors that rise during pregnancy are highlighted in red, and those that may decrease, in green.

9

Table 2.1 Changes in coagulation factors during pregnancy

		Comments
Factors that increase	VII	Levels have returned to pre-pregnancy levels by 4–6 weeks
	X	
	VIII	Factor VIII is carried by von Willebrand factor
	von Willebrand factor	Levels begin to fall 3 days following delivery, returning to baseline levels by 3 weeks
	Fibrinogen	Normal range in pregnancy increases to 4–6 g/L
	Plasminogen activator inhibitor (PAI) 1 and 2	PAI-2 is produced exclusively by the placenta. Levels are reflective of placental function – are reduced in babies of low birth weight
	α2-macroglobulin	A pregnancy-associated form of α2-macroglobulin has been reported, the levels of which rise significantly during the first trimester, persist throughout pregnancy, and fall 8 weeks post-partum
Factors that do not change	V	
	Thrombin (II)	
	Protein C	
	Antithrombin	
	Tissue factor pathway inhibitor (TFPI)	
	Thrombin activatable fibrinolysis inhibitor (TAFI)	
	α2-antiplasmin	May increase slightly
Factors that decrease	XI	May be unchanged or sometimes increase
	Protein S	Both free and bound protein S are reduced

While antithrombin and protein C are unchanged during pregnancy, protein S falls by up to 50% early in the second trimester, limiting the action of both activated protein C and tissue factor pathway inhibitor (TFPI) (Table 2.1).

Antithrombin by inhibiting thrombin, IXa, Xa, and XIa, serves to limit thrombin generation to the site of need. Antithrombin levels are unchanged during pregnancy[19].

Thrombin which is not clot-bound is also able to bind to thrombomodulin, which is expressed by the endothelium. This complex is then able to activate protein C which, in the presence of its cofactor protein S, inhibits both factor V and factor VIII. A proportion of protein S is bound to C4b-binding protein, and the activity of protein S is determined by the amount and activity of the free antigen. Protein C levels are unaffected by pregnancy but protein S levels fall early in the second trimester by as much as 50% due to altered binding to C4b-binding protein. Protein S levels remain low until delivery but return to baseline by 3 days following delivery[21]. Both free and bound protein S are reduced[22].

The activity of protein C can be measured in vitro by the activated protein C (APC) resistance

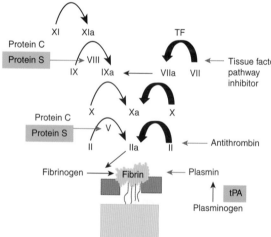

Figure 2.3 Natural anticoagulants and the normal changes during pregnancy. Thrombin generation is limited by the action of the natural anticoagulants, antithrombin, protein C, and its cofactor, protein S. Antithrombin binds free thrombin but also inactivates factors IX, X, and XI. Activated protein C inhibits factors V and VIII. Whilst antithrombin and protein C are unchanged during pregnancy, protein S falls by up to 50% early in the second trimester, limiting the action of both activated protein C and tissue factor pathway inhibitor (TFPI).

assay, which was originally used to detect the presence of genetic mutations in factor V, such as factor V Leiden, that caused a resistance to the effect of activated protein C and thus an increased tendency to venous thrombosis. APC resistance is increased during pregnancy. The reason for this is unclear; it does not appear to be due just to the reduction in protein S nor the rise in factor VIII that occurs in pregnancy[23].

The ability of tissue factor to activate factor X is limited by tissue factor pathway inhibitor. Levels of both tissue factor and TFPI are unchanged during normal pregnancy. However, elevated levels of TFPI have been associated with hypertensive disorders in pregnancy[24].

Assessment of Hemostasis during Pregnancy

Full Blood Count

There may be a mild thrombocytopenia. Blood film examination often shows platelet anisocytosis (variation in size) and it may be useful, when the platelet count is below 100×10^9/L, to accurately determine the platelet count by immunophenotyping in order to inform management plans for delivery.

Routine Coagulation Tests

Neither the prothrombin (PT time) nor the activated partial thromboplastin time (aPTT) are very sensitive during pregnancy. The aPTT is often shortened, due to the increased levels of clotting factors, in particular factor VIII[21]. They are unhelpful in assessing coagulopathy secondary to postpartum hemorrhage and become prolonged only in the event of catastrophic bleeds. Fibrinogen levels can be close to surprisingly low levels without any disturbance in either the aPTT or the PT[25]. Fibrinogen estimation should be performed using the Clauss method, since there is reduced precision with the PT-derived fibrinogen estimation with increasing fibrinogen levels[26]. Fibrinogen levels rise during pregnancy (normal range 4–6 g/L).

Tests of Global Hemostasis

A major limitation of laboratory assessment of fibrinogen is the turnaround time, due to time taken to transport samples to the laboratory and the speed of response of the laboratory technician; the assay itself only takes 10–15 minutes. There is currently much interest in the role of point-of-care testing in the delivery suite, to inform clinicians promptly of significant deterioration in hemostatic competence. The utility of both thromboelastography (TEG®) and rotational elastometry (ROTEM®) is being investigated. Both tests allow visualization of clot formation and subsequent lysis under conditions of low shear [27]. Both tests give a visual depiction of the ability of the clot to transmit a rotational force to an electromechanical transduction system. However, there are minor differences in the technology and in the terminology applied to the curves and the data from each test cannot be directly compared.

In a prospective, longitudinal study in healthy pregnant women, TEG demonstrated faster blood coagulation with increased strength of the fibrin clot and less fibrinolysis during the pregnancy compared to 8 weeks postpartum[28]. Indeed, the differences between TEG parameters of pregnant and non-pregnant women have led to the recommendation of a pregnancy-specific normal range for TEG [29]. During major obstetric hemorrhage, the TEG functional fibrinogen seems to correlate with fibrinogen levels, which in turn predict for ongoing hemorrhage[30]. Further studies are required to determine the normal parameters for TEG during pregnancy and its role in the management of obstetric hemorrhage.

Akin to TEG®, rotational ROTEM® demonstrates the hypercoagulability of pregnancy, with increased clot firmness and shortened clotting times[31], again raising the need for pregnancy-specific normal ranges for this assay. A modification of the ROTEM®, the FIBTEM®, is being used to assess fibrinogen requirements in a variety of situations, including cardiac surgery, trauma, and obstetric hemorrhage[27]. Since fibrinogen is often the first coagulation factor to fall to critical levels in massive hemorrhage it would appear to be an ideal marker for the integrity of hemostasis (Figure 2.4). Selective replacement of fibrinogen may reduce or avoid the need for transfusion of other allogeneic blood products thus reducing morbidity due to transfusion-associated circulatory overload. In the FIBTEM®, platelets are inactivated by the addition of cytochalasin D, so that the traces obtained are reflective of all the coagulation factors including fibrinogen and factor XIII activity. The amplitude of clot at either 5 minutes or 10 minutes following activation of the whole blood sample has been shown to correlate

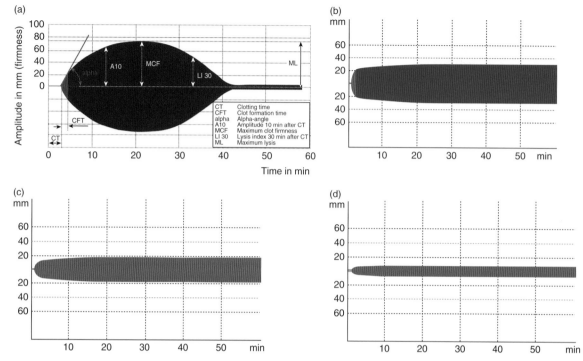

Figure 2.4 Rotational elastometry and its use in the assessment of global hemostasis at parturition. Standard clotting assays detect the starting time of clotting whereas thromboelastometry (TEM®) provides information on the whole kinetics of hemostasis: clotting time, clot formation, clot stability, and lysis. Clinically useful results are available within 5–10 min. Inhibition of platelets by cytochalasin D allows assessment of fibrinogen in the FIBTEM® assay. (a) Normal ROTEM® trace. (b) FIBTEM® trace taken following a postpartum hemorrhage of 1600 mL showing an A5 of 25 mm, suggesting adequate hemostasis. (c) FIBTEM® trace showing an A5 of 14 mm following a 2000-mL hemorrhage. (d) FIBTEM® trace showing an A5 of 8 mm following a 1300-mL hemorrhage. Fibrinogen replacement is likely to be required in both C and D in the presence of ongoing hemorrhage.

Case Studies

Case Study 1

A 31-year-old woman was referred to the hematology antenatal clinic at 16 weeks' gestation. She had a history of two first trimester miscarriages in 2015. She was found to have a borderline free protein S level of 57 IU/dL (63–127) at the time of the second miscarriage at 11 weeks' gestation. This had been repeated when she attended her booking appointment at 13 weeks' gestation and was reported to be further reduced at 45 IU/dL. There was no personal or family history of thrombosis.

The pregnancy was managed routinely. She delivered, by spontaneous vaginal delivery, a healthy girl weighing 3.8 kg. She received 2 weeks of postnatal thromboprophylaxis.

Repeat testing of the free protein S at 3 months postpartum showed normalization to 67 IU/dL.

Free protein S levels fall early in the second trimester, to approximately half of those seen in the non-pregnant state, contributing to the prothrombotic state seen in pregnancy. To avoid confusion and wasted resources, protein S levels should not be checked during pregnancy or the postpartum period.

Case Study 2

A 26-year-old woman presented to the delivery suite with vaginal bleeding at 36 weeks' gestation. She was tachycardic, with a pulse of 120 beats per minute and hypotensive, with a blood pressure of 80/40. Fetal ultrasound confirmed an intrauterine demise and placental abruption, with significant retroplacental hemorrhage.

Hemoglobin on blood gas analyzer was 72 g/L. FIBTEM® A5 was 3 mm. She was resuscitated with crystalloid, 2 units of red cells, and 6 g of fibrinogen concentrate.

Post-treatment FIBTEM A5 was 8 mm. Her blood pressure was stabilized at 100/60 and pulse lowered to 110. Although the ongoing vaginal loss was minimal, concern remained about the risk of bleeding at the time of delivery. So a further 4 g of fibrinogen and 2 units of red cells were given. Following treatment, the FIBTEM® A5 was 12 mm. The baby was delivered vaginally and there was no significant bleeding postpartum. No fresh frozen plasma (FFP) was transfused. She received thromboprophylaxis with enoxaparin (40 mg) 6 hours following delivery.

Subsequent results from the coagulation testing were as follows:

	PT (11.0–13.0 s)	aPTT (22–33 s)	Fibrinogen (g/L)
On arrival	11.4	24.6	0.9
Following 6 g fibrinogen	11.3	26.2	2.1
Following a further 4 g fibrinogen	11.6	25.7	3

This case illustrates the role of near patient testing with FIBTEM® to inform clinical management of major obstetric hemorrhage. Within minutes of arrival, a decision to transfuse fibrinogen could be made, allowing reduction of bleeding due to hemostatic failure. The average turnaround time for coagulation screens in hospital laboratories is over an hour, which makes real time management impossible. Note that even in the presence of a significantly low fibrinogen (normal range in pregnancy is 4–6 g/L and outside of pregnancy 2–4 g/L), the PT and aPTT are normal. Estimation of fibrinogen is essential for the management of major bleeding. The risk of venous thrombosis rises significantly in association with major bleeding and transfusion of blood products. It is important to administer pharmacological thromboprophylaxis once the cause of bleeding has been controlled.

with Clauss fibrinogen levels during obstetric hemorrhage[32]. Studies are needed to determine the role of TEG functional fibrinogen and FIBTEM® in the bedside management of major obstetric hemorrhage.

References

1. Khan RU, El-Refey H. Pathophysiology of postpartum hemorrhage and the third stage of labor. In Arulkumaran MKS, Keith LG, Lalonde AB, Lynch CB, (eds). *A Comprehensive Textbook of Postpartum Hemorrhage*, 2nd edn. The Global Library of Women's Medicine; 2012.

2. Wang Y. Vascular Biology of the Placenta. *Colloquium Series on Integrated Systems Physiology: From Molecule to Function* 2010; **2**(1): 1–98.

3. Harrison RL, McKee PA. Estrogen stimulates von Willebrand factor production by cultured endothelial cells. *Blood* 1984; **63**(3): 657–664.

4. Huq FY, Kulkarni A, Agbim EC et al. Changes in the levels of factor VIII and von Willebrand factor in the puerperium. *Hemophilia* 2012; **18**(2): 241–245.

5. Gernsheimer T, James AH, Stasi R. How I treat thrombocytopenia in pregnancy. *Blood* 2013; **121**(1): 38–47.

6. McLean KC, Bernstein IM, Brummel-Ziedins KE. Tissue factor-dependent thrombin generation across pregnancy. *American Journal of Obstetrics and Gynecology* 2012; **207**(2): 135.e1–6.

7. Hammerova L, Chabada J, Drobny J et al. Longitudinal evaluation of markers of hemostasis in pregnancy. *Bratisl Lek Listy* 2014; **115**(3): 140–144.

8. Comeglio P, Fedi S, Liotta A et al. Blood clotting activation during normal pregnancy. *Thrombosis Research* 1996; **84**(3): 199–202.

9. de Boer KW, ten Cate J, Sturk A et al. Enhanced thrombin generation in normal and hypertensive pregnancy. *American Journal of Obstetrics and Gynecology* 1989; **160**(1): 95–100.

10. Dahlman T, Hellgren M, Blomback M. Changes in blood coagulation and fibrinolysis in the normal puerperium. *Gynecologic and Obstetric Investigation* 1985; **20**(1): 37–44.

11. Hiippala ST, Myllyla GJ, Vahtera EM. Hemostatic factors and replacement of major blood loss with plasma-poor red cell concentrates. *Anesthesia and Analgesia* 1995; **81**(2): 360–365.

12. Charbit B, Mandelbrot L, Samain E et al. The decrease of fibrinogen is an early predictor of the severity of postpartum hemorrhage. *Journal of Thrombosis and Haemostasis* 2007; **5**(2): 266–273.

13. Sharief LT, Kadir R, Smith C et al. Changes in factor XIII level during pregnancy. *Hemophilia* 2014; **20**(2): E144–E148.

14. Brenner B. Hemostatic changes in pregnancy. *Thrombosis Research* 2004; **114**(5–6): 409–414.

13

15. Kruithof EK, Tran-Thang C, Gudinchet A *et al.* Fibrinolysis in pregnancy: a study of plasminogen activator inhibitors. *Blood* 1987; **69**(2): 460–466.

16. Choi JW, Pai SH. Tissue plasminogen activator levels change with plasma fibrinogen concentrations during pregnancy. *Annals of Hematology* 2002; **81**(11): 611–615.

17. Kovac M Mikovic Z, Rakicevic L *et al.* The use of D-dimer with new cutoff can be useful in diagnosis of venous thromboembolism in pregnancy. *European Journal of Obstetrics & Gynecology and Reproductive Biology* 2010; **148**(1): 27–30.

18. Bajzar L. Thrombin activatable fibrinolysis inhibitor and an antifibrinolytic pathway. *Arteriosclerosis Thrombosis and Vascular Biology* 2000; **20**(12): 2511–2518.

19. Hellgren M. Hemostasis during normal pregnancy and puerperium. *Seminars in Thrombosis and Hemostasis* 2003; **29**(2): 125–130.

20. Stimson WH, Farquharson DM, Lang GD. Pregnancy-associated alpha 2-macroglobulin – a new serum protein elevated in normal human pregnancy. *Journal of Reproductive Immunology* 1983; **5**(6): 321–327.

21. Saha P, Stott D, Atalla R. Hemostatic changes in the puerperium '6 weeks postpartum' (HIP Study) – implication for maternal thromboembolism. *British Journal of Obstetrics and Gynaecology* 2009; **116**(12): 1602–1612.

22. Comp PC, Thurnau GR, Welsh J *et al.* Functional and immunologic protein S levels are decreased during pregnancy. *Blood* 1986; **68**(4): 881–885.

23. Mahieu B, B, Jacobs N, Mahieu S *et al.* Hemostatic changes and acquired activated protein C resistance in normal pregnancy. *Blood Coagulation and Fibrinolysis* 2007; **18**(7): 685–688.

24. Godoi LC, Gomes K, Alpoim P *et al.* Preeclampsia: the role of tissue factor and tissue factor pathway inhibitor. *Journal of Thrombosis and Thrombolysis* 2012; **34**(1): 1–6.

25. de Lloyd L, Bovington R, Kaye A *et al.* Standard hemostatic tests following major obstetric hemorrhage. *International Journal of Obstetric Anesthesia* 2011; **20**(2): 135–141.

26. Mackie IJ, Kitchen S, Machin SJ *et al.* Guidelines on fibrinogen assays. *British Journal of Hematology* 2003; **121**(3): 396–404.

27. Whiting, D, DiNardo JA. TEG and ROTEM: technology and clinical applications. *American Journal of Hematology* 2014; **89**(2): 228–232.

28. Karlsson O, Sporrong T, Hillarp A *et al.* Prospective longitudinal study of thromboelastography and standard hemostatic laboratory tests in healthy women during normal pregnancy. *Anesthesia and Analgesia* 2012; **115**(4): 890–898.

29. Polak F, Kolnikova I, Lips M *et al.* New recommendations for thromboelastography reference ranges for pregnant women. *Thrombosis Research* 2011; **128**(4): E14–17.

30. Karlsson O, Jeppsson A, Hellgren M. Major obstetric hemorrhage: monitoring with thromboelastography, laboratory analyses or both? *International Journal of Obstetric Anesthesia* 2014; **23**(1): 10–17.

31. Armstrong S, Fernando S, Ashpole K *et al.* Assessment of coagulation in the obstetric population using ROTEM(R) thromboelastometry. *International Journal of Obstetric Anesthesia* 2011; **20**(4): 293–298.

32. Collins PW, Lilley G, Bruynseels D *et al.* Fibrin-based clot formation as an early and rapid biomarker for progression of postpartum hemorrhage: a prospective study. *Blood* 2014; **124**(11): 1727–1736.

Iron Deficiency in Pregnancy

Xiao-Yin Zhang and Sue Pavord

Definition

Anemia is defined as hemoglobin (Hb) less than two standard deviations below the mean for a healthy, matched population. The World Health Organization (WHO) defines iron deficiency anemia in pregnancy as iron deficiency (serum ferritin <12 µg/L) with an Hb level of less than 110 g/L and a hematocrit of <33%. However, studies in healthy Caucasian women on iron supplements found a lower reference value of 105 g/L during pregnancy[1,2]. This lower cut-off value has been adopted by the United States (US) Centers for Disease Control and Prevention (CDC) and the British Committee for Standards in Hematology (BCSH) from the second trimester of pregnancy[3]. There is also a racial difference in normal Hb levels, and the optimum Hb during pregnancy is lower in African and Asian populations compared to Europeans[4,5].

During pregnancy, physiological plasma expansion occurs, resulting in a plasma volume 30–50% above that found in non-pregnant women. This increased blood volume helps to compensate for blood loss at delivery – up to 1000 mL can be tolerated without a significant drop in Hb.

Postpartum, plasma volume decreases by diuresis and returns to pre-pregnant volumes. In iron-replete women, red cell mass begins to increase at 8 to 10 weeks of gestation and steadily rises by 20–30% above non-pregnant levels by the end of pregnancy. Healthy pregnancy is associated with a modest decrease in Hb levels, known as physiological or dilutional anemia of pregnancy. This is due to a greater expansion of plasma volume relative to the increase in red cell mass. Hemoglobin levels are typically lowest at 28 to 36 weeks. Nearer to term, plasma expansion ceases while Hb mass continues to increase, resulting in a small rise in Hb concentration.

Iron deficiency is found in a spectrum that can be categorized according to the effect on normal physiology. In iron depletion, the amount of stored iron (measured by serum ferritin concentration) is reduced but the amount of transport (measured by transferrin saturation) and functional iron may not be affected. Iron-deplete individuals have no iron stores to mobilize should the body require more iron. With further iron depletion, a shortage of stored, transport, and functional iron results in underproduction of iron-containing compounds such as hemoglobin, leading to anemia.

Epidemiology

Iron deficiency is the most common and widespread nutritional disorder in the world. It is unique in being the only nutrient deficiency that is also significantly prevalent in virtually all industrialized nations[6]. Iron deficiency is the most common cause of anemia during pregnancy and is particularly prevalent in women in developing countries, who have low iron stores due to poor nutritional intake, recurrent infections, menstrual blood loss, and repeated pregnancies.

Currently, there are no global figures for iron deficiency due to the high cost of the biochemical tests required to precisely define an individual's iron status. In the United States, the overall prevalence of iron deficiency and iron deficiency anemia in pregnancy was found to be 18 and 5.4%, respectively, in the 1999–2006 National Health and Nutrition Examination Survey. The prevalence of iron deficiency increased from 6.9 to 14.3 to 29.7% across the three trimesters [7]. A higher prevalence of iron deficiency and iron deficiency anemia has been found in the Korean population – 60 and 25.7%, respectively[8].

Pathophysiology

All cells need iron. It is found as iron porphyrin complexes in hemoglobin, myoglobin, and a variety of heme-containing enzymes (such as cytochrome, catalase, and peroxidase) and in metallo-flavoprotein enzymes (such as nicotinamide adenine dinucleotide – NAD). It is crucial for oxygen transport, energy production, and cellular growth and proliferation[9].

15

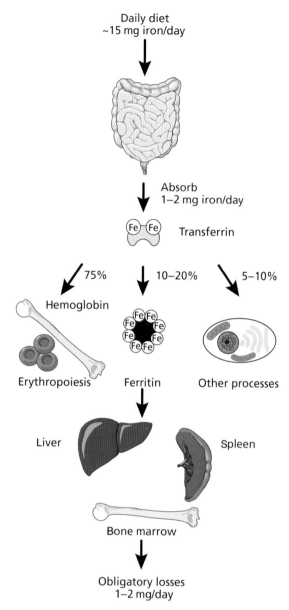

Figure 3.1 Iron homeostasis.

The human body has very limited capacity to absorb dietary iron. Absorption takes place in the duodenum and upper jejunum (Figure 3.1). The typical Western diet contains approximately 15 mg iron per day, of which less than 10% is absorbed (approximately 1–2 mg per day). Heme iron is 2–3 times more readily absorbed than non-heme iron. The main sources of dietary heme iron are hemoglobin and myoglobin from red meats, fish, and poultry. Elemental iron absorption is enhanced by reducing agents such as vitamin C (hence the recommendation to take iron supplements with orange juice or ascorbic acid tablets) and is inhibited by phytates in cereals, tannins in tea, and polyphenols in some vegetables. Iron homeostasis is closely regulated at the level of intestinal absorption, as once iron is absorbed there is no physiological mechanism for excretion of excess body iron other than blood loss. Obligatory losses take place from the skin and gastrointestinal and genitourinary tracts, and amount to up to 1 mg per day in a 70-kg man.

Once absorbed, iron is transported to virtually all tissues via the bloodstream where it is bound to the carrier protein transferrin. Normally, 20–45% of transferrin binding sites are filled (measured as percentage transferrin saturation). Excess iron is stored in the form of ferritin and hemosiderin, found mostly in the liver, spleen, and bone marrow. Adult women have less storage iron than men due to menstrual losses and pregnancies.

The normal iron content of the body is 3–4 g and is found in the following forms[10]:

- hemoglobin – approximately 2 g
- iron-containing proteins (e.g. myoglobin, cytochromes, catalase) – 400 mg
- iron bound to transferrin – 3–7 mg
- storage iron (ferritin and hemosiderin) – makes up the remainder

Iron Requirement during Pregnancy

Iron requirement rises sharply during the course of pregnancy by nearly 10-fold, from <0.8 mg/day in the first trimester to 4–5 mg/day in the second trimester, and to >6 mg/day in the third trimester[11]. This increased demand arises from the need to support placental and fetal growth, to fuel the increase in maternal red cell mass and to compensate for blood loss during delivery[12] (Figure 3.2). Accordingly, the recommended dietary allowance (RDA) for iron increases from 18 mg/day for non-pregnant females to 27 mg/day during pregnancy. However, the median dietary iron intake among pregnant women is only 15 mg/day [13]. To meet her requirements fully, a woman must enter pregnancy with an iron store of ≥300 mg – an amount which exceeds what most women possess, especially in developing countries [11]. This has led to major health organizations recommending iron supplementation during pregnancy. Postpartum, lactation requires 1.2 mg/day of iron [13].

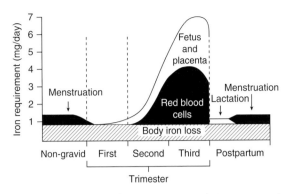

Figure 3.2 Estimated daily iron requirements during pregnancy in a 55-kg woman. From Bothwell (1979) with permission from Wiley-Blackwell[9].

Mechanism of Maternal–Fetal Iron Transfer

Maternal iron (Fe) is carried to the placenta bound to transferrin (Tf), where it binds to Tf receptors (TfR) on the apical surface of syncytiotrophoblasts (Figure 3.3). The Fe–Tf/TfR complex is endocytosed and Fe dissociates from maternal Tf when the vesicle acidifies. The released Fe is actively transported out of the vesicle into the cytosol, where it is used for cellular processes, stored in ferritin, or exported into the fetal circulation. TfR and Tf are recycled. Fe destined for export exits the basolateral membrane of the syncytiotrophoblast via ferroportin (Fpn), an iron exporter.

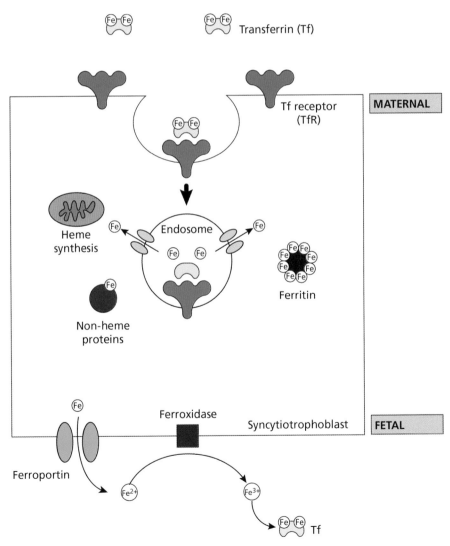

Figure 3.3 Mechanism of maternal–fetal iron transfer.

17

Ferroxidase then oxidizes Fe before it can be loaded onto fetal transferrin [14].

Iron transport to the fetus is strictly regulated. When the maternal iron store is low, the number of placental transferrin receptors increases so that more iron can be taken up by the placenta. Conversely, excessive iron transport to the fetus may be prevented by the placental synthesis of ferritin.

Hepcidin and Iron Homeostasis during Pregnancy

In the last decade, the peptide hormone hepcidin has emerged as the master regulator of iron absorption and tissue iron distribution. It acts by inducing degradation of the only known cellular iron transporter, ferroportin. Ferroportin exports iron from enterocytes that absorb dietary iron, from macrophages that recycle the iron of old erythrocytes, from hepatocytes that store iron, and from placental trophoblasts transferring iron to the fetus during pregnancy. When hepcidin concentration is high, ferroportin is depleted and iron is retained in iron-exporting cells. Conversely, when hepcidin concentration is low, stabilization of ferroportin promotes the absorption of dietary iron and the release of stored iron from macrophages and hepatocytes.

Hepcidin synthesis in the liver is regulated by the level of circulating and stored iron, erythropoietic activity, and inflammation[15]. Hepcidin production is increased in the context of inflammation, infection, and high body iron levels. In the event of blood loss, provision of additional iron for red cell production has obvious evolutionary advantage. Such an "erythroid regulator of iron" that links erythropoiesis with iron metabolism has long been sought after. This was recently identified as erythroferrone, a hormone that is produced by erythroblasts in response to erythropoietin and suppresses liver hepcidin synthesis in the event of blood loss[16].

During pregnancy, maternal hepcidin regulates iron availability to the developing fetus[12]. Hepcidin is lower in pregnant women compared to the non-pregnant healthy women and hepcidin levels decrease as pregnancy progresses. The lowest hepcidin levels are observed in the third trimester, which correlates with the time of greatest fetal demand for iron. It is currently unknown whether there are pregnancy-specific regulators of hepcidin production or whether hepcidin may be suppressed

in response to decreasing maternal iron levels during pregnancy. One study has shown that maternal transfer of iron to the fetus is inversely correlated with maternal hepcidin and was directly associated with neonatal hemoglobin[17]. In pregnancies associated with inflammatory conditions (such as obesity and pre-eclampsia), hepcidin levels were found to be elevated when compared to healthy pregnancies[18,19]. One would expect this to affect maternal–fetal iron transfer, but how this affects fetal and placenta development is currently unknown[12].

Causes of Iron Deficiency

There are many causes of iron deficiency anemia in the general population, all of which should be considered in the pregnant woman. The most common causes are inadequate dietary intake and depletion of iron stores from previous pregnancies or heavy menstrual losses.

The main causes are listed in Table 3.1.

Clinical Features

Iron deficiency anemia classically presents with symptoms of anemia, such as fatigue, weakness, headache, irritability, poor concentration, and exercise intolerance. Many patients are asymptomatic and may recognize that they have had these symptoms only after successful treatment with iron. Similar symptoms can also be present in non-anemic individuals who are iron depleted, with low serum ferritin[20,21].

Pagophagia, or pica for ice, has been recognized to be quite specific for the iron deficiency state. It may be present in patients who are not anemic and responds rapidly to iron replacement, often before any increase

Table 3.1 Causes of iron deficiency in pregnancy

Insufficient dietary intake	Vegetarian/vegan diet Malnutrition
Impaired intestinal absorption	Celiac disease Inflammatory bowel disease Atrophic gastritis Gastric bypass Food that impairs iron absorption: • Phytate in cereals • Tannin in tea
Blood loss	Heavy pre-pregnancy menstrual loss Frequent blood donation Occult blood loss, e.g. peptic ulcer, gastrointestinal malignancy Infections, e.g. hookworm
Pregnancy	Short interpregnancy interval Multiple previous pregnancies

in hemoglobin concentration. Iron deficiency has also been identified as a cause of restless legs syndrome, a marked discomfort in the legs that occurs only at rest and is immediately relieved by movement.

Severe iron deficiency is associated with pallor, glossitis, angular cheilitis, koilonychia, and nail ridging. Plummer–Vinson syndrome (iron deficiency anemia with post-cricoid web and dysphagia), which was relatively common in the first half of the twentieth century, has virtually disappeared.

Pregnancy Outcome

Although it is assumed that iron deficiency anemia during pregnancy negatively impacts on maternal and fetal outcome, the evidence available is often conflicting, or lacking altogether.

Birth Outcome

A U-shaped association has been observed between maternal Hb and birth weight. Maternal anemia in the first and second, but not the third trimester, is associated with a greater risk of low birth weight. The apparent loss or reversal of this association in the third trimester is probably because abnormally high Hb concentrations in the third trimester may reflect poor plasma volume expansion, which itself is a risk factor for poor birth outcome[22].

A similar relationship has been observed between maternal anemia and preterm delivery. In a study reported by Murphy and colleagues looking at the outcome of 54,382 singleton pregnancies in Wales, women found to be anemic in the second trimester had a 1.18- to 1.75-fold higher relative risk of preterm birth, low birth weight, and prenatal mortality[22]. In a large Californian study, Klebanoff showed an approximately doubled risk of preterm delivery with anemia during the second trimester but not during the third trimester[23]. In an analysis of 3728 deliveries in Singapore, 571 women who were anemic at the time of delivery had a higher incidence of preterm delivery than those who were not anemic[24].

Interestingly, some studies have shown that iron deficiency anemia but not anemia from other causes is associated with poor birth outcome. Scholl et al. showed that the odds of preterm delivery more than doubled with iron deficiency, but were not increased with anemia from other causes[25]. Similarly, in women from rural Nepal, anemia with iron deficiency in the first or second trimester was associated with a 1.9-fold higher risk of preterm birth, but anemia alone

was not[26]. A meta-analysis by Pratt found that iron deficiency without anemia is associated with low birth weight[21]. A recent systematic review of cohort studies looking at the association between anemia and birth outcomes did not find a significant association between maternal anemia and perinatal mortality. Association with neonatal mortality could not be evaluated owing to the paucity of data[27].

Infant Health

By increasing the risk of preterm birth, maternal iron deficiency anemia is likely to adversely affect infant health, as preterm infants are more likely to have perinatal complications. However, despite the important clinical implications, surprisingly little is known concerning the effects of maternal iron status during pregnancy on the subsequent health and development of the infant[26]. It was previously believed that the placenta is efficient at obtaining all the iron required by the fetus and that the iron status of the fetus, and subsequently the infant, is independent of maternal iron status during pregnancy[9]. Indeed, a number of studies conducted in diverse countries have shown that there is no significant association between maternal Hb at or near term and cord blood Hb concentrations[26,28–31]. However, on closer inspection, serum ferritin of the newborn is correlated with maternal Hb in several studies [29,30,32–37]. Preziosi et al. found that infants born to mothers who received iron supplementation had significantly higher serum ferritin at 3 months of age compared to those born to mothers who did not, even though there was no difference between the cord blood indices of the two groups[29]. Further research is needed to clarify the effect of maternal iron status on infant iron stores postpartum because of the known detrimental effects of iron deficiency anemia on the cognitive and motor development of infants.

Maternal Morbidity and Mortality

To date, no prospective studies have shown that anemia per se increases the risk of maternal mortality [26]. Observational studies have shown an association between severe anemia at, or close to, delivery and a higher risk of maternal mortality. However, as other conditions could have caused both the anemia and subsequent mortality, such data do not prove that maternal anemia causes higher mortality.

Large-scale, prospective, controlled trials are required to assess the efficacy of iron supplementation for reducing maternal mortality.

The influence of iron on immune function has long been appreciated. There is, however, currently a lack of information on the rates and severity of infection in pregnant women with iron deficiency anemia[26].

Diagnosis

Iron deficiency manifests in several stages – initially depletion of iron stores, followed by a fall in iron available for hemoglobin synthesis, and finally anemia ensues. Various tests exist to detect different stages of iron deficiency, which are outlined below.

Full Blood Count, Blood Film, and Red Cell Indices

A full blood count should be done routinely at booking and at 28 weeks of pregnancy. In iron deficiency anemia, this may show low Hb, mean cell hemoglobin (MCH), and mean cell hemoglobin concentration (MCHC). Despite the classic description of iron deficiency causing a hypochromic, microcytic picture (Figure 3.4), many iron-deficient patients in Western countries have normal red cell morphology. Furthermore, hypochromic microcytes are not pathognomonic of iron deficiency, with thalassemia and, less commonly, anemia of chronic disease being other common conditions encountered in clinical practice. In milder cases of iron deficiency, the MCV may be in the normal range.

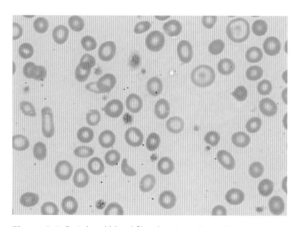

Figure 3.4 Peripheral blood film showing microcytic, hypochromic cells, target cells, and pencil cells typically seen in iron deficiency anemia.

With the advent of automated counting of reticulocytes, several reticulocyte parameters, including reticulocyte volume, hemoglobin content, and concentration, have become available, and their utility has recently been studied. Two studies, on children and hemodialysis patients treated with erythropoietin, respectively, found that a reticulocyte hemoglobin content <26 pg/cell was a stronger predictor for iron deficiency than serum ferritin and transferrin saturation[38,39]. Its utility in pregnant women has not yet been studied and it is not widely available.

Serum Ferritin

Serum ferritin level is an excellent indicator of iron stores in otherwise healthy adults. It has replaced assessment of bone marrow iron as the gold standard for the diagnosis of iron deficiency in most patients. It is the first laboratory test to become abnormal as iron stores decrease and it is not affected by recent iron ingestion. For ferritin levels in the range from 20 to 300 ng/mL, there appears to be a direct quantitative relationship between the ferritin concentration and iron stores. There is no clinical situation other than iron deficiency in which extremely low values of serum ferritin are seen.

During pregnancy in iron-replete women, the serum ferritin concentration initially rises, followed by a progressive fall at 32 weeks to about 50% of pre-pregnancy levels due to hemodilution and mobilization of iron. The levels increase again mildly in the third trimester[40]. Van den Broek et al. showed that serum ferritin is the best single indicator of storage iron in pregnant women when a cut-off point of 30 µg/L is used[41]. Treatment should be considered at this level as it indicates early iron depletion, which will worsen if not treated.

One caveat in using serum ferritin as an indicator of iron deficiency is that it is an acute phase reactant. Plasma levels are increased in liver disease, infection, inflammation, and malignancy. Inflammation elevates serum ferritin by approximately threefold and it has been suggested that in such patients, an estimation of iron stores can be achieved by dividing the patient's serum ferritin concentration by three[10].

Bone Marrow Iron

When demand exceeds requirement, tissue and bone marrow iron are depleted first. Iron stored in bone marrow macrophages and erythroid precursors can be detected with Prussian Blue stain on marrow samples. Lack of stainable iron is traditionally considered by most clinicians as the "gold standard" for the diagnosis of iron deficiency. However, bone marrow sampling is invasive and expensive, and has been replaced in practice by measurement of serum ferritin. Bone marrow examination is generally reserved for severe anemia when the cause cannot be determined by other means and when there is evidence of bone marrow failure.

Serum Iron and Transferrin Saturation

In iron deficiency anemia, serum iron concentration is reduced and transferrin level (also measured as total iron-binding capacity or TIBC) is elevated. This reflects the increase in transferrin expression in the presence of low serum iron. Pregnancy and oral contraceptives increase the plasma transferrin concentration, making it less accurate as a predictor of iron deficiency than serum ferritin. A low serum iron is also less specific, as it is seen in anemia of chronic disease. Furthermore, both serum iron and transferrin saturation show wide fluctuations in levels due to recent ingestion of iron, diurnal rhythm, and other factors such as concurrent infection[42].

Soluble Transferrin Receptor (STfR)

Transferrin receptors are transmembrane proteins that transport transferrin-bound iron into cells. A proportion of transferrin receptors circulate in the plasma in amounts proportional to the total. In response to a decrease in iron supply, more transferrin receptors are made, which circulate in the plasma and can be used as an indicator of iron deficiency. However, there is little change in the early stages of iron store depletion. It is not as sensitive or specific as serum ferritin and is also an expensive test, restricting its general availability. There is little data on its use in pregnancy.

Zinc Protoporphyrin (ZPP)

The last step in the biosynthesis of heme is the addition of iron to a protoporphyrin ring. When iron is unavailable, zinc is substituted, forming zinc protoporphyrin, which can be measured. This test shows that iron is not available, but not why, so the ZPP level is increased in both iron deficiency and anemia of chronic disease (in which iron is present but trapped in macrophages and thus not available for heme synthesis). Serum ZPP is affected by inflammation and infection, although to a lesser extent than serum ferritin. Red cell ZPP has greater sensitivity and specificity for iron depletion but is rarely performed[3].

Therapeutic Trial of Oral Iron

A time- and cost-effective way of diagnosing iron deficiency is assessing the response to a trial of oral iron. If the patient is known to have a hemoglobinopathy, ferritin should be checked first. A rise in Hb should be seen by 2 weeks after commencement of supplementation to confirm iron deficiency. If there is no response, further investigation is needed to distinguish between poor patient compliance, inability to absorb the iron preparation, incorrect diagnosis, ongoing bleeding, or a coexisting condition such as anemia of chronic disease or renal failure that reduces the erythropoietic response.

Management: Dietary Advice

All women should be counseled regarding how to optimize iron intake during pregnancy, including details of iron-rich food sources and factors that inhibit or promote iron absorption. While this may improve iron intake and enhance absorption, the degree of change achievable remains in question. Furthermore, once a woman becomes iron deficient in pregnancy, it is not possible to ensure repletion through diet alone and supplementation is needed.

Oral Iron

Oral iron is cheap, safe, and effective. Ferrous iron salts are the preparation of choice, as ferric irons are much less well absorbed. The various available ferrous salts differ in strength of elemental iron. The oral dose for iron deficiency anemia should not exceed 200 mg of elemental iron daily; higher doses saturate absorption and increase side effects. Indeed, lower doses, such as 60 mg once or twice daily, may be more effective when considering absorption, tolerance, and compliance altogether. Oral iron should be taken on an empty stomach, 1 hour before meals, with a source of vitamin C (ascorbic acid) such as orange juice to maximize absorption.

Gastrointestinal side effects are extremely common, leading to poor adherence to treatment. This can be particularly problematic in pregnant women, in whom bloating and constipation are already common due to high progesterone levels (which slow bowel movement) and increasing pressure of the gravid uterus on the rectum. Up to 70% of pregnant women on oral iron report adverse effects.

Due to our body's limited capacity to absorb iron from the gut, prolonged treatment over 6 to 8 weeks may be required to fully correct the anemia. Certain conditions, such as celiac disease, can also affect one's ability to absorb iron optimally.

Hb concentration is expected to rise by approximately 20 g/L over 3–4 weeks (British National Formulary, 2017: www.medicinescomplete.com/mc/bnf/current/PHP5839-ferrous-fumarate.htm#PHP54940-indicationsAndDose-topic). A repeat Hb at 2 weeks is required to assess response to treatment. Once the Hb is in the normal range, treatment should be continued for a further 3 months and until at least 6 weeks postpartum to replenish iron stores.

Parenteral Iron

The historical reluctance to use parenteral iron stems, at least partly, from the severe side effects (including anaphylaxis, shock, and death) associated with earlier preparations, such as high-molecular-weight iron dextran. Newer formulations of low-molecular-weight iron have a lower risk of anaphylaxis and improved toxicity profiles. A systematic review and meta-analysis of 103 randomized controlled trials found that there was no increase in the risk of serious adverse events or mortality with intravenous iron compared with controls[43].

Parenteral iron therapy is indicated in pregnancy when there is non-compliance with, or intolerance to, oral iron therapy or proven malabsorption. While the maximum amount of elemental iron that can be absorbed with an oral preparation is limited to about 25 mg/day, depending on the intravenous preparation used, up to 1000 mg of elemental iron can be administered in a single infusion. Contraindications include a history of anaphylaxis or reactions to parenteral iron therapy, first trimester of pregnancy, active acute or chronic infection, and chronic liver disease.

The intravenous iron preparations currently available in the UK are low-molecular-weight iron dextran (Cosmofer), iron sucrose (Venofer), iron isomaltoside (Monofer), and ferric carboxymaltose (Ferinject). Calculation of the required dose is based on the patient's ideal body weight and hemoglobin deficit.

Numerous studies have demonstrated the safety and efficacy of parenteral iron in pregnancy. Parenteral iron achieves a more rapid increase in Hb and replenishes iron stores faster than oral iron preparations[44–47]. Anaphylactic reaction to low-molecular-weight iron rarely occurs, although patients with a history of drug allergy may be at increased risk. Facilities and staff trained in the management of anaphylaxis should be available. For certain formulations, a small test dose is recommended when it is given for the first time. Premedication is generally not recommended except in those with asthma or more than one drug allergy. A small percentage of patients may experience a minor reaction with acute chest and back tightness without associated hypotension, tachypnea, wheezing, stridor, or periorbital edema. This is known as the Fishbane reaction. Pre-treatment with corticosteroids may be beneficial in preventing a recurrence, although it rarely occurs with re-challenge.

Only a small number of randomized, prospective trials have compared the relative safety of the various intravenous iron preparations. Currently, it is not possible to conclude that any one preparation is safer than another.

Intramuscular Preparations

Low-molecular-weight iron dextran can be given as a deep intramuscular (IM) injection in the gluteal muscle. However, the mobilization of iron from IM site is thought to be slow and variable. Reveiz et al. identified four randomized controlled trials (RCTs) conducted in India and Nigeria comparing IM to oral iron in a recent Cochrane review[48]. Three of the four studies showed that compared to oral iron, IM iron improved hematological indices. No conclusion could be drawn regarding the relative efficacy of IM versus IV administration from the few available studies. However, IM injection of iron is painful, has a significant risk of permanent skin staining, and has been associated with the development of gluteal sarcomas[49]. IM administration of iron dextran has not been shown to be safer or less toxic than the IV route. For all the above reasons, the use of IM iron is generally discouraged [50]. One advantage, however, is that following a test dose, IM iron can be administered in primary care, although facilities for resuscitation should still be available because of the small risk of systemic reaction.

Erythropoietin

Erythropoietin is a hormone produced in the kidney that stimulates erythropoiesis. Recombinant erythropoietin has been successfully used in pregnant women with iron deficiency anemia. Sifakis *et al.* treated 26 pregnant women (Hb <85 g/L and evidence of iron deficiency) who had been ineffectively treated with iron supplementation alone for at least 8 weeks with recombinant human erythropoietin combined with parenteral iron. Seventy-three percent of the women showed a quick response, with Hb reaching normal levels within the first 2 weeks of treatment[51]. Compared with parenteral iron alone, combination therapy with erythropoietin produces a quicker hemoglobin rise with a shorter median duration of therapy (18 days versus 25 days)[52].

Adverse effects of treatment with recombinant erythropoietin include mild flu-like symptoms. Uncommon but more serious adverse effects include hypertension, thromboembolic complications, seizures, and pure red cell aplasia. Several studies have shown that treatment of cancer-related anemia with erythropoietin is associated with accelerated tumor progression [53]. This led to a Food and Drug Administration (FDA) black box warning and the use of erythropoietin is now restricted to specific patient groups.

Blood Transfusion

There is currently greater scrutiny of blood transfusion practice than ever before, stemming from concerns about safety, high costs, and availability of donor blood. Potential dangers of transfusion are numerous but most commonly include transfusion-associated circulatory overload (TACO) or arise from clinical and laboratory errors. In women of childbearing age, there is the additional risk of fetal hemolytic disease in future pregnancies arising from transfusion-induced sensitization of red cell antigens.

Transfusion is rarely required or justified in women with iron deficiency anemia. It should be reserved for those who are hemodynamically unstable from active hemorrhage (such as in the setting of major obstetric hemorrhage) or who show evidence of end-organ ischemia secondary to severe iron deficiency anemia (very rare).

Management of Delivery in Women with Iron Deficiency Anemia

With good antenatal care, iron deficiency anemia at the time of delivery should generally be avoided. However, there will be instances when women book late, have recently come from abroad or have not engaged with antenatal care. Active measures should be taken to minimize blood loss at delivery, including delivery in hospital, preparation for possible transfusion with intravenous access and blood group and save, and active management of the third stage of labor. There is also ample evidence supporting delayed umbilical cord clamping during management of the third stage of labor to allow placental transfusion. RCTs have shown that delayed cord clamping reduces neonatal anemia and iron deficiency in infancy, and improves neurodevelopmental scores in young children[54–56]. Such effects may be particularly significant in the presence of maternal anemia.

Prevention: Iron Supplementation

There is little doubt that iron supplementation improves maternal iron status and hematological indices both during pregnancy and postpartum, even in industrialized countries and in women who enter pregnancy with adequate iron stores. Such benefit may be especially important when interpregnancy intervals are short because the supplemented mother will enter a subsequent pregnancy with a more favorable iron status[26]. However, while it is clear that iron supplementation significantly reduces the risk of maternal anemia and iron deficiency, the effect on pregnancy outcome is unclear[27,57,58]. Most studies looking at the effect of iron supplementation have focused on maternal hematological indices rather than fetal and maternal outcome.

A 2015 Cochrane review evaluated the effect of daily oral iron supplementation on pregnancy outcomes. Sixty-one trials were included, with 44 trials and a total of 43,274 women contributing data to the meta-analyses. Daily oral iron supplementation does reduce the number of women who are anemic (Hb <110 g/L) or iron deficient at term, but there was no convincing evidence supporting any effect on maternal or fetal outcome. Most of the studies focused on hematological indices. The overall quality of evidence was poor, with large heterogeneity between trials[58].

In contrast, another meta-analysis of RCTs published in the *British Medical Journal* in 2013 found that iron supplementation has a significant effect on increasing birth weight, but not on preterm birth, duration of gestation, small-for-gestational age births, and birth length [27]. Only a small number of trials reported effects on stillbirths, perinatal mortality, neonatal mortality, and maternal morbidity outcomes such as gestational diabetes, infection during pregnancy, puerperal sepsis, and malaria indicators, precluding further analyses for these outcomes.

Significant discrepancy exists between the impact of iron supplementation observed in the clinical trials' setting and in large-scale public health programs. Without the close supervision and careful counseling that patients receive in clinical trials, compliance is often inconsistent and poor, such that there is currently no good evidence of benefit[3].

Intermittent oral iron supplementation has been shown to produce similar maternal and fetal outcomes to daily supplementation and is associated with fewer side effects and reduced risk of women developing high Hb in mid and late pregnancy[59]. Moretti *et al.* recently revealed the possible mechanistic basis of this. They found that oral iron given to iron-depleted non-anemic non-pregnant women acutely increased plasma hepcidin at 24 but not 48 hours post-dose[60]. This was associated with a significant reduction in the fractional iron absorption from the dose administered within 24 hours, suggesting that a 48-hour spacing between doses is likely to result in higher fractional absorption.

The WHO strongly recommends the use of intermittent iron and folic acid supplements by non-anemic pregnant women to prevent anemia and improve gestational outcomes. The recommended scheme is 120 mg elemental iron once per week throughout pregnancy [61]. In the UK, the emphasis is on early detection and treatment of iron depletion and iron deficiency anemia, based on the results of blood count screening tests, as well as identification of women at increased risk[3].

Risk of Iron Supplementation

Observational studies suggest that high iron intake during pregnancy is associated with a risk of gestational diabetes[62,63]. A recent re-analysis of an RCT comparing selective (only in anemic patients and continued until Hb >110 g/L) to routine (regardless of Hb and throughout pregnancy) iron supplementation found that routine iron supplementation throughout pregnancy did not increase the risk of glucose intolerance during pregnancy[64]. Another large RCT (1164 women) comparing routine iron supplementation with placebo similarly found no significant difference in the incidence of gestational diabetes between the two groups[65].

Given the key role iron plays in host–pathogen interactions, the safety of routine iron supplementation in settings where infectious diseases such as malaria are endemic has been under scrutiny[66]. An early observational study found that parenteral iron infusion during pregnancy was associated with increased risk for perinatal malaria in primigravida but not multigravida[67]. In a prospective cohort study of 2112 pregnant women in Thailand, there was an association between recent iron supplementation and development of *Plasmodium vivax* (but not *Plasmodium falciparum*) malaria[68]. However, a randomized, double-blind, placebo-controlled community-based trial of oral iron supplementation administered to multigravid pregnant women by traditional birth attendants in rural Gambia found that iron supplementation did not increase the risk of malaria infection[69]. This is clearly an important area of ongoing research given the heavy burden of iron deficiency anemia in malaria endemic countries.

Screening for Iron Deficiency

No randomized trial or observational study compared clinical outcomes or adverse effects between pregnant women who were screened or not screened for iron deficiency anemia[70]. Routine serum ferritin is not recommended in the UK or the US[3,71]. However, this practice may be helpful in local populations where there is a particularly high prevalence of "at risk" women.

Postpartum Iron Deficiency Anemia

Postpartum anemia is defined by the WHO as Hb <100 g/L in the first 6 weeks after delivery. During pregnancy, a woman's circulating volume increases in preparation for blood loss at delivery. Bleeding and resorption of excess fluid during and after delivery vary in extent among individuals. This can have a major impact on postpartum Hb. Postpartum anemia is poorly defined and Hb level depends strongly on when it is measured.

Excessive bleeding during childbirth can cause or contribute to postpartum iron deficiency anemia. By causing the classical symptoms of weakness, fatigue, and breathlessness, it can impact on a woman's ability to breast-feed and care for her baby. One study estimated the incidence of postpartum iron deficiency and iron deficiency anemia to be 12.7 and 4.2%, respectively, in women in the USA within the first 6 months postpartum[72].

A recent Cochrane review analyzed the efficacy of the various treatment options (oral iron, parenteral iron, erythropoietin, and blood transfusion) available for postpartum iron deficiency anemia using data from 22 randomized controlled trials (2858 women) [73]. Clinical outcomes, such as maternal mortality, fatigue, and other anemia symptoms, were rarely reported, focusing instead on laboratory indices. The overall quality of evidence was poor with high risks of bias in most trials. Studies also differed in their treatment regimen (dose, formulation, route, schedule) and follow-up.

It was unclear which treatment modality is most effective in alleviating symptoms of postpartum anemia. Intravenous iron clearly causes fewer gastrointestinal symptoms compared to oral iron, but no conclusion could be drawn regarding its clinical efficacy as only 2 out of the 10 studies included in the analysis reported on fatigue and maternal mortality. Only one study compared red cell transfusion to no treatment (519 women). There was a small but statistically significant improvement in fatigue symptoms with red cell transfusion during the first week. However, the effect was transient and there was no significant difference at 6 weeks. The risk of transfusion does not appear to justify this transient improvement, in non-bleeding stable patients, but which mode of treatment provides the best response is not clear from the available body of evidence.

Summary

Iron deficiency is the most common cause of anemia in pregnancy worldwide. Iron requirement increases markedly during pregnancy and many women do not have sufficient iron stores to support this. Maternal iron deficiency anemia is associated with low birth weight and preterm delivery, but other effects on pregnancy are unclear. Routine iron supplementation is effective in improving maternal hematological indices and iron status, but studies so far have not shown a benefit to pregnancy outcome. Attention should be given to early detection and prompt management of iron deficiency, to minimize complications and avoid unnecessary blood transfusion.

Case Studies

Case Study 1

A 30-year-old woman presented to her midwife for booking of her third pregnancy. She had a history of menorrhagia prior to her pregnancies, all three of which have been within the last 3 years. She eats a typical Western diet, although she is not a fan of red meat. Her booking full blood count showed a mild anemia with an Hb of 95 g/dL and MCV of 80 fL. She was recalled for further blood tests and was found to have a serum ferritin of 10 ng/mL. She reported feeling exhausted, but had attributed this to looking after two young children. She was commenced on ferrous fumarate 200 mg three times daily and was advised to take it with orange juice 1 hour before meals. She found it difficult to tolerate due to nausea and epigastric discomfort, so the frequency was reduced to once daily. After 4 weeks, her Hb normalized and she had an otherwise uncomplicated pregnancy and delivery. She was advised to continue oral iron for at least 6 weeks postpartum to replenish her iron stores.

Case Study 2

A 25-year-old woman was reviewed on the ward round the day after an emergency cesarean section, performed because of prolonged labor and early signs of fetal distress. Estimated blood loss at surgery had been 800 mL and she said she felt exhausted. Her Hb was 78 g/L, having been 104 g/L before delivery. The surgery had otherwise been straightforward and no excess bleeding had occurred overnight. Examination showed normal pulse and blood pressure and her abdomen was soft, albeit with some tenderness following the surgery. Blood transfusion was considered in the light of her Hb and fatigue but given that there was no cardiovascular instability and there was no concern about bleeding, an infusion of total dose iron was given instead. She still felt fatigued 3 days later when she was discharged from hospital, but symptoms improved over the next few days and she was pleased she had not received a transfusion.

These cases illustrate how iron requirement increases markedly during pregnancy to support placental and fetal growth, to fuel the increase in maternal red cell mass and to compensate for blood loss during delivery. Iron deficiency anemia is common in pregnancy and may be associated with low birth weight and preterm delivery. Oral iron is the first-line treatment for iron deficiency +/− anemia, although routine screening and supplementation in pregnant women are not currently recommended in the UK. Iron supplementation reduces maternal anemia and iron deficiency, but the benefits for maternal and fetal outcomes are currently unclear.

References

1. Milman N, Bergholt T, Byg KE, Eriksen L, Hvas AM. Reference intervals for hematological variables during normal pregnancy and postpartum in 434 healthy Danish women. *European Journal of Haematology* 2007; **79**(1): 39–46.

2. Milman N, Byg KE, Agger AO. Hemoglobin and erythrocyte indices during normal pregnancy and postpartum in 206 women with and without iron supplementation. *Acta Obstetricia et Gynecologica Scandinavica* 2000; **79**(2): 89–98.

3. Pavord S, Myers B, Robinson S *et al.*; on behalf of the British Committee for Standards in Hematology. UK Guidelines on the Management of Iron Deficiency in Pregnancy. British Committee for Standards in Hematology. *British Journal of Haematology* 2012; **156**(5): 588–600.

4. Shen C, Jiang YM, Shi H *et al.* A prospective, sequential and longitudinal study of hematological profile during normal pregnancy in Chinese women. *Journal of Obstetrics and Gynecology* 2010; **30**(4): 357–361.

5. Akingbola TS, Adewole IF, Adesina OA *et al.* Hematological profile of healthy pregnant women in Ibadan, south-western Nigeria. *Journal of Obstetrics and Gynecology* 2006; **26**(8): 763–769.

6. WHO. *Iron Deficiency Anemia – Assessment, Prevention, and Control.* Geneva: WHO; 2001.

7. Mei Z, Cogswell ME, Looker AC *et al.* Assessment of iron status in US pregnant women from the National Health and Nutrition Examination Survey (NHANES), 1999–2006. *American Journal of Clinical Nutrition* 2011; **93**(6): 1312–1320.

8. Lee JO, Lee JH, Ahn S *et al.* Prevalence and risk factors for iron deficiency anemia in the Korean population: results of the fifth Korea National Health and Nutrition Examination Survey. *Journal of Korean Medical Science* 2014; **29**(2): 224–229.

9. Bothwell TH. *Iron Metabolism in Man.* Wiley-Blackwell; 1979.

10. Schrier S. Causes and diagnosis of iron deficiency anemia in the adult. *UpToDate* [online series]. 2015. Available from: http://www.uptodate.com/contents/causes-and-diagnosis-of-iron-deficiency-anemia-in-the-adult?source=search_result&search=iron±deficiency±anemia&selectedTitle=1~150#H12 (accessed 26 May 2017).

11. Bothwell TH. Iron requirements in pregnancy and strategies to meet them. *American Journal of Clinical Nutrition* 2000; **72**(1 Suppl): 257S–264S.

12. Koenig MD, Tussing-Humphreys L, Day J, Cadwell B, Nemeth E. Hepcidin and iron homeostasis during pregnancy. *Nutrients* 2014; **6**(8): 3062–3083.

13. Institute of Medicine (US) Panel on Micronutrients. *Dietary Reference Intakes for Vitamin A, Vitamin K, Arsenic, Boron, Chromium, Copper, Iodine, Iron, Manganese, Molybdenum, Nickel, Silicon, Vanadium, and Zinc.* Washington DC: National Academies Press (US); 2001.

14. McArdle HJ, Lang C, Hayes H, Gambling L. Role of the placenta in regulation of fetal iron status. *Nutrition Reviews* 2011; **69** (Suppl 1): S17–22.

15. Ganz T, Nemeth E. Hepcidin and iron homeostasis. *Biochimica et Biophysica Acta* 2012; **1823**(9): 1434–1443.

16. Kautz L, Jung G, Valore EV, Rivella S, Nemeth E, Ganz T. Identification of erythroferrone as an erythroid regulator of iron metabolism. *Nature Genetics* 2014; **46** (7): 678–684.

17. Young MF, Griffin I, Pressman E *et al.* Maternal hepcidin is associated with placental transfer of iron derived from dietary heme and nonheme sources. *Journal of Nutrition* 2012; **142**(1): 33–39.

18. Toldi G, Stenczer B, Molvarec A *et al.* Hepcidin concentrations and iron homeostasis in preeclampsia. *Clinical Chemistry and Laboratory Medicine* 2010; **48** (10): 1423–1426.

19. Dao MC, Sen S, Iyer C, Klebenov D, Meydani SN. Obesity during pregnancy and fetal iron status: is hepcidin the link? *Journal of Perinatology* 2013; **33**(3): 177–181.

20. Schrier S, Auerbach M. Treatment of the adult with iron deficiency anemia [Review]. *UpToDate* 2015. Available at: http://www.uptodate.com/contents/treatment-of-iron-deficiency-anemia-in-adults?source=search_result&search=iron+deficiency+anaemia&selectedTitle=2%7E150.

21. Pratt JJ, Khan KS. Non-anemic iron deficiency – a disease looking for recognition of diagnosis: a systematic review. *European Journal of Haematology* 2016; **96**(6): 618–628.

22. Murphy JF, O'Riordan J, Newcombe RG, Coles EC, Pearson JF. Relation of hemoglobin levels in first and second trimesters to outcome of pregnancy. *Lancet* 1986; **1**(8488): 992–995.

23. Klebanoff MA, Shiono PH, Selby JV, Trachtenberg AI, Graubard BI. Anemia and spontaneous preterm birth. *American Journal of Obstetrics and Gynecology* 1991; **164**(1 Pt 1): 59–63.

24. Singh K, Fong YF, Arulkumaran S. Anemia in pregnancy – a cross-sectional study in Singapore. *European Journal of Clinical Nutrition* 1998; **52**(1): 65–70.

25. Scholl TO, Hediger ML, Fischer RL, Shearer JW. Anemia vs iron deficiency: increased risk of preterm delivery in a prospective study. *American Journal of Clinical Nutrition* 1992; **55**(5): 985–988.

26. Allen LH. Anemia and iron deficiency: effects on pregnancy outcome. *American Journal of Clinical Nutrition* 2000; **71**(5 Suppl): 1280S–1284S.

27. Haider BA, Olofin I, Wang M *et al.* Anemia, prenatal iron use, and risk of adverse pregnancy outcomes: systematic review and meta-analysis. *BMJ* 2013; **346**: f3443.

28. Lao TT, Loong EP, Chin RK, Lam CW, Lam YM. Relationship between newborn and maternal iron status and hematological indices. *Biology of the Neonate* 1991; **60**(5): 303–307.

29. Preziosi P, Prual A, Galan P *et al.* Effect of iron supplementation on the iron status of pregnant women: consequences for newborns. *American Journal of Clinical Nutrition* 1997; **66**(5): 1178–1182.

30. Hokama T, Takenaka S, Hirayama K *et al.* Iron status of newborns born to iron deficient anemic mothers. *Journal of Tropical Pediatrics* 1996; **42**(2): 75–77.

31. Barton DP, Joy MT, Lappin TR *et al.* Maternal erythropoietin in singleton pregnancies: a randomized trial on the effect of oral hematinic supplementation. *American Journal of Obstetrics and Gynecology* 1994; **170**(3): 896–901.

32. Gaspar MJ, Ortega RM, Moreiras O. Relationship between iron status in pregnant women and their newborn babies. Investigation in a Spanish population. *Acta Obstetricia et Gynecologica Scandinavica* 1993; **72**(7): 534–537.

33. Agrawal RM, Tripathi AM, Agarwal KN. Cord blood hemoglobin, iron and ferritin status in maternal anemia. *Acta Pediatrica Scandinavica* 1983; **72**(4): 545–548.

34. Ajayi OA. Iron stores in pregnant Nigerians and their infants at term. *European Journal of Clinical Nutrition* 1988; **42**(1): 23–28.

35. Rusia U, Flowers C, Madan N *et al.* Serum transferrin receptor levels in the evaluation of iron deficiency in the neonate. *Acta Paediatrica Japonica* 1996; **38**(5): 455–459.

36. Colomer J, Colomer C, Gutierrez D *et al.* Anemia during pregnancy as a risk factor for infant iron deficiency: report from the Valencia Infant Anemia Cohort (VIAC) study. *Paediatric and Perinatal Epidemiology* 1990; **4**(2): 196–204.

37. Milman N, Agger AO, Nielsen OJ. Iron status markers and serum erythropoietin in 120 mothers and newborn infants. Effect of iron supplementation in normal pregnancy. *Acta Obstetricia et Gynecologica Scandinavica* 1994; **73**(3): 200–204.

38. Brugnara C, Zurakowski D, DiCanzio J, Boyd T, Platt O. Reticulocyte hemoglobin content to diagnose iron deficiency in children. *JAMA* 1999; **281**(23): 2225–2230.

39. Fishbane S, Galgano C, Langley RC, Jr., Canfield W, Mesaka JK. Reticulocyte hemoglobin content in the evaluation of iron status of hemodialysis patients. *Kidney International* 1997; **52**(1): 217–222.

40. Asif N, Hassan K, Mahmud S *et al.* Comparison of serum ferritin levels in three trimesters of pregnancy and their correlation with increasing gravidity. *International Journal of Pathology* 2007; **5**: 26–30.

41. van den Broek NR, Letsky EA, White SA, Shenkin A. Iron status in pregnant women: which measurements are valid? *British Journal of Haematology* 1998; **103**(3): 817–824.

42. Adams PC, Reboussin DM, Press RD *et al.* Biological variability of transferrin saturation and unsaturated iron-binding capacity. *American Journal of Medicine* 2007; **120**(11): 999.e1–7.

43. Avni T, Bieber A, Grossman A *et al.* The safety of intravenous iron preparations: systematic review and meta-analysis. *Mayo Clinic Proceedings* 2015; **90**(1): 12–23.

44. Al RA, Unlubilgin E, Kandemir O *et al.* Intravenous versus oral iron for treatment of anemia in pregnancy: a randomized trial. *Obstetrics and Gynecology* 2005; **106**(6): 1335–1340.

45. Bhandal N, Russell R. Intravenous versus oral iron therapy for postpartum anemia. *British Journal of Obstetrics and Gynaecology* 2006; **113**(11): 1248–1252.

46. Breymann C, Gliga F, Bejenariu C, Strizhova N. Comparative efficacy and safety of intravenous ferric carboxymaltose in the treatment of postpartum iron deficiency anemia. *International Journal of Gynecology and Obstetrics* 2008; **101**(1): 67–73.

47. Van Wyck DB, Martens MG, Seid MH, Baker JB, Mangione A. Intravenous ferric carboxymaltose compared with oral iron in the treatment of postpartum anemia: a randomized controlled trial. *Obstetrics and Gynecology* 2007; **110**(2 Pt 1): 267–278.

48. Reveiz L, Gyte GM, Cuervo LG, Casasbuenas A. Treatments for iron-deficiency anemia in pregnancy. *Cochrane Database of Systematic Reviews* 2011; (**10**): CD003094.

49. Greenberg G. Sarcoma after intramuscular iron injection. *British Medical Journal* 1976; **1**(6024): 1508–1509.

50. Solomons NW, Schumann K. Intramuscular administration of iron dextran is inappropriate for treatment of moderate pregnancy anemia, both in intervention research on underprivileged women and in routine prenatal care provided by public health services. *American Journal of Clinical Nutrition* 2004; **79**(1): 1–3.

51. Sifakis S, Angelakis E, Vardaki E *et al.* Erythropoietin in the treatment of iron deficiency anemia during

pregnancy. *Gynecologic and Obstetric Investigation* 2001; **51**(3): 150–156.

52. Breymann C, Visca E, Huch R, Huch A. Efficacy and safety of intravenously administered iron sucrose with and without adjuvant recombinant human erythropoietin for the treatment of resistant iron-deficiency anemia during pregnancy. *American Journal of Obstetrics and Gynecology* 2001; **184**(4): 662–667.

53. Blau CA. Erythropoietin in cancer: presumption of innocence? *Stem Cells* 2007; **25**(8): 2094–2097.

54. Hutton EK, Hassan ES. Late vs early clamping of the umbilical cord in full-term neonates: systematic review and meta-analysis of controlled trials. *JAMA* 2007; **297** (11): 1241–1252.

55. Andersson O, Lindquist B, Lindgren M *et al.* Effect of delayed cord clamping on neurodevelopment at 4 years of age: a randomized clinical trial. *JAMA Pediatrics* 2015; **169**(7): 631–638.

56. Andersson O, Hellstrom-Westas L, Andersson D, Domellof M. Effect of delayed versus early umbilical cord clamping on neonatal outcomes and iron status at 4 months: a randomised controlled trial. *BMJ* 2011; **343**: d7157.

57. Imdad A, Bhutta ZA. Routine iron/folate supplementation during pregnancy: effect on maternal anemia and birth outcomes. *Paediatric and Perinatal Epidemiology* 2012; **26** (Suppl 1): 168–177.

58. Pena-Rosas JP, De-Regil LM, Garcia-Casal MN, Dowswell T. Daily oral iron supplementation during pregnancy. *Cochrane Database of Systematic Reviews* 2015; **7**: CD004736.

59. Pena-Rosas JP, De-Regil LM, Dowswell T, Viteri FE. Intermittent oral iron supplementation during pregnancy. *Cochrane Database of Systematic Reviews* 2012; **7**: CD009997.

60. Moretti D, Goede JS, Zeder C *et al.* Oral iron supplements increase hepcidin and decrease iron absorption from daily or twice-daily doses in iron-depleted young women. *Blood* 2015; **126**(17): 1981–1989.

61. World Health Organization. *Intermittent Iron and Folic Acid Supplementation in Non-Anemic Pregnant Women.* 2015/06/26 ed 2012. http://www.who.int/nutrition/pub lications/micronutrients/guidelines/guideline_intermit tent_ifa_non_anaemic_pregnancy/en/

62. Qiu C, Zhang C, Gelaye B *et al.* Gestational diabetes mellitus in relation to maternal dietary heme iron and nonheme iron intake. *Diabetes Care* 2011; **34**(7): 1564–1569.

63. Helin A, Kinnunen TI, Raitanen J *et al.* Iron intake, hemoglobin and risk of gestational diabetes: a prospective cohort study. *BMJ Open* 2012; **2**(5).

64. Kinnunen TI, Luoto R, Helin A, Hemminki E. Supplemental iron intake and the risk of glucose intolerance in pregnancy: re-analysis of a randomised controlled trial in Finland. *Maternal and Child Nutrition* 2016; **12**(1): 74–78.

65. Chan KK, Chan BC, Lam KF, Tam S, Lao TT. Iron supplement in pregnancy and development of gestational diabetes – a randomised placebo-controlled trial. *British Journal of Obstetrics and Gynaecology* 2009; **116**(6): 789–797; discussion 97–98.

66. Sangare L, van Eijk AM, Ter Kuile FO, Walson J, Stergachis A. The association between malaria and iron status or supplementation in pregnancy: a systematic review and meta-analysis. *PLoS One* 2014; **9**(2): e87743.

67. Oppenheimer SJ, Macfarlane SB, Moody JB, Harrison C. Total dose iron infusion, malaria and pregnancy in Papua New Guinea. *Transactions of the Royal Society of Tropical Medicine and Hygiene* 1986; **80**(5): 818–822.

68. Nacher M, McGready R, Stepniewska K *et al.* Hematinic treatment of anemia increases the risk of *Plasmodium vivax* malaria in pregnancy. *Transactions of the Royal Society of Tropical Medicine and Hygiene* 2003; **97**(3): 273–276.

69. Menendez C, Todd J, Alonso PL *et al.* The effects of iron supplementation during pregnancy, given by traditional birth attendants, on the prevalence of anemia and malaria. *Transactions of the Royal Society of Tropical Medicine and Hygiene* 1994; **88**(5): 590–593.

70. McDonagh M, Cantor A, Bougatsos C, Dana T, Blazina I. *Routine Iron Supplementation and Screening for Iron Deficiency Anemia in Pregnant Women: A Systematic Review to Update the US Preventive Services Task Force Recommendation.* Rockville (MD); 2015.

71. McCarthy M. Evidence for iron deficiency screening "inadequate," US panel concludes. *BMJ* 2015; **350**: h1841.

72. Bodnar LM, Cogswell ME, Scanlon KS. Low income postpartum women are at risk of iron deficiency. *Journal of Nutrition* 2002; **132**(8): 2298–2302.

73. Markova V, Norgaard A, Jorgensen KJ, Langhoff-Roos J. Treatment for women with postpartum iron deficiency anemia. *Cochrane Database of Systematic Reviews* 2015; **8**: CD010861.

Vitamin B$_{12}$ and Folate Deficiencies in Pregnancy

Alesia Khan and Susan Robinson

Vitamin B$_{12}$ Deficiency

Epidemiology

Vitamin B$_{12}$ deficiency is relatively common, with significant and variable clinical consequences. Vitamin B$_{12}$ deficiency in pregnancy is associated with adverse outcomes such as neural tube defects (NTDs), preterm labor, intrauterine growth retardation (IUGR), and recurrent miscarriage[1,2].

Pathophysiology

The "normal" blood concentrations of vitamin B$_{12}$ fall in pregnancy, due to the altered physiology. Women have a state of hemodilution due to expanded blood volume, altered renal function[1],

rise in vitamin B$_{12}$-binding proteins, and transfer of materno-fetal vitamin B$_{12}$. It is not clear at what level the vitamin B$_{12}$ status becomes detrimental, particularly if pregnancy-specific reference ranges are not available.

Vitamin B$_{12}$ is an essential cofactor that is integral to methylation processes in reactions related to DNA and cell metabolism. Intracellular conversion of vitamin B$_{12}$ to two active coenzymes, adenosylcobalamin in mitochondria and methylcobalamin in the cytoplasm, is necessary for the homeostasis of methylmalonic acid and homocysteine, respectively (Figure 4.1)[3–5].

In serum, vitamin B$_{12}$ is bound to haptocorrin as holo-haptocorrin (holoHC) (formally transcobalamin III) and to transcobalamin as holo-transcobalamin (holoTC). HoloHC accounts for 80–94% of endogenous plasma vitamin B$_{12}$, whereas HoloTC

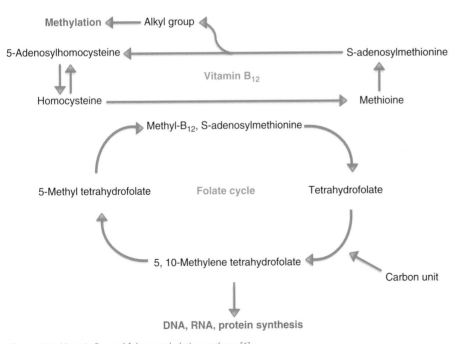

Figure 4.1 Vitamin B$_{12}$ and folate methylation pathway[6].

accounts for 6–20% of bound vitamin B_{12}. Only vitamin B_{12} bound as holoTC is presented for cellular uptake[7].

Causes of Vitamin B_{12} Deficiency

There are many causes of vitamin B_{12} deficiency among the general population. All causes should be considered when assessing the pregnant woman. Causes of deficiency can be related to the complex intake and absorption of vitamin B_{12}, as highlighted in Figure 4.2. This can be disrupted at various stages resulting in deficiency states, which may be reversible or irreversible.

Foods containing vitamin B_{12} are only derived from animal origin: meat, fish, and dairy. The daily western diet contains around 5–30 μg of vitamin B_{12} per day, of which 1–5 μg is absorbed. A developing fetus requires 50 μg per day. Body storage is relatively high, about 1–5 μg, and deficiency may not manifest for several months to years following diminished intake or absorption[3,8,9].

The most commonly seen cause of vitamin B_{12} deficiency in pregnant women relates to vegetarian or vegan diets. Demand increases in pregnancy;

therefore, deficiency may simply be related to inadequate intake. The main causes are listed in Table 4.1 [8–11].

Clinical Features

The clinical manifestations of vitamin B_{12} deficiency (see Figure 4.3) represent the effects of depletion upon multiple systems and vary greatly in severity. The clinical manifestations are heterogeneous but can also be different depending on the degree and duration of deficiency.

Manifestations in mild deficiency may include fatigue and anemia with indices suggesting B_{12} deficiency but an absence of neurological features. Anemia may range from mild to severe with symptoms of easy fatigue, dyspnea, palpitations, and pallor. Moderate deficiency may include an obvious macrocytic anemia with symptoms such as glossitis and stomatitis, and subtle neurological features, for example, distal sensory impairment. Severe deficiency will show evidence of bone marrow suppression with macrocytic anemia, neutropenia, and thrombocytopenia. There may be clear evidence of neurological features and risk of cardiomyopathy. It

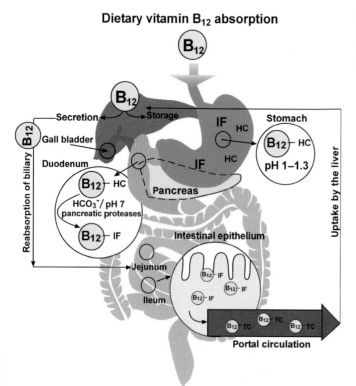

Figure 4.2 Intake and absorption of vitamin B_{12}. IF: intrinsic factor; TC: holo-transcobalamin; HC: holo-haptocorrin; B_{12}: vitamin B_{12}. With thanks to Renata Gorska from the Nutristasis Unit, Guy's and St Thomas' NHS Foundation Trust, London for figure preparation.

Table 4.1 Causes of vitamin B$_{12}$ deficiency

Impaired gastric absorption	Pernicious anemia
	Previous gastrectomy
	Zollinger–Ellison syndrome
Impaired intestinal absorption	Inflammatory bowel disease
	Previous gastrectomy or resection or terminal ileum
	Parasites
Pancreatic insufficiency	
Decreased intake	Malnutrition
	Vegetarian/vegan diet
Increased requirements	Hemolysis
	HIV
Drugs	Alcohol
	Proton pump inhibitors
	H2 receptor antagonists
	Metformin

is also important to recognize that clinical features of deficiency can manifest without anemia and also without a low serum vitamin B$_{12}$. In these cases, treatment should still be given without delay [5,10,12,13].

Pregnancy Outcomes

Evidence regarding the correlation between maternal vitamin B$_{12}$ deficiency and adverse pregnancy outcomes is not clear. In women with pernicious anemia there has been an observed association between vitamin B$_{12}$ deficiency and recurrent miscarriages[14]. It is likely that maternal vitamin B$_{12}$ status correlates with neonatal vitamin B$_{12}$ status. Low vitamin B$_{12}$ in the neonate is compounded by reduced concentration of the vitamin in breast milk[2].

Reproductive tissue can be affected, manifesting as infertility, recurrent miscarriage, intrauterine growth restriction, neural tube defects, and neurological developmental delay. In mild deficiency, there may be little effect upon the fetus but if the baby is exclusively breast-fed they may become progressively B$_{12}$ deficient resulting in failure to thrive, floppiness, and developmental delay[2,5].

Neurological Features

Neurological impairment includes motor disturbances, sensory loss, abnormal balance and reflexes, cognitive impairment, and memory loss. Extreme cases may present with stupor or psychosis. Subacute combined degeneration of the cord involves demyelination of the posterior and lateral tracts. Initial bilateral peripheral neuropathy can progress to axonal degeneration and neuronal death if left untreated. There may also be disturbances of proprioception, vibratory sense, and areflexia. The patient may complain of clumsiness, poor coordination, and difficulty walking. Without treatment, weakness and stiffness may develop, manifesting as spastic ataxia. Damage to peripheral nerves results in sleepiness, altered taste and smell, and optic atrophy. In severe deficiency or advanced stages, a dementia-like illness may be seen and frank psychosis with hallucinations, paranoia, and severe depression [6,10].

Diagnosis

There are no clearly available vitamin B$_{12}$ reference ranges for the different stages of pregnancy and still no "gold standard" test for measuring vitamin B$_{12}$ deficiency. Serum vitamin B$_{12}$ remains the first-line test. Second-line tests include looking for increased levels of plasma methylmalonic acid (MMA), which can help clarify uncertainties of underlying biochemical/functional deficiencies. Serum holo-transcobalamin has an indeterminate 'gray area' and therefore should be correlated with MMA [12]. Plasma homocysteine may be helpful, but is less specific than MMA. Furthermore, reference ranges for pregnancy should be established given the variation in levels throughout pregnancy[4].

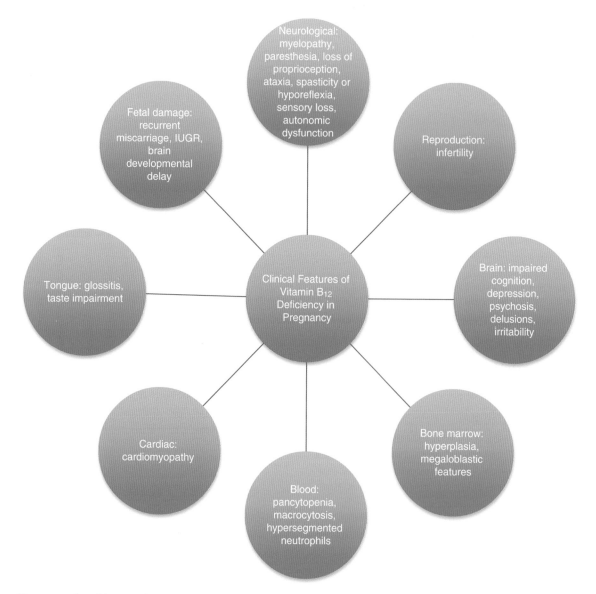

Figure 4.3 Clinical features of vitamin B$_{12}$ deficiency in pregnancy[5,8,9,10,11,13,15].

Investigations

The routine full blood count (mean cell volume [MCV] and hemoglobin) at the 12-week antenatal booking appointment may indicate B$_{12}$ deficiency. If there is evidence of macrocytic anemia, blood tests should include reticulocyte count, blood film (see Figure 4.4), and lactate dehydrogenase (LDH). Macrocytosis is the most common trigger to check vitamin B$_{12}$, folate, and thyroid status, although there is a physiological increase in MCV during pregnancy and an elevated MCV may

also be absent or masked by concomitant iron deficiency or thalassemia trait[8,9,11]. Pregnant women with a concomitant iron deficiency may not develop macrocytosis until the iron deficiency has been resolved.

Serum Vitamin B$_{12}$

Measurement of vitamin B$_{12}$ in serum is the most common assay used to evaluate vitamin B$_{12}$. However, false positives and negatives are common, failing to detect true deficiency or falsely implying a deficient state. It is widely available at low cost using automated methods

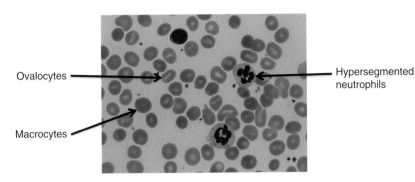

Ovalocytes

Macrocytes

Hypersegmented
neutrophils

Figure 4.4 Peripheral blood film illustrating a megaloblastic picture.

and competitive-binding immuno-chemiluminescence [4,12,16–19].

Serum vitamin B$_{12}$ levels fall in pregnancy. The physiological reduction can be up to 50%. Levels return to normal rapidly after delivery without supplementation. Levels greater than 130 ng/mL may be considered normal but levels of less than 130 ng/mL with macrocytosis and/or neurological symptoms should be considered for B$_{12}$ treatment.

Owing to the lack of pregnancy-specific reference ranges, the vitamin B$_{12}$ level is ideally only checked if there is a high suspicion of vitamin B$_{12}$ deficiency, as in the following scenarios:

1. A risk factor for vitamin B$_{12}$ deficiency, for example, gastrectomy or diseased terminal ileum as in Crohn's or tuberculosis
2. MCV >100 fL
3. Neurological features

HoloTC

HoloTC measures the metabolically active form of vitamin B$_{12}$ by immunoassay, with the reference range varying depending on the individual assay. The theoretical merits of measuring holoTC have been known for many years but it is only recently that an assay suited to routine use, known as "active B$_{12}$" has become available. Emerging evidence indicates that a low concentration of holoTC is a more reliable marker of impaired vitamin B$_{12}$ status than a low concentration of serum vitamin B$_{12}$. HoloTC may be the earliest marker for vitamin B$_{12}$ depletion. This test is increasingly being adopted; however, there remain discrepancies with regards to mode of application and assignment of cut-off values. It is recommended that a second confirmatory test, such

as MMA, should be used if the result is in the intermediate range. Once again, the reference ranges specific for pregnancy states are yet to be established[19,20].

Methylmalonic Acid (MMA)

The conversion of MMA to succinyl-CoA requires B$_{12}$ as a cofactor and hence accumulation of MMA occurs if B$_{12}$ is not available. Elevated MMA is an indicator of tissue vitamin B$_{12}$ deficiency and will persist for several days even after replacement is commenced. Measurement of MMA may be the most representative marker of metabolic vitamin B$_{12}$ insufficiency. However, the interpretation in those with impaired renal function is potentially challenging because it can be falsely elevated, although very high levels of plasma MMA are usually indicative of cobalamin deficiency. It is a high-cost test requiring gas chromatography mass spectrometry[4].

Total Homocysteine (THcy)

Plasma total homocysteine is elevated in B$_{12}$ deficiency and can increase early in the course of deficiency. It is a sensitive marker but non-specific and is also raised in folate, B$_6$ deficiency, renal failure, and hypothyroidism. Most laboratories regard >15 μmol/L as high, although it depends on the individual technique. The sample must be processed within 2 hours, which can inhibit its utility.

Bone Marrow Biopsy

Bone marrow biopsy is very rarely required but may be indicated in selective cases where the diagnosis is unclear or blood indices are not responding to adequate treatment (see Figure 4.5).

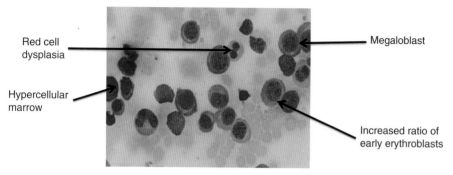

Figure 4.5 Bone marrow biopsy illustrating megaloblastic features.

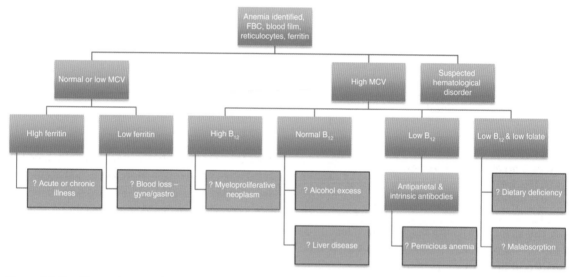

Figure 4.6 Algorithm to determine the cause of vitamin B_{12} deficiency[7–9,11].

Identifying the Cause of Vitamin B_{12} Deficiency

Once a diagnosis of vitamin B_{12} deficiency is identified, history and examination are important (see Figure 4.6). If there is no obvious dietary lack of vitamin B_{12} or malabsorptive cause, intrinsic factor and parietal cell antibodies should be performed to exclude pernicious anemia. Parietal cell antibodies were 80% sensitive and 90% specific, while intrinsic factor antibodies are highly specific (95%,) but have low sensitivity (40–60%)[12].

Management

It is usually acceptable to commence treatment within a few days of confirming the diagnosis. If there are neurological disturbances then treatment should be expedited and commenced without delay. Specialist input should be sought in the event of neurological features, including impaired cognitive state[21].

Parenteral Treatment

In the UK, current clinical practice is to commence parenteral therapy with intramuscular (IM) hydroxycobalamin. This bypasses the possibility of debate concerning whether the therapy will be adequately taken, absorbed, and metabolized. Standard initial therapy for patients without neurological involvement is 1000 µg IM three times a week for 2 weeks. If there are neurological symptoms then 1000 µg IM on alternate days should be continued for up to 3 weeks or until there is no further improvement[12,22]. In irreversible causes, for example pernicious anemia, the treatment should be continued life long at 3-monthly intervals. If the cause is temporary in pregnancy due to deficient diet, then the treatment can be reviewed postpartum and after completion of exclusive breast-feeding.

Hydroxycobalamin is safe to use in pregnancy and is generally well tolerated. Rare side effects include itching, exanthema, chills, fever, hot flushes, nausea, dizziness, and very rarely anaphylaxis. If there is a concern regarding this, then the drug should be administered in a place where hypersensitivity can be managed, with hydrocortisone and chlorphenamine cover available [12,15].

Oral Treatment

Cyanocobalamin is the oral preparation, which can be given at 50–150 μg daily. This is a pharmacological preparation requiring conversion to metabolically active cobalamins. Oral therapy may be considered in certain situations, for example in mild or subclinical deficiency with no clinical features and when there are no concerns about absorption and compliance [12,15].

Treating Concomitant Deficiencies

If there is concomitant vitamin B$_{12}$ and folate deficiency, then vitamin B$_{12}$ must be commenced first to avoid precipitating subacute combined degeneration of the cord. Giving folic acid alone results in the methylation of any remaining vitamin B$_{12}$, which cannot participate in fatty acid production; the result is degeneration of both central and peripheral nerves. In patients with isolated vitamin B$_{12}$ deficiency and anemia, additional folic acid supplementation is recommended until vitamin B$_{12}$ is replete to prevent subsequent folate deficiency following replenishment of B$_{12}$ stores. Iron deficiency can be treated with ferrous sulfate 200 mg three times daily orally (or alternative iron preparations can be tried) with vitamin C supplementation. Constipation and nausea in pregnancy may reduce tolerability[11,13,15,21,23]; see Chapter 3 for further information.

Summary

Vitamin B$_{12}$ demands increase in pregnancy, but normal body stores last up to 5 years, resulting in deficiency in pregnancy being relatively uncommon. This, coupled with changes in normal B$_{12}$ levels in pregnancy and the absence of pregnancy-specific reference ranges, means assay levels should be interpreted with caution.

Vitamin B$_{12}$ deficiency can have serious sequelae for both mother and fetus and therefore genuine deficiency should be treated appropriately. In cases where the diagnosis is missed, the neonate may exhibit failure-to-thrive, megaloblastic anemia, and neurological symptoms.

Folate Deficiency

Epidemiology

Folate deficiency in women of childbearing age and pregnant women varies considerably throughout the world. In developed countries, prevalence may be as low as 5% whereas in some developing countries this can rise to 50–73%. It has been estimated that between 700 and 900 pregnancies are affected by neural tube defects, such as spina bifida, each year in the UK. In pregnancy, demands for folate increase due to the requirement for growth and development of the fetus [24].

Pathophysiology

Folate (vitamin B$_9$) is an essential vitamin required for DNA replication and as a substrate for a range of enzymatic reactions involved in amino acid synthesis and vitamin metabolism. Dietary folate is a naturally occurring nutrient found in foods such as leafy green vegetables, legumes, egg yolk, liver, and citrus fruit. Folic acid is a synthetic dietary supplement. Both folate and folic acid are metabolically inactive, and must be reduced to l-5-methyltetrahydrofolate to participate in cellular metabolism.

The methylenetetrahydrofolate reductase (MTHFR) enzyme is required to metabolize folic acid into the biologically active form; however, MTHFR has a high prevalence of genetic polymorphisms in the general population. This may result in reduced enzymatic activity and, therefore, less biologically available l-methylfolate. Research is underway to investigate the need for supplementation with l-methylfolate rather than folic acid in people with variants of the *MTHFR* gene, which result in reduced enzymatic activity. However, this mechanism is not fully understood and the oral bioavailability of l-methylfolate is unclear.

Causes of Folate Deficiency

Folate deficiency may arise if there is decreased intake, increased demand, such as in pregnancy and impaired absorption. Concomitant disorders such as hemolysis,

Table 4.2 Causes of folate deficiency

Increased demand	Pregnancy
Impaired intestinal absorption	Malabsorption
	Bowel surgery
	Parasites
Hematological disorders	
Decreased intake	Malnutrition
	Vegetarian/vegan diet
Increased requirements	Hemolysis
	HIV
Drugs:	
Anticonvulsants	Phenytoin
	Penobarbital
	Primidone
	Carbamazepine
Folate inhibitors	Methotrexate
	Sulphasalazine
	Co-trimoxazole

drugs, and primary hematological disorders may increase folate demand[8] (see Table 4.2).

Clinical Features

In the mother, folate deficiency results in anemia and peripheral neuropathy.

There is strong evidence linking low blood folate concentrations and the risk of low birth weight. Folic acid supplementation increased birth weight in studies in Africa and India. Some evidence suggests that low folate concentrations during pregnancy may result in an increased risk of placental abruption and preterm delivery[25,26].

In mild folate deficiencies, fetal congenital abnormalities, such as neural tube defects (NTD), spinal dysraphism, and anencephaly may arise. Strong evidence from previous randomized control trials demonstrates the association between low maternal folate intake and status with an increased risk of NTDs. It is well established that supplementation of the diet with folic acid around the time of conception reduces the risk of NTDs. Women with the MTHFR 677C→T gene variant may have an increased risk of NTDs. Other birth defects, such as orofacial clefts and heart defects, may be associated with low folate intake[14,23,27,28].

Diagnosis

Full Blood Count

Folate deficiency causes a megaloblastic anemia, with macrocytic red cells and hypersegmented neutrophils.

Owing to a physiological increase in red cell size, using MCV in pregnancy may be an unreliable diagnostic method for diagnosing folate deficiency. Furthermore, in mixed diagnoses, for example concomitant iron deficiency, the MCV may be in the normal range. Advanced deficiencies may manifest with pancytopenia.

Folate Levels

Serum folate can be reduced in pregnancy even when tissue stores are adequate. Red cell folate also reduces physiologically in pregnancy, due to reduced glomerular filtration rate and inadequate plasma volume expansion. Assays have low sensitivity and specificity in pregnancy. Both assays are reduced in smokers, who also typically have poor vitamin status, high total homocysteine, and low-birth-weight babies. These issues highlight the need for specific reference ranges in pregnancy. It is also essential to check the vitamin B_{12} and iron status in these patients.

Total Homocysteine (tHcy)

The concentration of tHcy in plasma is a responsive marker of impaired folate status, which increases in deficiencies. Plasma tHcy is also influenced by pregnancy and levels may be related to factors in pregnancy. Plasma tHcy concentrations are 30–60% lower in pregnancy, with the lowest tHcy values observed in the second trimester. The concentrations of both maternal and fetal tHcy were lowered by folic acid supplementation[28].

Bone Marrow Biopsy

This is unlikely to be performed, and is not usually necessary, because the diagnosis is likely to be made following the blood tests described. If the patient is pancytopenic and the diagnosis is uncertain then in rare cases a bone marrow may be performed. It will demonstrate megaloblastic features, with hypercellularity, a hypercellular erythroid series with large erythroblasts, nucleocytoplasmic asynchrony, and irregular giant metamyelocytes. The features are identical to those of B_{12} deficiency and relate to impaired DNA synthesis, illustrated in Figures 4.4 and 4.5.

Management

Prevention and Prophylaxis of Folate Deficiency

General dietary intake of folate in the UK, without supplementation, is approximately 260 µg daily. It is well known that peri-conception folate supplementation reduces the occurrence and recurrence of NTDs. The neural tube closure occurs at 4 weeks' gestation, at which point many women may be unaware of the pregnancy as up to 50% of pregnancies in the UK are thought to be unplanned[29]. It is recommended that 400 µg of folic acid daily should be taken from 3 months pre-conceptually; however, this is only feasible in women attempting conception[26]. General supplementation with multivitamins is likely to contain at least 400 µg of folic acid (Table 4.3).

Table 4.3 Recommended folic acid doses depending on clinical state

Population	Folic acid dose
No medical conditions	Folic acid 0.4–1.0 mg o.d.
Concomitant medical problems	Folic acid 5 mg od or folate-rich foods and folic acid 0.4–1.0 mg o.d.
Family history of NTD High-risk ethnic groups Strict vegans High-risk women (poor compliance, no contraception, exposure to teratogenic substances, haemolysis, etc.)	Folic acid 5 mg o.d.

Women at high risk of having a child with a NTD, which includes those with a personal or family history of NTD, a previously affected pregnancy, or those on anticonvulsant medications and folate inhibitors, should receive 5 mg folic acid daily prior to conception[30].

As part of normal physiological changes in pregnancy, expansion of blood volume results in an increase in both plasma and erythrocytes of up to 420 mL. Folic acid is required for the increased erythropoiesis.

Dietary Folate and Food Fortification

Breakfast cereals in the UK are usually fortified voluntarily with folic acid, typically containing 50–100 µg per 40-g serving. The Food and Drug Administration (FDA) in the USA has mandated supplementation since 1998, which has reduced NTDs by 20%. The Food Standard Agency (FSA) in the UK is still debating the mandatory fortification of cereals, flour, pasta, and bread. They propose that the fortification will not only help reduce NTDs but also target other vulnerable groups such as the elderly. The addition is unlikely to cause harm to the wider population[29,31].

Treatment of Folate Deficiency

Folate deficiency should be treated with 5 mg three times daily of folic acid.

Case Studies

Case Study 1

A 36-year-old woman presented to her midwife at 27 weeks during her third pregnancy feeling exhausted. Initially she assumed it was the combination of looking after two small children while becoming increasingly more gravid. Then she started to experience loss of concentration and her husband said she looked pale. At booking her hemoglobin had been on the normal low side, 105 g/dL, MCV 101fL, so the midwife rechecked her full blood count, renal function, and glucose. The hemoglobin result was 86 g/dL, MCV 105 fL and she was recalled for hematinic testing. The vitamin B$_{12}$ level was found to be 18 ng/L (174–1132). Further testing found her to have positive intrinsic factor antibodies, at which time the patient recalled that her mother had regular B$_{12}$ injections. Pernicious anemia was diagnosed and she was commenced on hydroxycobalamin injections, with supplementary folic acid for the first week, with resolution of symptoms. At the time of delivery the baby was healthy and unaffected.

Case Study 2

A 28-year-old woman, in her first pregnancy, commented to her midwife at a routine 25-week antenatal appointment that she had persistent mouth ulcers. She had just recovered from 14 weeks of severe hyperemesis. Advice was given regarding oral hygiene. When she returned to her 28-week appointment the ulcers were worsening and she also commented on mild shortness of breath on exertion. The midwife added the hematinics to the week 28 full blood count, group, and antibody screen. The hemoglobin was found to be 96 g/dL, the MCV 102 fL, and the folate 0.8 µg/L (4.2–18.7). The ferritin and vitamin B$_{12}$ were within the normal range. Oral folic acid treatment was commenced at 5 mg t.d.s. and her symptoms resolved. She had been taking folic acid 400 µg supplements every morning until week 16 but this coincided with hyperemesis so the amount absorbed was unclear.

It is imperative to check the vitamin B_{12} status and iron studies at the time of folate deficiency diagnosis since in settings of low folate with concomitant deficiencies, anemia will likely ensue. Folate supplementation can mask vitamin B_{12} deficiency and caution should be taken with susceptible individuals to avoid missing this diagnosis.

Summary

Peri-conception folic acid supplementation protects against fetal structural anomalies, including NTD, orofacial abnormalities, and congenital heart defects. It may also protect against placental abruption and preterm birth. Existing data suggest that dietary folic acid supplementation is recommended for all women of reproductive age and especially those attempting conception or sexually active without contraception. Pregnancy-specific reference ranges for folate are not available and the development of these is likely to be beneficial.

References

1. Murphy MM, Molloy A, Ueland PM *et al.* Longitudinal study of the effect of pregnancy on maternal and fetal cobalamin status in healthy women and their offspring. *The Journal of Nutrition* 2007; **137**: 1863–1866.

2. Vanderjagt D, Ujah I, Ikeh EI *et al.* Assessment of the vitamin B12 status of pregnant women in Nigeria using plasma holotranscobalamin. *ISRN Obstetrics and Gynecology* 2011: 365894.

3. Green R. Physiology, dietary sources, and requirements. *Encyclopedia of Human Nutrition*, 3rd edn, Vol **4**. USA: Elsevier; 2013: 351–356.

4. Sobczyńska-Malefora A, Gorska R, Pelisser M *et al.* An audit of holotranscobalamin ("Active" B12) and methylmalonic acid assays for the assessment of vitamin B12 status: Application in a mixed patient population. *Clinical Biochemistry* 2014; **47**: 82–86.

5. Stabler S. Vitamin B_{12} deficiency. *New England Journal of Medicine* 2013; **368**:149–160.

6. Reynolds E. Vitamin B12, folic acid, and the nervous system. *The Lancet Neurology* 2006; **5**(11): 949–960.

7. Gauchan D, Joshi N, Singh Gill A, *et al.* Does an elevated serum vitamin B_{12} level mask actual vitamin B_{12} deficiency in myeloproliferative disorders? *Clinical Lymphoma, Myeloma & Leukemia* 2012; **12**(4): 269–273.

8. Harmening D. *Clinical Hematology and Fundamentals of Hemostasis*, 4th edn, Vol **7**. USA: The Taber's publisher; 2002: 112–119.

9. Provan D, Singer C, Baglin T, Dokal I. *Oxford Handbook of Clinical Hematology*, 3rd edn, Vol **2**. Oxford: Oxford University Press; 2009: 46–47.

10. Gröber U, Kisters K, Schmidt J. Neuroenhancement with vitamin B_{12} underestimated neurological significance. *Nutrients* 2013; **5**: 5031–5045.

11. Kaushansky K, Lichtman M, Beutler E *et al. Williams Hematology*, 8th edn, Vol 41. USA: McGraw Hill Medical; 2008: 538–545.

12. Devalia V, Hamilton M, Molloy A. Guidelines for the diagnosis and treatment of cobalamin and folate disorders. *British Journal of Hematology* 2014; **166**: 496–513.

13. Quadros E. Advances in the understanding of cobalamin assimilation and metabolism. *British Journal of Hematology* 2010; **148**: 195–204.

14. Black M. Effects of vitamin B12 and folate deficiency on brain development in children. *Food and Nutrition Bulletin* 2008; **29**(2 Suppl): S126–S131.

15. Carmel R. How I treat cobalamin (vitamin B_{12}) deficiency. *Blood* 2008; **112**: 2214–2221.

16. Lindenbaum J, Healton E, Savage D. Neuropsychiatric disorders caused by cobalamin deficiency in the absence of anemia or macrocytosis. *New England Journal of Medicine* 1988; **318**: 1720–1728.

17. Solomon L. Disorders of cobalamin (Vitamin B_{12}) metabolism: Emerging concepts in pathophysiology, diagnosis and treatment. *Blood Reviews* 2007; **21**: 113–130.

18. Clarke R, Sherliker P, Hin H. Detection of vitamin B12 deficiency in older people by measuring vitamin B12 or the active fraction of vitamin B12, holotranscobalamin. *Clinical Chemistry* 2007; **53**(5); 963–970.

19. Valente E, Scott J, Ueland P *et al.* Diagnostic accuracy of holotranscobalamin, methylmalonic acid, serum cobalamin, and other indicators of tissue vitamin B12 status in the elderly. *Clinical Chemistry* 2011; **57**(6): 856–863.

20. Sobczyńska-Malefora A, Harrington D, Voong K *et al.* Plasma and red cell reference intervals of 5-methyltetrahydrofolate of healthy adults in whom biochemical functional deficiencies of folate and vitamin B12 had been excluded. *Advances in Hematology* 2014: 465623. doi:10.1155/2014/465623.

21. Clinical Knowledge Summaries. Anemia – B12 and folate. https://cks.nice.org.uk/anaemia-b12-and-folate-deficiency#!topicsummary

22. British National Formulary (BNF). http://www.medicinescomplete.com/mc/bnf/current/PHP5867-drugs-used-in-megaloblastic-anemias.htm

23. Yakoob M, Bhutta Z. Effect of routine iron supplementation with or without folic acid on anemia during pregnancy. *BMC Public Health* 2011; **11**(Suppl 3): S21.

24. Short R. UK government consults public on compulsory folate fortification. *BMJ* 2006; **332**(7546): 873.

25. Rain J, Blot I, Tcherina G. Folic acid deficiency in developing nations. In Cooper BA *et al.* (eds) *Folates and Cobalamins*, Bertin, Heidelberg: spinger-verlag; 1989: 171–177.

26. De Benoist B. Conclusions of a WHO Technical Consultation on folate and vitamin B12 deficiencies. *Food and Nutrition Bulletin* 2008; **29** (2): S238–244.

27. Greenberg J, Bell S, Guan Y *et al.* Folic acid supplementation and pregnancy: more than just neural tube defect prevention. *Reviews in Obstetrics and Gynecology* 2011; **4**(2): 52–59.

28. Ueland PM, Vollset SE. Homocysteine and folate in pregnancy. *Clinical Chemistry* 2004; **50**(8): 1293–1294.

29. Fuller-Deets M, Dingwall R. The Ethical Implications of Options for Improving the Folate Intake of Women of Reproductive Age. Food Standards Agency report produced by the Institute for Science and Society, University of Nottingham. 2007; **17**: 1–56.

30. Wilson RD, Johnson JA, Wyatt P *et al.* Genetics Committee of the Society of Obstetricians and Gynecologists of Canada and The Motherrisk Program. Pre-conceptional vitamin/folic acid supplementation 2007: the use of folic acid in combination with a multivitamin supplement for the prevention of neural tube defects and other congenital anomalies. *Journal of Obstetrics and Gynaecology Canada* 2007; **29**: 1003–1026.

31. Castillo-Lancellotti C, Tur J, Uauy R. Impact of folic acid fortification of flour on neural tube defects: a systematic review. *Public Health Nutrition* 2013; **16**(5): 901–911.

Chapter 5

Autoimmune Cytopenias in Pregnancy

Hamish Lyall and Bethan Myers

Introduction

Autoimmune conditions are characterized by the production of antibodies against self-antigens (autoantibodies). Since these conditions can occur at any age, they may occur during or predating pregnancy. In these circumstances, the additional considerations of both the effect of pregnancy on the disease and the disease (and its treatment) on the pregnancy need to be taken into account.

It is recognized that pregnancy may influence the course of maternal autoimmune diseases. This can result in remissions, relapses, or new presentations of these disorders. The pathogenesis of this phenomenon is likely to be related to the hormonal and complex immunological changes that occur during pregnancy. Immunological changes in pregnancy are necessary to prevent rejection of the fetus, which expresses both paternal as well as maternal antigens. Placental immunology and modulation of the systemic immune response have been identified as important mechanisms of this immune tolerance. It is probable that these features have a significant influence on autoimmune hematological disorders that occur during pregnancy.

In this chapter, three autoimmune hematological conditions that may complicate pregnancy are discussed: immune/idiopathic thrombocytopenic purpura (ITP), autoimmune hemolytic anemia (AIHA), and autoimmune neutropenia (AIN). These disorders are characterized by the development of an autoantibody specific for a surface antigen on the platelet, erythrocyte, or neutrophil. Premature cellular destruction occurs by reticuloendothelial phagocytosis, T-lymphocyte cytotoxicity, or complement-mediated cell lysis. To date, the relationship between these immune mechanisms and the immunological changes in pregnancy is not fully understood.

Cytopenias occur when the enhanced clearance of the platelet, erythrocyte, or neutrophil from the peripheral blood is greater than the bone marrow's ability to produce new cells. ITP is by far the most frequently seen condition. AIN and AIHA rarely occur in pregnancy and few cases are reported in the published literature. The three conditions usually occur in isolation but occasionally may be seen together, e.g. Evans syndrome (ITP and AIHA).

About two-thirds of cases present prior to pregnancy with the diagnosis already established, but the remaining third present during pregnancy, either as an incidental finding or less commonly in the symptomatic state. For many women, pregnancy is the first time that a full blood count (FBC) is performed. Careful evaluation of any abnormal result is required before an immune cytopenia can be diagnosed.

The majority of autoantibodies implicated in these disorders are of the IgG subtype, and hence are able to cross the placenta. Consideration, therefore, needs to be given not just to the implications for the mother, but also for the developing fetus and, after delivery, the neonate.

Management can be challenging because where treatment is required, there are no agents that are universally efficacious and all carry the potential for adverse effects. As with all therapies in pregnancy, the benefits of treatment compared with the relative risks to mother and baby have to be considered. A multidisciplinary approach, combining expertise from obstetricians, hematologists, anesthetists, and neonatologists, is required for optimal care.

Idiopathic/Immune Thrombocytopenic Purpura

Introduction

ITP is usually a chronic condition in adults, often occurring in young women, and can be challenging to diagnose and manage in pregnancy. Although it is principally mediated by autoantibodies, the development of specific assays as a diagnostic tool has, to date, proved unsuccessful. Therefore, the diagnosis is predominantly one of exclusion with frequent difficulty in excluding alternative causes of thrombocytopenia. Fortuitously, the risk of major hemorrhagic complications is low. Successful management requires maintaining adequate platelet counts for pregnancy and delivery while minimizing the risks of treatment-related side effects for mother and baby. The potential risks of fatal thrombocytopenia need to be appreciated, with measures taken to prevent hemorrhagic complications at delivery.

Epidemiology

The annual incidence of acute and chronic ITP in adults from population-based studies is estimated to be 2–4 per 100 000, when defined using a platelet count of less than 100×10^9/L. These incidence figures are similar for Europe and the USA[1]. In keeping with other immune disorders, it is more common in women than men (F:M 1.7–1.9:1), and frequently occurs during the reproductive years, occurring in all ethnic groups. The incidence in pregnancy has been estimated at 0.11 per 1000 pregnancies[1,2], accounting for about 3%[3] of cases of thrombocytopenia in pregnancy. Approximately two-thirds of cases of ITP already have an established diagnosis prior to pregnancy, allowing the opportunity for pre-pregnancy counseling and planning for a future pregnancy.

Pathogenesis

Thrombocytopenia is predominantly caused by autoantibodies specific for platelet glycoproteins binding to platelets in the maternal circulation. This results in immune-mediated platelet destruction. In addition to increased destruction of platelets, suppression of megakaryopoiesis in the bone marrow has been observed. The cause of the immune dysregulation which permits these phenomena is not fully known. There is usually no apparent stimulus predating a diagnosis of ITP; however, occasionally a history of recent viral illness, vaccination, or drug exposure can be implicated. ITP usually occurs in isolation but may occur with other immune cytopenias or be secondary to a systemic autoimmune condition, e.g. systemic lupus erythematosus (SLE). The association with autoimmune thyroid disease is also quite striking, although there is no consistent relationship between the course of the ITP and treatment of the thyroid disease.

The spleen has an important role in ITP, being both a major source of antibody production and the predominant site for destruction of antibody-bound platelets. The antibodies are of the IgG subtype and therefore able to cross the placenta and potentially cause thrombocytopenia in the fetus/neonate. The risk of neonatal thrombocytopenia therefore persists after splenectomy, even when the maternal platelet count is normal.

Diagnosis

Thrombocytopenia in Pregnancy

The reference range for platelet counts in non-pregnant women is $150–400 \times 10^9$/L. The finding of mild thrombocytopenia in pregnancy is common, with approximately 8–10% of women having a platelet count below the laboratory normal range by the end of pregnancy [2,4]. The principal differential diagnoses of thrombocytopenia in pregnancy are discussed below and are summarized in Table 5.1.

Gestational Thrombocytopenia

The majority of cases of thrombocytopenia in pregnancy (74%) are attributable to gestational thrombocytopenia (incidental thrombocytopenia) of pregnancy[5]. This is a benign condition and is not considered to represent a bleeding risk to mother or fetus. It appears to be due to physiological hemodilution and increased platelet consumption[6]. It typically occurs in the third trimester and usually results in a mild thrombocytopenia. Platelet counts below 70×10^9/L should alert the physician to consider alternative diagnoses, although in rare cases the diagnosis has been subsequently confirmed in women with counts as low as 50×10^9/L[7]. A platelet count that has been normal before pregnancy and in the first and second trimesters is useful in helping to make the diagnosis. The FBC returns to normal within a few weeks of delivery. It may cause diagnostic difficulty with ITP when there are no pre-pregnancy counts.

Hypertensive Disorders

Hypertensive disorders of pregnancy complicate between 12% and 22% of pregnancies and are a common cause of thrombocytopenia in pregnancy, accounting for approximately 20% of cases. "Gestational hypertension," which includes "hypertension in pregnancy" (HIP), pre-eclampsia, and eclampsia, is responsible for

Table 5.1 Causes of thrombocytopenia in pregnancy

Thrombocytopenic condition	Pathogenesis of thrombocytopenia	Diagnostic characteristics
Gestational thrombocytopenia	Physiological dilution	Third trimester, plts >70 × 10^9/L
	Accelerated destruction	Incidental finding, no features of other disease
HIP/pre-eclampsia/eclampsia	Peripheral consumption	Unwell patient. Clinical features – hypertension, proteinuria, neurological signs/symptoms
Micoangiopathic hemolytic anemias (MAHA) – TTP, HUS, HELLP syndrome	Mechanical destruction and peripheral consumption (accumulation of microthrombi in small vessels)	Unwell patient. Clinical features – neurological signs, fever, renal impairment, deranged LFTs, hemolysis
ITP	Immune-mediated peripheral consumption and suppression of megakaryocytes	Absence of other causes of thrombocytopenia. Diagnosis of exclusion
Hereditary thrombocytopenia	Bone marrow underproduction Abnormal von Willebrand factor (type 2B von Willebrand disease)	Family history, somatic abnormalities, abnormal blood film Family history, bleeding symptoms. Diagnosis confirmed by specialist VWF investigations
Leukemia/Lymphoma	Bone marrow infiltration	Lymphadenopathy, hepatosplenomegaly, other FBC abnormalities
Pseudothrombocytopenia	EDTA artifact	Platelet clumping seen on blood film
Viral infection	Multifactorial	Recent viral illness. Risk factors
Drugs	Multifactorial	Timing of drug exposure

HIP: Hypertension in pregnancy; TTP: Thrombotic thrombocytopenic purpura; HUS: Hemolytic uremic syndrome; HELLP: Hemolysis with elevated liver enzymes and low platelets; LFT, liver function test; ITP: Immune thrombocytopenic purpura; VWF, von Willebrand factor.

the vast majority of these. Thrombotic thrombocytopenic purpura (TTP), hemolytic uremic syndrome (HUS), and Hemolysis, Elevated **Liver** Enzymes, and **Low Platelets** (HELLP) syndrome can share similar features with pre-eclampsia, and distinguishing between these conditions is sometimes problematic. Together, these rarer microangiopathic hemolytic anemia (MAHA) conditions cause less than 1% of pregnancy-related thrombocytopenia. Management of these conditions is described in Chapters 22 and 23. Hypertensive disorders may be associated with the disseminated intravascular coagulation (DIC), which will contribute to further platelet reduction.

Constitutional Thrombocytopenia

Hereditary causes of thrombocytopenia are rare, accounting for less than 1% of cases. This includes MYH-9 disorders characterized by giant platelets on the blood film and Dohle body inclusions in neutrophils. Of these, the May Hegglin anomaly is the most likely to be encountered in pregnancy. Rarely, hereditary bone marrow failure syndromes such as Fanconi's anemia may present with an isolated thrombocytopenia in pregnancy. These diagnoses may be suspected if there is a family history of thrombocytopenia, unexplained thrombocytopenia in more

than two first-degree relatives, or physical abnormalities suggestive of the disorder. Thrombocytopenia may also be a feature of type 2B von Willebrand disease. This rare subtype is characterized by the production of abnormal von Willebrand factor with a high affinity for binding platelets. A feature of this disorder is worsening of thrombocytopenia during pregnancy, particularly approaching term, in response to rising von Willebrand factor levels.

Drugs and Infections

Thrombocytopenia is a frequently occurring side effect of many medications. Heparin-induced thrombocytopenia (HIT), a potentially life-threatening condition, appears to have a very low incidence in pregnancy, especially when low-molecular-weight heparin is used[8]. As with the non-pregnant setting, viral infection is an important cause of thrombocytopenia. While this occurs as a transient phenomenon with many viruses, specific consideration should be given to hepatitis B and C, and HIV infection, particularly if risk factors are present. Thrombocytopenia in this setting is likely to be multifactorial with both an immune and non-immune pathogenesis. Diagnosing these infections early in pregnancy may allow treatment to be initiated, reducing the risk of related complications and vertical transmission.

Others

Hematological malignancies can present in pregnancy and the initial feature may be isolated thrombocytopenia. Occasionally, a bone marrow examination may be required to exclude these disorders.

Laboratory artifact from EDTA present in the sample tubes may account for some cases of apparent thrombocytopenia. Examination of the blood film is essential to exclude this possibility.

There are no specific diagnostic tests for ITP. Although platelet glycoprotein specific antibodies can be detected in the majority of cases, this test lacks the sensitivity and specificity to be of clinical use. Diagnostic parameters for ITP in pregnancy are: thrombocytopenia with a past history of ITP, or a platelet count during pregnancy of less than 70×10^9/L with other causes excluded. Mild thrombocytopenia presenting in the first or second trimesters may also represent ITP, but this is not clinically significant for the mother since no treatment is required. In all cases, a careful history and examination of the blood film are critical to the evaluation of thrombocytopenia and diagnosing ITP in pregnancy. The important clinical and laboratory points for diagnosis are discussed below and listed in Table 5.2.

History

- Where there is a preceding history of ITP, check diagnosis for accuracy.
- Documented response to corticosteroids or intravenous immunoglobulin (IVIG) is usually diagnostic of ITP. In addition, this information is valuable for deciding on future treatment.
- Previous pregnancy experience and any documented blood counts both during and outside of pregnancy are very useful.
- Neonatal platelet counts from previous successful pregnancies should be noted.
- Note any illnesses associated with ITP (e.g. SLE), or the occurrence of other autoimmune disorders in the patient.
- A family history of thrombocytopenia may suggest a hereditary disorder.
- Identify any risk factors for HIV and viral hepatitis, and include the relevant tests.
- Any current medications should be considered for the possibility of drug-induced thrombocytopenia.

Clinical Examination

- Clinical examination should be normal except for bleeding manifestations (e.g. purpura, mucosal bleeding).

Table 5.2 Evaluation of suspected ITP

	Specific point to elicit	Relevance
Current history	Is patient hemorrhagic?	Thrombocytopenia genuine. Indication for treatment
	Viral illness/risk factors for HIV or hepatitis	Viral cause for thrombocytopenia. Check serology, especially for HIV
Family history	Family history of unexplained thrombocytopenia	Consider hereditary causes
Past medical history	Known ITP	ITP likely causes thrombocytopenia. ? Previous response to steroids or immunoglobulin
	SLE, thyroid or other autoimmune disorders	ITP likely causes thrombocytopenia. Possibility of SLE-related complications
Past obstetric history	History of pre-eclampsia or previous thrombocytopenia in pregnancy	Increased likelihood of recurrence
		Establish cause
	Previous baby with neonatal thrombocytopenia	ITP likely. If not, consider possibility of neonatal alloimmune thrombocytopenia (NAIT)(see Chapter 10)
		May predict risk of future neonatal thrombocytopenia
Clinical examination	Mucocutaneous bleeding	Thrombocytopenia genuine; indication for treatment
	Lymphadenopathy, hepatosplenomegaly	Possible leukemia/lymphoma. Not consistent with ITP
Laboratory assessment	Platelets: clumping present?	Pseudothrombocytopenia; repeat FBC in citrate
	Giant platelets	Check platelet count by alternative method. Consider MYH-9 disorders
	Normal red cell and white cell numbers and normal morphology	Consistent with gestational thrombocytopenia or ITP
	Schistocytes/red cell fragments	Consider MAHA
	LFTs abnormal, coagulation screen abnormal	Consistent with HELLP syndrome. Consider DIC, hypertensive disorders of pregnancy

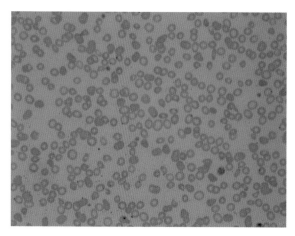

Figure 5.1 Blood film of ITP, showing variable platelet size and reduced number.

- Splenomegaly and/or lymphadenopathy are not characteristic of ITP.
- Physical abnormalities may suggest a hereditary disorder.
- **FBC:** Incidental finding of thrombocytopenia should prompt a recheck of the FBC.
- **Blood film** is essential to exclude alternative diagnoses (Figure 5.1):

  (a) Spurious thrombocytopenia is caused either by EDTA artifact (causing platelet clumps – if present, repeat count in citrate sample) or platelet satellitism. Both are readily seen on the film.

  (b) Check erythroid and leukocyte morphology and confirm within normal limits. Abnormal red cell fragmentation (requires urgent medical attention) or white cell morphology suggests alternative diagnosis.

  (c) Check platelet morphology. Giant platelets may be seen in ITP but, if this is the dominant finding, consider a MYH-9 disorder and examine the neutrophils for Dohle bodies. Giant platelets and thrombocytopenia may also be seen with Bernard–Soulier disease, but a lifelong history of abnormal bleeding would be expected. Abnormally small platelets may be seen with hereditary thrombocytopenia and bone marrow failure syndromes. Automated platelet counts may be erroneous if they are performed on an analyzer that relies on impedance counting and if the platelets are

very large. This should be suspected if the film appearances differ significantly from the analyzer result. An alternative method of platelet measurement available on some analyzers (e.g. flow cytometry platelet count) may give a more accurate measurement.

Some analyzers are able to measure reticulated platelets and this percentage increases significantly in ITP.

Other **routine investigations** that should be performed are listed in Table 5.2.

Bone Marrow Examination

- A bone marrow examination can confirm the presence of normal megakaryocytes, normal hematopoiesis, and the absence of bone marrow infiltration.
- This is not necessary where there are no other clinical or laboratory features to suggest bone marrow failure or infiltration.
- Consider performing a bone marrow examination in cases that do not respond to standard treatments.
- NB: bone marrow examination will not differentiate between ITP and gestational thrombocytopenia or other consumptive causes, which constitute the main differential diagnoses, only confirming that thrombocytopenia is due to peripheral consumption.

ITP Management

The aim of management is not to achieve a sustained normal platelet count but simply to maintain a platelet count which is adequate to avoid hemorrhagic complications during pregnancy, delivery, and immediately postpartum. This conservative approach minimizes the risks of maternal and fetal exposure to therapeutic agents. There are no universally accepted criteria for "safe" platelet counts in pregnancy. It is advisable that members of the team involved in managing these cases (obstetricians, hematologists, anesthetists) agree a consensus for minimum accepted platelet thresholds. Generally, these can be low in the antenatal period if the patient is not hemorrhagic. Thresholds typically need to be higher for delivery. Suggested platelet thresholds for ITP are stipulated in Table 5.3.

Monitoring during Pregnancy

Platelet counts in women with ITP need to be closely monitored through pregnancy: in general, monthly in

Table 5.3 Suggested platelet thresholds for intervention for ITP

Intervention	Platelet count
Antenatal, no invasive procedure planned	$>20 \times 10^9$/L
Delivery	$>50 \times 10^9$/L
Epidural anesthesia	$>80 \times 10^9$/L

Table 5.4A Advantages and disadvantages of corticosteroids

Advantages	Disadvantages
• Oral therapy	• Risk of gestational diabetes mellitus
• Most experience	• Immunosuppressive
• Can be used for extended periods if prolonged platelet count rise is required	• Slow response: 3–7 days for first response, maximal response 2–3 weeks
• Dose can be tapered to minimum required for desired effect	• Risk of osteoporosis with prolonged therapy
• Not a blood product	• Risk of hypertension
• Inexpensive	• Possible adverse effects on fetus (variable, depending on dose and type of steroid)

Table 5.4B Advantages and disadvantages of intravenous immunoglobulin (IVIG)

Advantages	Disadvantages
• Established therapy	• Intravenous therapy with long duration of administration
• Response to treatment is rapid (6–72 hours)	• Pooled plasma product therefore potential risk of pathogen transmission for mother and fetus
• No corticosteroid side effects	• Transient response (<1 month)
• Low risk to fetus	• Risk of infusional reactions
	• Risk of aseptic meningitis
	• Headache common
	• Expensive

the first and second trimesters, 2-weekly in the third, and weekly near term, although the frequency of monitoring will depend on the rate of change as well as absolute values.

Treatment

There are two decisions to be made in treating ITP in pregnancy: when to treat and what treatment to give. The majority of women will not require therapy throughout the whole duration of the antenatal

period[9,10]. Only women with very low platelet counts ($<20 \times 10^9$/L) who are hemorrhagic or require an invasive procedure will require treatment at this stage. By contrast, treatment is often required to raise the platelet count prior to delivery. The two treatment options for the initial management of ITP usually considered are corticosteroids and intravenous immunoglobulin (IVIG). The characteristics of these agents are summarized in Table 5.4A and 5.4B. The choice of which agent to use requires discussion with the individual about the relative risks and benefits of each treatment. Patients with contraindications to corticosteroids (diabetes mellitus, concurrent infections, history of steroid psychosis) can be managed with IVIG alone.

The choice of therapy depends on the following factors:

- the speed with which a platelet increment is required;
- the length of time for which a rise needs to be sustained; and
- which therapy carries the least potential risk for a given individual.

A suggested algorithm for initial therapy is shown in Figure 5.2. This algorithm is only suitable for uncomplicated cases. Suggested management for various scenarios are listed below.

Patients with Moderate/Severe Thrombocytopenia ($<20 \times 10^9$/L)

- Prednisolone 20 mg/day[6] (it is common practice to use less than the conventional dose of 1 mg/kg given outside pregnancy to avoid adverse effects)

Patients with Severe Thrombocytopenia ($<20 \times 10^9$/L) and Significant Bleeding

- Requires treatment to raise the platelet count urgently
- IVIG +/– high-dose corticosteroids (e.g. prednisolone 60 mg daily)
- Consider platelet transfusions if major hemorrhage

Patients with Life-Threatening Bleeding

- Platelet transfusion +
- IVIG + IV methylprednisolone

Where possible, the dose of prednisolone should be promptly reduced to the minimum effective dose. Unless hemorrhage is a major feature, prolonged

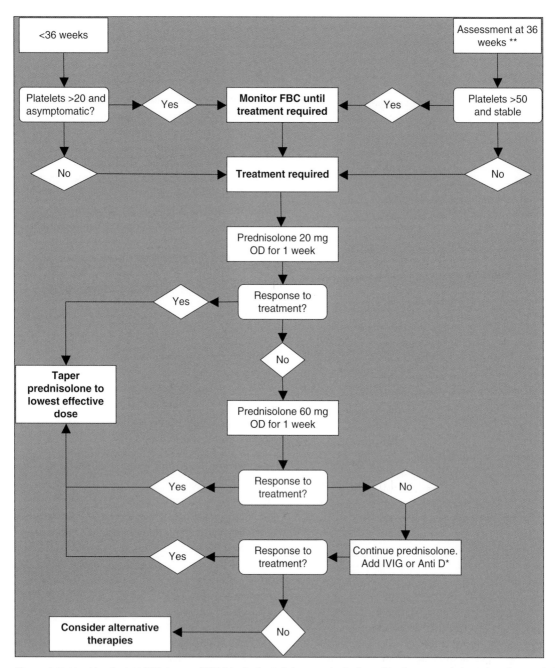

Figure 5.2 Algorithm for initial ITP therapy. *IVIG 0.4 g/kg for 2–5 days or a single dose of 1 g/kg repeated after 3 days if required. Consider methylprednisolone 1 g IV in addition to IVIG **Reassess earlier if there are obstetric indications that might need early delivery.

therapy (>6 weeks) with high doses of prednisolone is considered to carry too high a risk of adverse events for the mother. The response to IVIG is often transient. Patients receiving these treatments may require repeat infusions. The addition of methylprednisolone 1 g intravenously is used to speed up/improve the response as compared to standard prednisolone in difficult or refractory cases.

It is not always possible to achieve the desired platelet count in individuals with ITP. Many patients (35% in one series) diagnosed with ITP in pregnancy will not respond to corticosteroids or IVIG. In addition, responses to platelet transfusions are transient with poor increments as circulating antibody rapidly clears transfused platelets.

Management of Refractory Cases

- In considering other therapeutic options the balance of risks need to be considered between treatment-related toxic effects versus the risk of major bleeding with prolonged severe thrombocytopenia. In many circumstances, it may be preferable or necessary to accept the increased hemorrhagic risk of significant thrombocytopenia rather than use more aggressive therapies.
- **Azathioprine.** This is widely used as a second-line agent; it is safe for the fetus and is used frequently in the management of systemic lupus erythematosus in pregnancy. Thiopurine methyltransferase (TPMT) levels should be checked prior to its use to identify those at risk of severe side effects. It has a slow onset of action (6–8 weeks), which reduces its utility.
- **Splenectomy.** This procedure has a well-established, though diminishing, role in ITP. It can generally be performed safely in pregnancy but carries the risks of general surgery and of fetal loss. Where possible, it should be performed in the second trimester. This avoids the risks of teratogenicity associated with drugs in the first trimester. In the third trimester, the gravid uterus may make splenectomy technically more demanding, although laparoscopic splenectomy may make the procedure more feasible.
- **Tranexamic acid.** This is an antifibrinolytic, which in the past has been avoided in pregnancy because of concerns that it may increase thrombotic risk, although this seems unlikely from the current literature. Reproductive animal studies do not indicate risk to the fetus, but there are no adequate and well-controlled studies done on pregnant women (category B). It could be considered in the refractory patient with ongoing symptoms, after the first trimester.
- **Rituximab.** This agent is an anti-CD20 monoclonal antibody, which is used off label to treat non-pregnancy-related ITP. There are some anecdotal reports of its use in pregnancy. However, there is insufficient evidence regarding safety and efficacy to advocate its use in this setting. In the non-pregnant patient, it is currently advised to avoid pregnancy for 1 year.
- **Anti-D.** Experience with intravenous anti-D in pregnancy to treat ITP is limited. It is used in RhD positive, non-splenectomized patients. Significant fetal hemolysis from maternal antepartum prophylaxis has not been reported, but concerns regarding this and maternal hemolysis in addition to lack of availability have contributed to little usage.
- **Thrombopoietin agonists** (eltrombopag, romiplostim). Case reports of successful romiplostim use in pregnancy have been described. However, pregnancy experience with these drugs is limited, and the maternal and fetal adverse effects of these agents are not fully known.

Other agents, which are useful outside pregnancy, including mycophenolate, androgen analogs (e.g. danazol), and cytotoxic agents such as cyclophosphamide or vinca alkaloids, are contraindicated in pregnancy.

General Measures

The following should be avoided if there is significant thrombocytopenia (platelets $<50 \times 10^9$/L):

- Aspirin and non-steroidal medication
- Anticoagulants (unless benefits outweigh risks)
- Intramuscular injections
- Activities with a risk of traumatic injury

Planning for Delivery

Consideration of potential maternal and neonatal thrombocytopenia is required in addition to any obstetric factors that may be present when planning delivery.

Maternal Considerations

The principal concern is hemorrhage. This may be during delivery or postpartum. Postpartum hemorrhage is of particular concern due to the sharp fall in procoagulant factors that occurs at this time. As discussed above, there is no universally agreed safe platelet count; however, hemorrhage caused by thrombocytopenia occurring at a platelet count $>50 \times 10^9$/L would be considered unusual, especially with the increased fibrinogen levels of pregnancy.

Epidural analgesia is of particular concern, as even a small increase in venous hemorrhage could have the potential for spinal cord compression. The risk is considered to be greatest at the time of insertion and withdrawal of the catheter. There is controversy over the safe threshold for epidural anesthesia. There is a body of opinion that a platelet count of 50×10^9/L may be adequate; however, anesthetic practice is to use a threshold of at least 80×10^9/L. A pre-delivery anesthetic consultation is helpful to discuss alternative analgesia during labor. The role of spinal anesthetic is more difficult. This procedure may allow a cesarean section to be performed without the need for a general anesthetic. A decision may be taken that the risks of a single pass spinal needle could be less than those of a general anesthetic in some situations and, if an experienced obstetric anesthetist is available, a cut-off of 50×10^9/L is suggested.

Chronic immunosuppression antenatally for ITP may increase the risks of postpartum sepsis.

Twenty-five percent of those with ITP have antiphospholipid antibodies (aPL), so testing for aPL should be considered if the ITP is severe, resistant to treatment, or there are clinical features to suggest antiphospholipid syndrome.

Neonatal Considerations

The principal neonatal risk is intracranial hemorrhage due to severe thrombocytopenia and birth trauma. This is rare (<1% of ITP cases), although potentially devastating when it occurs. The overall incidence of thrombocytopenia in neonates born to mothers with ITP is reported in various studies as 14–37.5%[10,11,12]. However, only approximately 5% of babies born to mothers with ITP will have platelet counts $<20 \times 10^9$/L, with a further 5% having counts between 20×10^9 and 50×10^9/L[10,13].

Unfortunately, predicting which babies may be affected or directly assessing the fetal platelet count is difficult. No correlation has been established with the severity of maternal ITP or levels of circulating antibody. Although there are no reliable predictors of its occurrence or severity, neonatal thrombocytopenia is more likely if:

- There is a previous sibling with thrombocytopenia[13]
- The mother has had a splenectomy prior to this pregnancy (although not all studies confirmed this finding)
- Maternal ITP is severe (not confirmed in all studies)[13,14]

Where babies have been born previously with severe thrombocytopenia, testing for paternal platelet antigen incompatibility to exclude neonatal alloimmune thrombocytopenia (NAIT) is required.

There is no role for the routine measuring of fetal platelet counts by percutaneous umbilical blood sampling in ITP. Studies evaluating this technique have estimated the procedure-related risk to be greater than the risk of preventing neonatal hemorrhage. Platelet counts taken from fetal scalp samples are prone to erroneously low results and carry the risk of scalp hematoma, and are therefore best avoided.

Mode of Delivery

The exact mode and timing of delivery has many patient-specific variables and an individualized plan with multidisciplinary input is advised. Concerns regarding potential neonatal thrombocytopenia and birth trauma have previously led some clinicians to recommend cesarean section. However, there is currently no evidence that cesarean section reduces the incidence of intracranial hemorrhage in babies affected with ITP, compared with uncomplicated vaginal delivery. It is recommended that the mode of delivery is determined by obstetric indications rather than ITP. Instrumentation increases the risk of head trauma and should be avoided wherever possible. Early recourse to cesarean delivery may be needed. Low cavity forceps are reasonable to use, but if the baby is stuck in the second stage, the risks and benefits of instrumentation need to be assessed on an individual basis. For example, if the patient has chronic, mild ITP and previous pregnancies have had a normal cord platelet count, it may not be necessary to restrict instrumental aids to delivery. In contrast, where there has been previous severe neonatal thrombocytopenia, cesarean delivery may be preferred, depending on other comorbidities and risk/benefit balance.

Induction of labor may be required if platelet responses to treatment are transient, so that delivery can be timed to occur at the maximal platelet count.

Management of Labor When Platelet Count Has Not Been Corrected

In these cases, a pragmatic approach needs to be taken. Reassuringly, experiences suggest that normal delivery can occur without excess hemorrhage, even at very low platelet counts due to the increased fibrinogen levels seen in pregnancy. It is advisable to have platelet transfusions available on standby and to proceed with delivery. If time allows, IVIG may be used. Epidural anesthesia should be avoided as should non-steroidal anti-inflammatory drugs (NSAIDs) for postpartum pain relief.

Postpartum: Neonatal Care

The neonatal team should be alerted prior to delivery. A cord platelet count should be measured at birth. If the platelet count is normal, further neonatal platelet counts are not required. If thrombocytopenia is present, this should preferably be confirmed on a venous sample. Heel prick samples are best avoided due to the risk of preanalytical clot formation and falsely low platelet levels being obtained. Intramuscular injections should be avoided if severe thrombocytopenia is present. Vitamin K can be given orally.

If the cord platelet count is below $100 \times 10^9/L$, further full blood count measurements every 2–3 days over the next week are required to ensure that the neonate is not at risk of hemorrhage. The nadir platelet count is usually between days 2 and 5, when the neonatal spleen has developed. Most cases of thrombocytopenia will be resolving by day 7. However, some cases can last for several weeks or months.

Babies with severe thrombocytopenia of $<20 \times 10^9/L$ or clinical hemorrhage require treatment with IVIG. Life-threatening complications should be treated with immediate platelet transfusions and IVIG. Consideration should be given to using human platelet alloantigens (HPA) 1a 5b negative platelets if available until neonatal alloimmune thrombocytopenia (NAIT) is excluded.

Babies with severe thrombocytopenia ($<50 \times 10^9/L$) should have a cranial ultrasound, computerized tomography, or magnetic resonance to assess for evidence of intracranial hemorrhage.

Women should not be discouraged from breastfeeding as there is no firm evidence for its association with neonatal thrombocytopenia.

Prenatal Counseling

Women who have an established diagnosis of ITP may request prenatal counseling before deciding whether to embark on a pregnancy. There are few predictors of outcome that can be used to assess risk. Overall, the risks of maternal ITP to mother and baby during pregnancy are small and therefore pregnancy is not usually discouraged. However, it is suggested that the following points should be discussed:

- Circulating antiplatelet antibodies may still be present in the maternal blood despite a near normal platelet count. This is particularly relevant for women who have had a splenectomy. In these circumstances, ITP may appear in remission with normal platelet counts. However, this is primarily due to an inability to clear platelet–antibody complexes rather than a cessation of antibody production. There is therefore still a risk of neonatal thrombocytopenia or hemorrhagic complications in utero.
- ITP may relapse or worsen during pregnancy. Current evidence suggests the long-term effect of pregnancy on pre-existing ITP is fairly mild[15].
- If treatment of ITP is required it may carry both maternal and fetal risks.
- There is an increased risk of hemorrhage at delivery, but the risk is small even if the platelet count is low.
- Epidural anesthesia may not be possible.
- Although it is not possible to accurately predict if a neonate will be affected, the risk is highest if there was neonatal thrombocytopenia in an older sibling.
- Maternal death or serious adverse outcomes for mothers with ITP are rare.
- The risk of intracranial hemorrhage for the fetus/neonate is very low.

Autoimmune Neutropenia (AIN)

Introduction

Neutropenia is a common finding in routine FBC testing, and is defined as an absolute neutrophil count (ANC) of $<1.5 \times 10^9/L$ (or <1.2 for some ethnic groups – see below). The majority of cases are mild, transient, and no specific etiology is determined. By contrast, AIN is a rare disorder and can cause severe neutropenia associated with recurrent infection[15]. It may occur in isolation or in conjunction with ITP or AIHA. Many cases in adults are secondary, associated with other autoimmune disorders, e.g. SLE. The main complication of this condition is recurrent infection, which occurs if the neutropenia is severe (ANC $<0.5 \times 10^9/L$). Diagnosis can be problematic as laboratory investigation of neutropenia is limited, and usually restricted to specialist centers. Pregnancy poses an additional problem, as autoantibodies may cross the placenta resulting in neonatal neutropenia after delivery. Currently, published evidence on management of these cases is lacking.

Incidence and Pathogenesis

The true incidence of AIN is not known. Persistent neutropenia in adults is a common finding and is frequently not investigated if asymptomatic and mild (ANC 1.0×10^9–2.0×10^9/L). Cases are often labeled as chronic idiopathic neutropenia (CIN). It is probable that some cases with a presumptive diagnosis of CIN are immune mediated. The benign nature of asymptomatic CIN means that specialist investigation is often of little value and immunological studies are therefore not pursued. This may not be the case for women of childbearing age, as identification of immune-mediated cases may help with neonatal assessment.

The pathogenesis of AIN is similar to that of other immune cytopenias. It is an acquired disorder in which autoantibodies specific for neutrophil surface glycoproteins result in reduced neutrophil survival and neutropenia.

Diagnosis

Patients with symptomatic neutropenia (recurrent infections, severe neutropenia) are likely to present outside of pregnancy and have an established diagnosis. Difficulty occurs in the asymptomatic patient if an incidental finding of neutropenia is made following FBC testing during routine antenatal care. Assessment involves a careful history, examination of the other FBC indices, and inspection of the blood film.

The differential diagnosis includes: drugs, viral infections, immune-mediated disorders, large granular lymphocyte (LGL) disease (often associated with rheumatoid arthritis), benign ethnic neutropenia, and CIN. Important clinical and laboratory aids to diagnosis are listed in Table 5.5.

History

- History of SLE, rheumatoid arthritis, or other autoimmune disease suggests secondary immune neutropenia (more common than primary AIN in adults).
- Ethnic origin (ANC >1.2×10^9/L may be considered within normal limits for some African,

Table 5.5 Severity of neutropenia according to the ANC

ANC	Severity	Clinical effect
>1.0×10^9/L	Mild	Usually asymptomatic
0.5×10^9–1.0×10^9/L	Moderate	Usually asymptomatic
0.2×10^9–0.5×10^9/L	Severe	Infections possible
<0.2×10^9/L	Very severe	High risk of infection

Middle Eastern, and Yemenite Jewish populations).
- Ask about any recent viral illness.
- Assess risk factors for HIV.
- Assess for evidence of recurrent infections, particularly unusual infections, or mouth ulcers (if there is a temporal pattern – consider cyclical neutropenia).
- Take a careful drug history (especially antithyroid drugs, phenothiazines, and NSAIDs), which are known to cause neutropenia.
- Is there a known family history of neutropenia?
- Is there a history of ITP or AIHA?

Laboratory Assessment

- A blood film should be examined to confirm neutropenia. Severity (and hence possible risk of infection) may be graded using the criteria in Table 5.5. NB: Risk of infection is derived from observations of chemotherapy-induced neutropenia. Infection risks from immune neutropenia are generally less.
- Increase in large granular lymphocytes on the blood film should be noted.
- The presence of abnormalities other than neutropenia suggests an alternative diagnosis to AIN.
- Asymptomatic cases with ANC >0.5×10^9/L and where there is no apparent cause are best managed by repeating the test to determine the trend.
- A bone marrow examination is of value in cases of severe neutropenia. The bone marrow appearances in AIN may show normal hematopoiesis or an apparent arrest at the metamyelocyte stage with a reduction

in the number of mature neutrophils and band forms.

Management

There are two main risks during pregnancy – the maternal risk of sepsis and the risk of neonatal neutropenia. Sepsis in pregnancy may provoke miscarriage or premature labor and is the main concern, for example, a normally benign urinary infection may progress to pyelonephritis and septicemia.

Information on neonatal outcomes in women with AIN is limited. Neutropenia from all causes in neonates is common. Information from neonates affected by neonatal alloimmune neutropenia (NAIN) suggests that infections are, in the main, mild and death or serious morbidity from sepsis is very rare.

Sepsis

Sepsis in individuals with severe neutropenia is an emergency. Untreated sepsis in the setting carries a significant mortality for both mother and baby. Blood cultures should be taken and broad-spectrum intravenous antibiotics commenced promptly according to local protocols. Fetuses tolerate pyrexia poorly, and neurological damage may occur if the baby suffers prolonged fever.

Granulocyte Colony-Stimulating Factor (GCSF)

GCSF has significantly changed the management of severe chronic neutropenia. For many individuals, the administration of low doses of GCSF 2–3 times per week substantially reduces the incidence of infection. GCSF has replaced traditional therapies such as IVIG, corticosteroids, or splenectomy as first-line therapy outside of pregnancy. Although theoretical concerns exist, it is likely that GCSF is relatively safe in pregnancy. Published reports from the severe chronic neutropenia international registry have not demonstrated adverse effects of GCSF during pregnancy [16,17].

Postpartum

Women with proven AIN or where AIN is strongly suspected are at risk of delivering a neutropenic baby. The neutrophil count at birth should be measured and subsequent measurements performed according to the degree of neutropenia and the infection risk. Immune neutropenia may take several weeks to resolve.

Practical Approach to Pregnant Patients with Diagnosed AIN

- Individuals who are asymptomatic are unlikely to benefit from specific therapy.
- If the ANC is $<0.5 \times 10^9$/L, advice on treating sepsis promptly with intravenous antibiotics is required.
- Individuals who are symptomatic and already on GCSF may benefit from continuing therapy but a careful discussion of the risks of therapy is necessary. Consideration can be given to stopping GCSF, particularly for the first trimester.
- Monitoring FBC to tailor GCSF dose may be required.
- The neonatal team should be alerted prior to delivery.
- A cord blood sample should be taken.
- A postpartum FBC should be sent.

Management of a Newly Presenting Case of Neutropenia in Pregnancy

- Exclude other causes of neutropenia.
- Check hematinics (ferritin, vitamin B_{12}, and folate – see Chapter 2).
- Assess for evidence of associated autoimmune conditions.
- If severe neutropenia, warn patient of risk of life-threatening infection – ensure they understand that prompt treatment is necessary, and have clear, efficient self-referral route.
- Treatment options should be discussed if severe neutropenia is present and infections are problematic: GCSF or corticosteroids could be considered as initial therapeutic options.

Autoimmune Hemolytic Anemia

Introduction

Hemolysis is defined as shortened red cell survival, the average lifespan of an erythrocyte being 120 days. Mild hemolysis is compensated for by an increase in bone marrow erythropoiesis and may not affect the hemoglobin concentration. Anemia occurs when red cell survival is sufficiently shortened to exceed this increase in erythropoietic activity. Causes of hemolysis are listed in Table 5.6. AIHA is a common cause of hemolysis but rarely complicates pregnancy. Non-immune hemolysis

Table 5.6 Causes of hemolysis

Immune	• Autoimmune warm type	IgG mediated
	• Autoimmune cold type	IgM mediated
	• Autoimmune mixed type	IgG and IgM mediated
	• Alloimmune	Reaction to blood transfusion
Hereditary	• Disorder of hemoglobin synthesis	e.g. sickle cell anemia
	• Disorder of red cell enzymes	e.g. G6PD deficiency
	• Disorder of red cell membrane	e.g. hereditary spherocytosis
Mechanical	• Red cell fragmentation	• Mechanical heart valve
		• MAHA (TTP, HUS, HELLP syndrome, pre-eclampsia)
Paroxysmal nocturnal hemoglobinuria	• Clonal stem cell disorder	Increased susceptibility to complement lysis
Drugs	• Oxidative stress, immune	e.g. Dapsone
Infections	• Bacterial enzymes	e.g. *Clostridium perfringens*

occurs more frequently in pregnancy and is mostly associated with pre-eclampsia or other hypertension-related disorders. It is essential to distinguish between these types of hemolysis as the management is very different. AIHA may be further divided into "warm" and "cold" types. Warm AIHA is usually IgG mediated. Cold AIHA is mostly IgM and complement mediated. The blood film shows red cell agglutination and a direct antiglobulin test (DAT) is positive for C3d. Treatment of AIHA in pregnancy is similar to that outside pregnancy. Transplacental passage of IgG antibodies may occur, but neonatal hemolysis is rarely severe.

Epidemiology and Pathogenesis

AIHA in pregnancy is a rare disorder with an estimated incidence of 1:50 000 pregnancies[18]. Pregnancy appears to be a stimulus for AIHA with a fourfold higher incidence than outside pregnancy. Cases of AIHA may predate conception and relapse in pregnancy or occur as a new presentation. Secondary causes include lymphoproliferative disorders, infections (mycoplasma, Epstein–Barr virus), and connective tissue disorders. AIHA is caused by the production of autoantibodies directed against a red cell surface antigen, which on binding results in premature destruction of the erythrocyte. This is usually extravascular in the spleen or liver but occasionally may be intravascular. The antibodies are most frequently IgG followed by the IgM subtype. A spectrum of severity exists. In mild cases, a positive direct DAT is the only abnormality found. More severe cases have evidence of compensated hemolysis with the most severe resulting in significant anemia.

Diagnosis

Anemia during pregnancy is a common finding. For patients presenting during pregnancy, the diagnosis of AIHA requires careful exclusion of other causes of anemia, biochemical evidence of hemolysis, and serological evidence that the hemolysis is immune mediated. Important clinical and laboratory features for diagnosis are summarized below.

History

- Is the patient symptomatic of anemia?
- Is there a history of cardiovascular or pulmonary problems which may impair ability to cope with anemia?
- Is there evidence of a secondary cause, e.g. recent chest infection (mycoplasma) or autoimmune disorders?
- Is the patient on any drugs known to cause hemolysis (especially penicillins, methyldopa, NSAIDs)?
- Identify other potential causes of anemia (hematinic deficiency, hereditary disorders, etc.).

Examination

- Clinical examination may demonstrate evidence of a secondary disorder.

- Cases of chronic hemolysis (e.g. hereditary spherocytosis) can have mild splenomegaly present.

Laboratory

Hemolysis is characterized by:

- ↑bilirubin, ↑LDH, ↑reticulocytes, ↓haptoglobins
- blood film – polychromasia, spherocytes, red cell agglutination (cold AIHA)
- immune-mediated hemolysis – characterized by positive DAT (Coombs test)
- intravascular hemolysis – characterized by urinary hemosiderin, hemoglobinuria

Management

The principal risk is of a sudden fall in hemoglobin resulting in symptomatic anemia and spontaneous abortion. Successful management requires maintaining an adequate hemoglobin level with red cell transfusion and giving specific therapy (usually prednisolone) to arrest the hemolysis. Although transplacental passage of antibodies occurs, the risk of developing anemia in utero or significant neonatal anemia with associated hyperbilirubinemia is small. Published experience of AIHA in pregnancy is limited, but the majority of reports are favorable using this approach.

Blood Transfusion

The presence of autoantibodies can cause difficulty in identifying suitable units for transfusion. Autoantibodies may mask alloantibodies present in the maternal serum, with the possibility of causing a hemolytic transfusion reaction. Specialist investigation is required to exclude an alloantibody or identify the specificity of an alloantibody if present. This may delay the provision of suitable units. Many hospital transfusion laboratories refer this work to specialist transfusion centers, and the following points should be considered.

- Ensure close liaison with the transfusion laboratory to ensure that adequate samples have been provided for testing.
- Ensure that the time within which blood is required is clearly agreed with the transfusion laboratory.
- In cases requiring emergency transfusion, the risks of issuing blood without compatibility being fully

determined should be discussed between the hematologist and obstetrician.
- Patients with cold hemagglutinin disease (CHAD) should receive transfusions via a blood warmer.

Treatment of Hemolysis

Corticosteroids may be effective in reducing hemolysis. The risks of corticosteroid use are listed in Table 5.4A for ITP. Patients with warm AIHA are more likely to respond than those with cold AIHA. A similar treatment pattern to that for ITP may be used and as with ITP, the minimum dose possible to control hemolysis should be used.

Experience with other agents in pregnancy is limited. The benefit of IVIG is not clear, but its use may be justified in pregnancy if corticosteroids are ineffective or contraindicated. Rituximab is increasingly used outside of pregnancy but there are insufficient data currently available in pregnancy to advise its use.

Additional Measures

- Folic acid 5 mg daily should be given. This prevents folate deficiency occurring as a result of increased erythropoiesis. Increased dosage may occasionally be necessary.
- Thromboprophylaxis should be considered. Hemolysis is a prothrombotic condition and there is an increased risk of venous thromboembolism (VTE). Individual assessment of the degree of risk is necessary, and should include assessment of other risk factors for VTE. General measures should be emphasized, such as ensuring adequate hydration, and re-evaluation of degree of risk should continue through the pregnancy. The puerperium is a peak time for thrombotic events, and pharmacological thromboprophylaxis during the first 6 weeks postpartum is recommended.

Considerations for Fetus and at Birth

There is the potential for in utero hemolysis if transplacental passage of antibodies occurs. This applies only to cases of IgG-mediated hemolysis. Unlike hemolytic disease of the newborn, the role of monitoring maternal antibody titers has not been established. Non-invasive monitoring for anemia using ultrasonography may be of value.

The neonatal team should be alerted prior to delivery and neonates should have their hemoglobin and bilirubin measured at birth. Neonates born to mothers with AIHA frequently have a positive DAT; however, hemolysis is usually mild if present.

Significant anemia or elevated bilirubin level requiring treatment is unusual. This is in contrast to hemolytic disease of the newborn (HDN), which may result in very severe hemolysis requiring in utero transfusion or neonatal exchange transfusion.

Case Studies

Case Study 1

A 27-year-old primigravida was referred at 16 weeks' gestation for a hematology consultation. Routine full blood count performed at booking showed Hb 127 g/L, WBC 6.3×10^9/L, and platelets 93×10^9/L. Thrombocytopenia was confirmed on a repeat test. No previous blood tests had been performed for comparison. On clinical assessment, the patient was well with no bleeding symptoms. There was no significant medical history or history of familial thrombocytopenia. The patient was taking no medications. Blood film appearances confirmed the thrombocytopenia was genuine with large platelets present but no other diagnostic features. Routine testing for hepatitis B and C and HIV was negative. A presumptive diagnosis of ITP was made and monthly monitoring of the platelet count was agreed. Serial blood counts during pregnancy demonstrated a progressive fall in platelets with a nadir of 32×10^9/L by 34 weeks. The patient was counseled about the potential risks of maternal and neonatal thrombocytopenia. Prednisolone 20 mg daily was commenced aiming for a platelet count $>50 \times 10^9$/L for delivery. At 36 weeks, the platelet count was 67×10^9/L, which was maintained for the remainder of the pregnancy. The possibility of neonatal thrombocytopenia was discussed and measures to minimize head trauma by avoiding ventouse, rotational forceps, and scalp monitoring at delivery were agreed. A healthy baby was born by normal delivery at term. A cord sample showed a platelet count of 76×10^9/L, which fell to 22×10^9/L over the next few days. A USS of the head did not show any evidence of hemorrhage and the baby was treated with IVIG. The count was slow to respond and screening tests for fetal/neonatal alloimmune thrombocytopenia (FNAIT) and TORCH (Toxoplasmosis, Other [syphilis, varicella-zoster, parvovirus B19], Rubella, Cytomegalovirus [CMV], and Herpes) infections were performed as a precaution. By the fourth week, the platelet count was over 50×10^9/L and normalized by week 6 post-delivery.

This case illustrates the investigation of thrombocytopenia in pregnancy and neonatal thrombocytopenia.

Key Learning Points from this Case

1. The importance of distinguishing ITP from the more common gestational thrombocytopenia.
2. Neonatal thrombocytopenia detected on a cord sample should be followed up as it may worsen in the first few days following delivery.
3. Neonatal thrombocytopenia may take several weeks, and occasionally months, to resolve.
4. While neonatal thrombocytopenia secondary to maternal ITP is a likely cause, other causes of neonatal thrombocytopenia need to be considered, especially NAIT. If neonatal platelet transfusion is required, HPA 1a 5b negative platelets should be considered pending NAIT test results.

Case Study 2

A 26-year-old primigravida with known chronic ITP requested a consultation for pre-pregnancy counseling. Her platelet count was 32×10^9/L. The potential risks for mother and baby were discussed but pregnancy was not discouraged. She subsequently became pregnant and presented to her obstetrician at 16 weeks with mild vaginal bleeding. Ultrasound demonstrated a healthy pregnancy. The platelet count was 12×10^9/L. Treatment for ITP was advised based on her bleeding symptoms and the severity of thrombocytopenia. Prednisolone 20 mg daily was commenced resulting in an improvement of symptoms and was eventually discontinued at 26 weeks. For the remainder of the pregnancy the platelet count remained greater than 20×10^9/L with no further bleeding symptoms. At 34 weeks, a delivery plan was discussed. Measures to reduce neonatal head trauma were advised and an anesthetic opinion was sought for alternatives to epidural anesthesia. The patient was advised that an epidural anesthetic for pain relief would not be offered if the platelet count was less than 75×10^9/L. Prednisolone was recommended with weekly monitoring of the platelet count instituted. Despite escalating the dose, the platelet count did not increase beyond 40×10^9/L. Prednisolone was continued and a single dose of intravenous immunoglobulin (1 g/kg body weight) was given at 38 weeks with good effect resulting in a platelet count of 123×10^9/L. A repeat dose of immunoglobulin was required at 40 weeks due to falling platelet counts. Eight days beyond her due date a healthy baby was born by emergency cesarean section. The cord platelet count was normal. A routine thrombosis risk assessment at delivery advised low-molecular-weight heparin prophylaxis was indicated. This was administered but with careful monitoring of the platelet count. The patient's prednisolone dose was tapered over the following 6 weeks with only minor postpartum bleeding symptoms reported.

This case illustrates the management of maternal ITP.

Key Learning Points from this Case

1. Maternal and neonatal outcomes for women with ITP are usually good and pregnancy is not normally discouraged.
2. Treatment often needs to be escalated toward the end of pregnancy to achieve a safe platelet count for delivery.
3. Postpartum it is necessary to consider both bleeding and thrombosis risks.

References

1. Segal JB, Powe NR. Prevalence of immune thrombocytopenia: analyses of administrative data. *Journal of Thrombosis and Hemostasis* 2006; **4**: 2377–2383.

2. Sainio S, Kekomaki R, Riikonen S, Teramo K. Maternal thrombocytopenia at term: a population-based study. *Acta Obstetrica Gynecologica Scandinavica* 2000; **79**: 744–749.

3. Gill KK, Kelton JG. Management of idiopathic thrombocytopenic purpura in pregnancy. *Seminars in Hematology* 2000; **37**: 275–289.

4. Boehlen F, Hohlfeld P, Extermann P *et al.* Platelet count at term pregnancy: a reappraisal of the threshold. *Obstetrics and Gynecology* 2000; **95**: 29–33.

5. Verdy E, Bessous V, Dreyfus M *et al.* Longitudinal analysis of platelet count and volume in normal pregnancy. *Thrombosis and Hemostasis* 1997; **77**: 806–807.

6. Provan D, Stasi R, Newland AC. International consensus report on the investigation and management of primary immune thrombocytopenia. *Blood* 2010; **115**: 168–186.

7. Win N, Rowley M, Pollard C *et al.* Severe gestational (incidental) thrombocytopenia: to treat or not to treat. *Hematology* 2005; **10**: 69–72.

8. Watson H, Davidson S, Keeling D. Guidelines on the diagnosis and management of heparin-induced thrombocytopenia: second edition. *British Journal of Haematology* 2012; **159**(5): 528–540.

9. British Committee for Standards in Hematology General Hematology Task Force. Guidelines for investigation and management of idiopathic thrombocytopenic purpura in adults, children and in pregnancy. *British Journal of Hematology* 2003; **120**: 574–596.

10. Webert KE, Mittal R, Sigouin C *et al.* A retrospective 11-year analysis of obstetric patients with idiopathic thrombocytopenic purpura. *Blood* 2003; **102**: 4306–4311.

11. Veneri D, Franchini M, Raffelli R *et al.* Idiopathic thrombocytopenic purpura in pregnancy: analysis of 43 consecutive cases followed at a single Italian institution. *Annals of Hematology* 2006; **85**: 552–554.

12. Yamada H, Kato E, Kobashi G *et al.* Passive immune thrombocytopenia in neonates of mothers with idiopathic thrombocytopenic purpura: incidence and risk factors. *Seminars in Thrombosis Hemostasis* 1999; **25**: 491–496.

13. Christiens GC, Niewenhuis HK, Bussel JB. Comparison of platelet counts in first and second newborns of mothers with immune thrombocytopenic purpura. *Obstetrics and Gynecology* 1997; **90**: 546–552.

14. Burrows, R, Kelton J. Pregnancy in patients with idiopathic thrombocytopenic purpura: assessing the risks for the infant at delivery. *Obstetrical and Gynecological Survey* 1993; **48**: 781–788.

15. Loustau V. Effect of pregnancy on the course of immune thrombocytopenia: a retrospective study of 118 pregnancies in 82 women. *British Journal of Haematology* 2014; **166**(6): 929–935.

16. Boxer LA, Bolyard AA, Kelley ML *et al.* Use of granulocyte colony-stimulating factor during pregnancy in women with chronic neutropenia. Obstetrics and Gynecology 2015; **125**(1): 197–203.

17. Zeidler C, Grote UA, Nickel A. Outcome and management of pregnancies in severe chronic neutropenia patients by the European Branch of the Severe Chronic Neutropenia International Registry. Hematologica 2014; **99**(8): 1395–1402.

18. Sokol RJ, Hewitt S, Stamps BK. Erythrocyte autoantibodies, autoimmune hemolysis and pregnancy. *Vox Sanguinis* 1982; **43**: 169–176.

Chapter

6 Management of Sickle Cell Disease in Pregnancy

Karyn Longmuir and Jo Howard

Introduction

Sickle cell disease is a heterogeneous group of disorders with autosomal recessive inheritance. In adults without sickle cell disease, hemoglobin A (Hb A) is the predominant hemoglobin; it is made up of 2 alpha chains and 2 beta chains. Hemoglobin A_2 (2 alpha chains and 2 delta chains) and hemoglobin F (2 alpha chains and 2 gamma chains) make up the remainder. In sickle cell disease, mutations in the β-globin gene lead to the production of a structurally abnormal hemoglobin chain and in hemoglobin S (HbS), valine replaces glutaminic acid. Other mutations lead to the production of further abnormal hemoglobins, which can act synergistically with HbS; for example, if lysine replaces glutaminic acid, hemoglobin C (HbC) is produced.

Sickle cell anemia is the homozygous state with the inheritance of HbS from both parents but there are various compound heterozygous states (sickle cell disease) that result in a similar clinical picture but differ in severity, for example:

1. HbSC
2. HbSβ thalassemia
3. $HbSD_{Punjab}$
4. $HbSO_{Arab}$

Sickle cell disease is characterized by chronic hemolysis complicated by periods of acute pain crisis, which in the long term leads to a multitude of chronic complications and end-organ damage. HbS polymerizes and forms crystals when exposed to low oxygen tensions. These large polymers cause the red cells to become rigid and fragile resulting in vaso-occlusion and red cell hemolysis. Endothelial activation and increased adhesion of the leukocytes and red cells to the vascular endothelium also play a role in vaso-occlusion. Tissue damage is increased by ischemia/reperfusion injury and nitric oxide depletion (secondary to intravascular hemolysis) leading to free radical generation.

Epidemiology

Around 300 000 children are born with sickle cell disease each year. The vast majority are born in Africa but with increased migration and improved survival, sickle cell disease is of worldwide importance[1]. There are approximately 12 000–15 000 affected individuals in the UK, and currently around 300 infants are born with sickle cell disease every year [2,3], compared to 25–30 deliveries per annum in the 1970s. Around two-thirds of these deliveries are in London (south London has the highest density of sickle cell disease in Europe) with the majority of the rest occurring in other major cities, for example Manchester and Birmingham.

Sickle cell disease is now the most common serious genetic condition in England and as advised by the National Health Service (NHS) screening program it must be viewed as a mainstream issue for the NHS[4].

Clinical Features

Patients with sickle cell disease usually have a chronic anemia with a hemoglobin of 60–90 g/L in HbSS and slightly higher in the milder phenotypes.

Patients with HbSS tolerate this hemoglobin level well, in part because HbS has a lower oxygen affinity than HbA so oxygen is more readily released to the tissues, and hence patients do not routinely require transfusion for treatment of chronic anemia.

Painful vaso-occlusive crises are the most common clinical feature of sickle cell disease and severe episodes occur, on average, one to three times a year. They may be triggered by dehydration, hypoxia, infection, acidosis, cold weather, strenuous exercise, and menstruation, and while mild crises will be managed at home, severe pain will require hospital attendance for strong analgesia. Other acute complications include stroke, acute chest syndrome, and acute renal failure, and patients are at increased risk of septic complications. Sickle cell disease causes multiorgan damage and by the time patients reach adulthood they will often be troubled by chronic disease complications including neurological complications, chronic lung damage, renal dysfunction, retinopathy, pulmonary hypertension, avascular necrosis, and leg ulcers[5].

Pregnancy and Sickle Cell Disease

In the UK, there are between 100 and 200 pregnancies per year in women with sickle cell disease. The 2010–2011 UK Obstetric Surveillance System (UKOSS) Survey identified 109 pregnancies in women with sickle cell disease, 46.8% with HbSS and 40.4% with HbSC[6].

Historic data have shown that pregnancy in women with sickle cell disease is associated with increased maternal complications and poorer fetal/neonatal outcomes and these have persisted despite advances in therapy and modern medical care[7]. The rates of both sickle-related and pregnancy-related complications are higher in this group of women. Management must take into account the effect of the pregnancy on the sickle cell disease and the effect of the sickle cell disease on the pregnancy.

Maternal Complications

Sickle-Related Complications

Pregnancy is associated with an increased rate of painful crisis; 52.3% of women in the UKOSS survey experienced at least one painful crisis during the antenatal period[6]. The rates were significantly higher in women with sickle cell anemia (HbSS = 76.5%) compared to HbSC (27.3%). Rates of severe or extremely severe crisis were also higher in women with HbSS (17.6%) compared to HbSC (9.1%) although this did not reach statistical significance. Postnatal pain episodes were also common, being experienced by 21.6% of women with HbSS and 2.3% of women with HbSC[6].

Acute chest syndrome (ACS) was seen in 6.4% of women in the UKOSS survey[6] (9.8% in HbSS and 4.5% in HbSC). Intensive care admission was reported in 21.1% of the women in the survey and although more common in women with HbSS (29.4%), around one in ten women with HbSC (11.4%) also required intensive care level treatment.

A recent meta-analysis has confirmed increased maternal mortality in women with HbSS[7]. A review of maternal mortality figures from the triennial CEMACH[8,9] (Confidential Enquiry into Maternal and Child Health), CMACE[10] (Center for Maternal and Child Enquiries), and the recent MBRRACE-UK [11] (Mothers and Babies – Reducing Risk through Audits and Confidential Enquiries across the UK) reports, along with the 2008 NCEPOD[12] (National Confidential Enquiry into Patient Outcome and Death) report and the recent UKOSS survey[6] reveals that there have been two maternal deaths per year or less in women with sickle cell disease. Given the number of pregnancies in women with sickle cell disease (100–200 per year), maternal mortality in women with sickle cell disease in the UK is much higher than the overall mortality rate of 10.12 per 100 000 maternities reported in the latest triennial report[11].

- CEMACH 2000–2002[8] – three deaths in women with sickle cell disease. One death was secondary to pulmonary embolus, one was during hospital admission for treatment of sickle crisis, and the other was a woman who also had epilepsy.
- CEMACH 2003–2005[9] – no maternal deaths directly related to sickle but two deaths in women with sickle cell disease. One related to amniotic fluid embolism and one a sudden death in a woman who also had a history of epilepsy.
- NCEPOD 2008[12] – no maternal deaths.
- CMACE 2006–2008[10] – four deaths in women with sickle cell disease – three related to sepsis and one to cardiac complications.
- UKOSS 2010–2011[6] – no maternal deaths.
- MBRRACE-UK 2009–2011[11] – four deaths in women with sickle cell disease. Two were secondary to complications from sickle cell crisis in early pregnancy, one was secondary to sepsis, and one was due to an intracerebral hemorrhage.

Pregnancy-Related Complications

Pregnancy-related complications are also higher than in the non-sickle population with a recent meta-analysis showing an increased rate of preeclampsia and eclampsia[7]. In the UKOSS survey [6], urinary tract infection complicated 12% of the pregnancies and was more common in women with HbSS: 19.6% compared to 4.6% (HbSC). Hypertensive disease was reported in 9.2% and both pregnancy-induced hypertension and pre-eclampsia were increased. In addition, renal insufficiency (3.7%) and venous thromboembolism (5.5%) were increased in women with sickle cell disease. The difference in complication rates between those with HbSS and HbSC was not statistically significant.

Obstetric Outcome

Cesarean section rates for women with sickle cell disease have long been reported to be well above the national average. The UKOSS survey[6] revealed a 37.6% cesarean section rate, with a higher rate in women with HbSS (52.9%) compared to HbSC (29.6%). Fetal compromise was the most frequent indication, accounting for over half of all cesarean sections in women with HbSS and around a third of those in women with HbSC.

Postpartum hemorrhage complicated 16.5% of pregnancies in the UKOSS survey[6] and was three times more frequent in women with HbSC (25%) compared to HbSS (7.8%).

Fetal Complications and Fetal Outcome

Stillbirth, neonatal death, and premature delivery have all been reported as complications of pregnancy in women with sickle cell disease, with a reported perinatal mortality rate of 4–6%[7]. The 2010–2011 UKOSS [6] survey revealed that term delivery was reached in only 35.4% of women with HbSS (74.6% in those with HbSC), and 47.1% of women with HbSS delivered at less than 37 weeks and 5.9% at less than 34 weeks' gestation (compared to 20.5% and 4.6% in HbSC). These figures compare poorly with the 2.7% rate of delivery at less than 34 weeks from national hospital episode statistics (HES) data. From these data, it is difficult to differentiate between spontaneous premature delivery and prematurity due to induction. The stillbirth rate in the UKOSS study was reported at 2.8%, which is three times higher than the national rate of stillbirth in the black population and around five times that of the general population (CMACE data)[10].

Intrauterine growth restriction with resultant low birth weight is known to complicate pregnancies in women with sickle cell disease and is thought to be due to placental sickling and infarction[7]. Of the babies born to women with sickle cell disease in the 2010–2011 UKOSS survey[6], 23.3% weighed less than 2.5 kg (35.4% in HbSS and 14% in HbSC) compared to around 3% of all births nationally.

The UKOSS survey confirmed the previously held view that pregnancy in sickle cell disease is a high-risk time with higher rates of maternal and fetal complications compared to the non-sickle population[6]. Although the complication rates were lower in women with HbSC than HbSS, the rates were still higher than the non-sickle population. It was also noted that there was great variation in the severity of complications in those with HbSC with no reliable determinants of which women would be affected. As such the authors concluded that all pregnancies in women with sickle cell disease should be treated as high risk and require the same monitoring and care throughout the preconception, antenatal, intrapartum, and postpartum periods[6].

Fertility and Contraception

As the management of sickle cell disease has been optimized over the years, overall survival has improved with reduced morbidity and better quality of life. There are more pregnancies occurring in women with sickle cell disease, and management of fertility and reproduction is becoming a higher priority.

Infertility in men with sickle cell disease secondary to hypogonadism, sperm abnormalities, and erectile dysfunction due to priapism is well described but less is known about fertility in women with sickle cell disease[13].

Pregnancy rates cannot be used as a surrogate marker of fertility as historically women with sickle cell disease have been advised against pregnancy. Menarche is often delayed and while menstrual bleeding cycles are usually normal, menstruation may trigger sickle pain crisis[13]. The rates of unplanned pregnancies in women with sickle are higher than the national average and may be due to a reluctance to prescribe hormonal contraception to these women [13]. It should be remembered that all forms of contraception carry less risk than pregnancy.

Progesterone-only contraceptives are effective and may reduce the frequency of painful crisis in women of childbearing age. There is also evidence that HbF levels are higher when taking these preparations[13,14]. Although there are some disadvantages, including reduced reliability and irregular bleeding, the progesterone-only pill, depot preparations, and intrauterine systems are frequently prescribed in women with sickle cell disease and are rated as level 1 contraceptives by the UK Medical Eligibility Criteria (UKMEC), which recommends there is no restriction on their use[14,15].

Sickle cell disease is listed as a relative contraindication for the combined oral contraceptive pill (COCP) given the associated thrombotic risks but these risks are small especially if low-dose estrogen preparations are prescribed. UKMEC classify these as level 2 contraceptives, recommending that the benefits outweigh the risks and they should be used if progesterone-containing contraceptives are not suitable[14,15].

Preparing for Pregnancy and Preconception Care

Preconception care and discussions about contraception, pregnancy plans, and the inheritance of sickle cell disease should ideally begin around the time of transition from pediatric to adult services [14,15]. Partner screening should be discussed and arranged as appropriate and if the partner has sickle trait, the couple should be offered detailed discussion of reproductive options including pre-implantation genetic diagnosis (see Chapter 8)[14]. There should be education and discussion about the risks of pregnancy including the increased risks of maternal and fetal complications and optimization of any chronic disease complications[14,15].

All patients with sickle cell disease should be reviewed at least annually, and certainly prior to planning a pregnancy[15]. This should include an assessment of the clinical history (frequency and severity of crises, transfusion history, and review of known chronic complications/end-organ damage), a review of medications and vaccinations, a screen for red cell allo-antibodies, screening for chronic disease including blood pressure measurement, assessment of renal function (urinalysis for both microalbuminuria and proteinuria and U&Es), retinal screening for retinopathy, echocardiography screening for pulmonary hypertension, and T2*MRI and R2*MRI assessment of cardiac and hepatic iron status if there is a significant transfusion history, i.e. long-term transfusion program for stroke prevention or multiple transfusions for management of acute sickle crisis. Any required treatments should be initiated prior to pregnancy and monitored to allow discussions regarding the optimal timing of pregnancy.

Medications and Vaccinations

Women who are contemplating pregnancy should take regular folic acid supplements that should then continue throughout pregnancy. There is an increased risk of folate deficiency due to chronic hemolysis and 5 mg daily[14,15] (rather than the standard 400 µg dose) should be prescribed. Iron supplements should only be prescribed to women with sickle cell disease if there is definite evidence of iron deficiency[15].

Given the increased risk of infection due to the functional hyposplenism in sickle cell disease, it is recommended that penicillin 250 mg bd (erythromycin in penicillin allergic patients) should be continued throughout pregnancy to reduce the risk of infection [14,15]. Vaccinations should be reviewed prior to pregnancy ensuring they are up to date including pneumococcal vaccine polyvalent (pneumovax 23) and influenza (including swine flu – H1N1) vaccinations[15]. Serology for hepatitis viruses and HIV should be reviewed prior to pregnancy. Given the increased frequency of blood transfusion in this group, hepatitis B vaccination should be arranged if required[15] as well as other vaccinations recommended by "The Green Book" governmental advice in vaccination.

Angiotensin-converting enzyme (ACE) inhibitors and angiotensin receptor II blockers used for the treatment of proteinuria in sickle cell disease are not safe in pregnancy and should be stopped prior to conception[15].

Women should be counseled about the safety of analgesia in pregnancy and advised that anti-inflammatories should only be taken if medically advised and should not be taken before 12 weeks or after 28 weeks' gestation[15].

Hydroxycarbamide is potentially teratogenic, hence effective contraception is required while taking it, and men and women with sickle cell disease should be counseled that ideally hydroxycarbamide should be stopped 3 months prior to conception[14,15]. Counseling about the potential detrimental effects that cessation of this medication will have on the course of the sickle cell disease should be provided. A small number of pregnancies have occurred while taking this medication and no fetal abnormalities in humans have been reported. If a pregnancy is unplanned the medication should be stopped as soon as the pregnancy is recognized and the couple counseled regarding the potential risks. In our practice, we do not advise termination but would organize a detailed anomaly scan at 20 weeks' gestation.

Iron overload should ideally have been identified and intensively treated pre-pregnancy with iron chelation, and this too should be reviewed prior to pregnancy and stopped prior to conception. However, there is some evidence from patients with thalassemia that desferrioxamine could be reintroduced at low doses after 20 weeks' gestation and after a review of the risks versus benefits[16].

Confirmation of Pregnancy/Booking Appointment

When a pregnancy is confirmed the issues raised in preconceptual care should be recapped or given immediate attention if not reviewed previously, for example, if first presentation is at booking. If partner screening has not been addressed previously this should be arranged urgently so that the couple can receive genetic counseling within the first trimester.

General health education advice should be provided including the avoidance of known triggers of vaso-occlusive crisis. Financial and social support services may be required. Morning sickness should be adequately treated to reduce the risks of dehydration. Women should be advised to present early if they experience severe pain due to vaso-occlusive crisis and not try to manage at home[15].

A multidisciplinary approach (obstetrician, hematologist with an interest in sickle cell disease, and a midwife experienced in the provision of antenatal care to those with high-risk pregnancies) is required. An individualized care plan should be constructed including clear protocols for management of complications including escalation of care to specialist sickle cell centers if required[15].

Given the increased risks of pre-eclampsia in women with sickle cell disease, daily low-dose (75 mg) aspirin is advised, unless there is a contraindication to its use. Although there is no specific evidence that aspirin decreases pre-eclampsia in this subgroup, studies have shown that aspirin decreases pre-eclampsia in women at increased risk of pre-eclampsia and sickle cell disease could certainly be considered a risk factor. Royal College of Obstetricians and Gynecologists (RCOG) guidance[15] states that aspirin should start at 12 weeks but there is anecdotal evidence that many would advocate starting earlier (as soon as pregnancy is confirmed).

Antenatal Appointments

After the booking appointment the women should be seen at least every 4 weeks until 24 weeks, fortnightly until 38 weeks, and then every week until delivery. Blood pressure measurement and urinalysis for proteinuria should be undertaken at each visit given the increased risk of hypertensive disease. A midstream specimen of urine for culture and sensitivity should also be sent every 4 weeks to screen for asymptomatic urinary tract infection[15].

A full blood count should be performed every 4 weeks to monitor for maternal anemia. Iron supplementation should only be provided if there is evidence of definite iron deficiency[15].

Ultrasound Schedule

A viability scan should be performed at 7–9 weeks' gestation, the routine first trimester scan at 11–14 weeks, and a detailed anomaly scan at 20 weeks. Given the high risk of intrauterine growth restriction, serial growth scans should be performed at least every 4 weeks from 24 weeks' gestation[15]. If growth restriction is detected, more frequent scans should be arranged to help inform decisions about optimal timing of delivery.

Anesthetic Review

An anesthetic review should be scheduled for the third trimester to discuss analgesia at delivery[15]. Regional anesthesia can be undertaken as in those without sickle cell disease. Pethidine should be avoided due to the risks of seizure but other opioids can be used[15]. There should be careful monitoring of oxygen saturations to detect hypoxia if Entonox is used. Given the increased complication rates associated with general anesthesia in this patient group, regional anesthesia is preferred for cesarean section[15].

Blood Transfusion

The necessity of prophylactic transfusion during pregnancy should be considered on a case by case basis on the first antenatal visit, or at a preconceptual visit if possible. Transfusion should be continued throughout pregnancy if a woman is already on a regular transfusion program, e.g. for secondary stroke prevention or management of frequent chest crises [14]. Routine or universal prophylactic transfusion during pregnancy is not currently recommended for women with sickle cell disease[15]. A randomized controlled trial in the USA[17] and a retrospective study in the UK[18] demonstrated a reduction in episodes of painful crisis but did not show any improvement in either fetal or maternal outcomes. A recent retrospective study from Turkey of 37 women concluded that red cell exchange was a feasible and safe procedure for the prevention of complications[19]. Transfusion programs in the previous studies that showed no beneficial effect on pregnancy outcome began in the second trimester and, as such, placental function may have already been compromised and further randomized control trials in early pregnancy are required.

There are clear clinical indications for ad hoc transfusion in this patient group, and in the 2010–2011 UKOSS survey[6] 23.9% of women received at least one blood transfusion (43.1% in those with HbSS and 6.8% in women with HbSC). Indications for transfusion include acute chest syndrome, acute stroke, and management of acute severe anemia (Hb less than 60 g/L or more than 20 g/L below baseline or if causing cardiorespiratory compromise)[14]. Transfusion should also be considered for those women with a twin pregnancy and in those with a poor obstetric history and is an effective treatment for women with repeated painful crises in pregnancy. Once transfusion is required for treatment of an acute complication during pregnancy, continuation throughout pregnancy should be considered[15].

Transfusion is not without complication and the risks versus benefits must be considered, the main risks including the formation of alloantibodies, transfusion-transmitted infection, and iron overload[14]. Patients with sickle cell disease have an increased incidence of red cell alloantibodies, up to 36% in some studies[15], with the potential to cause both delayed transfusion reactions and hemolytic disease of the newborn. The majority of the red cell antibodies detected in this patient group are directed against the Rh antigens (C and E) and the Kell antigens. All patients with sickle cell disease should receive blood compatible for their Rh and Kell phenotype; it should be HbS negative and in addition, in pregnancy, blood should be cytomegalovirus (CMV) negative[14,15].

Pain Management/Management of Acute Complications

Acute pain crises are common during pregnancy and in the postnatal period and should be treated according to recommendations in the NICE guidelines[20]. This will include analgesia given within 30 minutes of presentation and supportive therapy including fluids and oxygen; if there is evidence of infection antibiotics should be administered. Most patients will have a standard pain plan, based on previous requirements for analgesia, but women with a previous mild phenotype may present with pain during pregnancy. Mild to moderate pain should be treated with oral analgesia as per the WHO analgesia ladder starting with paracetamol, then with the addition of mild opiates

(e.g. co-dydramol), and then stronger opiates (e.g. dihydrocodeine or oral morphine).

NSAIDs should be avoided in the first and third trimesters[14,15]. Most women will have self-administered weak opiates before arrival at hospital and may need injectable opiates on arrival in hospital, which can be given as intermittent dosages or via patient-controlled analgesia devices. This should be continued until pain is under control and then analgesia should be decreased before discharge. Clinical observations (including oxygen saturations) should be monitored hourly for the first 6 hours after admission or until pain is under control. Antiemetics and laxatives may be necessary to treat the side effects of opiates.

Fluid intake should be assessed and if oral fluid intake is less than 3 L per 24 hours, intravenous fluids should be prescribed. If oxygen saturations are ≤94% on air a diagnosis of acute chest syndrome should be considered and urgent medical review should be requested to include arterial blood gases. A high index of suspicion should be maintained for acute chest syndrome in any patients with chest symptoms, and this should be investigated and treated as in non-pregnant sickle patients[21].

Infection is more common in patients with sickle cell disease, due in part to their hyposplenism, and is a common precipitant of both acute pain and acute chest syndrome. Indicators of infection (including blood culture and urine cultures) should be performed as appropriate on hospital admission and care givers should have a low index of suspicion for treating with antibiotics.

Other acute complications, e.g. acute stroke and cholecystitis, should be treated as in the non-pregnant patient with sickle cell disease[5].

Thrombosis

Recent data indicate that the risk of venous thromboembolism (VTE) is increased during pregnancy in women with sickle cell disease[22], though well-designed large prospective studies are still needed to firmly establish this association[23]. This increased risk does not appear to extend to women with sickle cell trait[24], though general VTE prevention advice should be provided to all pregnant women.

RCOG Guidelines[25] include sickle cell disease as a risk factor for thromboembolism with an adjusted odds ratio of 1.7–6.7 and recommend that these women are at "intermediate risk" of thromboembolism and that antenatal prophylaxis with low-molecular-weight heparin (LMWH) should be considered. Risk assessment should be undertaken and certainly antenatal pharmacological thromboprophylaxis initiated if there are additional risk factors for VTE. Women should receive pharmacological thromboprophylaxis throughout any antenatal hospital admissions[25].

Postnatally women with sickle cell disease are also classified as 'intermediate risk' for thromboprophylaxis and should receive at least 10 days of postnatal prophylactic LMWH. This should be extended if they have additional risk factors, i.e. women who undergo cesarean section should have LMWH thromboprophylaxis for 6 weeks postnatally[25].

Sickle cell disease itself can be associated with elevated D-dimer levels[26], and as such, the usefulness of this test is limited in the investigation of potential VTE in pregnant women with sickle cell disease. The role of D-dimer in the investigation of suspected VTE in any pregnant woman has not been well established and the new RCOG Guidelines[27], for example, advise against the use of D-dimer in the investigation of VTE in any pregnant woman.

Delivery

Care during delivery, including timing and type of delivery, should be determined primarily by obstetric indications[15]. Spontaneous labor and normal vaginal delivery is recommended if possible. There is no clear evidence about optimal timing of delivery but in view of increased risks of complications both maternal (e.g. pain crisis) and fetal (e.g. IUGR), most obstetricians will monitor the clinical situation and growth scans intensively from 38 weeks and suggest induction at term. Delivery should take place in a unit prepared for high-risk pregnancies, preferably with experience of women with sickle cell disease [15]. The multidisciplinary team should be informed when labor is confirmed.

Given the higher rates of stillbirth, placental abruption, and reduced placental reserve, continuous electronic fetal heart monitoring is recommended to allow for early detection of fetal distress and the need for operative delivery[15]. Fluid balance and oxygenation should be carefully monitored, particularly with prolonged labor. Pethidine should be avoided because of the risk of seizure in patients with sickle cell disease[15].

Postnatal Management

Careful monitoring of fluid, oxygen, and analgesia requirements should continue into the postpartum period with at least daily review by the hematology team in addition to obstetric review. Thromboprophylaxis and advice regarding contraception should be considered/provided as above. In high-risk pregnancies, early sickle testing of the baby should be offered[14,15].

Case Studies

Case Study 1
A 26-year-old woman with known sickle cell anemia attends clinic to discuss potential pregnancy. Her husband is known to have sickle cell trait. They have received genetic counseling in the past and are aware of the 50% chance that the child would have sickle cell anemia. They have declined prenatal diagnosis.

She has previously had one episode of chest crisis associated with a hospital admission with pneumonia as a teenager but does not have frequent painful crises requiring hospitalization. She uses paracetamol and anti-inflammatory medication to manage her pain. She only received transfusion during the admission with chest crisis and has no evidence of iron overload but does have an Anti-Fya antibody.

Recent screening including an echocardiogram has not shown evidence of end-organ damage. She is compliant with her penicillin prophylaxis and folic acid and has recently stopped taking the progesterone-only pill in preparation for pregnancy.

The potential maternal and fetal complications are discussed and a plan for antenatal care is established. She is advised not to use anti-inflammatory medication in the first 12 weeks or after 28 weeks.

Twelve weeks later she contacts the department stating that she is pregnant and is experiencing significant "morning sickness." Review in the hematology/obstetric clinic is arranged. An ultrasound scan confirms a viable pregnancy. Management of nausea and vomiting is optimized and a schedule for antenatal care planned. Aspirin is commenced at 12 weeks to reduce the risks of pre-eclampsia.

A growth scan at 24 weeks raises possible concerns regarding intrauterine growth restriction, and ongoing scans every 4 weeks are arranged to monitor fetal growth.

She presents at 26 weeks with painful crisis possibly triggered by a urinary tract infection. She receives treatment with intravenous fluids, analgesia, antibiotics, and thromboprophylaxis and is able to be discharged 4 days later.

At 28 weeks thromboprophylaxis is commenced to reduce thrombotic risks. Her hemoglobin is stable at around 80 g/L with no evidence of iron deficiency.

Over the next 8 weeks there are detailed multidisciplinary discussions regarding plans for delivery. Given the concerns regarding growth restriction, induction of labor is arranged for 38 weeks. However, due to cardiotocographic (CTG) findings of fetal distress she delivers by cesarean section.

She requires supplemental oxygen for 24 hours in the high-dependency unit (HDU) post-delivery but is otherwise well. Testing shows that the baby is a carrier and does not have sickle cell anemia and they are both discharged home on day +3 with plans for her to complete 6 weeks of postnatal thromboprophylaxis.

Case Study 2

A 36-year-old woman with HbSC disease delivered vaginally at term. The pregnancy had been uncomplicated although labor was prolonged and she developed a urinary tract infection at 1 day postpartum, requiring oral antibiotics. At discharge, she was also continued on her prophylactic dalteparin at 5000 units daily.

On day 5 she was readmitted with pain and tenderness in the left upper-quadrant of her abdomen. Examination was otherwise unremarkable and after surgical review, conservative management was recommended; she was kept nil by mouth and given intravenous fluids and broad-spectrum antibiotics. Her blood results showed a stable Hb of 102 g/L and no biochemical evidence of increased hemolysis.

The next day, her spleen had become considerably enlarged, reaching the left iliac fossa. Ultrasound confirmed splenic arterial infarct and massive venous engorgement. More scrupulous review identified an occlusive thrombus at the junction of the superior mesenteric vein and the splenic vein. This was surprising given the prophylactic low-molecular-weight heparin she had been taking but it highlights the increased thrombotic risk in patients with sickle cell disorders, exaggerated in her case by her age, infection, prolonged labor, and dehydration.

She responded well to full anticoagulation and sickle prevention measures.

References

1. Angastiniotis M, Modell B, Englezos P, Boulyjenkou V. Prevention and control of hemoglobinopathies. *Bulletin of the World Health Organization* 1995; **73**: 375–386

2. UK NSC & UK Joint Committee on Medical Genetics Statement on Genetic Carrier Testing; 2012.

3. Streetley A, Latinovic R, Hall K, Henthorn K. Implementation of universal newborn bloodspot screening for sickle cell disease and other clinically significant hemoglobinopathies in England: screening results for 2005–7. *Journal of Clinical Pathology* 2009; **62**: 26–30

4. NHS Sickle Cell and Thalassemia Screening Programmes/Sicke Cell Society. *Sickle Cell Disease in Childhood: Standards and Guidelines for Clinical Care*, 2nd edn. London: NHS Sickle Cell and Thalassaemia Screening Programme in partnership with the Sickle Cell Society; 2010.

5. Howard J, Telfer P. *Sickle Cell Disease in Clinical Practice*. London: Springer; 2015.

6. Oteng-Ntim E, Ayensah B, Knight M, Howard J. Pregnancy outcome in patients with sickle cell disease in the UK – a national cohort study comparing sickle cell anemia (Hb SS) with Hb SC disease. *British Journal of Hematology* 2015; **169**(1): 129–137.

7. Oteng-Ntim E, Meeks D, Seed P. Adverse maternal and perinatal outcomes in pregnant women with sickle cell disease: systematic review and meta-analysis. *Blood* 2015; **125**(21): 3316–3325.

8. CEMACH. *Why Mothers Die 2000–2002. The Sixth Report of the Confidential Enquiries into Maternal Deaths in the United Kingdom*. London: RCOG Press; 2004.

9. CEMACH. *Saving Mothers' Lives: Reviewing Maternal Deaths to make Motherhood Safer: 2003–2005. The Seventh Report of the Confidential Enquiries into Maternal Deaths in the United Kingdom*. London: RCOG Press; 2007.

10. CMACE. *Saving Mothers' Lives: Reviewing Maternal Deaths to make Motherhood Safer: 2006–2008. The Eighth Report of the Confidential Enquiries into Maternal Deaths in the United Kingdom*. *British Journal of Obstetrics and Gynaecology* 2011; **118**: 1–203

11. MBRRACE-UK. *Saving Lives, Improving Mothers' Care. Lessons Learned to Inform Future Maternity Care from the UK and Ireland Confidential Enquiries into Maternal Deaths and Morbidity 2009-2012*. Oxford: National Perinatal Epidemiology Unit, University of Oxford; 2014.

12. NCEPOD. *A Sickle Crisis? A Report of the National Confidential Enquiry into Patient Outcome and Death*. London: NCEPOD; 2008.

13. Smith-Whitley K. Reproductive issues in sickle cell disease. *Blood* 2014; **124**(24), 3538–3543.

14. Sickle Cell Society. Pregnancy, contraception and fertility. In *Standards for the Clinical Care of Adults with Sickle Cell Disease in the UK*. London: Sickle Cell Society; 2008: pp. 59–68.

15. Royal College of Obstetricians and Gynecologists. *Management of Sickle Cell Disease in Pregnancy. Green-Top Guideline No. 61*. London: Royal College of Obstetricians and Gynecologists; 2011.

16. Royal College of Obstetricians and Gynecologists. *Management of Beta Thalassemia in Pregnancy. Green-Top Guideline No. 66*. London: Royal College of Obstetricians and Gynecologists; 2014.

17. Koshy M, Burd L, Wallace D *et al*. Prophylactic red cell transfusion in pregnant patients with sickle cell disease. a randomised comparative study. *New England Journal of Medicine* 1998; **319**: 1447–1452

18. Howard RJ, Tuck SM, Pearson TC. Pregnancy in sickle cell disease in the UK: results of a multicenter survey of the effect of prophylactic blood transfusion on maternal and fetal outcome. *British Journal of Obstetrics and Gynecology* 1995; **102**(12): 947–951.

19. Asma S, Kozanoglu I, Tarım E *et al*. Prophylactic red blood cell exchange may be beneficial in the management of sickle cell disease in pregnancy. *Transfusion* 2015; **55**: 36–44.

20. NICE. Sickle cell acute painful episode: management of an acute painful sickle cell episode in hospital. *NICE Clinical Guideline 143*, June 2012.

21. Howard J Hart N, Roberts-Harewood M *et al*. Guideline on the management of Acute Chest Syndrome in Sickle Cell Disease. General Hematology Task Force of the British Committee for Standards in Hematology (BCSH); 2015.

22. Seaman CD, Yabes J, Moore CG, Ragni MV. Venous thromboembolism in pregnant women with SCD: A retrospective database analysis. *Thrombosis Research* 2014; **134**(6): 1249–1252.

23. Noubouossie D, Key NS. Sickle cell disease and venous thromboembolism in pregnancy and the puerperium. *Thrombosis Research* 2015; **135**(S1): S46–S48.

24. Pintova S, Cohen HW, Billett HH. Sickle cell trait: is there an increased VTE risk in pregnancy and the postpartum? *PLoS One* 2013; **8**(5): 1–6.

25. Royal College of Obstetricians and Gynecologists. *Thrombosis and Embolism during Pregnancy and the Puerperium, Reducing the Risk. Green-Top Guideline No. 37a*. London: Royal College of Obstetricians and Gynecologists; 2015.

26. Kabrhel C, Mark Courtney D, Camargo CA Jr *et al*. Factors associated with positive D-dimer results in patients evaluated for pulmonary embolism. *Academic Emergency Medicine* 2010; **17**(6): 589–597.

27. Royal College of Obstetricians and Gynecologists. *Thromboembolic Disease in Pregnancy and the Puerperium: Acute Management. Green-Top Guideline No. 37b*. London: Royal College of Obstetricians and Gynecologists; 2015.

Management of Thalassemias in Pregnancy

Farrukh Shah, Emma Prescott, and Amma Kyei-Mensah

Background

Worldwide more than 70 000 babies are born with thalassemia each year, and there are 270 million individuals with asymptomatic thalassemia trait[1]. The α thalassemias are the most common single gene disorders worldwide. No robust figures are available on the number of patients affected by thalassemia syndromes, with estimates of around 200 000 patients with thalassemia major (TM) receiving treatment in designated centers globally (Figure 7.1). The number of patients with non-transfusion-dependent thalassemia (NTDT) is far greater than those with TM but is not actually quantifiable as the disease spectrum is wide with many patients being diagnosed incidentally.

Classification

Thalassemia syndromes are broadly subdivided according to the type of globin chain production that is defective. Beta thalassemia syndromes have reduced or absent β globin chains and α thalassemia syndromes have defective α globin production. This results in an excess of α or β globin chains, which will then form deposits of hemichromes on the membrane of developing red cells resulting in ineffective erythropoiesis.

The degree of imbalance between the α and the β globin genes results therefore in the clinical phenotype of anemia. The larger the degree of imbalance the more severe the anemia, hence ameliorating factors can change the phenotypic presentation of the genotype. Clinically, however, it is simpler to classify patients according to the clinical severity of the anemia and transfusion dependence (see Tables 7.1 and 7.2).

Non-Transfusion-Dependent Thalassemia

Thalassemia intermedia or NTDT are interchangeable terms used to define a group of patients with α

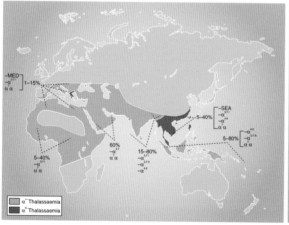
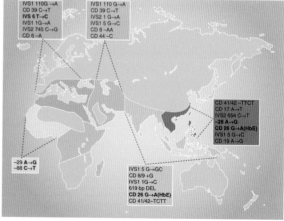

Figure 7.1 Worldwide distribution of α and β thalassemias.
Reprinted by permission from Macmillan Publishers Ltd, copyright 2001[2].

Table 7.1 Simplified effects of β globin gene mutations

Genotype	Outcome	Effect
β/β	Normal	Normal indices HbA2 normal
β/–	Heterozygous Thalassemia trait	Mild to moderate anemia Low MCV and MCH. HbA2 above 3.5%
–/δβ or δβγ	Thalassemia trait	Mild to moderate anemia Low MCV and MCH, HbA2 normal or low, raised HbF in δβ
β+/β+ β+/β⁰ E/β+ –/β and ααα variant –/– and HPFH or alpha trait variant	Non-transfusion-dependent thalassemia (NTDT)	Moderate to moderately severe anemia MCV<75, MCH <25
–/– Eβ⁰	β thalassemia major	Transfusion dependent

HPFH, hereditary persistence of fetal hemoglobin; MCV, mean cell volume; MCH, mean cell hemoglobin.

Table 7.2 Effect of α globin gene mutations

Genotype	Outcome	Effect
α α/α α	Normal	Normal
–α/αα	Heterozygous α+ thalassemia trait	Frequently silent or slight decrease in MCV/MCH
–α/–α	Homozygous α+	MCH <25 pg
–/α α	Heterozygous α0 thalassemia trait	MCH <25 pg
–/–α	Hemoglobin H disease	Hb 8–9 g/dL
–/–	Hemoglobin Barts hydrops	Death in utero

MCV, mean cell volume; MCH, mean cell hemoglobin.

or β thalassemia in whom the clinical severity of the disease is somewhere between the mild symptoms of thalassemia trait and the severe manifestations of TM. The diagnosis is a clinical one that is based on the patient maintaining a satisfactory hemoglobin (Hb) without the need for regular blood transfusions. In its severe form, patients present at a young age with moderate to moderately severe anemia that will impact on growth and quality of life, and may require either intermittent or more regular but low-frequency transfusion support. At the other end of the spectrum, patients may be completely asymptomatic and present with mild anemia often found incidentally during hematological examinations or family studies.

Patients with severe forms of NTDT and those patients with TM who had poor access to blood were previously offered splenectomy to help reduce transfusion requirements. Splenectomy is now rarely undertaken in β NTDT because of increasing evidence of poor clinical outcomes in patients who were splenectomized[3]. All NTDT patients may develop serious iron overload from increased gastrointestinal iron absorption or intermittent top-up transfusions. These patients by and large have normal fertility.

Thalassemia Major

The mainstay of modern treatment in TM is blood transfusion and iron chelation therapy[4]. A patient will gain 200 mg of iron with each unit of blood transfused and in the absence of iron chelation therapy, iron overload develops and will result in complications due to deposition of iron in organs. All regularly transfused patients will have started iron chelation therapy in childhood and will be on an established regime before pregnancy. Chelation therapy often needs to be modified prior to pregnancy to optimize iron burden.

Complications of Blood Transfusion during Pregnancy

Women with TM will already be established on transfusion regimens, which generally remain stable during pregnancy. In cases where lower pre-transfusion thresholds have been used pre-conceptually, the aim is to achieve a pre-transfusion Hb of 100 g/L. It is rare for new complications to develop during the pregnancy but if a patient has alloantibodies, these may rise during the pregnancy. This may genuinely reflect a worsening of the alloimmunization and a high risk of hemolytic disease (HDN) in the fetus but may also simply be a non-specific rising titer. In this situation, the father of the child should have a red cell phenotype undertaken looking specifically to see if the fetus may have inherited the relevant antigen. If there is evidence of HDN, that would need to be managed appropriately.

In women with NTDT who have only been minimally transfused there is an increased risk of alloimmunization and careful monitoring is required. All women should have a red cell phenotype done prior to first transfusion for the common antigens (Rh system and Kell as a minimum standard).

Complications from Transfusional Iron Overload

Multiple transfusions cause iron overload resulting in hepatic, cardiac, and endocrine dysfunction (Figure 7.2). The anterior pituitary is very sensitive to iron overload and evidence of dysfunction is common[5]. The commonest manifestation of this is delayed or absent pubertal development due to hypogonadotrophic hypogonadism. Aside from the failure of development of secondary sexual characteristics, patients can also develop problems with osteoporosis or osteopenia[6]. If a woman required hormonal support to transition into puberty then she is likely to be subfertile due to hypogonadotrophic hypogonadism and therefore requires ovulation induction therapy with gonadotrophins to achieve a pregnancy[7]. Many younger women undergo spontaneous puberty and have normal fertility [8]. Poorly controlled iron overload will also result in other endocrinopathies such as diabetes mellitus, hypothyroidism, and hypoparathyroidism.

Cardiac iron overload tends to develop as a result of inadequate chelation over a prolonged period of time. The commonest complications are either cardiac failure or a dysrhythmia. Cardiac complications accounted for death in over 50% of cases[9] until the development of MRI methods for monitoring cardiac and hepatic iron overload (T2* or R2 Ferriscan® Resonance Health, Australia). These methods are now available in most large centers looking after patients with hemoglobinopathies. TM women who are planning a pregnancy should undergo cardiac T2*

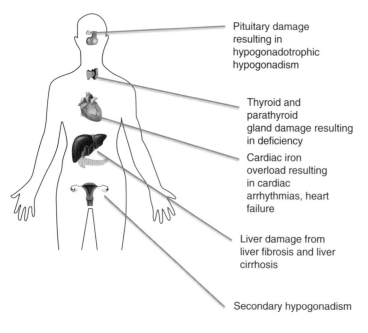

Pituitary damage resulting in hypogonadotrophic hypogonadism

Thyroid and parathyroid gland damage resulting in deficiency

Cardiac iron overload resulting in cardiac arrhythmias, heart failure

Liver damage from liver fibrosis and liver cirrhosis

Secondary hypogonadism

Figure 7.2 Sites of end-organ damage from iron overload.

assessment for cardiac and hepatic iron burden as part of pre-pregnancy optimization. Women who have had severe cardiac iron overload in the past may still develop cardiac complications in the absence of cardiac iron overload (predominantly dysrhythmias). A target cardiac T2 of greater than 20 ms with normal ejection fraction is the desired goal before embarking on a pregnancy but successful pregnancies have occurred with good outcomes with lower T2* values.

Patients may therefore present in a variety of ways to the obstetric teams. NTDT patients who are not transfused or intermittently transfused will generally present following spontaneous conception and may develop complications during a pregnancy from:

- anemia,
- unrecognized iron overload,
- thrombosis risk because of previous splenectomy, or
- complications because of an enlarged spleen.

TM patients may present following spontaneous conception or may require ovulation induction or in vitro fertilization (IVF) to help conceive. These patients may have poorly controlled iron overload and cardiac complications, concurrent endocrinopathies, and increased thrombotic risk because of splenectomy.

A multidisciplinary team should manage patients and pregnancies should be planned to ensure best maternal and fetal outcomes[10]. Care should be focused on preconception preparation, antenatal care, and peri/postpartum management.

Preconception and Antenatal Care

Thalassemia syndromes are associated with an increased risk to both mother and baby. Care has to be focused toward the underlying disorder because complications for both mother and fetus are often related to the splenectomy status, severity of anemia, or iron overload complications. In particular, in TM patients there are the issues surrounding cardiomyopathy in the mother and concurrent diabetes. Women with TM will also receive little or no chelation for 9 months of the pregnancy and may develop new endocrinopathies such as diabetes mellitus, hypothyroidism, and hypoparathyroidism due to the increasing iron burden[11].

Risk of an Affected Offspring: Partner Testing

Antenatal screening of partners should be carried out well before a pregnancy is underway for all women who have a thalassemia mutation. It is important that the risk

Table 7.3 Conditions requiring counseling where the mother is affected by a β thalassemia mutation

Carrier or sufferer condition in partner	Affected offspring
β thalassemia	Risk of serious hemoglobinopathy in offspring
HbS	
HbE	
Delta β thalassemia	
Hb Lepore	
HbO Arab	
Hb Constant Spring	
HbC	Risk of a mild to moderate disorder; counseling and further investigation needed
Other variant hemoglobin	

Table 7.4 Conditions requiring counseling where the mother is affected by α thalassemia trait or NTDT (–/αα or HbH)

Carrier or sufferer condition in partner	Affected offspring
α thalassemia trait (homozygous)	Risk of HbH or Barts hydrops in offspring
–/αα	
Hb Constant Spring	
Other α globin variant	Risk of a mild to moderate disorder; counseling and further investigation needed
Other variant hemoglobin	

of a clinically relevant hemoglobinopathy is clearly ascertained in the couple (Tables 7.3 and 7.4) and a discussion takes place on the methods and risks of prenatal diagnosis and termination of pregnancy[12]. In high-risk couples, pre-implantation genetic diagnosis (PGD) is an option and should be offered. In women who are already pregnant and if the partner is unavailable, an offer of invasive testing is appropriate.

Thalassemia Carriers/Trait/Minor

These patients tend to present to obstetric services after conception and pregnancy is relatively straightforward with little by way of thalassemia-specific issues. It is, however, important to remember that these women have a lower baseline Hb and are hypochromic and microcytic because of the thalassemia carrier status. Iron replacement therapy should be offered if there is evidence of genuine iron deficiency anemia with a low serum ferritin and a high total iron-binding capacity. Iron should not be administered for a period of longer than 3 months without careful monitoring of the serum ferritin and iron profile in order to prevent the development of iron overload. In addition, blood transfusions should rarely be required in these patients.

Non-transfusion-Dependent Thalassemia

These women may be known to the service because of moderate or moderately severe anemia and already under regular follow-up. Other women, in particular those with HbH, may be identified as part of the antenatal screening blood tests. These women are at an increased risk of complications from maternal anemia and should be monitored carefully[13]. They should also be immunized for hepatitis B as they may be exposed to this as a result of blood transfusion. Many women with NTDT are already on folic acid 5 mg daily as they have a much higher demand for folic acid for erythropoiesis. Folic acid 5 mg daily should be commenced 3 months prior to conception if the patient is not already taking it[14].

If already on transfusions, the patient should be managed as for any TM pregnancy. If not on transfusions, then careful assessment for anemia and its impact on mother and fetus is needed.

1. **The multidisciplinary team should review women with NTDT monthly.** These women should be carefully assessed for evidence of increasing anemia or fetal growth restriction (FGR). Monitoring of Hb values should be done at each visit. FGR in pregnant women with NTDT may be related to maternal anemia[11].

2. **Women should be offered an early scan at 7–9 weeks of gestation followed by regular scans.** Women should be offered the routine first trimester scan (11–14 weeks of gestation) and a detailed anomaly scan at 18–20 weeks of gestation. In addition, women should be offered serial fetal biometry scans every 4 weeks from 24 weeks of gestation to assess and monitor for FGR.

3. **Consider blood transfusions if worsening maternal anemia or evidence of FGR.** Severe maternal anemia predisposes to FGR because chronic anemia affects placental transfer of nutrients. Regular transfusions if initiated should aim for a pre-transfusion Hb of around 100 g/L.

Each woman's Hb falls at different rates after transfusion so close surveillance of pre-transfusion Hb concentrations is required.

4. **Asymptomatic women with normal fetal growth and low hemoglobin should have a formal plan outlined in the notes with regard to blood transfusion in late pregnancy.** Generally if the hemoglobin is above 80 g/L at 36 weeks of gestation, transfusion can be avoided before delivery. Postnatal transfusion can be provided as necessary. If the hemoglobin is less than 80 g/L, then a top-up transfusion of 2 units can be considered at 37–38 weeks of gestation.

5. **Women with NTDT have a prothrombotic tendency** due to the presence of abnormal red cell fragments in their blood, especially if they have undergone splenectomy. These red cell fragments combined with a high platelet count significantly increase the risk of venous thromboembolism (ranges between 4% and 29%)[15,16]. This risk is highest in splenectomized women who are not receiving transfusions as a good transfusion regimen suppresses endogenous erythropoiesis [17]. Women with NTDT who have had a splenectomy or a platelet count greater than 600 × 10^9/L should therefore be offered aspirin and LMWH.

Please see Figure 7.3 for an outline of obstetric care in NTDT.

Women with Thalassemia Major

Pregnancies in TM patients have to be carefully planned to reduce the risks of complications in the mother from iron overload and risks to the fetus from maternal medications and endocrine complications. During clinical reviews, the patient should be asked about plans for pregnancy because optimization is important in ensuring good outcomes. This should be done well in advance of the proposed pregnancy as it can take several years to improve cardiac iron loading and a year or longer to optimize the liver iron burden. A prolonged period of iron chelation therapy may be required before both induction of ovulation and pregnancy. All patients should be assessed for evidence of end-organ damage before embarking on a pregnancy.

In sexually active TM women contraception should be advised despite the reduced fertility associated with iron overload. There is no contraindication to the use of hormonal methods such as the combined oral

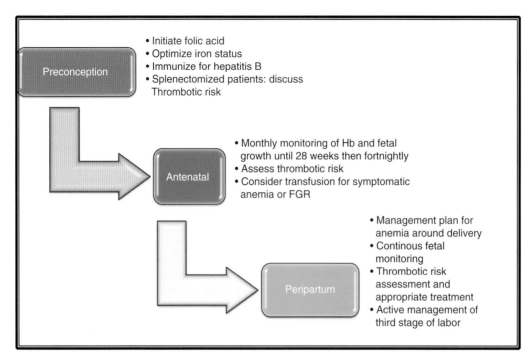

- Preconception
  - Initiate folic acid
  - Optimize iron status
  - Immunize for hepatitis B
  - Splenectomized patients: discuss Thrombotic risk

- Antenatal
  - Monthly monitoring of Hb and fetal growth until 28 weeks then fortnightly
  - Assess thrombotic risk
  - Consider transfusion for symptomatic anemia or FGR

- Peripartum
  - Management plan for anemia around delivery
  - Continous fetal monitoring
  - Thrombotic risk assessment and appropriate treatment
  - Active management of third stage of labor

Figure 7.3 Women with NTDT: outline of obstetric care.

contraceptive pill, the progesterone-only pill, or IUS in women with thalassemia[18].

In TM patients, reduced fertility is often because of hypogonadotrophic hypogonadism, and these women will require ovulation induction using injectable gonadotrophins to conceive.

Preconceptual care should include advice to start folic acid (5 mg) daily to prevent neural tube defects.

Women with thalassemia are best cared for in a multidisciplinary team setting, including an obstetrician with expertise in managing high-risk pregnancies and a hematologist.

1. Iron overload should be optimized prior to embarking on a pregnancy: There is evidence from clinical trials that optimizing body iron reduces end-organ damage and can reverse cardiac iron loading. Longitudinal data from registries show that patients who have been optimally chelated are less likely to suffer from endocrinopathies or cardiac problems[8,19].

2. Iron chelation with deferasirox or deferiprone should be stopped 12 weeks prior to a planned pregnancy or as soon as a pregnancy test is positive in an unplanned pregnancy. Deferiprone is known to be teratogenic but animal studies with

deferasirox did not show teratogenicity; however, there are only limited safety data on its use in pregnancy. Deferasirox and deferiprone therefore should be discontinued 3 months before conception and women converted to deferoxamine iron chelation. Deferoxamine is the only chelation agent with a body of evidence for use in the second and third trimester[20–22].

3. All women should be assessed by a cardiologist prior to embarking on pregnancy. The impact of iron overload on the heart should be assessed before embarking on a pregnancy. A cardiac iron assessment should be undertaken (T2*). The aim is for no cardiac iron, but this can take years to achieve so care should be individualized to the woman. The goal is for a cardiac T2* >20 ms wherever possible as this reflects minimal iron in the heart. However, pregnancies have occurred with successful maternal and fetal outcomes with lower cardiac T2* values. A T2* <10 ms is associated with an increased risk of cardiac failure [23]. A reduced ejection fraction is a relative contraindication to pregnancy and may be life threatening if it is found during a pregnancy. Cardiac arrhythmias are more likely in older

71

patients who have previously had severe myocardial iron overload.

4. Women with myocardial iron loading should undergo regular cardiology review with careful monitoring of ejection fraction during the pregnancy as signs of cardiac decompensation require intervention with chelation therapy. As the cardiac T2* value falls below 20 ms there is an increasing risk of cardiac decompensation[23]. Cardiac MRI is safe in pregnancy and should be undertaken in women who have not had preconceptual assessment, or where there is concern about cardiac function. Presentation with cardiac decompensation in the first trimester is associated with adverse clinical outcome. A falling ejection fraction or increasing ventricular volumes on echocardiography will suggest increasing risk of developing heart failure. If the woman complains of palpitations then a detailed history, ECG, and Holter monitor assessment is needed to confirm a pathological cause. In either circumstance, deferoxamine infusions may be indicated if there are concerns[22].

5. Women should be assessed for liver iron concentration using an MRI technique before pregnancy. Ideally the liver iron should be <7 mg/g dry weight. A liver iron of less than 7 mg/g (dw) is desirable as iron chelation is discontinued during pregnancy. If the initial liver iron burden is high, the 9 months of no chelation during pregnancy will result in an increased risk of iron overload complications. If liver iron exceeds the target range, a period of intensive preconception chelation is required to optimize liver iron burden. At very high liver iron values, the risk of myocardial iron loading increases so iron chelation with low-dose deferoxamine may be commenced between 20 and 28 weeks under guidance from the hemoglobinopathy team. Anecdotally, ovulation induction is more likely to be successful when iron burden is well controlled.

6. Women with diabetes should be referred to a diabetes physician. Good glycemic control is essential prior to and during the pregnancy. Women with established diabetes mellitus should ideally have serum fructosamine concentrations <300 nmol/L for at least 3 months before conception. This is equivalent to a HbA1c of 43 mmol/L. Similar to women with diabetes without thalassemia a HbA1c of less than 43 mmol/L is associated with a reduced risk of congenital abnormalities[24]. Glycosylated hemoglobin is not a reliable marker of glycemic control as this is diluted by transfused blood and results in underestimation, so monthly serum fructosamine is preferred for monitoring[25].

7. Thyroid function should be appropriately monitored both prior to and during pregnancy. Hypothyroidism is frequently found in patients with thalassemia as a consequence of iron overload. Untreated hypothyroidism can result in maternal morbidity, as well as perinatal morbidity and mortality. Patients should be assessed for thyroid function as part of the preconceptual planning and if known to be hypothyroid, treatment initiated to ensure that they are clinically euthyroid[26]. Patients may develop hypothyroidism during the pregnancy or be inadequately treated and hence careful monitoring is essential.

8. Cholelithiasis, evidence of liver cirrhosis due to iron overload, or the presence of viral hepatitis should be identified. Cholelithiasis is common in women with thalassemia due to the underlying hemolytic anemia, and they may develop cholecystitis in pregnancy. Liver cirrhosis and active hepatitis C (HCV) may run a more complex clinical course during pregnancy. Women who are HCV RNA positive should be reviewed by their hepatologist pre-conceptually. Women who have any evidence of cirrhosis either due to previous hepatitis or as a consequence of severe hepatic iron loading should be reviewed by a hepatologist.

9. All women should be offered a bone density scan before pregnancy to document pre-existing osteoporosis. Osteoporosis is a common finding [6] and the underlying pathology is multifactorial including underlying thalassemia bone disease, chelation of calcium by chelation drugs, hypogonadism, and vitamin D deficiency[27]. All women should have vitamin D levels optimized before pregnancy and thereafter maintained in the normal range.

10. All bisphosphonates should be discontinued 3–6 months before pregnancy.

11. ABO and full blood group genotype and antibody titers should be measured. Alloimmunity occurs

in 7.7% to 21% of thalassemia patients[28]. Red cell antibodies may indicate a risk of hemolytic disease of the newborn.

12. Women with thalassemia major should be reviewed monthly until 28 weeks of gestation and fortnightly thereafter. The multidisciplinary team should provide routine as well as specialist antenatal care. The pattern of care should be individualized depending on the degree of end-organ damage, and women with diabetes or cardiac dysfunction may be reviewed more frequently.

13. Women with thalassemia should have a management plan for delivery documented in the obstetric medical record. The plan should cover proposed method of delivery, anesthetic review re analgesia and management of cesarean delivery if planned, cardiac risks relating to iron overload, and management of diabetes during delivery if the patient is diabetic.

Tables 7.5 and Figure 7.4 outline the obstetric care at booking and in the preconceptual, antenatal, and peripartum periods.

Table 7.5 Antenatal booking appointment review for women with NTDT and TM

Offer information, advice, and support in relation to optimizing general health

Discuss information, education, and advice about how thalassemia will affect pregnancy

Primary care or hospital appointment – offer partner testing if not already done; review partner results if available and discuss prenatal diagnosis (chorionic villus sampling, amniocentesis, or cell free fetal DNA) if appropriate

Take a clinical history to establish extent of thalassemia complications. Women with diabetes referred to joint diabetes pregnancy clinic with hematology input

Review medications and stop chelation if not already stopped

Women should be taking 5 mg folic acid

Women who have had a splenectomy should receive antibiotic prophylaxis

Review and optimize vaccination status in those women who have had a splenectomy

Offer MRI heart and liver (T2* and Ferriscan) if these have not been performed in the previous year for thalassemia major patients only

Determine presence of any red cell antibodies and consider phenotyping the partner

Document blood pressure

Send MSU for culture

Confirm viability with ultrasound

Plan transfusion program for the pregnancy

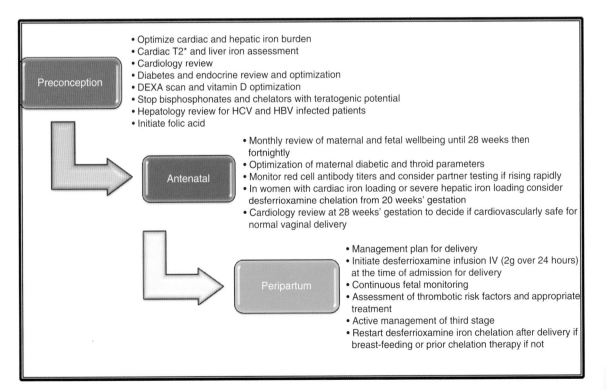

Figure 7.4 Women with TM: outline of obstetric care.

Labor and Delivery

Timing of delivery should be in line with national guidelines if the fetus is well grown.

The presence of a thalassemia syndrome in itself is not an indication for cesarean section. A delivery plan formulated by the multidisciplinary team should be in the woman's notes; this plan should include an anesthetic plan as well as a plan for management of diabetes if the patient is diabetic. The multidisciplinary team should be informed when the woman is admitted. Continuous electronic fetal monitoring is recommended in labor to monitor for fetal distress. In women with TM, intravenous deferoxamine 2 g over 24 hours should be administered for the duration of labor.

Active management of the third stage of labor is recommended to minimize blood loss.

Postpartum

Women with NTDT and TM are at high risk for venous thromboembolism and each should be risk assessed according to national guidelines and postnatal heparin thromboprophylaxis given accordingly. Breast-feeding is safe and should be encouraged while the patient is on deferoxamine.

Conclusion

Pregnancy in women with thalassemia syndromes carries significant risks for both mother and baby. However, advances in the management of transfusion and iron chelation therapy have greatly improved the life expectancy of these individuals so that embarking on pregnancy carries realistic prospects of success providing the care is carried out in a multidisciplinary setting with expertise in both hematological and obstetric management of thalassemia.

Case Studies

Case Study 1

This case report describes a 31-year-old patient with β thalassemia major. Her history included primary hypogonadotrophic hypogonadism secondary to pituitary iron damage and splenectomy. Pregnancy was achieved following one cycle of ovulation induction (OI).

Prior to the pregnancy the patient was transfused 3 units of red blood cells every 3 weeks (181 mL/kg). maintaining a pre-transfusion Hb of 103 g/L, with a rate of transfusional iron loading of 0.45 mg/kg/day. Iron chelation therapy historically consisted of deferasirox 19 mg/kg/day, switched to deferoxamine 3 months prior to OI, due to risk of teratogenicity. She had mild liver iron loading determined by Ferriscan (2.9 mg/g dry weight) but no cardiac iron measured by MRI T2* (36 ms), LVEF 66%. Her serum ferritin was 1986 μg/L. She was known to be anti-K positive but the antibody was no longer detectable.

Deferoxamine was stopped during OI and the first cycle resulted in successful conception. During the pregnancy, her transfusion requirements increased to 219.5 ml/kg, with a subsequent increase in transfusional iron loading to 0.56 mg/kg per day (20% increment). Mean pre-transfusion hemoglobin was maintained at 101 g/L. During pregnancy, no iron chelation therapy was needed as initial iron burden was in the optimal range. Her anti-K antibody remained non-detectable.

The delivery was planned as a normal vaginal delivery but she required help during the third stage and a ventouse-assisted delivery at 38+5/40 resulted in a healthy baby with a birth weight of 2.89 kg.

As a result of the pregnancy, her ferritin increased to 3967 μg/L (50% increment) and subsequent MRI assessment found severe hepatic iron overload at 24.2 mg/g dry weight but no increase in cardiac iron (T2* 29 ms); LVEF remained stable at 66%.

This case illustrates that blood transfusion requirements significantly increase during pregnancy in TM patients, with a subsequent rise in transfusional liver iron loading. However, in the absence of previous cardiac iron, patients will not significantly load iron into the heart and cardiac function remains unchanged.

Case Study 2

This case report describes a 39-year-old patient with β-thalassemia major. Her history included insulin-dependent diabetes mellitus, hypogonadotrophic hypogonadism, splenectomy, and previous cardiac iron loading. Pregnancy was achieved following egg donation.

She had suffered from severe cardiac iron loading (T2* 7 ms) with low LVEF (54%), at the age of 31 years and following intensive chelation therapy had successfully cleared the iron from her heart. Prior to egg implantation, cardiac MRI T2* showed no cardiac iron (T2* 29 ms) and cardiac function had significantly improved (LVEF 75%).

Liver iron was excellent at 3.3 mg/g dry weight. Deferoxamine therapy stopped on the day prior to egg implantation.

Her diabetes control was optimal during pregnancy using a basal bolus regime. However, she presented to the emergency department at 36/40 weeks' gestation with bilateral leg and facial edema, shortness of breath, and palpitations. Echocardiogram confirmed paroxysmal atrial fibrillation (AF) and enlarged left atrium; LVEF remained normal (64%). She spontaneously converted to sinus rhythm after 2 hours but was commenced on continuous intravenous deferoxamine (30 mg/kg) and labetalol 50 mg.

An elective cesarean section was performed at 37/40 weeks' gestation, delivering a healthy baby with a birth weight of 2.7 kg.

Intravenous desferrioxamine continued after discharge, combined with deferiprone once breast-feeding stopped. Cardiac MRI T2* showed mild cardiac iron loading (20 ms) with good LV function (71%); however, bi-atrial dilatation was noted. Eight years post pregnancy she continues to have intermittent episodes of paroxysmal AF.

This case illustrates that where there is a history of previous cardiac iron loading, cardiology review +/– cardiac MRI should be incorporated into the antenatal management plan. Low-dose desferrioxamine should be considered (second/third trimester) where indicated.

References

1. Cappellini MD, Cohen A, Porter J, Taher A, Viprakasit V, eds. *Guidelines for the Management of Transfusion Dependent Thalassemia (TDT)*. Nicosia (CY): Thalassemia International Federation. ©2014 Thalassemia International Federation; 2014.

2. Weatherall DJ. Phenotype—genotype relationships in monogenic disease: lessons from the thalassaemias. *Nature Reviews Genetics* 2001; **2**(4):245–255.

3. Taher AT, Musallam KM, Karimi M, *et al*. Overview on practices in thalassemia intermedia management aiming for lowering complication rates across a region of endemicity: the OPTIMAL CARE study. *Blood* 2010; **115**(10):1886–1892.

4. Weatherall DJ. Thalassemia in the next millennium. Keynote address. *Annals of the New York Academy of Sciences* 1998; **850**: 1–9.

5. Skordis N, Christou S, Koliou M, Pavlides N, Angastiniotis M. Fertility in female patients with thalassemia. *Journal of Pediatric Endocrinology and Metabolism* 1998; **11** (Suppl 3): 935–943.

6. Jensen CE, Tuck SM, Agnew JE et al. High incidence of osteoporosis in thalassemia major. *Journal of Pediatric Endocrinology and Metabolism* 1998; **11** (Suppl 3): 975–977.

7. De Sanctis V, Vullo C, Katz M et al. Hypothalamic-pituitary-gonadal axis in thalassemic patients with secondary amenorrhea. *Obstetrics and Gynecology* 1988; **72**(4): 643–647.

8. Borgna-Pignatti C, Rugolotto S, De Stefano P et al. Survival and complications in patients with thalassemia major treated with transfusion and deferoxamine. *Hematologica* 2004; **89**(10): 1187–1193.

9. Modell B, Khan M, Darlison M. Survival in beta-thalassemia major in the UK: data from the UK Thalassemia Register. *Lancet* 2000; **355**(9220): 2051–2052.

10. Tolis GJ, Vlachopapadopoulou E, Karydis I. Reproductive health in patients with beta-thalassemia. *Current Opinion in Pediatrics* 1996; **8**(4): 406–410.

11. Origa R, Piga A, Quarta G et al. Pregnancy and beta-thalassemia: an Italian multicenter experience. *Hematologica* 2010; **95**(3): 376–381.

12. Fiorentino F, Biricik A, Nuccitelli A et al. Strategies and clinical outcome of 250 cycles of preimplantation genetic diagnosis for single gene disorders. *Human Reproduction* 2006; **21**(3): 670–684.

13. Voskaridou E, Balassopoulou A, Boutou E et al. Pregnancy in beta-thalassemia intermedia: 20-year experience of a Greek thalassemia center. *European Journal of Hematology* 2014; **93**(6): 492–499.

14. MRC Vitamin Study Research Group. Prevention of neural tube defects: results of the Medical Research Council Vitamin Study. *Lancet* 1991; **338**(8760): 131–137.

15. Taher AT, Musallam KM, Cappellini MD, Weatherall DJ. Optimal management of beta thalassemia intermedia. *British Journal of Haematology* 2011; **152** (5): 512–523.

16. Cappellini MD, Robbiolo L, Bottasso BM et al. Venous thromboembolism and hypercoagulability in splenectomized patients with thalassemia intermedia. *British Journal of Haematology* 2000; **111**(2): 467–473.

17. Cappellini MD, Poggiali E, Taher AT, Musallam KM. Hypercoagulability in beta-thalassemia: a status quo. *Expert Review of Hematology* 2012; **5**(5): 505–511; quiz 12.

18. Faculty of Reproductive and Sexual Health Care. *UK Medical Eligibility Criteria for Contraceptive Use*. London: FRSHC; 2009.

19. Voskaridou E, Ladis V, Kattamis A et al. A national registry of hemoglobinopathies in Greece: deducted

demographics, trends in mortality and affected births. *Annals of Hematology* 2012; **91**(9): 1451–1458.

20. Nick H, Wong A, Acklin P *et al*. ICL670A: preclinical profile. *Advances in Experimental Medicine and Biology* 2002; **509**: 185–203.

21. Khoury S, Odeh M, Oettinger M. Deferoxamine treatment for acute iron intoxication in pregnancy. *Acta Obstetricia et Gynecologica Scandinavica* 1995; **74**(9): 756–757.

22. Singer ST, Vichinsky EP. Deferoxamine treatment during pregnancy: is it harmful? *American Journal of Hematology* 1999; **60**(1): 24–26.

23. Kirk P, Roughton M, Porter JB *et al*. Cardiac T2* magnetic resonance for prediction of cardiac complications in thalassemia major. *Circulation* 2009; **120**(20): 1961–1968.

24. National Institute for Health and Care Excellence (NICE). Diabetes in pregnancy: management of diabetes and its complications from pre-conception to the postnatal period. Clinical Guideline CG63; 2008.

25. Spencer DH, Grossman BJ, Scott MG. Red cell transfusion decreases hemoglobin A1c in patients with diabetes. *Clinical Chemistry* 2011; **57**(2): 344–346.

26. Abalovich M, Amino N, Barbour LA *et al*. Management of thyroid dysfunction during pregnancy and postpartum: an Endocrine Society Clinical Practice Guideline. *Journal of Clinical Endocrinology and Metabolism* 2007 **92**(8 Suppl): S1–47.

27. Walsh JM, McGowan CA, Kilbane M, McKenna MJ, McAuliffe FM. The relationship between maternal and fetal vitamin D, insulin resistance, and fetal growth. *Reproductive Sciences* 2013; **20**(5): 536–541.

28. Thompson AA, Cunningham MJ, Singer ST *et al*. Red cell alloimmunization in a diverse population of transfused patients with thalassemia. *British Journal of Haematology* 2011; **153**(1): 121–128.

Screening for Hemoglobinopathies

Shirley Henderson and Josh Wright

Screening

Structure of Hemoglobin and the Hemoglobinopathies

Adult hemoglobin is formed from two α and two β globin chains with four molecules of iron-containing heme (Figure 8.1). The α and β globin contain 141 and 146 amino acids, respectively. The α and β globin genes are situated on chromosomes 16 and 11, respectively. The linking of the individual amino acids is referred to as the primary structure but these globin chains also coil, cross-link, and interact with other chains to provide the completed hemoglobin molecule with a secondary, tertiary, and quaternary structure. Changes to the DNA encoding the chains may lead to reduced production of individual globin chains or production of a structurally altered globin.

Genetic change leading to a quantitative deficiency in globin chain production may result in globin chain imbalance and a thalassemic phenotype whereas structural or qualitative change results in variant hemoglobin such as HbS. The majority of variant hemoglobins arise from amino acid substitutions and there are over 1000 described on the globin gene server[1]. The vast majority of these are clinically

silent or lead to very mild phenotypic expression, with only a handful of variants of clinical significance.

Hemoglobinopathies are generally recessive conditions. Heterozygotes are symptom free with disease states resulting from either homozygosity or combined heterozygosity. Hemoglobinopathy screening programs have been established in many locations and aim to detect couples who are heterozygotes for interacting abnormalities. These couples are therefore at a 1:4 risk of having a child with a significant hemoglobin disorder. Identification of such at-risk couples will permit access to antenatal diagnostics and hence informed parental choices.

What Are the Significant Hemoglobin Disorders?

Variant Hemoglobins

The sickling disorders arise from either homozygosity for HbS or a variety of combined heterozygotic states (Table 8.1). SS disease and Sβ0 thalassemia are the most phenotypically severe conditions. These are both multiorgan diseases associated with significant morbidity and reduced life expectancy, even with availability of good medical care. Descriptions of the diseases are beyond the scope of this chapter but for further information the reader is directed to the Serjeants' comprehensive description[2].

β Thalassemia Syndromes

These represent a spectrum of disease described by the phenotypic behavior of a variety of genotypic interactions (Table 8.2). Clinical syndromes range from the asymptomatic carrier states through to thalassemia major where sufferers require transfusion in order to survive beyond childhood. In between these two extremes sit the thalassemia intermedias; patients with these diseases may not require lifelong transfusion but many need periods of therapy and are prone to a variety of significant complications including bone disease,

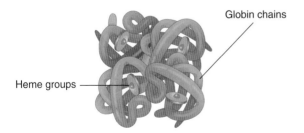

Figure 8.1 Hemoglobin structure. The hemoglobin molecule is a tetrameric protein made up of four 16-kDa subunits, of which two polypeptides are α globin chains and two are β globin chains. Each globin chain contains one heme molecule (purple disc), which is made up of a porphyrin ring and an iron ion (blue spheres). The function of hemoglobin, to carry oxygen, is directly dependent on this iron, to which it binds.

Globin chains

Heme groups

Table 8.1 Sickle cell disorders: interactions and indications for prenatal diagnosis

Genotype interaction	Clinical phenotype	PND offered
Homozygous		
β^0 or severe β^+-thal	Thal major	Yes
Mild β^+-thal	Thal intermedia	Occasionally[a]
$\delta\beta$-thalassemia	Thal intermedia	Occasionally[a]
Hb Lepore	Thal intermedia to major (variable)	Occasionally[a]
HPFH	Not clinically relevant	No
HbC	Not clinically relevant	No
Hb D-Punjab	Not clinically relevant	No
HbE	Not clinically relevant	No
Hb O-Arab	Not clinically relevant	No
Compound heterozygous		
β^0/severe β^+-thal	Thal major	Yes
Mild β^+/β^0 or severe β^+-thal	Thal intermedia to major (variable)	Occasionally[a]
$\delta\beta$/β or severe β^+-thal	Thal intermedia to major (variable)	Occasionally[a]
$\delta\beta$/mild β^+-thal	Mild thal intermedia	Occasionally[a]
$\delta\beta$/Hb Lepore	Thal intermedia	Occasionally[a]
Hb Lepore/β^0 or severe	Thal major	Yes
HbC/β^0 or severe β^+-thal	β-thal trait to intermedia (variable)	Occasionally[a]
HbC/mild β^+-thal	Not clinically relevant	No
Hb D-Punjab/β^0 or severe β^+-thal	Not clinically relevant	No
HbE/β^0 or severe β^+-thal	Thal intermedia to major (variable)	Yes
Hb O-Arab/β^0-thal	Severe thal intermedia	Yes

[a] Occasionally, depending upon parental choice following genetic counseling.

Table 8.2 β thalassemia: interactions and indications for prenatal diagnosis

Genotype interaction	Clinical phenotype	PND offered
Homozygous		
α^0-thalassemia (–/–)	Hb Barts hydrops fetalis	Yes
α^+-thalassemia (–α/–α)	Not clinically relevant	No
α^+-thalassemia ($\alpha^T\alpha$/$\alpha^T\alpha$)[b]	Severe α-thal carrier to severe HbH disease	Occasionally[a]
Compound heterozygous		
α^0-thal/α^+-thal (–/–α)	HbH disease	No
α^0-thal/α^T-thal (–/$\alpha^T\alpha$)[b]	Severe Hb disease to HbH hydrops fetalis	Occasionally[a]

[a] Occasionally, depending upon parental choice following genetic counseling.
[b] $\alpha^T\alpha$ denotes a carrier of non-deletional α thalassemia.

pulmonary hypertension, venous thromboembolism, and iron overload even in the absence of regular transfusion.

α Thalassemia Syndromes

Although carriage of α thalassemia is extremely common in selected populations (Figure 8.2), clinically significant α thalassemia is rare and most commonly seen in the Far East and Eastern Mediterranean. The most severe forms present during pregnancy with fetal hydrops (Table 8.3). Screening strategies are aimed at the detection of couples at risk of these severe forms.

Demographics and Geography

Populations affected by thalassemia occupy a great swathe of countries across the Mediterranean, Africa, Arabian Peninsula, Indian Subcontinent, and Far East. Individuals heterozygotic for α and β

Table 8.3 α thalassemia: interactions and indications for prenatal diagnosis

Genotype interaction	Clinical phenotype	PND offered
Homozygous		
HbS	Sickle cell disease	Yes
Compound heterozygous		
HbS/β⁰ or severe β⁺-thal	Sickle cell disease	Yes
HbS/mild β⁺-thal	Mild sickle cell disease	Occasionally[a]
HbS/δβ-thal	Mild sickle cell disease	Occasionally[a]
HbS/Hb Lepore	Mild sickle cell disease	Occasionally[a]
HbS/HbC	Sickle cell disease (variable severity)	Yes
HbS/Hb D-Punjab	Sickle cell disease	Yes
HbS/Hb O-Arab	Sickle cell disease	Yes
HbS/HbE	Mild to severe sickle cell disease	Occasionally[a]
HbS/HPFH	Sickle cell trait	No

[a] Occasionally, depending upon parental choice following genetic counseling.

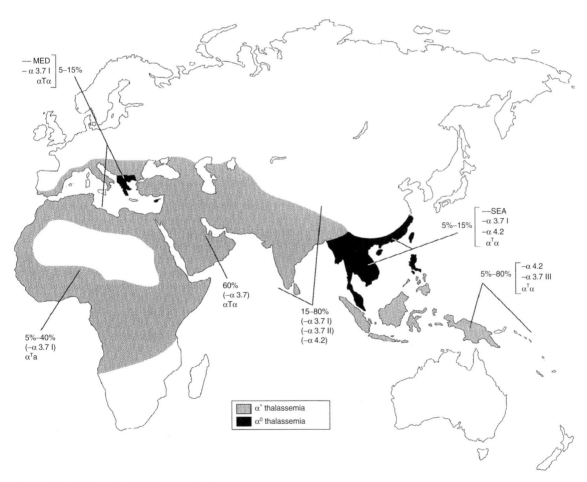

Figure 8.2 α thalassemia distribution worldwide.

thalassemia are protected from the effects of *Falciparum* malaria. With increasing migration, countries with a low indigenous incidence of these conditions now have growing at-risk populations[3].

In a similar way to thalassemia, carriers of sickle cell and other variant hemoglobins such as HbC are also at a survival advantage in malarial areas. The populations affected by sickle cell are found throughout equatorial Africa, the Americas, Caribbean, the Arabian Peninsula, and South India. Small populations also exist in Greece and Southern Italy.

Rationale for Screening

Antenatal screening aims to allow informed reproductive choice by identifying couples at risk of an affected infant at an early stage in pregnancy. Options include prenatal diagnosis with either termination or continuation of affected pregnancies.

It has long been known that morbidity and mortality in children with sickle cell disease are high in the first 5 years of life. The protective effects of high levels of HbF in the newborn decline over the first 4–6 months of life, thereafter much of the mortality is due to pneumococcal septicemia and acute splenic sequestration. Successful antibiotic prophylaxis, vaccination, and education programs have all but eliminated these problems and are perhaps the single most important steps in the improved survival of sickle cell disease.

Since these severe complications are often the presenting features of sickle cell disease, a screening program is required to identify at-risk couples and/or affected newborns.

In β thalassemia major, the failure of β globin chain production results in a severe transfusion-dependent anemia, which is manifest as HbF levels reduce in the first few months of life. From this point on, the management of thalassemia is based upon regular transfusion and iron chelation to reduce the risk of organ damage, particularly cardiac. Care of the patient with thalassemia involves collaboration of hematologists, endocrinologists, diabetologists, and cardiologists, with occasional input from other specialities such as hepatology. With appropriate care and good compliance, life expectancy may be normal; however, early cardiac death remains common in those who do not comply with iron chelation.

Methods of Screening

As is evident from the algorithms (Figures 8.3 and 8.4), screening relies on the combination of reliable information about family origins, red cell indices, and the use of techniques such as high-performance liquid chromatography (HPLC), electrophoresis, and sickle solubility testing. In the majority of situations, interpreting these data provides sufficient information to guide partner testing, risk assessment, and referral for prenatal diagnosis.

Hemoglobin tetramers (2α and 2β chains) readily separate into dimers during the production of a hemoglobin solution (hemolysate) for analysis. The various hemoglobin dimers are of differing charge and will pass at differing rates across a column (in the case of HPLC) or a gel (electrophoresis). The hemoglobin dimers, such as Hb A and HbS in a sickle carrier, will be seen as two peaks (HPLC) or bands (electrophoresis) the position of which is a feature of the charge of the Hb dimer. Laboratories should use a primary method and a different confirmatory test plus a sickle solubility test. The sickle solubility test denotes the presence of HbS but does not differentiate carriers from homozygotes or combined heterozygotes. Further testing on selected samples may be performed by molecular means (see section "UK NHS Sickle and Thalassemia Screening: an Example of a Linked Antenatal and Neonatal Program").

β thalassemia carriage is detected by measuring HbA2 levels and red cell indices; the majority of thalassemia carriers have reduced red cell indices. α thalassemia is more difficult to detect and relies upon a strategy of patient selection for molecular testing by red cell indices and at-risk family origin[4].

UK NHS Sickle and Thalassemia Screening: an Example of a Linked Antenatal and Neonatal Program

The UK NHS hemoglobinopathy screening program came into being following the NHS plan of 2000. Over the ensuing years it has been recognized internationally as a beacon of high-quality practice. The newborn program screens all births in England, with samples collected by heel prick onto a Guthrie card. The regional screening laboratories use HPLC or capillary electrophoresis or mass-spectrometry to detect the presence of significant variant hemoglobins; second-line confirmation is

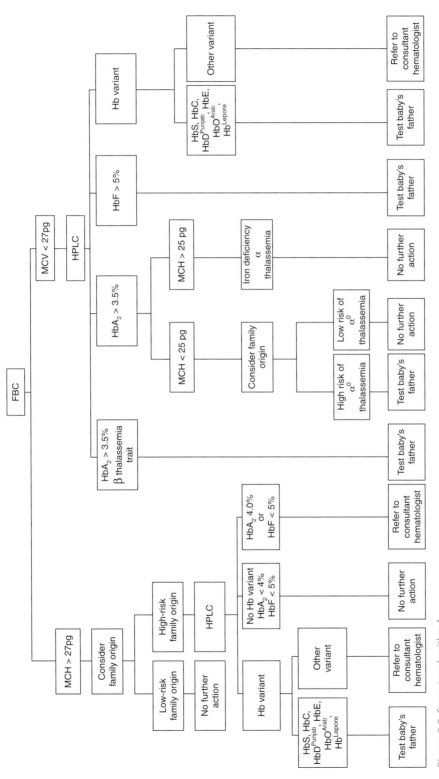

Figure 8.3 Screening algorithm 1.

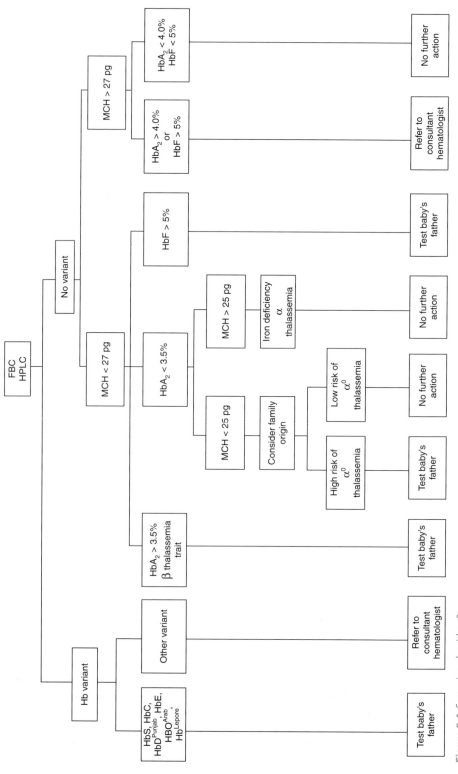

Figure 8.4 Screening algorithm 2.

performed by a technique with a different principle than the first. The program has close links with Child Health, to allow appropriate referral of those requiring further follow-up, and the antenatal laboratories to highlight mothers at risk of an affected child. The main aim of the program is the detection of children with sickling disorders, although those at risk of thalassemia major will be highlighted for further investigation. Further information about the NHS screening program and its associated literature and operating procedures can be obtained from sct.screening.nhs.uk

With the aim of the antenatal program being choice, there is considerable time pressure to obtain results of the patient and partner and to counsel and arrange antenatal diagnostic procedures if required. Since termination is one option, early diagnosis is crucial, and a target for identification of at-risk couples is set at 10 weeks.

All couples at risk of having an affected child should be offered prenatal diagnosis, although many will decline.

If prenatal testing results confirm a fetus affected with a major hemoglobin disorder, the couple will need further counseling about living with an affected child. The earlier a diagnosis of a hemoglobinopathy is made, the higher the likelihood that termination is acceptable. In a study examining prenatal testing in thalassemia among British Pakistanis, 70% accepted prenatal diagnosis if offered in the first trimester, with over 90% of pregnancies being terminated. However, if testing was offered in the second trimester, only 40% of couples accepted prenatal testing with fewer affected pregnancies terminated.

Antenatal screening for hemoglobin disorders is universal in areas of high prevalence and, where prevalence is low, the selection for screening is on the basis of family origin using an ethnicity questionnaire and red cell indices (see screening algorithms in Figures 8.3 and 8.4).

Prenatal Diagnosis

Background

Prenatal diagnosis for thalassemia was originally carried out by measuring the ratio of α-globin to β-globin chains in fetal blood. However, once the molecular basis of the globin genes and the hemoglobinopathies had been established, prenatal diagnosis swiftly moved to molecular analysis of fetal mutations, firstly in amniotic fluid and subsequently in DNA extracted from chorionic villi. This approach, first developed in the early 1980s[5], is still in mainstream use today as part of numerous national prevention programs worldwide. The main disadvantages of this tactic are the risk of fetal loss from invasive sampling (0.5–1.0%)[6] and the requirement for termination of an affected fetus. Either or both of these issues are unacceptable for many couples. Consequently, there has been considerable impetus to find alternative strategies for the prevention of these disorders. The two main routes that have been investigated with varying degrees of success are pre-implantation genetic diagnosis and non-invasive diagnosis, both of which will be considered briefly later in this chapter.

Conventional Invasive Prenatal Diagnosis

When Should Prenatal Diagnosis Be Offered?

The selective pressure exerted by the protective effect of the hemoglobinopathy carrier state to the malarial parasite has meant that a diverse range of hemoglobin mutations have undergone positive selection[7]. These are present in some populations at high frequencies and it is therefore common for individuals to harbor more than one type of hemoglobin mutation or for partners to have different hemoglobin mutations. This diversity of possible interactions and potentially different outcomes inevitably makes the decision of when to offer prenatal diagnosis more challenging.

There is also considerable clinical heterogeneity within each condition; individuals with apparently identical genotypes can have quite different phenotypes. The reasons for this are not clear but most likely relate to interaction of other genetic determinants. For example, co-inheritance of hereditary persistence of fetal hemoglobin (HPFH) or α^+ thalassemia can ameliorate the phenotype of β thalassemia major and co-inheritance of a triplicated α-globin gene can increase the severity of the disease[8]. However, the majority of modifying factors are as yet unknown, which means that it is not always possible to predict the precise clinical outcome in individual cases. However, the likely degree of severity (or range of severity) can usually be forecast with a reasonable degree of certainty for most hemoglobin disorders. The probable outcomes for sickle cell disorders, β thalassemia, and α thalassemia are summarized in Tables 8.1 to 8.3.

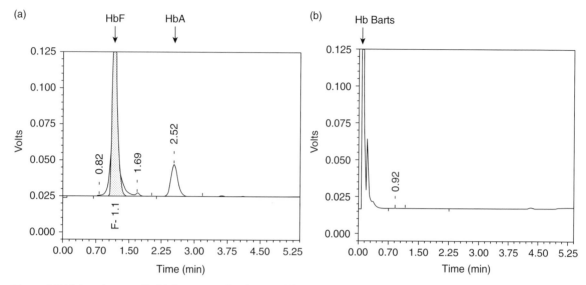

Figure 8.5 High-performance liquid chromatography of neonatal/fetal blood samples. (a) Normal neonate at birth. Chromatogram shows the predominant hemoglobin is HbF with a minor fraction of HbA. (b) Fetus affected with Barts hydrops fetalis. Chromatogram shows the complete absence of HbF, the predominant hemoglobin is Hb Barts (tetramer of γ globin).

β thalassemia and Sickle Cell Disease

The molecular basis of β thalassemia is heterogeneous with more than 100 different reported mutations giving rise to the condition; the majority of these are point mutations occurring within the β-globin gene[1]. These mutations are classified as β^+ or β^0 mutations depending on whether they partially or completely block expression of the β-globin gene. Sickle cell disease most commonly results from homozygosity for the sickle cell mutation but can also result from a variety of different compound heterozygous genotypes. The most common of these are HbS-β thalassemia, HbS/C disease, HbS/D-Punjab disease, and HbS/O-Arab.

Hb Barts Hydrops Fetalis Syndrome

In this condition, all four α-globin genes are deleted and therefore the affected fetus is unable to synthesize α-globin chains to produce HbF or HbA. Only tetramers of γ-globin (Hb Barts) and low levels of residual embryonic hemoglobins are present in the fetal blood [9]. This results in severe anemia and fetal hydrops; without intrauterine transfusion the condition is usually fatal. The fetal hydrops can typically be detected by ultrasound scan; therefore, unlike β thalassemia major or sickle cell disease, the disorder can potentially be detected in utero without invasive testing. It will be necessary to confirm that the observed hydrops is caused by homozygous α° thalassemia. This can be

achieved by HPLC analysis of a fetal blood sample; if the hydrops is due to homozygous α° thalassemia, large quantities of Hb Barts will be present and Hb F will be absent (Figure 8.5). The disadvantage of relying solely on ultrasound to detect the condition is that it may not be detected until later in the pregnancy. If the parents have been identified as being carriers for α° thalassemia from antenatal screening, then it may be possible to offer them first trimester prenatal diagnosis, allowing the parents the choice of termination before the fetal symptoms become apparent.

Hb H Hydrops Fetalis

Rarely, fetal hydrops can also be caused by unusually severe types of Hb H disease (Hb H hydrops fetalis)[10]. This results from the interaction of α° thalassemia with a severe type of non-deletion α^+ thalassemia allele. One example of this is the combination of the Southeast Asian deletion mutation with the hyper-unstable α-globin variant Hb Adana [11]. Carriers for Hb Adana and other severe non-deletional α thalassemia mutations will often be missed by antenatal screening as the carriers will usually only have a mild reduction in MCH (or possibly a normal MCH), therefore the potential risk to the pregnancy will not be identified. Consequently, the possibility of this condition should be considered if fetal hydrops is identified and the parents' families originate from areas of the world where α° thalassemia is common.

Confirmation of Risk

Fetal sampling should only be carried out when risk to the pregnancy is confirmed[12]. In some instances, this is straightforward, e.g. HbSS disease, as the sickle carrier status of the parents can easily be confirmed by most diagnostic/screening hematology laboratories using conventional protein-based techniques. As sickle hemoglobin always arises from the same mutation (HBB codon 6 Glu-Val), confirmation of the parental carrier status by DNA testing is not usually required. Most cases of β thalassemia are also detectable by routine diagnostics but as it can be caused by many different mutations, the parental mutations will need to be identified by DNA tests prior to prenatal diagnosis. Rarely, it may not be clear from the hematological indices whether an individual is a carrier for β thalassemia, particularly where the Hb A2 level is borderline; these cases will require confirmation by DNA testing so that the parents can be counseled appropriately.

It is not possible to reliably distinguish between the conditions of homozygous α+ thalassemia and α° thalassemia trait by hematological techniques. Therefore, if the parental family origins are from an area with significant risk of α° thalassemia and their hematological indices are consistent with homozygous α+ or α° thalassemia, then DNA confirmation of the parental carrier status must always be carried out so that the parents can be counseled appropriately. If there is any doubt about the parental genotypes or whether further testing is required prior to fetal sampling, the molecular laboratory carrying out the prenatal diagnosis should be contacted for advice prior to fetal sampling.

Fetal Samples

Chorionic villus sampling (CVS), amniotic fluid, or fetal blood can be used to extract fetal DNA for prenatal diagnosis. In most instances, sufficient DNA can be obtained from un-cultured fetal material to obtain a diagnosis, allowing results to be turned around within a few days. However, when it is only possible to obtain a very small fetal sample, it may need to be cultured in order to obtain enough DNA to carry out the diagnosis. Parents and health professionals must be aware that this eventuality will result in a considerably longer turnaround time for results, as cultures normally require 10–14 days to grow.

CVS samples must be cleaned by microscopic dissection to remove any contaminating maternal tissue before being used for fetal diagnosis. This is usually carried out in a cytogenetics laboratory prior to testing in the molecular genetics laboratory. It is good practice for the cytogenetics laboratory to set up CVS back-up cultures in case there is insufficient DNA in the un-cultured material to carry out the diagnosis. If the fetal diagnosis is to be carried out on amniotic fluid then obstetric departments should aim to take sufficient fluid so that it can be split between the two laboratories: the molecular laboratory for hemoglobinopathy testing and the cytogenetics laboratory for back-up cultures and any other required testing such as karyotyping. On very rare occasions, fetal blood sampling may be performed and a fetal blood sample sent in EDTA for analysis.

Ideally blood samples from both parents should be sent with each prenatal diagnosis sample. These can either be sent to the molecular hemoglobinopathy laboratory ahead of the fetal sampling or in cases where the parental mutations are known (e.g. carriers of sickle cell), can be sent with the fetal sample. If the paternal genotype is known (i.e. the father has been previously tested in another laboratory) but he is currently unavailable for blood sampling, a copy of the father's laboratory results should be sent to the prenatal diagnosis laboratory so they can assess the fetal risk.

If the paternal genotype is unknown and he is unavailable for testing, prenatal diagnosis can still be carried out but the conditions that can and cannot be excluded will be complex and depend on factors such as maternal genotype and family origins. The potential risk to the fetus in such cases should be discussed carefully with the molecular laboratory prior to fetal sampling being undertaken. Results will usually be presented on a risk basis and extended testing may be required, which could delay the turnaround time.

Molecular Diagnostic Strategy

The β-globin and α-globin gene clusters (situated on chromosomes 11 and 16, respectively) are relatively small and usually amenable to most standard DNA testing techniques[13]. Currently these are almost invariably PCR based. Whenever possible it is good practice to use two different diagnostic methods to confirm the diagnosis. For point mutations, Sanger sequencing is usually the method of choice, closely followed by allele-specific methods such as ARMS (amplification

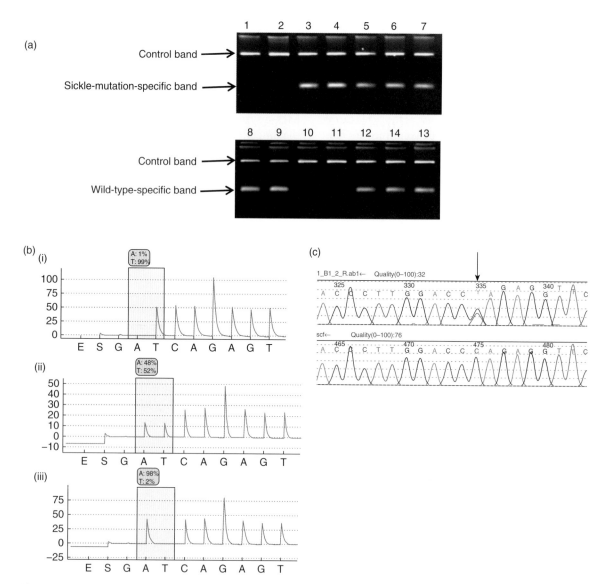

Figure 8.6 Some techniques which can be used to detect point mutations in fetal DNA. (a) Primer-specific amplification for the sickle cell mutation. The fetal DNA is tested using two ARMS primers, one of which is complementary to the sickle mutation and the other is complementary to the wild-type allele. DNA amplification will only occur for the sickle primer when the sickle mutation is present and for the wild-type primer when the wild-type allele is present. Lanes 1–7: results using the sickle-mutation-specific primer. Lanes 8–14: results using the wild-type-specific primer. Lanes 1–2 and 8–9: wild-type control showing normal amplification band only. Lanes 3–4 and 10–11: HbSS control showing sickle amplification band only. Lanes 5–7 and 12–14: Fetal DNA sample showing sickle and wild-type amplification bands which indicate the fetus is a sickle cell carrier. (b) Pyrosequencing. Three pyrograms showing sequencing (reverse primer) of the sickle mutation site and nearby nucleotides: (i) normal sequence at the sickle mutation site; (ii) heterozygous substitution of an A for a T nucleotide indicating sickle carrier status; (iii) homozygous substitution of an A for a T nucleotide indicating sickle disease status. (c) Sanger sequencing of fetal DNA. Arrow on upper panel shows heterozygosity for the β thalassemia mutation HBB Codon 39 (CAG-TAG). Lower panel shows wild-type sequence.

refractory mutation system). Pyrosequencing is another excellent technique which can be used to detect point mutations. ARMS and pyrosequencing have the particular advantage of speed in that for both techniques results can be obtained within a few hours. In the past, the method of choice for deletion detection was Southern blotting, but this has now been almost completely superseded by other methodology. The usual techniques of choice are Gap-PCR or MLPA (multiple ligation-dependent probe amplification). Further details and examples of these techniques can be seen in Figures 8.6 and 8.7.

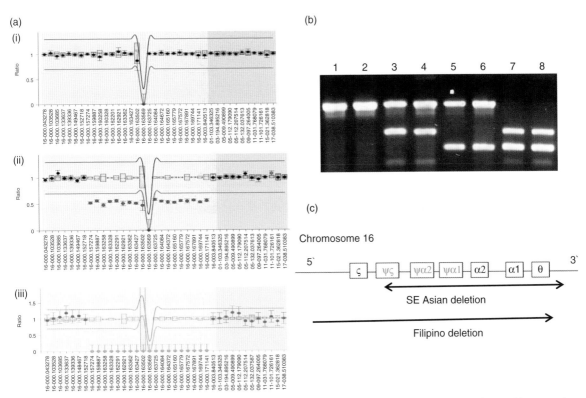

Figure 8.7 Examples of techniques which can be used to detect deletion mutations in fetal DNA. (a) MLPA analysis of the α-globin gene cluster in (i) a normal individual, (ii) an individual heterozygous for the Southeast Asian α⁰ thalassemia deletion mutation, and (iii) a fetus with Barts hydrops fetalis. MLPA (multiplex ligation-dependent probe amplification) is a multiplex PCR method for detecting chromosomal DNA copy number changes in multiple targets. The method depends on the hybridization of multiple probes against the target DNA which are subsequently ligated and amplified. Amplification only occurs if the target DNA is present in the sample; the quantity of PCR product produced is proportional to the amount of target DNA present in the sample. The results are analyzed using PCR peak height analysis software. In analysis (i), each black ellipse represents a probe with a different target over the gene cluster, whereas in analysis (ii), red ellipses specify probes from which the PCR amplification has been reduced by 50% indicating the presence of a heterozygous deletion. Finally, the red ellipses in analysis (iii) designate probes from which PCR amplification is absent, indicating the presence of a homozygous deletion mutation. (b) Analysis of fetal and parental DNA for α thalassemia deletion mutations by Gap-PCR. Lanes 1–2: normal control. Lanes 3-4: maternal DNA showing heterozygosity for the Southeast Asian deletion mutation. Lanes 5–6: paternal DNA showing heterozygosity for the Filipino deletion mutation. Lanes 7–8: fetal DNA showing compound heterozygosity for both parental deletions indicating the fetus is affected with Barts hydrops fetalis. PCR primers are designed which flank the deletion being tested for. If the deletion is present, then a PCR product will be obtained. If it is absent, then the primers will be too far apart for successful amplification and no PCR product will be produced. A primer pair with target sequence located within the boundaries of the deletion is also included to confirm the presence or absence of normal sequence. (c) Diagram showing the position of two common alpha zero deletion mutations (Southeast Asian and Filipino) in the α-globin gene cluster on chromosome 16.

Exclusion of Maternal Contamination

A major potential pitfall of prenatal diagnosis is contamination of the fetal sample with maternal DNA. Molecular techniques are often very sensitive and even the presence of a low level of contamination could result in a potential fetal misdiagnosis. Therefore, before issuing a fetal diagnosis report the laboratory must be confident that the sample being tested is all fetal.

Chorionic villi at fetal sampling are more prone to this problem than amniotic fluid samples due to the possible presence of maternal decidua in the sample. Usually careful dissection and removal of the maternal decidua under a phase-contrast microscope by a cytogenetic laboratory will result in a pure fetal sample. However, some maternal tissue may remain and tests are required to exclude this possibility; usually analysis of short tandem repeat (STR) polymorphisms. The fetus only inherits one allele from its mother; therefore, if a second is observed this usually indicates the presence of maternal contamination (Figure 8.8). Comparison of fetal and maternal STR patterns is essential.

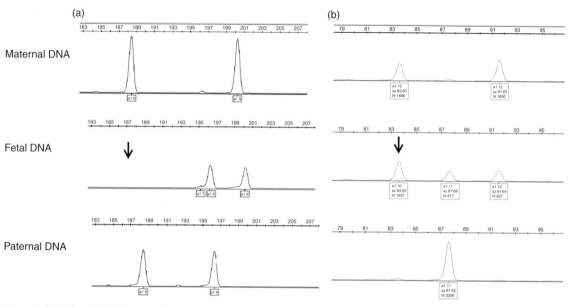

Figure 8.8 DNA analysis of short tandem repeats (STRs) in the fetal sample. This is required to exclude the possibility that the fetal sample is contaminated with maternal DNA, which could give rise to a misdiagnosis. The STR pattern in the fetal sample is compared with the STR patterns in parental DNA. (a) Analysis of the TH01 STR shows that the fetus has inherited one allele from its mother and the other from its father. There is no evidence of a 3rd allele (marked with an arrow) which would indicate the presence of contaminating maternal DNA. (b) Analysis of the D2S441 STR in another fetal sample shows the presence of a 3rd allele in the fetus (marked with arrow) indicating presence of maternal contamination.

Preimplantation Genetic Diagnosis (PGD)

PGD is now used for a wide range of monogenic genetic conditions and offers couples the chance to avoid having to terminate an affected fetus. Assisted reproductive techniques are used to create embryos which are tested for a genetic condition and only unaffected embryos are then implanted. The procedure was first used 20 years ago and is now an established technique in many countries[14]. Procedures and success rates have improved significantly in that time; however, the process remains complex and technically challenging with the requirement for a skilled multidisciplinary team, which includes gynecologists, embryologists, and geneticists. Also, as is usual for conventional assisted conception, it is likely that couples will need to undergo multiple cycles of treatment. Overall success rates vary among centers but are still comparatively low with only about 30% of couples having a baby following treatment[15]. Factors such as maternal age and weight significantly influence the chances of success.

PGD for Hemoglobin Disorders

Prevention of hemoglobin disorders has been one of the most common conditions for use of PGD. Initially carried out for β thalassemia in 1998, it is now also available for sickle cell disease and α thalassemia. Another application is human leukocyte antigen (HLA) typing of embryos, to provide HLA matched siblings for hemopoietic stem cell transplant to a child affected with a serious hemoglobinopathy, such as β thalassemia major. This was first carried out in 2001. The ethics has been widely debated but it is now considered acceptable in a number of countries. However, the number of suitable embryos is limited; only 25% will be HLA matched for the affected sibling and of these 25% will be affected with the hemoglobin disorder.

Non-invasive Prenatal Diagnosis (NIPD)

Circulating cell-free fetal DNA (cfDNA) in maternal plasma, which originates from trophoblastic cells, has the potential to act as a source of fetal material and allow fetal diagnosis from a simple blood test, thus avoiding the need for invasive procedures[16].

This cfDNA constitutes 5–15% of total plasma DNA [17] and is now used routinely for a variety of purposes such as fetal sex determination and fetal Rhesus typing (Chapters 10 and 21). These clinical applications are relatively straightforward as they rely on identification of alleles which have been paternally inherited by the fetus and are therefore not present in the mother. However, diagnoses of recessive conditions such as sickle cell disease and thalassemia are much more technically challenging as the fetus shares half its alleles with the mother. The principle that has been used successfully to detect fetal trisomies is that of allelic imbalance. For example, if a fetus is affected with trisomy 21 then the presence of the circulating DNA from the fetus in the maternal circulation will result in an over-representation of chromosome 21 in the maternal plasma relative to the other chromosomes. The detection of this disturbance can then be used to diagnose the trisomy in the fetus. However, the allelic imbalance produced will be very small and its accurate and reproducible detection is technically challenging. The techniques which have been used so far are digital PCR and more recently next generation sequencing (NGS)[16]. The NGS approach involves the random sequencing of millions of DNA molecules in maternal plasma. Individual sequence tags are aligned to the human genome to determine the chromosome of origin of a particular sequence tag. An increase in representation of sequence tags aligned to a particular chromosome indicates a potential trisomy. This approach, although shown to be effective, is currently expensive and requires access to high-throughput NGS platforms and complex bioinformatics. Nonetheless, the power of this technology is enormous and it is now possible to perform whole genome sequencing on maternal plasma and decipher the whole fetal genome[18]. As the cost of whole genome sequencing falls and if the power of bioinformatics continues to increase, it is conceivable that this approach will become more widely adopted and allow the non-invasive diagnosis of all inherited disease.

NIPD for Hemoglobinopathies

Most early reports for NIPD of hemoglobinopathies were aimed at the detection or exclusion of the paternal mutant allele. The proposed strategy was to reduce (but not remove) the need for invasive testing. If the paternal mutant allele is not present in the maternal plasma (or paternal single nucleotide polymorphisms linked to the mutant allele) then this implies the fetus does not carry the paternal mutation and therefore cannot be affected by the condition. Conversely, if the paternal mutation is detected then invasive testing will be required to ascertain whether the fetus is affected or a carrier for the disease in question. A number of different technical approaches of varying complexity have been described[19] but currently there are no reports of their use in routine diagnostic pathways. NIPD for sickle cell disease (and other homozygous hemoglobinopathies) can theoretically be achieved in a similar fashion to trisomy detection, i.e. by measuring disturbances in the wild-type to mutation allelic ratio produced by the presence of affected fetal DNA in maternal plasma. There is one report of digital PCR being used in this way to detect sickle cell mutation imbalances in maternal plasma to achieve NIPD for sickle cell disease[20]. Recent development has seen the launch of bench-top NGS sequencers. which are scaled down more cost-effective platforms that can be used for targeted rather than whole genome sequencing. This technology has the sensitivity to detect these minor allelic disturbances rapidly and economically and therefore has the potential to deliver the elusive goal of reliable and robust NIPD for hemoglobin disorders.

Laboratory Guidelines for Screening

The UK laboratory handbooks for screening antenatal women and neonates were updated in September 2017[21, 22].

Case Studies

Case Study 1
A 26-year-old woman of Thai origin presented at 9 weeks' gestation for antenatal screening. This was her first pregnancy. Her partner was also of Far Eastern origin. Her results showed Hb 112 g/L, MCV 62 fL, MCH 22 pg, and blood film showed target cells. HPLC showed a single major peak in the A2 window. Acid and alkaline electrophoresis suggested this band to be hemoglobin E (Figure 8.9).

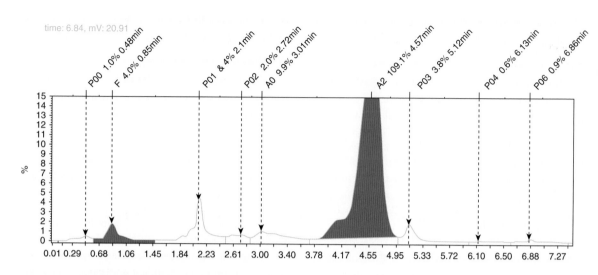

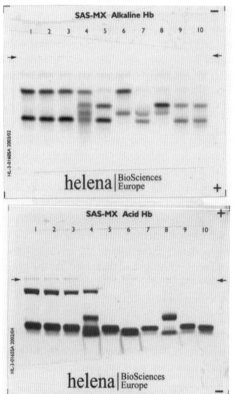

Lane 6 shows a single major band on the alkaline gel in the position of CEO with a second, smaller HbF band.

Similarly on the acid gel in lane 6 the band migrates in the position of ADE.

Figure 8.9 HPLC of patient sample. HPLC shows a single major peak in the A2 window. Acid and alkaline electrophoresis suggested the band to be hemoglobin E.

The report issued by the laboratory stated that the patient had homozygous HbE. Her partner attended for screening and his results showed Hb 128 g/L, MCV 64 fL, and MCH 24 pg. The HPLC trace was normal with a single major band in the A window.

This result may be regarded as reassuring since the partner is not a carrier of thalassemia. HbE thalassemia is a significant hemoglobinopathy. On the other hand, both of these individuals have MCH <25 and their family origin puts them both at risk of carrying α⁰ thalassemia. **The hidden risk here is the possibility of a pregnancy affected by fetal hydrops.** This case highlights the importance of combining family origin data with routine hematological indices alongside the results of hemoglobin analysis when evaluating risk. α^0 thalassemia is prevalent in the Eastern Mediterranean and Far East; MCH in carriers is always <25. Since there is no widely available, simple laboratory test for α^0 thalassemia, screening relies heavily on an MCH <25 in a patient of appropriate family origin.

Case Study 2
A 31-year-old woman of African origin presented in her first pregnancy for antenatal screening. Her results showed Hb 116 g/L, MCV 67 fL, and MCH 26 pg. The laboratory issued a report stating HbA2 1.6% and a summary statement "Cannot exclude carriage of α thalassemia." Since the patient was not regarded to be of an at-risk ethnic group, her partner (of Indian origin) did not require testing.

Neonatal screening shows a single major HbF peak with no detectable HbA, consistent with a possible diagnosis of thalassemia major.

What Has Gone Wrong?
The explanation lies with the A2 peak of 1.9% (Figure 8.10). HbA2 consists of 2 α chains and 2 δ chains. A small number of patients, usually of African origin, have a δ chain variant and therefore may have an A2 peak and an A2' peak. These may be easy to overlook. In this case, total HbA2= A2(1.6)+A2'(1.9)= 3.5%. Therefore, this woman is a carrier of thalassemia. Had her partner been tested he too would have had a raised HbA2 consistent with carriage of thalassemia. This case highlights some of the difficulties around interpretation of HbA2 levels.

Case Study 3
A 36-year-old female presented late for screening at 16 weeks' gestation. A family origin questionnaire suggested she was Northern European. Full blood count was normal. An HPLC trace was performed as she was in an area of universal screening. The result was normal.

Her male child was born at 36 weeks and transferred to the neonatal unit because of respiratory difficulties. A blood count and film revealed mild anemia, microcytic hypochromic indices, marked poikilocytosis, target cells, and nucleated red blood cells. HPLC showed Hb Barts peak 28% with HbA 19% and F 45%. The appearances are consistent with a 3 gene deletion (HbH disease in adults).

Direct questioning of the mother revealed that she had IVF using an ova donated in another UK city; the father had a blood count consistent with carriage of thalassemia. The donor, from Cyprus, had declared a family history of thalassemia at the IVF clinic and therefore underwent screening. This was reported as showing possible iron deficiency and a card issued stating she had no significant hemoglobinopathy. Two further screens over a period of years had failed to comment on the significance of thalassemic indices in the presence of a normal hemoglobin and HbA2.

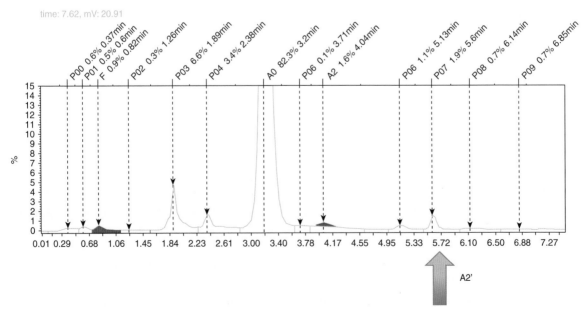

Figure 8.10 HPLC of patient sample.

DNA analysis showed the natural mother to have a Mediterranean α^0 deletion ($-^{MED}/\alpha\alpha$), the father a 3.7 kb α^+-thalassemia deletion ($-\alpha^{3.7}/\alpha\alpha$), and the baby hemoglobin H disease ($-\alpha^{3.7}/-^{MED}$).

The donated ova from the same woman had also been used in other pregnancies, including a pregnancy using the donated ova and a sperm donor of Asian origin. This sperm donor had not had a hemoglobinopathy screen and had to be recalled.

Although the family origin questionnaires have a section for IVF pregnancies, this is not always filled in and laboratories may make inaccurate risk assessments on the basis of poor information. If the correct box on the family origin questionnaire is ticked, then the mother's screen will not be informative, and the partner should be screened and results interpreted in conjunction with those of the egg donor (if available). This case highlights the importance of accuracy when completing family origin questions.

References

1. Globin Gene Server; 2015. Available from: http://globin.cse.psu.edu/.

2. Serjeant GH, Sergeant B. *Sickle Cell Disease*, 3rd edn. Oxford: Oxford Medical Publications; 2001.

3. Henderson S, Timbs A, McCarthy J *et al*. Incidence of hemoglobinopathies in various populations – the impact of immigration. *Clinical Biochemistry* 2009; **42**(18): 1745–1756.

4. Sorour Y, Heppinstall S, Porter N *et al*. Is routine molecular screening for common alpha-thalassemia deletions necessary as part of an antenatal screening programme? *Journal of Medical Screening* 2007; **14**(2): 60–1.

5. Old JM, Ward RH, Petrou M *et al*. First-trimester fetal diagnosis for hemoglobinopathies: three cases. *Lance* 1982; **2**(8313): 1413–1416.

6. Tabor A, Alfirevic Z. Update on procedure-related risks for prenatal diagnosis techniques. *Fetal Diagnosis and Therapy* 2010; **27**(1): 1–7.

7. Weatherall DJ. The role of the inherited disorders of hemoglobin, the first "molecular diseases," in the future of human genetics. *Annual Review of Genomics and Human Genetics* 2013; **14**: 1–24.

8. Thein SL. Genetic modifiers of beta-thalassemia. *Hematologica* 2005; **90**(5): 649–660.

9. Harteveld CL, Higgs DR. Alpha-thalassemia. *Orphanet Journal of Rare Diseases* 2010; **5**: 13.

10. Chui DH. Alpha-thalassemia: Hb H disease and Hb Barts hydrops fetalis. *Annals of the New York Academy of Sciences* 2005; **1054**: 25–32.

11. Henderson S, Pitman M, McCarthy J, Molyneux A, Old J. Molecular prenatal diagnosis of Hb H hydrops fetalis caused by hemoglobin Adana and the implications to antenatal screening for alpha-thalassemia. *Prenatal Diagnosis* 2008; **28**(9): 859–861.

12. Treger-Synodinos J, Harteveld CL, Old JM *et al*. EMQN Best Practice Guidelines for molecular and hematology methods for carrier identification and prenatal diagnosis of the hemoglobinopathies.

European Journal of Human Genetics 2015; **23**(4): 426–437.

13. Old J, Henderson S. Molecular diagnostics for hemoglobinopathies. *Expert Opinion on Medical Diagnostics* 2010; (**3**): 225–240.

14. Brezina PR, Brezina DS, Kearns WG. Preimplantation genetic testing. *BMJ* 2012; **345**: e5908.

15. Mastenbroek S, Twisk M, van der Veen F, Repping S. Preimplantation genetic screening: a systematic review and meta-analysis of RCTs. *Human Reproduction Update* 2011; **17**(4): 454–466.

16. Lo YM. Non-invasive prenatal diagnosis by massively parallel sequencing of maternal plasma DNA. *Open Biology* 2012; **2**(6): 120086.

17. Lun FM, Chiu RW, Chan KC *et al*. Microfluidics digital PCR reveals a higher than expected fraction of fetal DNA in maternal plasma. *Clinical Chemistry* 2008; **54**(10):1664–1672.

18. Fan HC, Gu W, Wang J *et al*. Non-invasive prenatal measurement of the fetal genome. *Nature* 2012; **487**(7407): 320–324.

19. Phylipsen M, Yamsri S, Treffers EE *et al*. Non-invasive prenatal diagnosis of beta-thalassemia and sickle-cell disease using pyrophosphorolysis-activated polymerization and melting curve analysis. *Prenatal Diagnosis* 2012; **32**(6): 578–587.

20. Barrett AN, McDonnell TC, Chan KC, Chitty LS. Digital PCR analysis of maternal plasma for noninvasive detection of sickle cell anemia. *Clinical Chemistry* 2012; **58**(6): 1026–1032.

21. Public Health England. NHS Sickle Cell and Thalassaemia Screening: handbook for antenatal laboratories; Sept 2017 https://www.gov.uk/government/uploads/system/uploads/attachment_data/file/647349/Antenatal Laboratory Handbook.pdf (accessed Oct 27, 2017)

22. Public Health England. NHS Sickle Cell and Thalassaemia Screening: handbook for antenatal laboratories; Jan 2017 https://www.gov.uk/government/uploads/system/uploads/attachment_data/file/585126/NHS_SCT_Handbook_for_Newborn_Laboratories.pdf (accessed Oct 27, 2017).

Management of Other Inherited Red Cell Disorders in Pregnancy

Noemi Roy and Sue Pavord

Introduction

While sickle cell disease and thalassemia are the most well-recognized inherited red cell disorders, a number of other inherited anemias occur and carry significant implications for both mother and fetus during pregnancy and delivery. The incidence of these conditions ranges from 1:2000 to 1:million and the rarity of them results in poor knowledge and lack of appreciation for the particular considerations necessary in caring for pregnant patients. This chapter focuses on some of these rare inherited disorders and the specific issues for mother and baby.

Severe phenotypes are diagnosed in childhood, but for milder cases, pregnancy can be the first presentation. This may involve an incidental finding of anemia on the routine booking blood count, or the development of anemia following the additional physiological stress of pregnancy, leading to a requirement for blood transfusion. As fetal outcomes can be adversely affected by some of these conditions, improved knowledge should allow appropriate monitoring strategies and early intervention, where indicated.

Patients suffering from these conditions have a spectrum of severity ranging from mild/asymptomatic anemia to lifelong transfusion dependence. Regardless of the etiology, patients with transfusion-dependent anemias will be subject to the complications of iron overload and management implications similar to those seen in patients with thalassemia major.

Erythropoiesis

Red blood cells (erythrocytes) are highly specialized cells whose function is to carry oxygen from the pulmonary vasculature to all tissues in the body. Oxygen is bound to hemoglobin, the most abundant protein in erythrocytes. Hypoxia may result from poor oxygenation of blood from the lungs or reduction in red cell numbers, caused either by inadequate production, such as hematinic deficiency and primary bone marrow failure syndromes, or excess loss from bleeding or hemolysis.

Red cells develop in the bone marrow, where hematopoietic stem cells differentiate down the erythroid lineage (Figure 9.1). There are numerous levels of control of erythroid differentiation, but one key element is erythropoietin (Epo). Epo is synthesized in the kidneys, where specialized O_2-sensing cells increase its

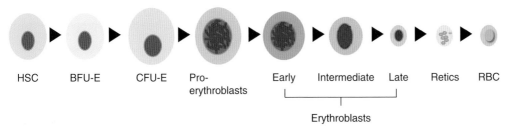

HSC BFU-E CFU-E Pro-erythroblasts Early Intermediate Late Retics RBC

Erythroblasts

Figure 9.1 Stages of erythropoiesis. Hematopoietic stem cells (HSCs) differentiate initially into multipotent progenitors able to produce all blood lineages, but the first fully committed erythroid precursors are the BFU-E (burst-forming units – erythroid) and CFU-E (colony-forming units – erythroid). Pro-erythroblasts are the earliest erythroid precursors that can be identified morphologically in bone marrow. These further differentiate into early, intermediate, and late erythroblasts. Differentiation is associated with decrease in cell size, nuclear condensation, and the appearance of pink cytoplasm, reflecting the rise in hemoglobin production. Once the nucleus has fully condensed, it is extruded, producing reticulocytes (Retics), which retain ribosomes and continue globin translation. Once these have been exhausted, fully mature biconcave disc red blood cells (RBCs) are released into the circulation. In cases of severe anemia due to peripheral loss of red cells (e.g. bleeding, hemolysis), red cell production is greatly increased under the control of erythropoietin, and reticulocytes are found in the peripheral blood in greater numbers.

production in response to hypoxia. Erythroid differentiation through a sequence of precursors and progenitors leads to the formation of cells (late erythroblasts) which extrude their nuclei but retain protein synthesis capacity due to the presence of high amounts of ribosomes and globin mRNA. These so-called reticulocytes appear in increased numbers in the circulation in conditions of marrow hyperactivity in response to peripheral loss or destruction of red cells. Once protein synthesis ceases, fully mature erythrocytes exit the bone marrow into the circulation, where they have a lifespan of 120 days. They are phagocytosed in the spleen and the iron is recycled.

In addition to containing hemoglobin, a key aspect of red cells is their specialized cytoskeleton, which gives them their characteristic biconcave shape and allows them to become deformable to pass through capillaries. Furthermore, red cells, in their absence of nuclei and protein synthesis, are entirely reliant on the ATP generated through glycolysis for normal function, highlighting the crucial role of glycolytic enzymes in their homeostasis. Congenital abnormalities in these structures and processes gives rise to anemia.

Transfusion-Dependent Anemias

Transfusion requirements often increase in pregnancy. At steady state, most transfusion-dependent adults require 2–3 units every 3–4 weeks. In pregnancy, the frequency often increases to 2–3 weeks. A significant complication of frequent blood transfusions is the development of alloantibodies conferring a risk of hemolytic disease of the newborn, if the corresponding antibody is inherited from the father. Other important risks include administrative errors, leading to incorrect transfusion with potentially fatal consequence, mild febrile reactions, transfusion-related acute lung injury, and risk of infection. There are no data regarding fetal outcomes following transfusions of mothers during pregnancy.

Patients receiving lifelong transfusion invariably require iron chelation. This can take the form of desferrioxamine (S/C), deferiprone (PO), or deferasirox (PO), the latter being better tolerated. Data on the use of chelation in pregnancy are limited to a few case reports but animal studies have shown teratogenicity and they should be avoided in pregnancy, unless it is felt that the benefits will outweigh the risks[1].

Enhanced erythropoiesis causes a high demand for folate. Normal requirements are 400 μg/day, rising to 600 μg/day in pregnancy. Requirements for patients with chronic hemolysis are estimated to be 1 mg/day and in pregnancy 5 mg/day is sufficient for adequate replacement.

Most of these conditions have autosomal recessive inheritance and the baby will be heterozygous unless the father is also affected. For autosomal dominant conditions such as Diamond–Blackfan anemia, the risk of an affected fetus is 50%; however, there is phenotypic variability even with identical genotypes and the need for intrauterine transfusion (IUT) is rare. Risks of IUTs are covered in Chapters 10 and 11. The abnormal erythrocytes have a shortened survival and the increased hemolysis may lead to significant maternal hyperbilirubinemia. However, bilirubin cannot cross the placenta and the fetus is not at risk of kernicterus during gestation.

Red Cell Membrane Disorders

The biconcave disk shape of red blood cells is critical to their ability to deform and squeeze through capillaries, the diameter of which is smaller than an erythrocyte. Their structure is maintained by a spectrin-based cytoskeleton which is anchored to the lipid bilayer of the cell membrane through a network of proteins. Membrane disorders are due to mutations either in the genes coding for key cytoskeletal proteins or for proteins that anchor the cytoskeleton to the cell membrane. There are a variety of molecular lesions which are typically inherited in an autosomal dominant manner and result in defects in the protein structure and interaction between various red cell membrane components, leading to loss of membrane surface area and reduced deformability. These cells have a reduced lifespan, resulting in a hemolytic anemia. The conditions are named after the morphological features of the abnormal cells. The commonest type is hereditary spherocytosis, followed by hereditary elliptocytosis, and hereditary pyropoikilocytosis (Figure 9.2).

Hereditary Spherocytosis

Hereditary spherocytosis (HS) occurs in all ethnic and racial groups. There is considerable heterogeneity reflecting the wide range of molecular lesions. Most patients have anemia, with hemoglobin between 90 and 120 g/L associated with a reticulocytosis and other biochemical evidence of hemolysis, such as reduced haptoglobin, and raised lactate dehydrogenase (LDH) and bilirubin. Approximately 10% of patients may have a more severe anemia, with hemoglobin between 60 and 80 g/L[2]. The diagnosis is made by

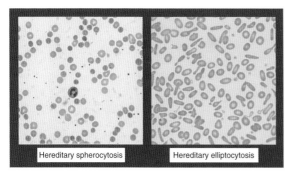

Hereditary spherocytosis   Hereditary elliptocytosis

Figure 9.2 Blood films showing spherocytes and elliptocytes at 400x magnification light microscopy.

the typical blood film appearances (Figure 9.2) and can be confirmed by an incubated osmotic fragility test or flow cytometry, or by sequencing the appropriate genes. Many patients lead normal lives and indeed the diagnosis may be an incidental finding.

Antenatal Management

For the most part, there are few implications for pregnancy and the outcome is good, for those with and without previous splenectomy[3]. Some women experience anemia greater than would be expected from the expanded plasma volume due to higher hemolytic rate. Patients should be encouraged to take preconception folic acid supplements and continue these throughout their pregnancy. In the more severe cases intermittent transfusion may be required.

Neonatal Management

A cord sample should be taken for hemoglobin and bilirubin levels. Neonates who have inherited HS themselves may require transfusion, but the degree of anemia at birth does not correlate with the hemoglobin level in later life and follow-up for the baby should be arranged at 4 months[4].

Hereditary Elliptocytosis and Hereditary Pyropoikilocytosis

Elliptocytosis has no significant implications for pregnancy, though folate supplementation throughout is prudent. Hereditary pyropoikilocytosis is a related condition and is associated with typical blood film appearances and a more severe degree of anemia. In addition to folate supplementation, such patients may require transfusion. The need for intervention with transfusion in all red cell membrane disorders should

be judged individually and based upon hemoglobin level, symptoms, and assessments of fetal wellbeing.

Enzymopathies

Glucose 6 Phosphate Dehydrogenase (G6PD) Deficiency

Deficiencies in red cell enzymes often lead to shortened red cell lifespan. G6PD deficiency was the first of such abnormalities to be discovered and is the most common, occurring in up to 20% of certain African and Mediterranean populations. The presence of G6PD is crucial to protect the red cell from oxidative damage. The deficiency is X-linked, with males being affected. Heterozygote females have two populations of red cells, one normal and one G6PD deficient, and may also be susceptible to hemolysis and have clinical manifestations. This is more severe when lyonization is unbalanced and there is greater inactivation of normal X chromosomes than mutated ones, leading to relatively higher proportions of G6PD-deficient red cells.

A large number of mutations within the gene for G6PD may result in a deficient phenotype. The majority cause mild deficiency and only result in significant hemolysis in "stress" situations such as infection and as a complication of certain drugs. Rarely, individuals have a more severe chronic non-spherocytic hemolytic anemia. Hemolysis is characterized by the presence of denatured hemoglobin within the red cell, which can be seen on supravital staining (Heinz bodies). Diagnosis may be made using G6PD deficiency screening tests available in the majority of hematology laboratories or by direct quantification, available in specialist centers.

Antenatal Management

For the most part, mild deficiency has little effect on pregnancy but the history of hemolytic episodes and precipitating factors should be determined, as well as a full blood count, blood film for characteristic red cell changes, serum folate, G6PD assay if not already known, reticulocyte count, LDH, and bilirubin. Heinz body preparation is helpful during active hemolysis. The patient should be advised against oxidant drugs (listed in the British National Formulary) and consumption of fresh or lightly cooked broad (fava) beans[5]. If a drug is felt to be indicated and there is no alternative, then the risks and benefits must be taken into account.

95

G6PD deficiency is heterogeneous and patients with a significant history of hemolytic crises or chronic hemolysis are more likely to react adversely than those with a milder phenotype. Folate status should be checked and folic acid, 5 mg daily, prescribed for all patients with chronic hemolysis. Patients should be made aware of the symptoms and signs of acute hemolytic anemia. Hemolysis is usually self-limiting, as reticulocytes have higher enzyme activity. However, red cell transfusion may be required in severe cases. Occasionally, renal failure can complicate acute severe intravascular hemolysis and should be treated as required. Caution should be taken with all drugs prescribed to the mother, to ensure there is no associated risk of hemolysis. There is some evidence from a small study in The Gambia that G6PD deficiency is associated with a poorer outcome with an increase of stillbirths and recurrent miscarriages, although whether this would be applicable to countries with good access to healthcare is not clear[6].

Management of the Neonate

As the condition has X-linked inheritance, a male baby has a 50% chance of inheritance from the carrier mother. Female babies have a 50% chance of being a carrier and may have low G6PD levels if lyonization is skewed. Neonatal erythrocytes have an increased susceptibility to oxidative hemolysis and immaturity of hepatic enzyme systems may enhance the risk of jaundice and kernicterus. Hemolysis is usually self-limiting but exchange transfusion, with G6PD screened blood, may be required for those cases with severe jaundice. A cord sample should be taken at birth for hemoglobin and bilirubin. G6PD assays should also be performed, although this may be difficult to interpret. Phytomenadione (a fat-soluble preparation of vitamin K) can be administered to the baby in accordance with normal procedures. Water-soluble preparations of the vitamin K should be avoided in view of the possible risk of hemolysis in newborns. Observations for jaundice should be continued for the first 4 days of life.

Breast-feeding

The mother should be advised that certain drugs may be excreted in breast milk and may trigger hemolysis in a G6PD-deficient baby.

Pyruvate Kinase (PK) Deficiency

Pyruvate kinase (PK) is the last enzyme in the glycolytic pathway, producing a pyruvate and a molecule of

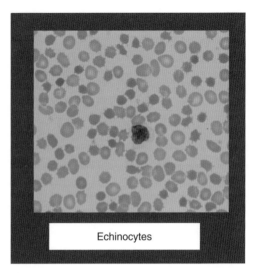

Echinocytes

Figure 9.3 Blood film showing spiculated echinocytes at 400x magnification light microscopy. These arise in pyruvate kinase deficiency as the resulting inadequacy of ATP production leads to a loss of potassium and water from the red cells.

ATP, on which the red cell is critically dependent for energy. There are different isoforms, including an erythroid-specific form. PK deficiency is an autosomal recessive condition, with most cases due to compound heterozygosity of missense mutations. The overall activity of the PK enzyme is reduced, and without adequate ATP, the red cells are unable to maintain their shape and damaged red cells are removed by the spleen. This, extravascular hemolysis causes a rise in reticulocytes, bilirubin, and LDH. The presence of echinocytes on the blood film is a clue to the diagnosis (Figure 9.3), but this is not invariably seen and confirmation requires enzyme levels or genetic tests.

Antenatal Management

There is no correlation between the in vitro enzyme activity and the severity of hemolysis and the clinical condition can range from asymptomatic chronic compensated hemolysis, which accounts for the majority, to transfusion dependence[7]. Patients may also develop gallstones. Pregnancy may worsen the anemia. Additionally, episodes of acute hemolytic exacerbations may occur, usually secondary to infections. Recovery is often rapid and spontaneous but may occasionally require blood transfusion. Patients may benefit from splenectomy, preferably outside of pregnancy, to reduce the destruction of abnormally shaped red cells and prolong red cell lifespan. All patients require supplementation with folic acid 5 mg/day, in and out of pregnancy. There are no large series reported in the literature of pregnant PK patients although some small series have described pre-eclampsia[8].

High-Affinity Hemoglobinopathies

Common disorders of α- or β-globin chain production (thalassemia) and structural Hb variants (sickle) are covered in Chapters 6 to 8. However, some β- and α-chain variants arise from mutations in the oxygen-binding regions of Hb, resulting in hemoglobin molecules with increased affinity to O_2 compared to HbA. This renders O_2 delivery to the tissues suboptimal, compensated for by cardiovascular adjustments and an increase in EPO production from the kidneys, with enhanced red cell production and erythrocytosis.

These conditions are invariably autosomal dominant. The diagnosis is usually made once other causes of erythrocytosis have been excluded. While oxygen tension curves can be carried out to identify high-affinity hemoglobins, more often the α and β genes are sequenced to look for evidence of a genetic lesion.

Management

Patients may suffer from the consequences of erythrocytosis and the increased plasma viscosity that ensues, such as headaches, fatigue, and blurred vision. Treatment is difficult and while venesection offers temporary relief from the hyperviscosity, this leads to an increase in EPO and further rise in hematocrit.

In pregnancy, the physiological increase in plasma volume leads to an improvement in the erthrocytosis and associated symptoms. There is no evidence for a detrimental effect on the fetus, either from a carrier mother with normal fetus, or a carrier fetus (paternal inheritance) with a normal mother [9]. It appears that compensatory cardiovascular and erythropoietic changes and possibly enhanced uterine and fetal blood flow, provide protection for the fetus. Animal models have shown increased fetal losses due to high-affinity Hb, but this has not been reported in humans.

Congenital Dyserythropoietic Anemia

Congenital dyserythropoietic anemia (CDA) refers to a group of related conditions characterized by ineffective erythropoiesis and abnormal maturation of the erythroid lineage (dyserythropoiesis). They are rare, autosomal recessive conditions, with an estimated prevalence of ~2–3/million. The subtypes (CDA-I, CDA-II, CDA-III, etc.) are defined on a morphological basis[10] (Table 9.1). The mutated genes causing each of these conditions have been discovered but their precise mechanisms remain unexplained.

Clinical Manifestations

Disease severity in CDA is extremely variable. The anemia is normo- or macrocytic and the reticulocyte count is inappropriately low. The diagnosis is based on bone marrow findings. Where light microscopy is suggestive of CDA, electron microscopy is diagnostic, due to the striking morphological features of spongy heterochromatin (Figure 9.4). Genetic testing is also available.

Most patients are not transfusion dependent but behave like thalassemia intermedia, with splenomegaly

Table 9.1 Description of the main subtypes of congenital dyserythropoietic anemia

	Bone marrow morphology	Clinical presentation	Molecular abnormality	Specific therapy
CDA-1	Erythroid hyperplasia, internuclear chromatin bridges, "Swiss cheese heterochromatin" on electron microscopy	Anemia (may be transfusion dependent) Iron overload Splenomegaly	Autosomal recessive due to mutations in CDAN1 or c15orf41	IFN-α
CDA-2	Erythroid hyperplasia with binuclear erythroblasts	Anemia (may be transfusion dependent) Jaundice, gallstones Splenomegaly, iron overload	Autosomal recessive due to mutations in SEC23B	Nil
CDA-3	Erythroid hyperplasia with multinuclear erythroblasts (up to 12 nuclei per cell)	Mild anemia No iron overload	Autosomal dominant due to mutations in KIF23	Nil

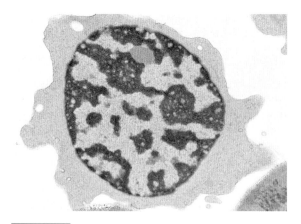

1 μm

Figure 9.4 Electron microscopy (x 8000 magnification) of a cultured erythroblast showing pale-colored euchromatin in the nucleus, and dark heterochromatin containing the characteristic moth-eaten appearance which is pathognomonic of CDA-1. This is sometimes also referred to as "Swiss cheese heterochromatin" on account of the abnormal "holes" in the heterochromatin. Photo courtesy of Professor David Ferguson.

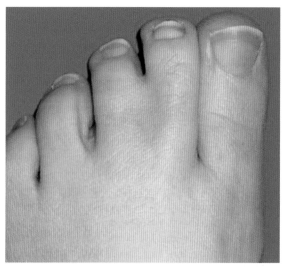

Figure 9.5 Approximately half of patients with Diamond–Blackfan anemia have non-hematological features such as cleft palate or limb or digit anomalies. Pictured here is a mild digit abnormality of partially fused toes.

due to extramedullary hematopoiesis and requirement for intermittent transfusions. Most women with CDA need transfusions during pregnancy. Iron overload may arise from repeated transfusions and excess oral iron absorption incurring need for iron chelation, although this should be avoided in pregnancy due to potential teratogenicity. Alpha interferon may be used to stabilize the hemoglobin and reduce production of abnormal erythroblasts. The risks and benefits need to be weighed up in the setting of pregnancy.

Owing to the rarity of the disease, there is not much data on outcome of pregnancy in CDA. One small series followed 28 pregnancies in a group of Bedouin women. The results were compounded by the migratory nature of the population and their poor access to healthcare and in particular poor attendance at regular antenatal appointments. Nevertheless, there were high rates of complications (64%): 42% of the newborns were of low birth weight and there was a higher rate of cesarean deliveries[11]. Fetal distress, pre-eclampsia, and preterm delivery were not increased.

Fetal disease ranges from mild anemia to hydrops fetalis. Exchange transfusions may be necessary for affected neonates. Outcomes are generally better with CDA-I.

Diamond–Blackfan Anemia

Diamond–Blackfan anemia (DBA) is a pure red cell aplasia. The marrow functions normally for the production of white blood cells and platelets but is unable to produce red blood cells. The estimated prevalence is 5–10/million. It is due to mutations in genes that code for ribosomal proteins. The gene most commonly implicated is *RPS19*. Ribosomal proteins are expressed in every cell type, but it is intriguing that the major defect is restricted to the erythroid lineage, although 40% of DBA patients have associated congenital malformations (Figure 9.5).

Clinical Features

DBA is inherited in an autosomal dominant manner, although it often occurs *de novo*, with neither parent carrying the mutation. Ribosomal proteins play a key role in protein translation. Although the exact mechanism is not clear, it appears that the p53 pathway is triggered and the erythroid precursors undergo apoptosis in cells with defective ribosomal protein processing; the patients are also at increased risk of malignancy. Most patients present in infancy and although 25% respond to steroids or resolve spontaneously, the majority are transfusion dependent. Some patients require bone marrow transplant. Diagnosis is usually made upon bone marrow examination, and genetic testing is available.

Case series have been published which examine the pregnancy outcome for mother and baby in patients with DBA. These are high-risk pregnancies, with 66% being complicated. Adverse outcomes included fetal loss (62%), pre-eclampsia (12%), and preterm delivery (9.5%). One series showed that only 56% of the pregnancies led to live births, 41% of which were also affected by DBA. Complications occurred in equal proportions in the affected and unaffected pregnancies. Interestingly, 23% of children born to DBA mothers had malformations. These occurred in affected and unaffected babies, suggesting maternal/placental effects. Where placentas could be examined, these showed significant infarcts[12,13].

Use of aspirin and LMWH has been described in a DBA mother who had previously suffered two fetal deaths. This led to the birth of a live infant[13]. It was noted that transfusion-dependent DBA mothers had an increased requirement for transfusions and steroids during pregnancy and it is felt that hemoglobin levels should be kept above 100 g/L[14].

The high risk associated with DBA pregnancies makes it essential that these patients are followed up in a specialized unit. Patients will need frequent ultrasound scans, with monitoring of fetal and placental development.

Bone Marrow Failure Syndromes

Bone marrow failure syndromes are caused by molecular defects at hematopoietic stem cell level, giving rise to a multilineage defect with varying degrees of anemia, neutropenia, and thrombocytopenia. Examples include Fanconi's anemia, Schwachman–Diamond syndrome, and dyskeratosis congenita. Severity varies but blood and/or platelet transfusions are often required and infections should be treated promptly. All are associated with an increased risk of hematological malignancies and solid tumors.

The median age of survival is 35 years. Fertility is reduced in Fanconi's anemia (FA), but not abolished, and some cases have only come to light during pregnancy itself. The pregnancies which have been reported in FA patients have occurred in those with milder forms of the disease. They were all associated with decreased blood counts during the pregnancy, which recovered following delivery and were considered to be hormonally induced myelosuppression. The incidence of pre-eclampsia was increased but neonates have been unaffected and the mode of delivery should be chosen for obstetric reasons[15].

The presence of aplastic anemia in early pregnancy is associated with poor outcome and the option of termination should be discussed.

Pregnancy in Splenectomized Patients

Splenectomy is a treatment modality used in some of the disorders mentioned above (CDA, membrane and enzyme disorders), as well as certain hemoglobinopathies. It carries significant implications during pregnancy, due to the risk of infection from encapsulated bacteria (*Hemophilus influenzae* b, *Streptococcus pneumoniae*, *Neisseria meningitidis*). These patients should be vaccinated regardless of pregnancy, but it is advisable to ensure the 36 vaccines have been given and that Pneumovax has been given in the previous 5 years[16]. There are no contraindications to inactivated viral and bacterial vaccines in pregnancy.

Parvovirus B19

This widespread infection can affect pregnant women, with potentially devastating consequences. All pregnant women may be affected but those with hemolytic anemia may develop aplastic crisis due to viral involvement of erythroid precursors. The inability to maintain erythropoiesis sufficient to balance the increased demands from pregnancy and hemolysis leads to a sudden drop in hemoglobin level and requirement for transfusion. This occurrence should alert the treating physician to the possibility of parvovirus B19 infection. The presence of specific IgM in serum confirms an acute infection.

Parvovirus B19 infection has potentially fatal consequences for the fetus. Viral transfer across the placenta with infection of fetal erythroid precursors leads to severe anemia and hydrops fetalis. Intrauterine transfusions have been shown to reduce fetal death by sevenfold. Fetal cardiac myocytes are also susceptible to infection by parvovirus B19, causing myocarditis and aggravation of cardiac failure. Fetal loss is more likely following infection in the first two trimesters (~15% vs 2% in the third trimester). Neonatal complications include transfusion-dependent anemia, myocarditis, neurological abnormalities, and hepatic insufficiency. However, these do not tend to cause long-term sequelae[17].

Case Studies

Case Study 1

A 28-year-old woman with known CDA-1 has hepatosplenomegaly due to extramedullary hematopoiesis. She spontaneously maintains a hemoglobin level of 80 g/L, from which she is not symptomatic. She has received occasional blood transfusions for worsening anemia during intercurrent infections and her ferritin level is 2000 µg/L. She wishes to become pregnant and in view of the association between iron overload and subfertility, agrees to commence iron chelation with deferasirox until ferritin <1000 µg/L and delay pregnancy until chelation is finished, due to the lack of evidence concerning teratogenicity and deferasirox. However, within 4 weeks of commencing therapy she becomes pregnant and deferasirox is stopped. Her hemoglobin levels fall to 70 g/L and she becomes symptomatic with fatigue and shortness of breath. Interferon alfa therapy is considered but the patient prefers not to start this therapy as risks to the fetus cannot be ruled out by current evidence. Intermittent transfusions are commenced to keep the patient's hemoglobin level above 80 g/L. Monitoring of the baby reveals that it is small for dates but a healthy infant is delivered at 39 weeks' gestation by an uncomplicated delivery.

Case Study 2

A 35-year-old woman who is not previously known to be anemic is found to have a hemoglobin of 75 g/L at booking. Hematinic deficiency is ruled out and she is referred for further investigation. Tests confirmed evidence of hemolysis with a raised serum bilirubin, LDH, and reticulocyte count. A blood film is unremarkable apart from the presence of occasional echinocytes. Family history reveals consanguinity (parents are first cousins) and a cousin with two stillbirths. An ultrasound confirms splenomegaly. Red cell enzyme assays show low levels of pyruvate kinase. Owing to symptoms of anemia, in addition to starting folic acid 5 mg/day, the patient is transfused 2 units of blood; however, 2 weeks later her hemoglobin is 70 g/L with evidence of ongoing hemolysis. A second transfusion is given and the option of a splenectomy is discussed with the patient, with an explanation that this is most safely performed during the second trimester. The patient agrees to this course of action and is vaccinated against meningococcus, pneumococcus, and *H. influenzae*. Two weeks later, at 20 weeks, a laparoscopic splenectomy is successfully performed. The rest of the pregnancy is uneventful, with the patient maintaining a hemoglobin level of 85 g/L. In view of the patient's partner being a second cousin, the couple is counseled about the possibility of their child being affected. At term, a healthy male infant is delivered; however, he is deeply jaundiced, requiring phototherapy, but not exchange transfusion. PK deficiency is confirmed in the child and daily folic acid commenced. The child is referred to a pediatric hematologist for follow-up and the risk of aplastic crises discussed; however, they are reassured that the child's clinical course is likely to follow his mother's moderate course.

References

1. Singer ST, Vichinsky EP. Deferoxamine treatment during pregnancy: is it harmful? *American Journal of Hematology* 1999; **60**(1): 24–26.

2. Gallagher PG. Abnormalities of the erythrocyte membrane. *Pediatric Clinics of North America* 2013; **60**(6): 1349–1362.

3. Pajor A, Lehoczky D, Szakács Z. Pregnancy and hereditary spherocytosis: Report of 8 patients and a review. *Archives of Gynecology and Obstetrics* 1993; **253**(1): 37–42.

4. Perrotta S, Gallagher P, Mohandas N. Hereditary spherocytosis. *Lancet* 2008; **372**(9647): 1411–1426.

5. Molad M, Waisman D, Rotschild A *et al.* Nonimmune hydrops fetalis caused by G6PD deficiency hemolytic crisis and congenital dyserythropoietic anemia. *Journal of Perinatology* 2013; **33**: 490–491.

6. Sirugo G, Schefer EA, Mendy A *et al.* Is G6PD A-deficiency associated with recurrent stillbirths in The Gambia? *American Journal of Medical Genetics A* 2004; **128A**(1): 104–5.

7. Zanella A, Fermo E, Bianchi P, Chiarelli LR, Valentini G. Pyruvate kinase deficiency: The genotype-phenotype association. *Blood Reviews* 2007; **21**: 217–231.

8. Wax JR, Pinette MG, Cartin A, Blackstone J. Pyruvate kinase deficiency complicating pregnancy. *Obstetrics and Gynecology* 2007; **109**(2 Pt2): 553–555.

9. Bard H, Rosenberg A, Huisman TH. Hemoglobinopathies affecting maternal-fetal oxygen gradient during pregnancy: molecular, biochemical and clinical studies. *American Journal of Perinatology* 1998; **15**(6): 389–393.

10. Iolascon A, Heimpel H, Wahlin A, Tamary H. Congenital dyserythropoietic anemias: molecular insights and diagnostic approach. *Blood* 2013; **122**(13): 2162–2166.

11. Shalev H, Avraham GP, Hershkovitz R, *et al.* Pregnancy outcome in congenital dyserythropoietic anemia Type 1. *European Journal of Haematology* 2008; **81**: 317–321.

12. Da Costa L, Chanoz-Poulard G, Simansour M *et al.* First de novo mutation in RPS19 gene as the cause of hydrops

fetalis in Diamond-Blackfan anemia. *American Journal of Hematology* 2013; **88**(4): 340–341.

13. Faivre L, Meerpohl J, Da Costa L *et al.* High-risk pregnancies in Diamond-Blackfan anemia: a survey of 64 pregnancies from the French and German registries. *Hematologica* 2006; **91**: 530–533.

14. Vlachos A, Ball S, Dahl N *et al.* Diagnosing and treating Diamond Blackfan anemia: results of an international clinical consensus conference. *British Journal of Haematology* 2008; **142**(6): 859–876.

15. Alter BP, Frissora CL, Halpérin DS *et al.* Fanconi's anemia and pregnancy. *British Journal of Haematology* 1991; **77**(3): 410–418.

16. Rubin LG, Schaffner W. Clinical practice: Care of the asplenic patient. *New England Journal of Medicine* 2014; **371**(4): 349–356.

17. Crane J, Mundle W, Boucoiran I *et al.* Parvovirus B19 infection in pregnancy. *Journal of Obstetrics and Gynecology Canada* 2014; **36**(12): 1107–1116.

Fetal/Neonatal Alloimmune Thrombocytopenia

Michael Murphy

Introduction

Fetal and neonatal alloimmune thrombocytopenia (FNAIT) is the commonest cause of severe neonatal thrombocytopenia, and is analogous to the fetal/neonatal anemia caused by hemolytic disease of the fetus and newborn (HDFN)[1]. Fetal platelet antigens are expressed on platelets in normal amounts from as early as the 16th week of pregnancy. Fetomaternal incompatibility for human platelet alloantigens (HPAs) may cause maternal alloimmunization, and fetal and neonatal thrombocytopenia may result from placental transfer of IgG antibodies. Many HPA systems have been described[2]. The majority of HPA antigens such as HPA-1a are located on the β3 subunit of the aIIbb3 integrin (GPIIb/IIIa, CD41/CD61) which is present at high density on the platelet membrane. Others such as HPA-5b are on α2β1 (GPIa/IIa, CD49b), the primary platelet receptor for collagen. Incompatibility for HPA-1a is found in about 80% of cases of FNAIT in Caucasians, and for HPA-5b in virtually all the remainder. In contrast to HDFN, up to 50% of cases of FNAIT occur in first pregnancies.

Considerable progress has been made in the laboratory investigation of FNAIT since it was first recognized in the 1950s[1]. There have also been improvements in its management, particularly in the antenatal management of women with a history of one or more pregnancies affected by FNAIT, resulting from a better understanding of the risk of severe hemorrhage and advances in fetal and transfusion medicine.

Epidemiology

The normal platelet count in the fetus and the neonate is the same as in adults. Neonatal thrombocytopenia has many causes and is the commonest hematological problem in the newborn infant. A platelet count of $<150 \times 10^9$/L occurs in about 1% of unselected neonates, and is $<50 \times 10^9$/L in about 0.15%[3]. FNAIT is the most important cause of severe fetal and neonatal thrombocytopenia, because of both its frequency and

the severity of the bleeding associated with it. For example, FNAIT is associated with more severe fetal/neonatal bleeding than with maternal autoimmune thrombocytopenic purpura for reasons which are not entirely clear but could be due to associated platelet and/or endothelial dysfunction. About 27% of the cases in which the neonatal platelet count is $<50 \times 10^9$/L and most cases where the fetal or neonatal platelet count is $<20 \times 10^9$/L are caused by FNAIT[3].

The most common entities in the differential diagnosis of severe fetal and neonatal thrombocytopenia are:

- congenital infections such as toxoplasmosis, rubella, and cytomegalovirus;
- maternal autoimmune thrombocytopenic purpura;
- chromosomal abnormalities;
- congenital heart disease; and
- disseminated intravascular coagulation (DIC).

Incidence

Prospective studies in Caucasian populations for FNAIT due to anti-HPA-1a indicate that about 2% of women are HPA-1a negative, and that about 10% of HPA-1a negative women develop anti-HPA-1a[4]. Alloimmunization to HPA-1a is HLA class II restricted. There is a strong association with HLADRB3*0101 (HLADRw52a), which is present in 1 in 3 of Caucasian women, and HPA-1a alloimmunization is rare in HPA-1a negative women who lack this antigen.

Severe FNAIT (platelet count $<50 \times 10^9$/L) occurs in 31% of pregnancies where the mother is HPA-1a negative with anti-HPA-1a, and perinatal intracranial hemorrhage (ICH) occurs in 10% of those with severe FNAIT[4].

Pooling the data from studies of antenatal and postnatal screening indicates an overall incidence of severe FNAIT of 63 per 100 000 and an incidence of

103

ICH of 6 per 100 000 with the majority of the cases of ICH occurring antenatally[3,4].

FNAIT is underdiagnosed in routine clinical practice. The evidence for this is the mismatch in the incidence of FNAIT between prospective studies involving laboratory screening for HPA antibodies and the identification of clinically diagnosed cases. It is estimated that only 7–23% of cases of FNAIT, and only 37% of severe cases, are detected clinically.

Clinical Diagnosis

FNAIT is usually suspected in neonates with bleeding or severe, unexplained, and/or isolated postnatal thrombocytopenia. The clinical diagnosis is one of exclusion:

- the infant has no signs of DIC, infection, or congenital anomalies known to be associated with thrombocytopenia;
- the mother has had a normal pregnancy with no history of autoimmune disease, thrombocytopenia, or drugs which may cause thrombocytopenia.

Specific criteria which distinguish cases of FNAIT from other causes of unexplained thrombocytopenia include:

- severe thrombocytopenia (platelet count $<50 \times 10^9/L$);
- no additional, non-hemorrhagic neonatal medical problems;
- ICH associated with one or more of:

  –Apgar score at 1 minute >5;

  –birth weight >2.2 kg;

  –documented antenatal or postnatal bleeding.

Laboratory Diagnosis

Detailed laboratory investigations are required for confirmation of a provisional clinical diagnosis, and should be performed by an experienced reference laboratory. The diagnosis is based on:

- detection and identification of the maternal HPA antibody;
- determination of the HPA genotype of mother, father, and, if needed, the child (or fetus).

In the past, it was difficult to differentiate between HLA and HPA antibodies in standard serological assays. The description of the monoclonal antibody-specific immobilization of platelet antigens (MAIPA) assay overcame this problem. Rather than working with intact platelets, the assay involves capture of specific GPs using monoclonal antibodies enabling analysis of complex mixtures of platelet antibodies. However, it requires considerable operator expertise in order to ensure maximum sensitivity and specificity, and the selection of appropriate screening cells is critical.

Immunization against HPA-1a and HPA-5b is responsible for up to 95% of cases of FNAIT[1]. Antibodies against other HPAs are more frequently detected in recent large series of FNAIT. In some of these cases, testing against standard donor platelet panels may be negative. To pursue further investigation requires strong clinical suspicion of FNAIT. Possible approaches include:

- cross-match of maternal serum and paternal platelets using MAIPA;
- identification of a mismatch between maternal and paternal (or neonatal) genotypes for low-frequency HPA antigens, and then screening maternal serum for the corresponding HPA antibodies.

Clinical Significance of FNAIT

ICH is the major cause of mortality and long-term morbidity in FNAIT. The long-term outcome may be devastating, with blindness and major physical and mental disability (Figure 10.1). ICH was reported in a large review of the literature to occur in 74/281 (26%) of cases of FNAIT due to anti-HPA-1a with a mortality of 7%[5].

Although there is a risk of hemorrhage due to severe thrombocytopenia at the time of delivery, 80% of cases of ICH associated with FNAIT occur in utero, with 14% occurring before 20 weeks and a further 28% occurring before 30 weeks[5]. There may also be unusual presentations such as isolated fetal hydrocephalus, unexplained fetal anemia, or recurrent miscarriages.

Bleeding is more severe with FNAIT due to anti-HPA-1a than, for example, anti-HPA-5b, possibly due to the higher density of HPA-1a antigen sites on platelets. Animal models found impaired angiogenesis in anti-HPA-1a-mediated FNAIT, which may contribute to ICH and fetal growth restriction[6].

Prediction of the Severity of FNAIT in Subsequent Pregnancies

Laboratory Testing

Unfortunately, there is no reliable laboratory method to predict severe clinical disease, which might be used to

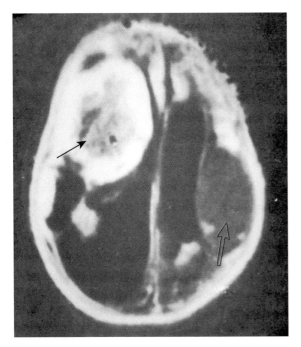

Figure 10.1 Intracranial hemorrhage in FNAIT: MRI scan showing subacute hematoma (black arrow) and chronic hematoma (open arrow).

Reproduced with permission from De Vries et al. Br J Obstet Gynaecol 1988;95:299-302.

identify pregnancies at risk of severe thrombocytopenia and ICH. Some studies have observed an association between high levels of maternal anti-HPA-1a and the severity of neonatal thrombocytopenia, but this is not a sufficiently reliable association to be clinically useful. Reliable methods for quantifying the other antibodies are not yet available. The lack of laboratory parameters predictive of severe disease remains one of the major barriers to optimizing antenatal management for FNAIT, and is an important area for future research.

History of FNAIT in Previous Pregnancies

Subsequent pregnancies of HPA-1a alloimmunized women with a history of a previously affected infant with FNAIT are well recognized to be associated with a high risk of recurrence of FNAIT and poor outcome[7].

These data provide the justification for antenatal intervention in women with a past history of pregnancies affected with FNAIT, particularly where there has been fetal or neonatal ICH in a previous pregnancy, to reduce the risk of morbidity and mortality from severe hemorrhage.

If there is paternal heterozygosity for the relevant HPA, fetal platelet genotyping should be considered using a sample obtained by amniocentesis. Chorionic villus sampling is unsuitable for this purpose but recently it has become possible to determine the HPA-1a genotype using cell-free fetal DNA isolated from maternal blood.

Consideration of Antenatal Screening for FNAIT

Advances in the laboratory diagnosis and antenatal management of FNAIT have drawn attention to the fact that the first affected fetus/neonate is usually only recognized after bleeding has occurred or severe thrombocytopenia detected by chance. This raises the question of whether routine screening for FNAIT should be considered. It is recognized that there are significant shortcomings in the knowledge about FNAIT necessary for the introduction of an antenatal screening program[8].

More research is required, for example, on the clinical outcome of first affected pregnancies, the identification of laboratory measures predictive of severe disease where antenatal intervention might be justified, and the optimal approach for the antenatal management of pregnant women with HPA antibodies but with no previous history of affected pregnancies, as antenatal treatment carries significant risks and costs.

Management of FNAIT

Postnatal Management

The thrombocytopenia in FNAIT usually resolves within 2 weeks, although it may last as long as 6 weeks. A cerebral ultrasound should be carried out to determine if ICH has occurred because of the changes in management that would occur if there had been a hemorrhage.

The optimal postnatal management of FNAIT depends on its rapid recognition, and prompt correction by transfusion of platelet concentrates to neonates who are severely thrombocytopenic (platelet count $<30 \times 10^9$/L) or bleeding. It is not appropriate to wait for the laboratory confirmation of the diagnosis in suspected cases. There is general agreement that if there has been ICH, that the platelet count should be maintained $>100 \times 10^9$/L for 1 week.

While there has been debate about the value of random donor platelets in the immediate postnatal management of FNAIT, two recent studies reported that random donor (i.e. not HPA-matched) platelets were often effective in increasing the platelet count in FNAIT. However, in some of the cases, spontaneous recovery of the neonatal platelet count may have been the reason for the apparent response to random donor platelet transfusions. Compatible platelet concentrates were shown in another study to produce a larger increase in platelet count and twice the length of survival of the transfused platelets compared to random donor platelets[9].

Compatible platelet concentrates, for example from HPA-1a- and 5b-negative donors, should be used initially, if they are available, on the basis of the certainty of their effectiveness in the more than 90% of cases of FNAIT that are due to anti-HPA-1a or anti-HPA-5b. Unfortunately, the routine availability of such HPA-1a- and HPA-5b-negative platelets for immediate use in suspected cases of FNAIT is limited to only a minority of countries, including England.

Although intravenous immunoglobulin (IVIG) is effective in at least 75% of cases, the platelet count does not increase in responders for 24–72 hours so it should not be used for the initial therapy of FNAIT. Its role in the management of postnatal FNAIT should be limited to those few cases with very prolonged and severe thrombocytopenia.

The platelet count will usually increase to a level where no further treatment is needed after 1 week. Thrombocytopenia may persist for 4–6 weeks, but alternative diagnoses should be considered if there is thrombocytopenia after 2–4 weeks.

Provision of Information to the Mother

The parents should be provided with information about FNAIT once the platelet antigen typing and antibody results are complete, specifically to provide:

1. an explanation of the cause of FNAIT;
2. the risk of recurrence in subsequent pregnancies;
3. the options for antenatal management as well as the fact that this is an evolving field;
4. a request that the mother should notify the fetal medicine center as soon as she becomes pregnant;
5. her risk for the future of transfusion reactions, and potentially post-transfusion purpura (PTP), although it appears that the risk of PTP is very low with leukocyte-reduced blood components, which are now standard in the UK; and
6. an opportunity to suggest HPA typing of female relatives of the mother.

Antenatal Management

Major advances in the antenatal management of FNAIT have been made in the last 25 years[1,10].

Early Antenatal Treatment Strategies

In 1984, the use of ultrasound-guided fetal blood sampling (FBS) was described to obtain the fetal platelet count at 32 weeks' gestation in the second pregnancy of a woman whose first child had ICH due to FNAIT; the fetal platelet count was 15×10^9/L. There was no ultrasound evidence of ICH by 37 weeks, and an in utero transfusion of maternal platelets was given 6 hours prior to delivery by cesarean section. As a result, the cord platelet count was 95×10^9/L and there were no signs of bleeding.

The use of in utero platelet transfusion (see Figure 10.2) immediately before delivery was described in greater detail in a series of nine cases, where FBS was carried out at 21 weeks' gestation to confirm the diagnosis of FNAIT[1]. FBS was repeated at 37 weeks with an in utero platelet transfusion if the fetal platelet count was $<50 \times 10^9$/L followed by delivery 6–36 hours later. However, over the next 10 years, it became clearer that an affected fetus is at risk of ICH in utero, even before 20 weeks' gestation, indicating

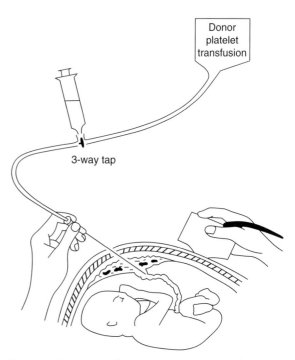

Donor platelet transfusion

3-way tap

Figure 10.2 Schematic diagram of ultrasound-guided fetal blood sampling and platelet transfusion.

that earlier antenatal intervention is required in cases likely to be severely affected. During this period, different groups began to explore alternative approaches to antenatal management, one based around serial weekly fetal platelet transfusion, and the other around medical treatment of the mother with IVIG and/or steroids.

Serial Fetal Platelet Transfusions

Early studies with intrauterine fetal transfusions, with compatible platelets, highlighted the short survival of transfused platelets, and the difficulty of maintaining the fetal platelet count at a "safe" level. Further experience indicated that it was possible to maintain the count above 30×10^9/L using transfusions at weekly intervals (Figure 10.3). This was achieved by increasing the dose of platelets, while avoiding an unacceptable increase in the transfused volume, by concentrating the platelet collection by centrifugation and removal of plasma. Later improvements in apheresis technology allowed the preparation of leukocyte-depleted concentrated platelets suitable for fetal transfusion without the need for further processing.

The main risks of FBS are severe cord bleeding, cardiac arrhythmias, and miscarriage. Pooling data

from several studies indicates a fetal loss rate of 3/223 (1.3%)/procedure and 3/55 (5.5%)/pregnancy.

Maternal Treatment

One of the main drivers for the development of maternally directed antenatal treatment for FNAIT was concern about the risks of FBS and platelet transfusion.

Steroids – – There is considerable experience from North America with the combined use of steroids and IVIG[11]. Although low-dose steroids did not add significantly to the effect of IVIG, high-dose steroids (prednisolone 60 mg and later 1 mg/kg) added substantially to the effect of IVIG. The use of 0.5 mg/kg prednisolone in the lowest risk cases (no previous sibling ICH, initial fetal count $>20 \times 10^9$/L) demonstrated efficacy comparable to that of IVIG in this group of patients.

Intravenous Immunogloblin (IVIG) – – The first protocol involving maternal administration of IVIG was described in 1988. Initial FBS was carried out at 20–22 weeks' gestation to confirm the diagnosis of FNAIT and its severity. IVIG (dose 1 g/kg body weight/week) was administered to the mother, and FBS was repeated 4–6 weeks later to assess the effect of IVIG.

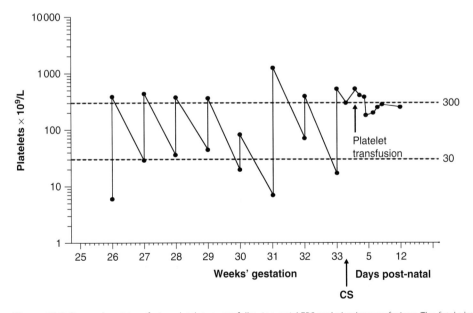

Figure 10.3 Pre- and post-transfusion platelet counts following serial FBS and platelet transfusions. The fetal platelet count was $<10 \times 10^9$/L at 26 weeks. The aim was to maintain the fetal platelet count above 30×10^9/L by raising the immediate post-transfusion platelet count to above 300×10^9/L after each transfusion. The fetal platelet count fell below 10×10^9/L on one occasion when there were problems in preparing the fetal platelet concentrate and the dose of platelets was inadequate. CS, cesarean section.

Reproduced with permission from Murphy MF, Heddle N & Pamphilon D (eds) Practical Transfusion Medicine, 4th edition; Wiley-Blackwell Publishing, 2013.

None had ICH in contrast to three of their respective untreated siblings, two of whom had antenatal ICH, and there were no serious complications of treatment. Overall, there was an increase of 36×10^9/L between the first and second FBS, and an increase of 69×10^9/L between the first FBS and birth. Sixty-two to 85% of fetuses responded to therapy depending on the definition of response used, and there were no cases with ICH. However, other reports described cases in which IVIG was ineffective in raising the fetal platelet count, and antenatal ICH was reported during maternal treatment with IVIG.

Complications of Maternal Treatment –– The use of IVIG is expensive, and both IVIG and prednisolone can cause adverse maternal effects. IVIG appears to be a safe blood product when administered to otherwise healthy young women. The risks of renal disease, hemolysis, fluid overload, and transmission of infection are extremely low, and none of these have been reported in a patient undergoing antenatal treatment for FNAIT. Headaches occur but usually lessen with time. Prednisolone has been widely used in pregnancy, and is known to cause fluid overload, high blood pressure, diabetes mellitus, irritability, and osteoporosis.

Recent Studies of Maternal Treatment –– A collaborative study between European centers reported in 2003 on the antenatal management of FNAIT in 56 fetuses managed with either maternal treatment or platelet transfusions. Maternal therapy, predominantly IVIG, resulted in a platelet count exceeding 50×10^9/L in 67%. The most serious complications encountered were associated with FBS and platelet transfusion, and the results supported the use of maternal therapy as first-line treatment for the antenatal management of FNAIT. The association of lower pre-treatment platelet counts in cases with a sibling history of antenatal ICH or severe thrombocytopenia favors stratification of antenatal management on the basis of the history of FNAIT in previous pregnancies.

In 2006, a North American team reported two randomized controlled trials of maternal treatment stratified according to the previous history of FNAIT[12]:

1. *High-risk* patients had either a sibling with peripartum ICH or one with an initial fetal platelet count $<20 \times 10^9$/L. Patients underwent FBS at 20 weeks or later, and were randomized to receive IVIG alone (1 g/kg per week) or in combination with prednisolone 1 mg/kg per day. There was a satisfactory increase in the fetal platelet count in 89% of pregnancies receiving combination treatment compared to 35% receiving IVIG alone ($P \leq 0.05$). In those with initial fetal platelet counts $< 10 \times 10^9$/L, 82% had a satisfactory response to IVIG and prednisolone compared to only 18% treated with IVIG alone ($P \leq 0.03$). There was one ICH; this occurred in a pregnancy managed with IVIG alone.

2. *Standard risk* patients were those with a sibling who had not had an ICH and a fetal platelet count between 20 and 100×10^9/L. These patients underwent FBS at around 20 weeks and were randomized to receive IVIG (1 g/kg per week) or prednisolone 0.5 mg/kg per day. Subsequent FBS was carried out in all patients at 3- to 8-weekly intervals. There were no significant differences in the responses to the two treatments. There were two cases of ICH; one in a fetus born at 38 weeks' gestation with a platelet count of 172×10^9/L, and one in an infant with a birth platelet count of 68×10^9/L delivered at 28 weeks because of bradycardia following FBS.

There were 11 serious complications out of a total of 175 (6%) FBS, confirming the dangers of FBS and platelet transfusion in FNAIT. This study demonstrates that effective antenatal treatment can be stratified according to the previous history of FNAIT.

The Search for Less Invasive Strategies for the Antenatal Management of FNAIT

Concern regarding the safety of FBS and platelet transfusion has led to a search to develop less invasive treatment strategies involving maternal administration of IVIG while reducing or even avoiding FBS for monitoring the fetal platelet count and administering platelet transfusions.

Some studies suggested that the pre-treatment platelet count had predictive value for the response to maternal treatment. A review of patients treated in North America found that the response rate in fetuses with a pre-treatment platelet count of $>20 \times 10^9$/L was 89%, but was only 51% in those with an initial fetal platelet count of $<20 \times 10^9$/L. The authors suggested that additional FBS might not be warranted in those cases with an initial fetal platelet count $>20 \times 10^9$/L; any gain from identifying and intensifying treatment in "poor responders" would be offset by the complications of additional FBS.

The Leiden group have evaluated less intensive antenatal treatment strategies over a number of years and found that a non-invasive strategy based on treatment with IVIG without FBS appears to be effective when there is no history of ICH in a previous pregnancy[13]. The same group extended this approach to the management of seven high-risk pregnancies where there had been a previous sibling history of ICH. IVIG was administered from 16 to 19 weeks' gestation in the six pregnancies where there had been previous antenatal ICH, and from 28–29 weeks in the case where ICH was postnatal. The total number of weekly IVIG infusions ranged from 8 to 21. The platelet count at birth ranged from 10 to 49×10^9/L. No ICH was seen on antenatal or postnatal ultrasound examinations, and all infants were doing well at follow-up at 3 months.

Optimal Approach for the Modern Antenatal Management of FNAIT

There has been huge progress in the antenatal management of FNAIT over the last 20 years. However, the ideal effective treatment without significant side effects to the mother or fetus has yet to be determined.

There are some basic principles to consider in the management of an individual case[2]:

1. Obtain as much information as possible about the clinical history of previously affected pregnancies with FNAIT focusing on the neonatal thrombocytopenia to exclude other causes of thrombocytopenia. It is important to determine as conclusively as possible if an ICH has occurred and if so, when.
2. Ensure that comprehensive laboratory investigations have been carried out in a reference laboratory, including testing for HPA antibodies and the identification of their specificity and HPA genotyping of the mother and her partner. If the partner is heterozygous for the relevant HPA, the fetal HPA genotype should be established.
3. Affected fetuses should be managed in referral centers with experience in the antenatal

management of FNAIT. Close collaboration is required between specialists in fetal medicine, obstetrics, hematology/transfusion medicine, and pediatrics.
4. The mother and her partner should be provided with detailed information about FNAIT and its potential clinical consequences, and the benefits and risks of different approaches to antenatal management.
5. Maternally administered therapy should be the first-line approach in all cases. This is based on data describing the effectiveness and safety of maternal treatment. Different centers have different strategies based on their own experience and those of published studies. Stratification of antenatal treatment based on the history of FNAIT in previous pregnancies is usual.
6. An example algorithm of the antenatal management of FNAIT is shown in Figure 10.4 [14]. No FBS is carried out so the maternal treatment is very intensive and is based on a "worst case" assumption that the fetal platelet count will be the lowest possible for each category of affected pregnancy (no sibling history of ICH, sibling with ICH after 28 weeks' gestation, and sibling with ICH before 28 weeks' gestation).

Summary

There have been considerable advances in the clinical and laboratory diagnosis of FNAIT and its postnatal and antenatal management. The antenatal management of FNAIT has been particularly problematic, because severe hemorrhage occurs as early as 16 weeks' gestation and there is no non-invasive investigation that reliably predicts the severity of FNAIT in utero. The strategies for antenatal treatment have included the use of serial platelet transfusions, which, while effective, are invasive and associated with significant morbidity and mortality. Maternal therapy involving the administration of intravenous immunoglobulin and/or steroids is also effective and associated with fewer risks to the fetus. Significant recent progress has involved refinement of maternal treatment, stratifying it according to the likely severity of FNAIT based on the history in previous pregnancies.

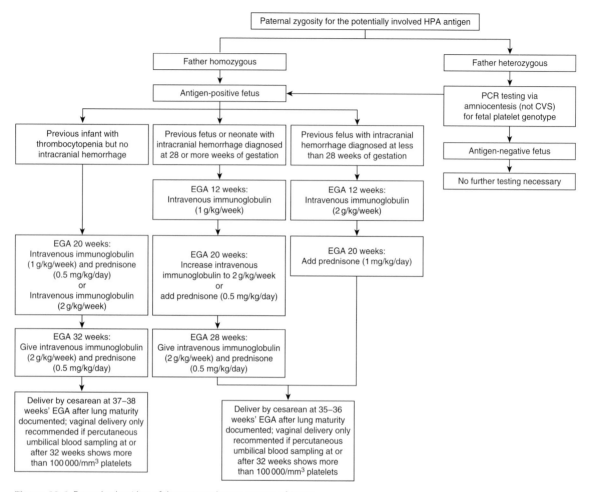

Figure 10.4 Example algorithm of the antenatal management of FNAIT.

Case Studies

Case Study 1
This case report describes the antenatal management of very severe FNAIT due to anti-HPA-1a. The patient's past history was the loss of her first three pregnancies due to ICH at 28, 19, and 16 weeks' gestation. Maternal treatment with intravenous immunoglobulin and steroids was started from 14 weeks in the third pregnancy. The fourth pregnancy was managed by administering weekly intraperitoneal injections of immunoglobulin to the fetus from 12 to 18 weeks. At 18 weeks' gestation, fetal blood sampling was carried out and the fetal platelet count was 12×10^9/L. Serial weekly fetal platelet transfusions were administered but there were poor responses because of immune destruction of the transfused platelets by maternal HLA antibodies. There were improved responses to transfusions prepared from the mother and from HLA-compatible HPA-1a-negative donors. At 35 weeks' gestation, a normal infant was delivered by cesarean section. This case illustrates several important points about FNAIT: its severe clinical consequences; how early ICH can occur; and the need to tailor management according to the specific clinical circumstances and to change it if it becomes necessary. This case report has been published[15].

Case Study 2
This case report describes the postnatal management of FNAIT due to an HPA antibody of undetermined specificity. The past history was of a first uncomplicated full-term pregnancy. The second pregnancy was also uncomplicated but skin bleeding was noted after birth and the neonatal platelet count was 4×10^9/L. The baby was otherwise well

110

and a provisional diagnosis of FNAIT was made. HPA-1a/5b-negative platelets were transfused on several occasions with no effect and intravenous immunoglobulin (1 g/kg) was administered, but the highest platelet count was only 25×10^9/L. Investigations found that the mother was HPA-1a positive and only maternal HLA antibodies were detected on routine testing. Cross-match of the mother's plasma versus the father's platelets was positive in the platelet immunofluorescence test (PIFT) but negative in MAIPA. It was considered that FNAIT might be due to a "private" HPA antibody. Transfusions of unwashed maternal platelets produced excellent and sustained responses with immediate post-transfusion platelet counts of >200×10^9/L. There was persistent thrombocytopenia possibly due to infusion of maternal HPA antibody with the platelet transfusions. The platelets were unwashed as it was considered to be more important to avoid additional manipulation and possible damage to the maternal platelets than the infusion of maternal antibody and prolongation of the neonatal thrombocytopenia. Further investigations are being carried out to determine the specificity of the HPA antibody. This case report illustrates the need to monitor responses to postnatal platelet transfusions and to change the management if there are poor responses to standard treatment, i.e. HPA-1a/5b-negative platelets.

References

1. Murphy MF, Bussel JB. Advances in the management of alloimmune thrombocytopenia. *British Journal of Haematology* 2007; **136**: 366–378.

2. Curtis BR, McFarland JG. Human platelet antigens – 2013. *Vox Sanguinis* 2014; **106**: 93–102.

3. Kamphuis MM, Paridaans NP, Porcelijn L, Lopriore E, Oepkes D. Incidence and consequences of neonatal alloimmune thrombocytopenia: a systematic review. *Pediatrics* 2014; **133**: 715–721.

4. Kamphuis MM, Paridaans NP, Porcelijn L *et al.* Screening in pregnancy for fetal or neonatal alloimmune thrombocytopenia: a systematic review. *British Journal of Obstetrics and Gynaecology* 2010; **117**: 1335–1343.

5. Spencer JA, Burrows RF. Feto-maternal alloimmune thrombocytopenia: a literature review and statistical analysis. *Australian and New Zealand Journal of Obstetrics and Gynecology* 2001; **41**: 45–55.

6. Heyu N. Fetal and neonatal alloimmune thrombocytopenia: lessons learned from animal models. *Blood Journal* 2013; **122**: SCI 50

7. Radder CM, Brand A, Kanhai HH. Will it ever be possible to balance the risk of intracranial hemorrhage in fetal or neonatal alloimmune thrombocytopenia against the risk of treatment strategies to prevent it? *Vox Sanguinis* 2003; **84**: 318–325.

8. Murphy MF, Williamson LM, Urbaniak SJ. Antenatal screening for fetomaternal alloimmune thrombocytopenia: should we be doing it? *Vox Sanguinis* 2002; **83** (Suppl 1): 409–416.

9. Allen D, Verjee S, Rees S, Murphy MF, Roberts DJ. Platelet transfusion in neonatal alloimmune thrombocytopenia. *Blood* 2007; **109**; 388–389.

10. Rayment R, Brunskill SJ, Soothill PW, *et al.* Antenatal interventions for fetomaternal alloimmune thrombocytopenia. *Cochrane Database of Systematic Reviews* 2011; **5**: CD004226. doi: 10.1002/14651858.

11. Bussel JB, Berkowitz RL, Lynch L *et al.* Antenatal management of alloimmune thrombocytopenia with intravenous gammaglobulin: a randomized trial of the addition of low dose steroid to IVIg in fifty-five maternal–fetal pairs. *American Journal of Obstetrics and Gynecology* 1996; **174**: 1414–1423.

12. Berkowitz RL, Kolb EA, McFarland JG *et al.* Parallel randomized trials of risk-based therapy for fetal alloimmune thrombocytopenia. *Obstetrics and Gynecology* 2006; **107**: 91–96.

13. Radder CM, Brand A, Kanhai HHH. A less invasive treatment strategy to prevent intracranial hemorrhage in fetal and neonatal alloimmune thrombocytopenia. *American Journal of Obstetrics and Gynecology* 2001; **185**: 683–688.

14. Pacheco LD, Berkowitz RL, Moise KJ, Jr *et al.* Fetal and neonatal alloimmune thrombocytopenia: a management algorithm based on risk stratification. *Obstetrics and Gynecology* 2011; **118**: 1157–1163.

15. Murphy MF, Metcalfe P, Waters AH *et al.* Antenatal management of severe feto-maternal alloimmune thrombocytopenia: HLA incompatibility may affect responses to fetal platelet transfusions. *Blood* 1993: **81**: 2174–2179.

Red Cell Alloimmunization

Alec McEwan

Introduction

Hemolytic disease of the fetus and newborn (HDFN) describes a process of rapid red blood cell breakdown, which puts the baby at risk of anemia and kernicterus (bilirubin-induced cerebral damage) within the first few days of life. A variety of etiologies are recognized; however, this chapter focuses on red cell alloimmunization, i.e. the immune-mediated destruction of erythrocytes initiated by maternal red cell antibodies which reach the fetal circulation by transportation across the placenta, onwards from approximately 12 weeks' gestation.

Pathogenesis

Antibodies recognizing red cell surface antigens usually arise secondary to a blood transfusion, or following the birth of a baby with a different blood group to the mother. Fetal red blood cells "traffick" into the maternal circulation throughout pregnancy, but "isoimmunization" against foreign antigens occurs most frequently around the time of delivery when the size of fetomaternal hemorrhage (FMH) tends to be greatest. Other events associated with FMH are listed in Table 11.1. These red cell antibodies can, in a subsequent pregnancy, reach the fetal circulation and cause immune-mediated destruction of fetal red blood cells. This transplacental transportation of maternal immunoglobulin G begins in the early second trimester and red cell antibodies recognizing certain erythrocyte antigens may bind and bring about premature destruction of the fetal red cells by the reticuloendothelial system. One of the breakdown products of heme is bilirubin, and levels rise within the fetus and amniotic fluid, although placental transfer limits this accumulation. Progressive anemia initially stimulates the bone marrow first but, as its capacity to maintain the hemoglobin levels is exceeded, extramedullary hematopoiesis becomes increasingly important. This hyperactivity of the reticuloendothelial system results in fetal hepatosplenomegaly. A degree of portal hypertension and hypoalbuminemia secondary to liver dysfunction may contribute to extracellular fluid accumulation within the

Table 11.1 Clinical scenarios associated with FMH and risk of isoimmunization

Any birth (including by cesarean section)
Manual removal of retained placenta
Stillbirths and intrauterine deaths
Abdominal trauma in the third trimester
Delivery of twins
Unexplained hydrops fetalis
Invasive prenatal diagnostic procedures such as amniocentesis or CVS
Antepartum hemorrhage
External cephalic version
Hydatidiform mole
Termination of pregnancy (prophylaxis is recommended at all gestations and with all methods)
Ectopic pregnancy (regardless of mode of treatment)
Spontaneous miscarriage ≥12 weeks (see below)

Adapted from RCOG Green-Top Guideline No. 22[1].

fetus (hydrops fetalis); however, cardiac dysfunction is more likely to be the main explanation for hydropic change. Fetal anemia induces a high-output cardiac state and a degree of hypoxia may directly impair myocardial contractility. Hydrops is characterized by skin edema, pleural and pericardial effusions, cardiomegaly, atrioventicular valve dysfunction, ascites, polyhydramnios, and placentomegaly, all of which can be detected by ultrasound scanning (Figures 11.1–11.3). These changes are seen only when fetal hemoglobin levels decline well below the normal range and are a late feature of *erythroblastosis fetalis*. Intrauterine death will ensue in severe cases if the problem is not treated or the baby delivered.

HDFN describes the consequences of this antenatal pathogenic process as it continues on into the newborn period. Maternal immunoglobulin G (IgG) remains with the baby for 4–6 months after birth and top-up blood transfusions may be needed by the infant while hemolysis continues. Far more concerning than this semi-chronic postnatal anemia, however, is the risk of kernicterus, which occurs within the first few days of

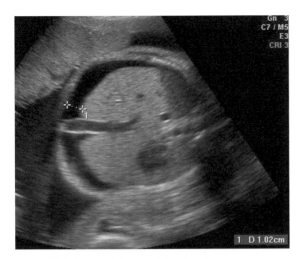

Figure 11.1 Antenatal ultrasound showing a transverse section through the upper fetal abdomen at the level of the stomach and liver. The calipers are measuring a 10-mm rim of ascites. There are numerous etiologies for fetal ascites, but fetal anemia (from any cause) is one of the more common explanations.

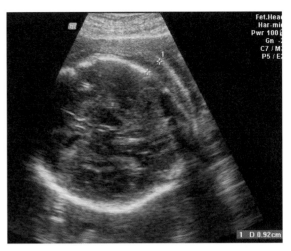

Figure 11.2 Antenatal ultrasound showing a transverse section through the fetal cranium. The calipers are measuring 9 mm of scalp edema. Edema can collect throughout the skin of the fetus in severe anemia. This results from a combination of high-output cardiac failure and also possible hepatic dysfunction and hypoproteinemia.

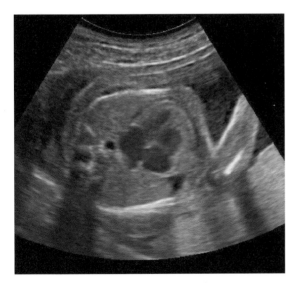

Figure 11.3 Antenatal ultrasound showing a transverse section through the fetal chest. A slender fetal pericardial effusion and a small left-sided pleural effusion behind the heart can be seen. The heart is also subjectively enlarged. These features are all consistent with, but are non-specific signs of, fetal anemia.

life. The immature fetal liver is unable to conjugate the excessive circulating bilirubin and, as serum levels rise, it permeates the blood–brain barrier. The globus pallidus of the basal ganglia and the brain stem nuclei are the structures most at risk of damage from the unconjugated bilirubin, which is thought to uncouple phosphorylation from oxidation, resulting in reduced ATP synthesis and impairment of energy-dependent metabolism. Athetoid cerebral palsy, other movement disorders, deafness, and impaired eye movements may all be long-term sequelae of kernicterus.

Repeated exposure of an isoimmunized woman to the same red cell antigen, as occurs in successive pregnancies, will further stimulate antibody production. Subsequent pregnancies, which express the blood group in question, have a tendency to show more severe hemolysis, and at earlier gestations.

Genotype and Phenotype

There are almost 30 different blood grouping systems, but the ABO and Rhesus groups are arguably the most important clinically. The Rhesus D (RhD) antigen was discovered in 1939, but the full complexity of this blood group system has only become evident much more recently with the advent of molecular biology.

Sixteen percent of white Europeans, 5% of West Africans, and virtually no Chinese are RhD negative. Of all deliveries in the UK, 10% are of RhD positive babies born to RhD negative women. In the absence of preventive measures, 1 in 6 RhD negative women will isoimmunize if they deliver a term RhD positive baby, and in the 1950s, 1 in 2000 babies died of HDFN, principally due to RhD isoimmunization.

The Rhesus proteins are coded for by two genes which share a major degree of homology. *RHD* and *RHCE* lie very close to one another, back-to-back, on

113

chromosome 1 and are thought to have arisen from a duplication event involving the original ancestral Rhesus gene, which can still be found in rodents and most other mammals. The Rhesus proteins are characterized by 12 intramembranous segments and 6 extracellular "surface" loops. Their function remains unclear, although ammonium ion transportation and gas exchange across the erythrocyte cell membrane have been postulated.

The RhD negative phenotype is recognized in the laboratory by failure of red cells to agglutinate with standard anti-D reagents (antibodies). The underlying genetic explanation for this phenotype is more complex. In Europeans, 90% of RhD negative individuals have a complete deletion of *RHD*, with the remaining cases being explained by nonsense and frameshift mutations which truncate the protein. However, in the majority of African individuals typed as RhD negative the genotype is very different. The two common *RHD* variants resulting in the D negative phenotype are the RHD pseudogene, *RHDψ*, which codes for a non-functional protein, and the *Cde^s* allele, which contains segments from both the *RHD* and the *RHCE* genes.

The situation is confused even further by alleles of *RHD*, which cause subtle *qualitative* changes in the extracellular surface loops of the RhD protein, meaning that serological tests are only weakly positive with standard anti-D reagents. Furthermore, missense mutations causing single amino acid substitutions in the intramembranous or cytoplasmic portions of the RhD protein may impair integration of the protein into the membrane, so bringing about a *quantitative* reduction in the number of cell-surface antigen sites per red blood cell. This too may reduce the agglutination response of these cells to standard laboratory anti-D

antibodies. These "partial D" and "weak D" phenotypes, as they are respectively known, can be important from a clinical perspective and will be discussed in greater detail later.

The DNA sequence of the *RHCE* gene shows far less variation, and differences at just five amino acid positions result in the four different antigens C, c, E, and e. Each allele expresses only C or c, in combination with E or e, and, among Europeans, the Ce haplotype is most common.

Prevention of RhD Isoimmunization

Antibodies against all the Rhesus proteins, and other red cell antigens, can cause erythroblastosis and HDN; however, anti-D has historically been of greatest significance. Prevention of RhD isoimmunization, and improvements in the antenatal and neonatal care of isoimmunized women and their babies, has all but eradicated serious morbidity and mortality associated with this condition. Some of the key landmarks in the evolution of this success story are listed in Table 11.2. By the early 1960s, Stern had demonstrated that exogenous anti-D given to RhD negative individuals could prevent immunization occurring when RhD positive blood was transfused into them.

Exogenous anti-D is produced by exposing RhD negative volunteers to the RhD antigen. These individuals are either men or women who have completed their families. They regularly donate their blood, and cold-ethanol precipitation is used to separate the immunoglobulins from their hyperimmune plasma. Following the emergence of variant Creutzfeldt-Jakob disease in the UK, only plasma from US volunteers has been used more recently, although it is not known for certain if prions can be transmitted via transfused immunoglobulins. A solvent/detergent

Table 11.2 Key events in the history of prevention of RhD isoimmunization

1938	Darrow concludes that "erythroblastosis fetalis" results from the formation of a maternal antibody against some component of fetal blood
1939	Levine and Stetson postulate that maternal immunization is caused by a fetal antigen inherited from the father which is lacking in the mother
1940	Landsteiner and Wiener discover the Rhesus antigen
1948	Wiener suggests that the initiating process is occult placental hemorrhage
1957	Kleihauer devises a test able to detect fetal cells in the maternal circulation
1961	Stern gives RhD positive red blood cells to RhD negative volunteers, both with and without anti-D, and shows that alloimmunization can be prevented
1966	Freda demonstrates that isoimmunization can be prevented by giving anti-D to recently delivered RhD negative women
1969	Widespread introduction of routine postnatal prophylaxis with anti-D following multicenter trials

treatment inactivates HIV, hepatitis B, and hepatitis C. BPL, one of the major manufacturers of anti-D, estimates a risk of viral infection of 1 in 10 000 billion doses of their product and, to date, there have been no recorded cases.

There were theoretical concerns that passive anti-D might itself cause hemolysis within the fetus. There is certainly no doubt that it can cross the placenta. Although a small number of babies were born in the anti-D trials with a weakly positive direct antiglobulin test (DAT), the reaction was insufficiently strong to cause significant hemolysis or anemia.

Delivery was recognized to be the time of greatest risk for FMH and by the end of the 1960s widespread postnatal prophylaxis had been introduced. A Cochrane review of six eligible trials of routine postpartum anti-D prophylaxis gives a relative risk of 0.12 for RhD alloimmunization in the subsequent pregnancy, i.e. a tenfold reduction in the incidence of isoimmunization[2]. Various doses of anti-D have been tried, and indeed protocols still vary around the world today. Doses of less than 500 IU are associated with a greater risk of isoimmunization; however, higher doses do not seem to confer any obvious benefit. A dose of 125 IU anti-D is able to neutralize 1 mL of fetal red blood cells. Fetomaternal hemorrhage (FMH) of ≥30 mL occurs in only 0.6% of all deliveries. A dose of 1500 IU has been adopted in the USA to cover the possibility of larger hemorrhages. In the UK and France, a smaller dose of 500 IU is routinely used; however, a test is also performed to quantify the size of the FMH (Table 11.3). Occasional bleeds exceeding 4 mL are recognized and a higher dose of anti-D is administered.

The anti-D is usually given by intramuscular injection (although intravenous preparations are available) and ideally should be given within 72 hours of delivery (or any other possible sensitizing event). There may, however, be benefit in giving anti-D as much as 9–10 days following potential isoimmunizing events.

Later came the recognition that a variety of events during pregnancy might cause or be associated with FMH, other than delivery, and that these might subsequently also lead to isoimmunization (Table 11.1). The RCOG Green-Top Guideline (No. 22) lists these situations and recommends the use of anti-D prophylaxis in these scenarios also[1]. The RhD antigen is thought to be expressed as early as 7–8 weeks' gestation and there is no doubt that FMH can be demonstrated during the first trimester. As little as 0.25 mL of fetal RhD positive blood may be sufficient to cause isoimmunization and older studies have shown that this value is often exceeded with FMH occurring after 8 weeks. The studies examining the risk of first trimester isoimmunization are old and few in number[3]. The risk probably lies between 0 and 3%, but does seem to be higher when the uterus is instrumented.

The RCOG have recommended anti-D only for miscarriages prior to 12 weeks if the uterus is instrumented. After 12 weeks, and before 20 weeks, 250 IU of anti-D should be given for all threatened and actual miscarriages. Miscarriages and other potential sensitizing events after 20 weeks should be covered by 500 IU of anti-D and a Kleihauer should be taken to identify those cases where the size of the FMH exceeds 4 mL[1].

Routine Antenatal Prophylaxis

Even in the absence of defined events known to be associated with FMH, leakage of fetal red blood cells into the maternal circulation is known to occur throughout pregnancy. Beyond 28 weeks' gestation the quantity of trafficked cells can be great enough to bring about alloimmunization. Indeed, "silent" FMH will cause RhD isoimmunization in 1–2% of all RhD negative women with RhD positive pregnancies.

There is good-quality evidence supporting the use of routine antenatal anti-D prophylaxis (RAADP) to prevent these isoimmunizations. A consensus conference hosted by the RCOG and Royal College of Physicians in 1997 came out strongly in favor of routine antenatal prophylaxis. Crowther subsequently published a systematic review in the Cochrane database, although only two trials were deemed of high enough quality to be included. This review reported a relative risk of isoimmunization of 0.4 in the women receiving RAADP. More recently, a Technology Appraisal Guidance (No. 41), produced by NICE[4],

Table 11.3 Tests used to quantify the size of a FMH

Kleihauer: Fetal hemoglobin (HbF) is more resistant to acid or alkaline elution than adult hemoglobin. After treatment, any erythrocytes containing HbF retain their hemoglobin and can be stained and recognized. Unfortunately, some adults have persistent HbF production and this can confuse matters. Furthermore, quantification is less precise with bigger bleeds.

Flow cytometry: This uses immunofluorescently stained antibodies to recognize fetal erythrocytes, which can then be flow-sorted and quantified. This method is often preferred for larger bleeds.

has reviewed the wider evidence from nine trials. Although the trials varied in design and methodology, they gave remarkably consistent results. Without RAADP the isoimmunization rate ranged from 0.9 to 1.6%. This fell to approximately 0.3% in the groups receiving RAADP.

A number of attempts at estimating the cost-effectiveness of this intervention have been made. The number of HDFN-related deaths would be reduced from approximately 30 to 10 per year in the UK if all women received RAADP. The cost–benefit seems clear for women in their first pregnancy, but less so for parous women. Ultimately, however, both the RCOG and NICE have recommended RAADP for all RhD negative women, irrespective of parity.

The following dosage schedules are currently in use in the UK:

- A – 500 IU at 28 weeks' and 34 weeks' gestation
- B – a single dose of 1500 IU at 28 weeks' gestation

Schedule A was used in the only randomized controlled trial of RAADP (Hutchet) and was most widely adopted in the UK[4]. The half-life of anti-D is 24 days and theoretically there is less circulating anti-D left at 40 weeks' gestation with schedule B than with A. The trials using this regime however did not show significantly poorer results. Commercially available preparations of 1500 IU anti-D are now available in the UK, and schedule B is now supported by NICE guidance. It is more cost-effective and more convenient (one injection rather than two).

Refusal of Anti-D Prophylaxis

A small minority of women will refuse anti-D, either as part of RAADP or following potentially sensitizing events (including delivery), perhaps due to safety fears or "needle phobia." The woman should be provided with good-quality information to ensure that this choice is truly informed. Declining anti-D prophylaxis carries no risk when:

1. the woman is confident she is not going to have further children (e.g. requesting sterilization); or
2. when the father of the baby, or the fetus itself, is known with certainty to be RhD negative.

Widespread non-invasive prenatal fetal RhD testing is possible (see later) and means that RAADP and the use of anti-D following sensitizing events will be reserved for women carrying a fetus which is RhD positive or of unknown status[5].

Traditional Management of Isoimmunization

Despite effective prophylaxis programs, new cases of RhD isoimmunization do arise, either because guidelines are not followed appropriately, women fail to seek medical advice around the time of potentially sensitizing events, or because of "silent" isoimmunizations, perhaps occurring prior to 28 weeks' gestation. Management of these pregnancies has become limited to a relatively small number of centers. Preventing morbidity and mortality in these cases necessitates the identification of pregnancies at risk, subsequent monitoring of disease severity, and timely intervention in the form of intrauterine transfusion and/or delivery of the baby. Modern management is quite different to that of even just 10 years ago and, to best appreciate the recent advances made, a brief review of traditional methods is included here.

Historical Perspectives

Routine maternal blood typing and serological testing was introduced in the 1950s. RhD negative women with anti-D antibodies were recognized as being at risk of having their pregnancies complicated by hydrops, stillbirth, and hemolytic disease of the newborn. Approximately 85% of the white European and North American population is RhD positive, and just over half are heterozygous. The offspring of RhD heterozygous males and RhD negative women are at 50% risk of being RhD positive themselves, and 50% will be RhD negative. The RhD negative fetus is at no risk of hemolysis, however high the levels of maternal anti-D. Although RhD negativity in male partners could be determined with certainty, predicting whether a RhD positive man was homo- or heterozygous was imprecise prior to the advent of molecular biology and relied on the results of serological testing with anti-sera to the D, C, c, E, and e antigens and racially specific incidence charts. However, this prediction was inexact and, when a male partner was thought to be heterozygous, the status of the fetus remained unclear. An RhD negative pregnancy could be exposed to invasive testing when there was no actual risk.

With the development of molecular genetic techniques, and improved understanding of the Rhesus gene cluster, it became possible to determine RhD status precisely using DNA amplification techniques [6]. These are able to sensitively distinguish between homozygotes and heterozygotes and can be applied to DNA from amniocytes to precisely assign RhD positive or negative status to the fetus of a couple where the male partner is heterozygous. A single amniocentesis meant that further testing could be avoided in 50% of cases (those found to be RhD negative). Surveillance and invasive testing could then be appropriately focused on the RhD positive pregnancies.

A number of different factors have been used to time interventions in Rhesus disease. The simplest and least sensitive of these is previous obstetric history. Walker showed how, in an RhD isoimmunized pregnancy, the risk of stillbirth was 8% if there was no previous history of HDFN. This rose to 18% if a previous child had been moderately affected and to 58% if there was a previous history of stillbirth caused by hemolytic disease. The tendency for the disease to become more severe, and at progressively earlier gestations, was well recognized. Recent retrospective reviews of isoimmunized pregnancies have confirmed these historical conclusions. However, relying on previous history to guide intervention was imprecise and hazardous.

Coombs demonstrated that the strength of anti-D isoimmunization could be measured by serially diluting maternal serum until agglutination of RhD positive red blood cells no longer occurred. The more doubling dilutions were required to lose this reaction, the more anti-D must have been there to begin with. Serial dilutions of 1/2, 1/4, 1/8, 1/16, 1/32, 1/64, and 1/128 indicated progressively higher starting levels of anti-D. More recently, levels of anti-D have been quantified more precisely in "international units per mL" (IU/mL) using different techniques. Significant hemolysis is unlikely at levels below 4 IU/mL and is unlikely to be severe at levels below 15 IU/mL. However, this threshold too is insensitive and the relationship between absolute anti-D levels and disease severity weakens in pregnancies beyond the first where antibodies are detected.

Nevertheless, these factors have been used (and still are to some degree) to decide when to investigate further with amniocentesis, perform fetal blood sampling, or indeed deliver.

Amniocentesis

Immune-mediated hemolysis within the fetus generates bilirubin, which is excreted by the fetal kidneys into the amniotic fluid. Ballantyne, at the end of the nineteenth century, recognized that yellow staining of amniotic fluid was associated with the subsequent development of severe jaundice in the newborn. Bevis recognized that the degree of yellow pigmentation of amniotic fluid samples taken during pregnancy offered a guide to the final outcome; however, reliable measurement of bilirubin concentrations proved difficult and the alternative technique of measuring the optical density shift caused by the bilirubin was adopted. Using a spectrophotometer, the optical density of amniotic fluid is assessed across a wide spectrum of wavelengths. Bilirubin causes a shift in absorption at the 450 nm wavelength and the degree of this shift (ΔOD450) is proportional to the concentration of bilirubin. In the early 1960s, Liley published a chart which could be used to estimate the risk of severe anemia in an isoimmunized pregnancy based on the ΔOD450 of amniotic fluid collected by amniocentesis after 27 weeks' gestation; the higher the ΔOD450, the greater the chance of severe fetal anemia. Results falling above a certain threshold ("Zone 3") would prompt intrauterine blood sampling and a subsequent transfusion if the fetus was found to be significantly anemic. When managing a RhD isoimmunized pregnancy, the timing of the first amniocentesis was decided by a number of factors, including previous history and anti-D titer (or concentration). If the ΔOD450 fell below these thresholds, repeated amniocenteses were subsequently required at intervals of 1 to 4 weeks, depending on the initial result, the rate of rise between successive samplings, the Rhesus history, and the anti-D level. In a group of pregnancies with a high incidence of fetal anemia, the sensitivity for detection of severe anemia (Hb of less than 5 SD below the mean) was found to be approximately 80%[7], meaning that 1 in 5 severely anemic fetuses would be missed by the amniocentesis. Reducing the ΔOD450 threshold above which fetal blood sampling would be performed did improve the sensitivity to nearly 100% but went together with a drop in the specificity (below 50%) and positive predictive value, meaning that a significant number of fetal blood samplings were being prompted by the ΔOD450 when, in fact, the fetus was not severely affected (false positives). Other studies quote somewhat different sensitivities and specificities but the overall message remains the same. Later, the Liley charts were extrapolated backward to 20 weeks' gestation but this too was associated with a reduction in the sensitivity, as demonstrated by Nicolaides. These were not the only weaknesses of amniocentesis used in this way (Table 11.4).

Table 11.4 The disadvantages of amniocentesis and ΔOD450 measurements in the assessment of immune-mediated fetal anemia

- 0.5–1.0% risk of miscarriage/preterm delivery/ chorioamnionitis/perinatal loss with each procedure
- Limited performance as a screening test, particularly at gestations <28 weeks
- Cause of fetomaternal hemorrhage and subsequent rise in antibody levels in 50% of cases
- A surrogate marker for fetal anemia. Particularly problematic in Kell isoimmunized pregnancies (see pp. 125)
- Unpleasant for the woman

Table 11.5 Historical landmarks in the development of fetal blood transfusion

1963	(Liley)	X-ray guided intraperitoneal IUT
1964	(Freda and Adamsons)	Direct IUT through hysterotomy incision
1981	(Rodeck)	Fetoscopically guided intravascular IUT
1981	(Berkowitz and Hobbins)	Ultrasound-guided intraperitoneal IUT
1986	(Nicolaides and Rodeck)	Ultrasound-guided intravascular IUT

Nevertheless, when the procedure-related risks associated with amniocentesis (0.5–1.0%) were compared with those of fetal blood sampling (1–4%) the benefit in "screening" by ΔOD450 prior to fetal blood sampling seemed clear. The optimum timing of first, and repeated, amniocentesis required significant experience but it soon became adopted as standard practice in most centers. Some questioned whether, with improvements in fetal blood transfusion techniques, it should be abandoned; however, the practice continued until newer non-invasive methods became more widespread at the beginning of the new millennium (see pp. 120). It is rare now for amniocentesis to be performed in the management of RhD isoimmunization.

Fetal Blood Transfusion

Prenatal treatment options for RhD hemolytic disease, other than preterm delivery, really began in the 1960s when Liley showed that the fetus could be transfused in utero by injection of blood into the fetal peritoneal cavity under X-ray guidance. A radio-opaque dye was injected into the amniotic cavity and taken up by the fetus. On reaching the bowel, it outlined the peritoneal cavity, into which the blood was injected. Erythrocytes were then absorbed directly across the bowel wall into the fetal intravascular compartment. This hazardous procedure was later superseded by ultrasound-guided transfusions into the peritoneal cavity and then directly into the fetal circulation. The timeline of the evolution of this remarkable fetal therapy is detailed in Table 11.5.

Intraperitoneal transfusion (IPT) had a number of drawbacks. No pre- or post-transfusion fetal hemoglobin level or hematocrit was available, so the volume to be transfused was, at best, an educated guess. Absorption of the donated red cells was slow and this was of particular concern for the very anemic fetus where immediate and rapid correction was needed.

The presence of edema could interfere with absorption completely. Furthermore, overdistension of the fetal abdomen by the donated blood possibly endangered the fetus by interfering with venous return and cardiac output. As intravascular transfusion (IVT) became more popular, comparative studies suggested a sixfold greater risk of fetal death following IPT.

Ultrasound-guided direct intravascular transfusions are performed via a number of different routes. Direct intracardiac transfusion is possible but, for understandable reasons, is not ideal. The majority of fetal IVT are performed into the umbilical vein at the insertion of the umbilical cord into the placenta or percutaneously into the intrahepatic portion of the umbilical vein[8]. A free loop of cord can be used if the placental insertion cannot be accessed. There is little evidence to suggest any one method is superior to the others. Whichever route is favored, the uterine wall, amniotic membrane, and sometimes the placenta, must be breached by the needle. The risk of fetal loss, membrane rupture, bradycardia, or fetal bleeding requiring delivery is quoted to be between 2.0% and 4.0% per procedure[9], but this depends on gestation, operator experience, and fetal condition prior to the transfusion. Transfusions below 20 weeks' gestation are a particular challenge and fetal loss rate is at least 10% if there is hydrops.

The blood used for a fetal transfusion is cross-matched against the maternal blood and should be fresh, cytomegalovirus (CMV) negative, and irradiated. The cross-matched unit ideally has a hematocrit of 75–80%, so as to minimize the volume load of the transfusion on the fetus. A degree of "overtransfusion" to a hematocrit of 40–50% will prolong the interval between subsequent transfusions. However, the transfused blood is acidotic and this and the volume load can be hazardous to the compromised hydropic fetus. In these cases, a hematocrit of 25% should be aimed for with the first transfusion, which can be followed 2 or 3 days later with a second "top-up." The total volume (in milliliters) to be transfused (V_T) is determined by the fetoplacental blood volume (V_{Fet}), which increases with gestation, the hematocrit of the fetal and donated blood (Hct_{Fet} and Hct_{Don}), and the target "desired" hematocrit (Hct_{Des}) according to the equation:

$$V_T(mL) = V_{Fet}(mL) \times \frac{Hct_{Des} - Hct_{Fet}}{Hct_{Don} - Hct_{Des}}$$

There is a steady increase in the total blood volume of the fetoplacental circuit (V_{Fet}) with advancing gestation, from approximately 25 mL at 20 weeks' gestation to 100 mL at 28 weeks', and 210 mL at 34 weeks' gestation. Nomograms and online calculators, which use fetal weight, are available to more precisely estimate V_{Fet}.

Maternal sedation is usually employed because the procedure can be uncomfortable and may last more than 30 minutes. These sedative drugs may also help to reduce fetal movement. Fetal paralysis using pancuronium has been described, but has not been adopted universally. Antibiotics and oral tocolytics are used by some operators, but there is no evidence to support or refute this practice. The maternal abdomen is sterilized and draped and strict aseptic technique is followed. Local anesthetic is injected into the maternal abdominal wall. Under ultrasound guidance, a 20 gauge needle is inserted through the uterine wall into the umbilical cord, or the vessels within the fetal liver. A small sample of blood is taken to confirm correct positioning and the hematocrit measured immediately, so that the total volume required can be calculated rapidly. Pancuronium is given at this point, if desired. Transfusion of blood at 5 mL per minute is usually tolerated well by the fetus. A post-transfusion hematocrit is taken to help guide the interval between transfusions. The hematocrit drops by approximately 1% per day, but this rate may decline as subsequent transfusions replace the fetal RhD positive blood with donated RhD negative blood, which survives longer. The interval is usually 2–3 weeks and newer scanning techniques may help to fine-tune this (see pp. 120). Serial transfusions are usually performed until 34–36 weeks' gestation, after which delivery is organized. Severe, early onset hemolytic disease may necessitate more than five transfusions in a single pregnancy. A vaginal birth should be the aim, unless there are other obstetric factors or the fetus is compromised.

Current Management

Despite the declining incidence of RhD isoimmunization, recent estimates suggest that 1 in 250 pregnancies is complicated by clinically significant red cell antibodies. The management of affected pregnancies has moved on, employing new technologies and therapeutic interventions, and the need for invasive assessment of the "at risk" pregnancy can be directed now with greater precision. Newer treatment options have shown promise in helping to avoid the need for transfusions at very early gestations.

Antibody Testing and Subsequent Care

Guidelines from the British Committee for Standards in Hematology[10], Royal College of Obstetricians and Gynecologists[11], and NICE all advocate testing all women for red cell antibodies at booking, and again at 28 weeks' gestation. Approximately 1% of pregnant women will be found to have a clinically significant red cell antibody which may carry a risk of cross-matching problems, hemolytic disease of the fetus and newborn, or both.

Women with red cell antibodies should be referred for consultant-based obstetric care and an explanation should be given regarding the potential implications. If there has been a previous history of HDFN, this care should be provided by a specialist in fetal medicine from the outset. Anti-D is the most frequent antibody responsible for serious HDFN and Rhesus D antibody levels should be measured every 4 weeks until 28 weeks' gestation, and fortnightly thereafter. Levels below 4 IU/mL are very unlikely to cause significant HDFN, whereas levels between 4 and 15 IU/mL carry a moderate risk, and levels of more than 15 IU/mL a high risk. Referral to a fetal medicine specialist should certainly occur when anti-D levels reach 4 IU/mL and a prior history of HDFN should prompt immediate review, whatever the level of antibody. Once a red cell antibody with the potential for causing HDFN is discovered, a sample of blood should be obtained from the father of the baby to ascertain his red cell antigen status. If he is negative for the antigen in question, determined through confidential enquiry of the mother, then the fetus will not be at risk. If paternity is unknown, or uncertain, or if the partner is heterozygous, then fetal Rhesus status should be determined using free fetal DNA studies. If the fetus is found to be Rhesus D positive then surveillance should begin using middle cerebral artery

119

peak systolic velocities on a weekly or fortnightly basis, depending on the actual scenario. Fetal blood sampling and intrauterine transfusions should begin when the middle cerebral artery (MCA) PSV exceeds 1.5 multiples of the median (MoM).

Anti-D given prophylactically can be detected in maternal serum for a number of weeks following administration and is indistinguishable from endogenously produced immune anti-D. However, the level will not exceed 1.0 IU/mL and if concern exists regarding the exact nature of anti-D detected on maternal sampling, a repeat sample 2 or 4 weeks later should help to determine its origin. A falling anti-D level suggests that it was exogenous prophylactic anti-D, and this does not cause HDFN.

Non-invasive Testing for Fetal RhD Status

The plasma of pregnant women contains free (i.e. non-cell-associated) fetal DNA (ffDNA) in significant quantities, from the early first trimester. The main source of this DNA is debated, but it probably originates from trophoblastic cells at the maternal–fetal interface. This DNA is fragmented and is degraded rapidly. Maternal free DNA is present in much larger quantities. Lo, in 1997, demonstrated how ffDNA could be used for the non-invasive prenatal diagnosis of fetal RhD status[12] and, since then, the same principles have been applied to non-invasive fetal sexing and the inheritance of paternally derived disease-causing mutations. This technology is strongly promoted by "SAFE" (The Special Non-invasive Advances in Fetal and Neonatal Evaluation Network), a multinational European group established in 2004 and funded by monies from the European Union[13].

An RhD negative woman should have no RhD DNA sequences in her plasma because her negative status is usually caused by a deletion of the RhD gene. There are rare exceptions (see pp. 124). If DNA probes designed to recognize RhD gene exons are added to her plasma, along with DNA polymerase, then no product should form if the fetus is also RhD negative, because there are no binding sites for the probes. If the fetus is RhD positive, then the probes will bind to the ffDNA and a PCR product will be produced, which can be detected easily using standard molecular techniques. Three separate exons from RHD are amplified, and if only one or two of the PCR products is generated then the result is considered equivocal and further investigation is required before a result can be given.

Use of this technology has become almost routine practice in the UK in Rhesus D isoimmunized pregnancies, where the father of the baby is a RhD positive heterozygote, where his status is unknown, or if paternity is uncertain[14]. The accuracy of the test is independent of gestation beyond 11 weeks; however, the rate of inconclusive results is higher at gestations below 16 weeks and the test must be repeated in a proportion of cases when the test is done in the first and early second trimesters. It avoids the need for amniocentesis to determine fetal RhD status when the father is heterozygous, or his blood group is unknown. This, in turn, bypasses the 1% risk of miscarriage associated with the amniocentesis and the likely fetomaternal transfusion of red cells, which may cause a subsequent rise in anti-D levels in already isoimmunized women. A RhD negative result provides welcome relief and reassurance without having put the pregnancy under any risk at all.

Middle Cerebral Artery Blood Flow

Since the late 1980s the relationship between fetal anemia and the velocity of blood flow in the middle cerebral artery (MCA) has been clearly documented. This can be measured using ultrasound, and a collaborative group, led by Mari[15], is usually credited with enhancing the profile of this technique so that today it has effectively replaced amniocentesis in the monitoring of pregnancies complicated by red cell antibodies.

A decrease in total red cell mass results in a reduction in blood viscosity and an increase in cardiac output. The effect on viscosity is thought to be the principal mechanism causing an increase in fetal peak systolic blood flow velocities (PSV). The vessel where this can be measured most easily and reliably is the middle cerebral artery.

The technique is not difficult; however, a number of factors influence the MCA PSV (see Table 11.6) and guidelines must be adhered to strictly. The angle of insonation of the pulse wave Doppler must be as close to 0 degrees as possible, or angle correction must be used. The vessel must be insonated within the first 2 mm of the proximal portion of the vessel as it arises from the circle of Willis (see Figures 11.4 and 11.5). Measurements taken at a distal point in the vessel may be 6–10 cm s^{-1} less than values taken proximally. Usually the MCA closest to the transducer is chosen, for ease, but the far-field vessel gives similar results. The fetus must be quiescent as fetal movement and

Table 11.6 Factors influencing the MCA PSV value

Fetal

Gestational age

Fetal activity

Cardiac status

Gender

Uterine contractions

Technical

Angle of insonation of Doppler wave

Positioning of the Doppler gate along the MCA

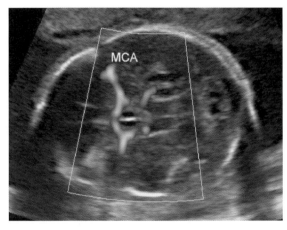

Figure 11.4 Power Doppler study showing the fetal circle of Willis and the near-field middle cerebral artery (MCA).

breathing can have a significant impact on the values obtained.

Normal ranges and charts (Figure 11.6) are available to plot the values onto and these show a normal gradual increase in the MCA PSV as gestation advances. Although the trend in values is important in any particular case, the most valuable indicator of significant fetal anemia has proven to be a threshold of 1.5 MoM (multiples of the median). Below this level, it is highly unlikely that the fetus will be more than just mildly anemic. The higher the value lies above this line, the more likely moderate or severe anemia becomes. If the MCA PSV in an "at risk" pregnancy is found to fall above this threshold, the study will usually be repeated within 24 hours. If the finding is persistent, then fetal blood sampling (with or without transfusion) will usually be performed soon after. MCA PSV studies are usually performed at intervals varying from 3 days to 4 weeks, depending on the perceived degree of risk, and previous values.

The collaborative group found a 100% sensitivity for the prediction of moderate-to-severe anemia, with a false-positive rate of 28%[16]. This compares very favorably with amniocentesis. Other studies have failed to achieve quite such impressive results, finding a sensitivity of 88% and a positive predictive value of 53%, i.e. approximately 1 in 10 cases of moderate–severe

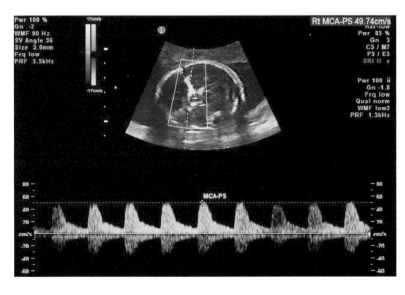

Figure 11.5 Color Doppler measurement of middle cerebral artery peak systolic velocity (MCA PSV). This study was performed at 22 weeks' gestation. A PSV of almost 50 cm s−1 in the MCA at this gestation is well above 1.5 multiples of the median and did indeed indicate fetal anemia in this case. Although the circulation is hyperdynamic in fetal anemia, the actual cause of the rise in blood velocity is thought to be a reduction in blood viscosity secondary to a falling fetal hematocrit. The fetal hemoglobin was found to be 4 g/dL on subsequent testing.

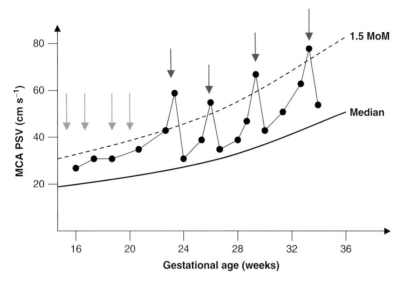

Figure 11.6 A chart showing median fetal middle cerebral artery peak systolic velocities (MCA PSV) throughout the second and third trimesters. An imaginary line has been drawn at 1.5 multiples of this median value and acts as an action line to prompt fetal blood sampling +/− transfusion. Superimposed is a fictitious case of severe RhD isoimmunization with a RhD positive fetus. The blue arrows show where maternal IVIG was given and the red arrows represent fetal blood transfusions. The MCA PSV can be seen to fall immediately following a fetal blood transfusion, but gradually increases again as hemolysis continues. As the fetal RhD positive blood becomes replaced by successive donations of RhD negative blood, the interval between transfusions increases. However, this donated blood also has a limited lifespan, even though it is not subject to the antibody-mediated hemolysis.

anemia were missed and half of all cases with a PSV greater than 1.5 MoM required transfusion. They recommended that this technique should not be used after 35 weeks' gestation, when the false-positive rate is higher. Other studies have suggested that the MCA PSV operates well in the second trimester, in contrast to ΔOD450[13]. Even if MCA PSV only matches the predictive abilities of liquor ΔOD450 measurements, the advantage remains clear; the technique is non-invasive. Indeed, by adopting MCA PSV measurements as the method of determining when fetal blood sampling is required, the number of invasive procedures can be reduced by two-thirds. Furthermore, reducing the time interval between MCA studies should improve the sensitivity of the test. Recent studies show that it remains a useful tool for timing second, third, and subsequent fetal blood transfusions.

Adjunctive Antenatal Treatments

Targeting the maternal immune response is a tempting strategy for tackling severe cases of isoimmunization. The knowledge that disease severity is, at least in part, related to absolute anti-D levels led to the proposal that plasmapheresis might help ameliorate the disease. Anti-D levels can be kept under control with this technique, but it is not without maternal risk, causes a rebound of antibody levels when treatment comes to an end, and was never convincingly shown to make a difference in erythroblastosis fetalis. For these reasons, its use as an adjunct to well-established

management techniques had fallen out of favor until more recently when it has been used in combination with a second form of immunomodulation which itself has shown greater promise. The use of intravenous immunoglobulin (IVIG) to prevent/treat fetal and neonatal alloimmune thrombocytopenia is described in Chapter 5 and there is more evidence of its value in this condition than there is for Rhesus isoimmunization. Nevertheless, non-randomized studies provide support for its use in cases of severe RhD isoimmunization. A dose of 1 g/kg is administered on a weekly or fortnightly basis from 13 to 20 weeks' gestation, the aim being to delay the onset of moderate–severe hemolysis to a point in the pregnancy where IVT can be more readily and reliably performed. The number of cases of hydrops can be reduced, as can the number of fetal blood transfusions needing to be performed. Table 11.7 lists some of the possible mechanisms by which IVIG might work. Good pregnancy outcomes have been achieved using a combination of IVIG with serial plasmapheresis from 12 weeks' gestation for women with the most severe histories[17]. The contribution of the two different methods of immunomodulation is not possible to assess. IVIG is expensive, and prepared from multiple donors. Rarely, it may cause unpleasant and potentially serious side effects, including:

- pyrexia and rigors;
- headache, backache, and myalgia;
- hypotension and tachycardia;

Table 11.7 Possible mechanism of action of IVIG in Rhesus D isoimmunization

Increased catabolism of maternal IgG
Competitive blockade of placental IgG transport mechanisms
Fc receptor blockade within the fetal reticuloendothelial system
Precipitation of immune complexes by excess antibody
Antigen neutralization
Binding of exogenous anti-idiotypic Ab to endogenous Ab

Table 11.8 Management strategies where moderate-to-severe HDN is expected

Close communication with neonatal team
Planned delivery (induction or cesarean section)
Cord blood analysis for bilirubin, Hb, group, and direct antiglobulin test (DAT)
Drainage of effusions and ascites in the hydropic infant
Phototherapy
Intravenous immunoglobulin
Exchange transfusion
Recombinant erythropoietin
Top-up blood transfusions

- tachypnea and chest tightness;
- alopecia;
- hemolytic anemia; and
- renal impairment.

Figure 11.6 illustrates how serial MCA PSV monitoring, early IVIG administration, and multiple fetal blood transfusions can support a pregnancy at risk of early and severe erythroblastosis fetalis through to a gestation where induction can be expected to bring about the normal birth of a non-hydropic baby with adequate hemoglobin levels.

Pediatric Management

It is rare now for a baby to be born at risk of HDN without the prior knowledge of maternity and pediatric staff. A multidisciplinary approach is vital for optimizing outcomes. Infants born with only a low risk of significant hemolysis should, at the very least, have cord blood sent for Coombs test (DCT), blood group, and hemoglobin and bilirubin levels. Close observation over the next 2–3 days is necessary and repeat bilirubin estimations may be required, as may phototherapy.

Management strategies for more significant cases of HDN are listed in Table 11.8.

It is far preferable to treat a hydropic fetus in utero than it is to deliver the baby in such poor condition. However, complications from an intrauterine transfusion may precipitate the unplanned delivery of such a baby in which case intubation, ventilation, and drainage of pleural effusions and ascites will be required. These babies are volume overloaded, making transfusion hazardous (although still necessary). They are at risk of hypoglycemia, hypocalcemia, hyponatremia, hyperkalemia, hyperbilirubinemia, acidosis, and renal failure. Mortality rates are high.

With modern antenatal and fetal management, this situation is fortunately rare. Nevertheless, planning delivery is important for the cases of moderate or severe erythroblastosis fetalis, even if intrauterine transfusions have minimized the risk. Bilirubin levels will rise sharply after birth and phototherapy must begin immediately.

Light from the blue–green region of the spectrum (425–490 nm) is most effective at converting non-polar bilirubin to water-soluble photoisomers and fluorescent tubes producing irradiance of >30 $\mu W/cm^2/nm$ are optimal. The surface area of the baby exposed to the light is crucial, and fiber-optic pads placed under the neonate, or the use of specifically designed "bili-beds," ensure that this is maximized. Bilirubin levels must be measured regularly and phototherapy may need to continue for a number of days. Gestation-specific charts are available for bilirubin levels and thresholds for exchange transfusion are recognized. A rise in serum bilirubin beyond these levels puts the newborn at increasing risk of kernicterus.

Severe anemia, high absolute bilirubin levels, excessive rise in bilirubin concentration, and unsafe bilirubin-to-albumin ratios are all indicators for exchange transfusion. An intravenous catheter is placed into the inferior vena cava via the umbilical vein through the cord stump and the entire blood volume of the neonate is usually replaced twice ("double-volume" exchange) by removing neonatal blood and replacing it with RhD negative blood in 5–10 mL aliquots. This process removes bilirubin and antibody-coated red blood cells and at the same time provides new albumin with unoccupied bilirubin binding sites and RhD negative erythrocytes. Between 70% and 90% of all fetal red blood cells are removed, but because most of the bilirubin is in the extravascular compartment, 75% of total body bilirubin remains and can cause a rebound rise in serum levels soon after the exchange, necessitating a repeat procedure. The inherent risks of exchange transfusion are substantial, however (Table 11.9)[18], and experience with the technique is declining. As many as 1 in 20 infants undergoing exchange

Table 11.9 Potential complications of exchange transfusion

Hematological: Over-anticoagulation with hemorrhage, anemia, neutropenia, thrombocytopenia

Cardiac: Volume overload, congestive heart failure, hypertension, arrhythmia, arrest

Metabolic: Acidosis, hypocalcemia, hypoglycemia, hyperkalemia, hypernatremia

Vascular: Thromboembolic events, necrotizing enterocolitis, vessel perforation

Infectious: Bacterial, viral, malarial

Other: Hypothermia, apnea, bowel perforation

transfusion may die and 1 in 4 suffer non-fatal complications. Much of this morbidity and mortality is found in preterm babies, emphasizing again the massive impact that antenatal management has had on this condition by delaying the gestation at which the baby needs to be born. Furthermore, intrauterine transfusions provide the fetus with red blood cells not at risk of immune-mediated hemolysis. By the third IUT, the fetal blood will be almost entirely RhD negative. At birth, therefore, these babies paradoxically are less likely to need exchange transfusion.

Avoiding exchange transfusion is clearly beneficial. The use of intravenous immunoglobulin is well established now in the treatment of neonatal alloimmune thrombocytopenia and HDFN. Although a number of mechanisms are possible, the main action is thought to be a blockade of Fc receptors in the reticuloendothelial system. IVIG reduces carboxyhemoglobin levels, a sensitive indicator of hemolysis. Although IVIG is prepared from multiple donors, and is extremely expensive, its use as an adjunct in moderate-to-severe HDFN seems justified. A Cochrane systematic review in 2002 concluded that IVIG significantly reduces the need for exchange transfusion (RR = 0.28), and reduces the number of exchanges needed when they cannot be avoided[19]. However, better quality studies are few in number and there has been a call for larger randomized trials. It should be used only as an adjunct to phototherapy and 0.5–1.0 g/kg is usually given as a single dose soon after delivery.

The baby remains at risk of developing anemia for some months, for two reasons. Firstly, maternal antibodies circulate for 4–6 months and continue to cause low-grade hemolysis. Secondly, intrauterine and newborn transfusions may suppress normal erythropoiesis and it may be a number of months before reticulocytes appear. During this time, "top-up" blood transfusions may be required, although these carry minimal risk in comparison with exchange transfusion. Regular

recombinant erythropoietin (EPO) injections can be used during this time to limit the number of top-up transfusions required.

Rhesus D Variants

RHD is a complex gene and much variation exists within it, particularly between racial groups. Understanding this is crucially important for a number of reasons. Phenotypic tests of RhD status examine how blood from an individual behaves when it is added to serum containing anti-D antibodies. Agglutination indicates that the individual is RhD positive. Genotypic tests of RhD status look for key DNA sequences from *RHD*. The entire gene cannot be examined, so sections from a variety of coding exons are chosen for multiplication, using the polymerase chain reaction. If a PCR product is produced, then the assumption is made that the individual is phenotypically RhD positive.

RhD variants can confuse this. The common cause for RhD negativity in Africans is an allele called the *RHD* pseudogene (*RHD*ψ) which contains a 37-base-pair insert in exon 4 and a nonsense mutation in exon 6, which effectively make the protein non-functional. Phenotypically, these individuals are RhD negative, but genetic tests might, for example, amplify exon 7 successfully and give a false-positive result for RhD status. Amplifying more exons, such as exon 5, would allow clarification because this exon is amplified from the normal *RHD* but not *RHD*ψ. This has relevance to non-invasive prenatal RhD testing. Knowledge of the racial origin of the woman's partner is clearly important. A second common African variant is the *RHD/CE* hybrid allele, of which there are more than 20. In these alleles, entire segments of the *RHCE* gene have been substituted into *RHD*. These red blood cells will agglutinate with polyclonal serum, but fail to react with monoclonal antibodies raised specifically against the extracellular loops coded by the missing exons. Although certain *RHD* exons will amplify with standard *RHD* probes, not all will (because they are missing), and this allows them to be distinguished from true RhD positive individuals using genetic rather than serological tests.

These RHD/CE hybrids are usually known as "partial D" alleles. The changes usually affect a long string of amino acids which is always located on the erythrocyte surface. The protein is altered so dramatically in these external "antigenic" portions that it is not recognized by anti-D and these individuals are prone to true RhD isoimmunization if exposed to normal RhD positive red cells. In the majority of cases, women with these alleles should be treated like RhD negative women and offered RhD negative blood if it is required and anti-D if the fetus is possibly or definitely RhD positive. It is very important that genetic tests in this group do not falsely classify them as RhD positive and a variety of strategies are in place in most laboratories to prevent this happening. The most common European partial D variant is *DNB*, caused by a missense mutation, which alters one amino acid in the sixth extracellular loop of the protein.

The second group of *RHD* variants is known as "weak D." The changes within these alleles substitute amino acids in the transmembranous portions of the protein. The surface antigenic sites are unaltered; however, integration of the weak D protein into the cell membrane is hindered or rendered unstable, effectively reducing the number of *RHD* antigenic sites expressed per red cell. The effect is quantitative rather than qualitative. Blood from these individuals will eventually show agglutination with anti-D if given more time and assisted by the addition of anti-human globulin reagent. Weak D type 1 is the most common European weak D variant and is caused by a single missense mutation at amino acid 270. Most women with weak D variants (types 1–3) can be given RhD positive blood and do not need prophylactic anti-D, although there are a few exceptions.

The term "Du" was previously applied to variants of *RHD*. In view of the complexity of the situation, and the consequences of treating women as RhD positive when in fact they carry a variant which puts them at risk of isoimmunization against RhD, it is recommended that advice is taken from the laboratory performing the serological and molecular tests in each case where a variant is identified.

Other Red Cell Antibodies

Table 11.10 lists some of the other red cell antigens, which have been documented to be the target of maternal antibodies, resulting in hemolytic disease. Those highlighted are the most significant from a clinical perspective. Certain red cell antibodies never cause hemolysis. Regional blood transfusion services will advise where rare antibodies are discovered on antenatal screening. National guidelines recommend 4-weekly antibody levels for anti-c and anti-Kell, and fortnightly from 28 weeks, as with anti-D. Anti-c levels below 7.5 iu/mL are unlikely to cause HDN and levels exceeding 20 iu/mL carry a high risk. Anti-E antibodies potentiate the effect of the anti-c, so a lower threshold for beginning ultrasound surveillance should be adopted

Table 11.10 Other red cell antigens implicated in fetal/neonatal hemolytic disease

Kell

Rhesus **c**, C, and **E**

A and B

Fy^a (Duffy) and Fy^b

Jk^a (Kidd) and Jk^b

S, M and U

Lu^a

Bold indicates most significant from a clinical perspective.

if both are present together. All other red cell antibodies are still quantified using the dilutional method, and the level of these will be given as a titer. Significant HDN is unlikely with a titer below 32, and measurement of these antibody levels need only occur at booking and 28 weeks.

Isoimmunization against the Kell antigen deserves special mention. Although there are four separate Kell antigens, Kell $_1$ causes most concern. Anti-Kell$_1$ antibodies are the second most common cause of fetal immune-mediated hemolysis, and early onset anemia and hydrops have been well documented. Nine out of 10 of the general population are Kell$_1$ negative and only 1 in 20 babies of Kell$_1$ negative women are Kell$_1$ positive. The Kell antigen is expressed on red cell progenitors in the bone marrow and it is via these cells that anti-Kell$_1$ antibodies are able to suppress hematopoiesis, as well as causing hemolysis. This made antenatal surveillance with amniocentesis unreliable because ΔOD450 of amniotic fluid acts only as a surrogate for hemolysis and cannot estimate the impact that the antibodies have on erythropoiesis. Fortunately, this problem is not shared by MCA PSV, which is used in exactly the same way as in RhD isoimmunization. In approximately half of all cases of Kell isoimmunization the cause is a previous blood transfusion where cross-matching did not take account of Kell status of the woman, or donor. The remainder result from FMH occurring at the delivery of a previous Kell positive baby. Absolute levels of anti-Kell antibodies are less useful in the prediction of disease severity. Non-invasive prenatal diagnosis (NIPD) for fetal Kell status is available through the Blood Transfusion Service (BTS) laboratory in Bristol and is particularly helpful because most Kell positive individuals are heterozygous. Fetal surveillance using middle cerebral artery Doppler studies should be offered irrespective of the anti-Kell level if the fetus is Kell positive. NIPD is also possible for the Rhesus c, C, E, and e antigens, although currently relatively few tests have been performed, when compared with RhD, meaning that the degree of diagnostic certainty is less. Anything more than mild disease is very unlikely with isolated RhE antibodies.

Women who have the blood group O quite commonly have antibodies to the A- and B-antigens, although these are more likely to be of the IgM class which does not cross the placenta. Anti-A and anti-B IgGs can reach the fetal circulation, but only mild hemolysis is the general rule for two reasons. Firstly, these antigens are expressed on a wide variety of cell types, effectively diluting their effect on red blood cells. Secondly, cell-surface expression is incomplete during gestation and develops gradually, thus limiting the risk before birth. Jaundice caused by ABO incompatibility is usually mild and readily treated with phototherapy.

The Future

The successes of recent years have not prevented further research and progress in the prevention and management of RhD hemolytic disease. Although polyclonal anti-D is a safe product, it is pooled from various donors and anxieties about viral and prion disease transfection remain. The infection of hundreds of Irish women with hepatitis C in 1977–1978 following the administration of contaminated anti-D illustrates this point all too well and currently 4 out of 10 women in the UK receiving anti-D will in fact be carrying a RhD negative fetus. The anti-D for these women is unnecessary, unpleasant, expensive, and not without a degree of risk.

Limiting the administration of anti-D to only those RhD negative women carrying a RhD positive fetus is a worthy goal. The techniques used for non-invasive prenatal fetus RhD testing (see above) are time consuming and expensive, although very accurate. Application of this technology to all pregnant RhD negative women is impractical. Mass screening requires an automated test, and robotic systems have been developed and tested recently with very promising results. Results from a recent UK study have given a detection rate for fetal RhD positive status after 11 weeks' gestation of >99 for a false-positive rate of 0.4%[5]. These false positives represent a group of RhD negative women who would continue to receive anti-D unnecessarily, but this is a tiny number compared with the 40% of RhD negative women currently receiving unnecessary anti-D prophylaxis. Of greater concern are the false-negative results (i.e. failure to detect fetal RhD positivity) of which there were only three cases from approximately 4000 tested pregnancies. Although these women would be at a threefold greater risk of isoimmunization because they would not receive antenatal prophylactic anti-D (they would still receive postnatal anti-D), mathematical modeling shows that this actually equates to only one extra case of hemolytic disease in 100 000 future pregnancies. Routine use of free fetal DNA studies to ascertain fetal RhD status in RhD negative women has already been instituted in Denmark[20], Sweden[21], and more recently, some centers in the UK. There are strong ethical arguments, if not financial ones, in support of this[22,23].

An alternative approach to improve on the safety of anti-D prophylaxis is to use recombinant monoclonal antibodies (mAb) produced from hybridoma or human B-cell lines, instead of polyclonal antibodies collected from human serum. A number of these cell lines exist and progress to date has recently been summarized by Kumpel[24]. Results with some of the mAb are encouraging and D-immunization can be prevented in RhD negative volunteers transfused with RhD positive cells. A "clean" and effective recombinant anti-D mAb may be on the horizon, but hurdles still exist, not least obtaining ethical approval for large-scale trials.

More distant are further exciting possibilities[25]. Mutated recombinant anti-D monoclonal antibodies have been designed and produced that are able to bind to the RhD antigen but have a much lower affinity for the Fcγ receptor on macrophages than normal anti-D [26]. These mutated antibodies would displace endogenous anti-D from its binding sites on the RhD antigen. Complement mediated lysis, hemolysis, and phagocytosis could all be reduced. There are many difficulties to overcome. The lifespan of these antibodies is limited and very high and frequent maternal administrations might be needed for transplacental transfer to maintain sufficient levels in the fetus.

A welcome move in neonatal care would be the avoidance altogether of exchange transfusion. The use of IVIG seems to have made some headway with this; however, a further option is close at hand. Competitive heme-oxygenase inhibitors, such as tinmesoporphyrin, have recently undergone phase III trials and are already available for certain conditions. This structural analog of heme competitively blocks heme-oxygenase, a rate-limiting enzyme in bilirubin production. Heme is left unaltered to be excreted in bile. It does not pass through the blood–brain barrier and does not accumulate in tissues. Several randomized trials have confirmed that these substances can prevent and block jaundice progression in the newborn. In the future, these drugs may result in a reduction in the need for phototherapy, and exchange transfusion for HDN may become a procedure confined to the history books.

Case Studies

Case Study 1

A 24-year-old woman delivered her first baby by emergency cesarean section during which she sustained a heavy postpartum hemorrhage and subsequently received a 3 unit blood transfusion. Two years later, in her second pregnancy, her routine screening bloods identified anti-K antibodies. The father of the baby was K negative and the baby was born normally at term. Her third pregnancy, with a new partner, occurred 8 years later, during which her anti-K titer was found to be 1 in 4 at booking, and 1 in 8 at 28 weeks. Her routine 20-week scan commented on a low placenta and a repeat was recommended for 32 weeks' gestation at which the fetus was found to be markedly hydropic, with ascites, pleural effusions, and widespread subcutaneous edema. Review by a fetal medicine specialist found the middle cerebral artery peak systolic velocity to be elevated at 76 cm s^{-1}. Fetal blood sampling the following day gave a fetal Hb of 29g/L and found the baby to be K positive. An intrauterine transfusion was performed into a fetal intrahepatic vein, with a post-transfusion value of 115g/L. A second IUT was performed later the same week, bringing the fetal Hb to 140g/L. Meanwhile, testing of the father of this baby found him to be heterozygous for K. The hydrops settled over the course of 2 weeks but at 35 weeks' gestation the MCA PSV became elevated once again, precipitating the delivery of the baby by semi-urgent cesarean section (induction of labor was advised against in view of the previous CS). The newborn Hb was 131 g/L and a mild rise in the bilirubin level settled with only 24 hours of phototherapy. This case emphasizes the importance of ascertaining paternal and fetal red cell antigen status when there are maternal antibodies, instituting appropriate surveillance for fetal anemia, and the poor relationship between anti-K titer and fetal hemoglobin.

Case Study 2

A 34-year-old woman in her first pregnancy was found to have developed low level RhD antibodies by the time of the delivery of her RhD positive baby, despite giving no history of potentially isoimmunizing events. This predated routine antenatal anti-D prophylaxis. The newborn had a positive direct Coombs test but required only 1 day of phototherapy.

In her second pregnancy, the anti-D levels rose sharply during the second and early third trimester. Fetal blood sampling at 29 weeks' gestation was performed in response to elevated OD450 levels at amniocentesis. The fetal Hb was found to be 110 g/L and an IUT was performed, followed by a further one at 32 weeks' gestation. Labor was induced at 34 weeks and the neonate did well following a single exchange transfusion and prolonged phototherapy.

She booked with anti-D levels of 12 iu/mL at 12 weeks in her third pregnancy. Serial MCA Doppler measurements suggested significant fetal anemia by 22 weeks' gestation. Fetal blood sampling and attempted intrauterine transfusion were complicated by fetal bradycardia and intrauterine fetal death at 23 weeks.

In her fourth pregnancy, the decision was made to administer weekly intravenous human immunoglobulin from 14 weeks' gestation, following confirmation using free fetal DNA studies that this fetus was also RhD positive. Anti-D levels increased less quickly than expected and the MCA peak systolic velocities only rose above 1.5 MoM at 27 weeks' gestation. Four IUTs were performed in total, and labor was induced at almost 36 weeks' gestation. IVIG was administered to the newborn and only 1 day of precautionary phototherapy was required. Three top-up transfusions were needed at 1, 2, and 4 months of life.

References

1. Royal Institute for Clinical Excellence. Guidance on the Use of Routine Antenatal Anti-D Prophylaxis. Green-Top Guideline no. 22. RCOG Press, 2002.

2. Crowther C, Middleton P. Anti-D administration after childbirth for preventing Rhesus alloimmunization. *Cochrane Database of Systematic Reviews* 1997; (**2**): CD000021.

3. Jabara S, Barnhart KT. Is Rh immune globulin needed in early first-trimester abortion? A review. *American Journal of Obstetrics and Gynecology* 2003; **188**: 623–627.

4. National Institute for Clinical Excellence. Guidance on the Use of Routine Antenatal Anti-D Prophylaxis for RhD-negative Women. Technology Appraisal Guidance no. 41. http://www.nice.org.uk; 2002.

5. Chitty LS, Finning K, Wade A *et al.* Diagnostic accuracy of routine antenatal determination of fetal RHD status across gestation: population based cohort study. *BMJ* 2014; **349**: g5243. doi: 10.1136/bmj.g5243.

6. Bennett PR, Le Van Kim C, Colin Y *et al.* Prenatal determination of fetal RhD type by DNA amplification. *New England Journal of Medicine* 1993; **329**: 607–610.

7. Sikkel E, Vandenbussche FPHA, Oepkes D *et al.* Amniotic fluid Δ OD450 values accurately predict severe fetal anemia in D-alloimmunization. *Obstetrics and Gynecology* 2002; **100**: 51–57.

8. Nicolaides KH, Soothill PW, Clewell W, Rodeck CH. Rh disease: intravascular fetal blood transfusion by cordocentesis. *Fetal Therapy* 1986; **1**: 185–192.

9. Dodd JM, Windrim RC, van Kamp IL. Techniques of intrauterine fetal transfusion for women with red cell isoimmunization for improving health outcomes (Review). *Cochrane Database of Systematic Reviews* 2012; (**9**): CD007096.

10. Milkins C, Berryman J, Cantwell C *et al.* Guidelines for pre-transfusion compatibility procedures in blood transfusion laboratories. *Transfusion Medicine* 2013; **23**(1): 3–35.

11. RCOG. *The Management of Women with Red Cell Antibodies During Pregnancy. Green-Top Guideline No. 65.* London: Royal College of Obstetricians and Gynecologists; 2014.

12. Lo YMD, Corbetta N, Chamberlain PF *et al.* Presence of fetal DNA in maternal plasma and serum. *Lancet* 1997; **350**: 485–487.

13. Chitty LS, van der Schoot CE, Hahn S, Avent ND. SAFE – The special non-invasive advances in fetal and neonatal evaluation network: aims and achievements. *Prenatal Diagnosis* 2008; **28**: 83–88.

14. Daniels G, Finning K, Martin P, Summers J. Fetal blood group genotyping. Present and future. *Annals of the New York Academy of Sciences* 2006; **1075**: 88–95.

15. Mari G, Deter RL, Carpenter RL *et al.* Non-invasive diagnosis by Doppler ultrasonography of fetal anemia due to maternal red-cell alloimmunization. Collaborative Group for the Assessment of the Blood Velocity in Anemic Fetuses. *New England Journal of Medicine* 2000; **342**: 9–14.

16. Pereira L, Jenkins TM, Berghella V. Conventional management of maternal red cell alloimmunization compared with management by Doppler assessment of middle cerebral artery peak systolic velocity. *American Journal of Obstetrics and Gynecology* 2003; **189**: 1002–1006.

17. Ruma MS, Moise KJ, Kim E *et al.* Combined plasmapheresis and intravenous immune globulin for the treatment of severe maternal red cell alloimmunization. *American Journal of Obstetrics and Gynecology* 2007; **196**: 138.e1–138.e6.

18. Jackson JC. Adverse events associated with exchange transfusion in healthy and ill newborns. *Pediatrics* 1997; **99**: E7.

19. Alcock GS, Liley H. Immunoglobulin infusion for isoimmune hemolytic jaundice in neonates. *Cochrane Database of Systematic Reviews* 2002; (**3**): CD003313.

20. Clausen FB, Christiansen M, Steffensen R *et al.* Report of the first nationally implemented clinical routine screening for fetal RHD in D-pregnant women to ascertain the requirement for antenatal RhD prophylaxis. *Transfusion* 2012; **52**: 752–758.

21. Tiblad E, Wikman AT, Ajne G *et al.* Targeted routine antenatal anti-D prophylaxis in the prevention of RhD immunization: outcome of a new antenatal screening and prevention program. *PLoS One* 2013; **8**: e70984.

22. Kent J, Farrell AM, Soothill P. Routine administration of Anti-D: the ethical case for offering pregnant women fetal RHD genotyping and a review of policy and practice. *BMC Pregnancy and Childbirth* 2014; **14**: 87.

23. Szczepura A, Osipenko L, Freeman K. A new fetal RHD genotyping test: Costs and benefits of mass testing to target antenatal anti-D prophylaxis in England and Wales. *BMC Pregnancy and Childbirth* 2011; **11**: 5.

24. Kumpel BM. Efficacy of RhD monoclonal antibodies in clinical trails as replacement therapy for prophylactic anti-D immunoglobulin: more questions than answers. *Vox Sanguinis* 2007; **93**: 99–111.

25. Urbaniak SJ. Noninvasive approaches to the management of RhD hemolytic disease of the fetus and newborn. *Transfusion* 2008; **48**: 2–5.

26. Nielson LK, Green TH, Sandlie I *et al.* In vitro assessment of recombinant, mutant anti-D immunoglobulin G devoid of hemolytic activity for treatment of on-going hemolytic disease of the fetus and newborn. *Transfusion* 2008; **48**: 12–19.

12
Acute Management of Suspected Thromboembolic Disease in Pregnancy

Andrew Thomson, Beverley Hunt, and Ian Greer

Introduction

Antenatal and postnatal venous thromboembolism (VTE) is around 10 and 25 times more common, respectively, than in non-pregnant women of the same age and is the major cause of direct maternal mortality in the developed world. European studies have consistently found the pregnancy-related VTE mortality to be 8.5–14 per million live births.[1,2] A recent study by Sultan *et al.*[3] showed that in women in the UK with pre-eclampsia, BMI >30 kg/m^2, infection, or those having cesarean delivery, VTE risk remained elevated for 6 weeks postpartum. For women with postpartum hemorrhage or preterm birth, the relative rate of VTE was only increased for the first 3 weeks postpartum. Kamel *et al.*[4] reported that the increased risk of VTE extended to 12 weeks postpartum: the odds ratio of having a VTE in a Californian multi-ethnic population was 12 (95% CI, 7.9–18.6) in the first 6 weeks postpartum and 2.2 (95% CI, 1.4–3.3) for period between 7 and 12 weeks postpartum. In the UK, sequential reports from Confidential Enquiries into Maternal Deaths have demonstrated that VTE remains the main direct cause of maternal death and have highlighted failures in obtaining objective diagnoses and employing adequate treatment[5,6]. The rate of maternal mortality due to VTE peaked between 1996 and 1998 at 2.18 deaths per 100 000 maternities. It gradually fell to 0.79 for the period of 2006–8 but there has been a reversal of the trend between 2009 and 2011 with a rate of 1.26 deaths per 100 000 maternities and declining further to 1.08 per 100 000 in the most recent data for 2010–12[5]. The cause for this is unclear: some consider that the increased prevalence of obesity and the rising average age of mothers may be factors that have not been counterset by an increased use of thromboprophylaxis.

Fatal pulmonary embolism (PE) arises from deep venous thrombosis (DVT), many cases of which are not recognized clinically and are only identified at postmortem following a maternal death[6]. The subjective, clinical assessment of DVT and PE is particularly unreliable in pregnancy and a minority of women with clinically suspected VTE have the diagnosis confirmed when objective testing is employed[7]. Acute VTE should be suspected during pregnancy in women with symptoms and signs consistent with possible VTE[7–8], particularly if there are other risk factors for VTE (see Tables 8.1 and 8.2) [9–14]. The symptoms and signs of VTE include leg pain and swelling (usually unilateral), lower abdominal pain, low-grade pyrexia, dyspnea, chest pain, hemoptysis, and collapse.

Epidemiology of VTE during Pregnancy

Virchow's triad for VTE consists of alterations in normal blood flow (stasis), trauma or damage to the vascular endothelium, and alterations in the constitution of blood (hypercoagulability), and describes the three broad categories of factors that contribute to thrombosis. During normal pregnancy, hypercoagulability results from increases in the levels of factor VIII and fibrinogen, reduction in protein S levels, a resistance to activated protein C and altered fibrinolysis, partly due to the production of plasminogen activator inhibitor-2 (PAI-2) from the placenta. Studies assessing blood flow velocity in the lower limbs in pregnancy have shown an extensive reduction in flow of up to 50% by 29 weeks' gestation, reaching its nadir at 36 weeks. The changes in both blood flow velocity and coagulation factors may persist for up to 6 weeks after delivery. The third component of Virchow's triad, damage to the vascular endothelium, arises during the course of vaginal or abdominal delivery – while VTE can occur at any stage of pregnancy, the puerperium is the time of greatest risk.

Almost 90% of cases of DVT occur in the left leg in pregnancy, in contrast to the non-pregnant situation, where only 55% occur on the left[7,15]. This may reflect compression of the left iliac vein by the right iliac artery and the ovarian artery, which cross the vein only on the left side. Over 70% of DVTs in pregnancy arise in the iliac and femoral veins rather than the calf veins, whereas in non-pregnant patients only about 9% arise in the ilio-femoral area. This is of importance since ilio-femoral DVTs are more likely to result in PE than are calf vein thromboses.

Assessment and Diagnosis of Acute VTE in Pregnancy

Clinical diagnosis of both DVT and PE is unreliable. In non-pregnant patients where DVT is suspected, the diagnosis is confirmed in about 20–30% of cases when objective testing is performed. Outside of pregnancy, 80% of DVTs produce no clinical signs[16], i.e. no swelling or change of color, but they do cause pain. In contrast, during pregnancy, clinical assessment is unreliable since many of the symptoms and signs of VTE, such as leg swelling, chest pain, and dyspnea, are commonly found in normal pregnancy (Table 12.1). As a consequence, the accuracy of clinical diagnosis falls to about 8% for DVT and to less than 5% for suspected PE [7–8,15].

It is therefore essential that objective testing is performed in women with suspected VTE. Failure to identify VTE will place the mother's life at risk, while unnecessary treatment is associated with risks, inconvenience, and costs during the pregnancy and may also have implications for her future healthcare (including future use of oral contraception and hormone

Table 12.1 Symptoms and signs of VTE in pregnancy

Deep venous thrombosis
- leg pain or discomfort alone or with:
  - tenderness
  - swelling
  - lower abdominal pain
  - increased temperature and edema
  - elevated white cell count

Pulmonary thromboembolism
- chest pain
- dyspnea
- hemoptysis
- tachycardia
- focal signs in the chest
- raised jugular venous pressure
- collapse
- abnormalities on the chest X-ray
- symptoms and signs associated with DVT

replacement therapy, and thromboprophylaxis in future pregnancies). However, this policy has led to CT pulmonary angiography (CTPA) being performed liberally in many pregnant women with chest symptoms. This is an important consideration as fewer than 2% of all scans performed are positive and therefore the majority of women with suspected pulmonary emboli will be exposed to potentially unnecessary radiation. As yet, there are no well-designed large clinical trials to support the management of suspected VTE in pregnancy and guidelines are therefore empirical and based on extrapolation from studies performed in non-pregnant patients[2,7,15].

Currently it is considered that if there is a delay in obtaining objective tests, the woman should be commenced on anticoagulant therapy, unless contraindicated, until testing can be performed[7].

Diagnosis of DVT

Compression Duplex ultrasound of the entire proximal venous system is the optimal initial diagnostic test for DVT in pregnancy. If the initial ultrasound shows an abnormality in the popliteal or femoral veins, the diagnosis of proximal DVT is confirmed and anticoagulant treatment should be commenced or continued. A "normal" ultrasound does not exclude a calf DVT and, therefore, if ultrasound is negative and a high level of clinical suspicion exists, the anticoagulation (if already started) should be stopped and repeat scans performed on days 3 and 7, or an alternative diagnostic test employed. If repeat testing is negative, anticoagulant treatment can be discontinued[7,15].

For the diagnosis of iliac vein thrombosis, which may present with back pain and/or swelling of the entire limb, pulsed Doppler, magnetic resonance direct thrombus imaging or venography or conventional contrast venography should be considered[7].

Diagnosis of PE

If the patient has signs and/or symptoms of DVT then Doppler ultrasound leg studies should be performed. A diagnosis of DVT may indirectly confirm a diagnosis of PE and since anticoagulant therapy is the same for both conditions, further investigation is not usually necessary.

In the absence of clinical features of DVT, a chest X-ray (CXR) should be performed. This may identify other pulmonary disease such as pneumonia, pneumothorax, or lobar collapse. While the CXR is normal in over half of pregnant patients with objectively proven PE, abnormal features caused by PE include atelectasis, effusion, focal opacities, regional oligemia, or pulmonary edema. The radiation dose to the fetus from a CXR performed at any stage of pregnancy is negligible. If the CXR is abnormal, planar ventilation-perfusion (V/Q) scanning is unreliable and either V/Q SPECT or CTPA should be performed[7–8].

Where the CXR is normal, the choice of technique for definitive diagnosis (V/Q planar or SPECT scan or CTPA) may depend on factors such as local availability and guidelines, and should usually be made after discussion with a radiologist. During pregnancy, the ventilation component of the V/Q scan can often be omitted, thereby minimizing the radiation dose for the fetus. In the UK, the British Thoracic Society[7] recommended CTPA as first-line investigation for non-massive PE in non-pregnant patients in 2003. At the time, this technique had potential advantages over radionuclide (V/Q) imaging including better sensitivity and specificity (in non-pregnant patients) and a lower radiation dose to the fetus. In addition it can identify other pathology such as aortic dissection. The main disadvantage of CTPA is the high radiation dose to the maternal breasts associated with an increased lifetime risk of developing breast cancer. This is particularly relevant when it is known that only around 5% at most of such investigations will have a positive result. In addition, conventional CTPA may not identify small peripheral PEs, although this is overcome by the latest multidetector row spiral CT techniques. In contrast to CTPA, in some centers V/Q scanning may be delayed because of availability of isotope. A new form of V/Q scanning is available, known as V/Q SPECT. This involves exposure to the same type and doses of isotopes that are used in planar V/Q, but with SPECT the camera rotates round the patient to produce better imaging which has similar sensitivity and specificity to CTPA, but a lower exposure of the mother to radiation. This is available from at least four centers in the UK and has been further enhanced by being combined with low-dose CT–CT V/Q SPECT so that a combination picture is produced[17].

Many authorities, including the authors, continue to recommend V/Q scanning, where possible, as first-line investigation in pregnancy because of its high negative predictive value in this situation, its substantially lower radiation dose to pregnant breast tissue, and because most pregnant women in the UK will not have comorbid pulmonary pathology[7,15,17–19].

Radiation Exposure Associated with Diagnostic Tests

CTPA delivers less radiation to the fetus than V/Q scanning during all trimesters of pregnancy. It has been estimated that the risk of fatal cancer to the age of 15 years is <1/1 000 000 after in utero exposure to CTPA and 1/280 000 following a perfusion scan. While CTPA is associated with a lower risk of radiation for the fetus, this must be offset by the relatively high radiation dose (20 mGy) to the mother's thorax and in particular breast tissue. The delivery of 10 mGy of radiation to a woman's breast increases her lifetime risk of developing breast cancer. It has been estimated that the increased risk is 13.6% (background risk 1/200), a figure that has been cited widely[7,15]. More recently, authorities have suggested that this risk is an overestimate. Further, bismuth breast shields can substantially reduce the radiation exposure[20]. Nevertheless, breast tissue is especially sensitive to radiation exposure during pregnancy, and it therefore seems sensible to recommend that lung perfusion scans should be considered the investigation of first choice for young women, especially if there is a family history of breast cancer or the patient has had a previous chest CT scan. Radiation exposure from pulmonary angiography is approximately 0.5 mSv to fetus, and 5 to 30 mSv to mother.

Well's Score and D-dimer Testing in Pregnancy

Outwith pregnancy, a low Well's score and normal plasma D-dimer level has been shown to have excellent negative predictive value in patients with a low clinical probability score for VTE. However despite a study suggesting it may be useful[18], the Well's score has never been validated in pregnancy, and D-dimer levels increase physiologically throughout pregnancy, becoming elevated at term and in the postnatal period in most healthy pregnant women. Furthermore, D-dimer levels are increased if there is a concomitant problem such as pre-eclampsia, preterm labor, and placental abruption. Thus, the probability of a negative result is lower and objective testing is more often required. For this reason guidelines produced by the Royal College of Obstetricians and Gynecologists in the UK[7] do not currently recommend that the Well's score and D-dimer levels are evaluated in pregnant women with suspected VTE. In contrast, the European Society of Cardiology[21] recommends that D-dimer levels should be measured, as a proportion of patients will have a normal result and be able to avoid unnecessary imaging. It should be noted, however, that although the SimpliRED test has been reported to have a negative predictive value of 100% in pregnancy, false-negative results have been reported.

A large UK-based multicenter study (DiPEP) assessed the utility of expert derived clinical decision tools such as the Wells and Geneva scores and candidate biomarkers, including D-dimers, from women with suspected PE and unfortunately showed they were all unreliable in pregnancy (unpublished data).

Thrombophilia Testing for Acute VTE in Pregnancy

Almost half of all women who have an episode of VTE in pregnancy will have a recognizable underlying heritable or acquired thrombophilia[22]. The prevalence rates for inherited thrombophilias in European populations are shown in Table 17.2 and the relative risk of each condition, shown by meta-analysis, in Table 12.2. The risk for protein C, S, and antithrombin deficiencies may be underestimated due to the low prevalence of these conditions, as data are drawn from inadequately sized populations. Performing thrombophilia testing in the acute stages of thrombosis gives misleading results and is not recommended. Levels of antithrombin, protein C, and protein S may fall, particularly if thrombus is extensive. In addition, protein S levels fall in normal pregnancy and an acquired activated protein C resistance (APC) is found with the APC sensitivity ratio test in around 40% of pregnancies, due to the physiological changes in the coagulation system. Clearly, genotyping for factor V

Table 12.2 Risk of pregnancy-associated VTE in women with underlying inherited thrombophilia[13]

Thrombophilic defect	Relative risk of thrombosis
Factor V Leiden (**heterozygote**)	8.32
Factor V Leiden (**homozygote**)	34.4
Prothrombin 20210A (**heterozygote**)	6.8
Prothrombin 20210A (**homozygote**)	26.4
Protein C deficiency	4.76
Protein S deficiency	3.19
Antithrombin deficiency	4.69

Leiden and prothrombin G20210A will not be affected by pregnancy or thrombus. The results of thrombophilia testing will not influence the immediate management of acute VTE unless the patient has antithrombin deficiency.

The value of thrombophilia testing is in providing information that can influence the duration and intensity of anticoagulation, such as when antiphospholipid syndrome is identified. However, modern management is changing and even those with persistent antiphospholipid syndrome would not usually be offered long-term anticoagulation where their first thrombotic event is in pregnancy, because outside of pregnancy they will be less prothrombotic. Diagnosis of heterozygous factor V Leiden would not change management as the risk of a second VTE is not greater in those with factor V Leiden than in those without a thrombophilia.

Initial Treatment of VTE in Pregnancy

Before anticoagulant therapy is initiated, blood should be taken for a full blood count and coagulation screen. Urea, electrolytes, and liver function tests should also be checked to exclude renal or hepatic dysfunction, which are cautions for anticoagulant therapy.

The treatment of VTE in pregnancy is heparin. Vitamin K antagonists are rarely employed in this setting as they cross the placenta and are associated with increased pregnancy loss, a specific embryopathy, and other abnormalities in the first trimester, as well as fetal hemorrhagic complications and central nervous system anomalies at any stage of pregnancy. Although for many years unfractionated heparin (UFH) was the standard anticoagulant used during and outwith pregnancy, it has now largely been replaced by low-molecular-weight heparin (LMWH). Meta-analyses of randomized controlled trials (RCTs) in non-pregnant patients indicate that LMWHs are more effective and are associated with a lower risk of hemorrhagic complications and lower mortality than unfractionated heparin in the initial treatment of DVT. A meta-analysis of RCTs has shown equivalent efficacy of LMWH to unfractionated heparin in the initial treatment of PE. A systematic review of LMWH in pregnancy has confirmed its efficacy and safety in the management of acute thrombosis and in the provision of thromboprophylaxis[23]. Furthermore, compared with UFH, LMWH is associated with a substantially lower risk of hemorrhage and osteoporosis[2,7,9,15]. Neither UFH nor LMWH crosses the placenta and both are safe for breast-feeding mothers.

While several LMWH preparations are available, most experience currently exists with enoxaparin, dalteparin, and tinzaparin. In non-pregnant patients with acute VTE, LMWH is usually administered in a once daily dose. In view of recognized alterations in the pharmacokinetics of dalteparin and enoxaparin during pregnancy, a twice daily dosage regimen has been recommended for these LMWHs in the treatment of VTE in pregnancy (enoxaparin 1 mg/kg twice daily; dalteparin 100 units/kg twice daily). However, there are increasing data supporting once daily dosing and it is uncertain whether once daily or twice daily dosing is most appropriate for treatment as pharmacokinetic and observational data suggest similar efficacy and safety[7,15]. Whichever preparation of LMWH is employed, the woman should be taught to self-administer the drug by subcutaneous injection, allowing further management on an outpatient basis until delivery[7].

In the early management of DVT, the leg should be elevated and where a graduated elastic compression stocking can be applied comfortably, it can reduce edema and help reduce symptoms. Once full anticoagulation has been commenced, the woman should be encouraged to mobilize while wearing compression hosiery as this has been shown to reduce pain and swelling in the affected leg. Studies in non-pregnant patients have shown that early mobilization, with compression therapy, does not increase the likelihood of developing PE. While post-thrombotic syndrome is common following gestational DVT[24], recent data from the non-pregnant situation have shown that long-term use of compression stockings following DVT does not prevent the development of post-thrombotic syndrome[25]. For patients with persisting leg edema after DVT, class II compression hosiery is more effective than class I stockings. Where DVT threatens leg viability through venous gangrene, the leg should be elevated, anticoagulation given, and strong consideration given to thrombolytic therapy and/or surgical embolectomy[7].

Monitoring of LMWH Therapy

Experience indicates that satisfactory anti-Xa levels (peak anti-Xa activity, 3 hours post-injection, of 0.5–1.2 units/mL) are obtained using a weight-based regimen and monitoring of anti-Xa is not routinely required in patients with VTE on therapeutic doses of LMWH, particularly as there are concerns over the standardization and accuracy of anti-Xa monitoring. There may be a case for monitoring levels at extremes of body weight (<50 kg and ≥90 kg), and women with other complicating factors including renal disease and recurrent VTE[7].

Guideline documents from North America[2] recommend that routine platelet count monitoring is not required in obstetric patients who have received only LMWH as heparin-induced thrombocytopenic thrombosis has not been seen in pregnancies managed exclusively with LMWH.

If unfractionated heparin is employed, or if the obstetric patient is receiving LMWH after first receiving unfractionated heparin, or if she has received unfractionated heparin in the past, the platelet count should ideally be monitored every 2–3 days from day 4 to day 14, or until heparin is stopped, whichever occurs first.

Maintenance Treatment of VTE

Women with antenatal VTE can be managed for the remainder of the pregnancy using LMWH administered subcutaneously. It is our practice to continue with the initial dose regimen throughout pregnancy despite the pregnancy-associated weight gain (since LMWH does not cross the placenta and therefore the weight of the fetoplacental unit is not relevant). If LMWH therapy requires monitoring, for example in extremes of body weight or renal impairment, the aim is to achieve a peak anti-Xa activity, 3 hours post-injection, of 0.5–1.2 units/mL.

It is not yet established whether the initial dose of LMWH can be reduced to an intermediate dose after an initial period of several weeks of therapeutic anticoagulation, although this practice has been successfully employed in some centers. Outwith pregnancy in patients with underlying malignancy, a reduction in dose has been shown to be safe after 4 weeks of therapeutic anticoagulation. Although there have been no studies directly comparing these two types of dosing strategies in pregnant women, this type of modified dosing regimen may be useful in pregnant women at increased risk of bleeding or osteoporosis[26].

Management at the Time of Delivery

For women on therapeutic anticoagulation, a planned delivery, either through induction of labor or elective cesarean section, allows accurate timing of events and minimizes the risk of the woman having to deliver on full anticoagulation. The dose of LMWH can be reduced to a once daily thromboprophylactic dose on the day before induction of labor or cesarean section. When a woman presents while on a therapeutic, twice daily regimen of LMWH, regional techniques should not usually be employed for at least 24 hours after the last dose of LMWH. LMWH should not be given for at least 4 hours after the epidural catheter has been removed and the cannula should not be removed within 12 hours of the most recent injection[7].

For delivery by elective cesarean section, the treatment doses of LMWH should be omitted for 24 hours prior to surgery. A thromboprophylactic dose of LMWH (enoxaparin 40 mg; dalteparin 5000 IU; tinzaparin 75 IU/kg) should be given by 3 hours postoperatively (>4 hours after removal of an epidural catheter) and the treatment dose recommenced that evening. There is an increased risk of wound hematoma following cesarean section with both unfractionated heparin and LMWH of around 9%[7]. For this reason, wound drains should be considered at cesarean section, and the skin incision should ideally be closed with staples or interrupted sutures to allow easy drainage of any hematoma.

If the thrombosis occurred in the last week of pregnancy, consideration should be given to the use of unfractionated heparin (since it can be relatively easily reversed using protamine sulfate and has a short duration of action). If spontaneous labor occurs in women receiving therapeutic doses of subcutaneous unfractionated heparin, careful monitoring of the anticoagulant effect by measuring the activated partial thromboplastin time (aPTT) is required. Subcutaneous unfractionated heparin should be discontinued 12 hours before and intravenous unfractionated heparin stopped 6 hours before induction of labor or regional anesthesia. It should be noted, however, that the aPTT is less reliable in pregnancy due to increased levels of FVIII and heparin-binding proteins, which can lead to an apparent heparin resistance: in this setting, monitoring anti-Xa levels is recommended[7,26].

Duration of Postpartum Anticoagulation Therapy

In the UK, it is recommended that in non-pregnant patients, anticoagulant therapy should be continued for 3 months for proximal DVT or PE when VTE has been provoked, i.e. occurred in relation to a temporary risk factor, or unprovoked[7]. The presence of ongoing risk factors and the safety of LMWH have led authorities to propose that anticoagulant therapy should be continued for the duration of the pregnancy and until at least 6 weeks postpartum and to allow a total duration of treatment of at least 3 months. Both heparin and warfarin are satisfactory for use postpartum. Warfarin can be difficult to stabilize in the postpartum period and in our experience, most women prefer to use LMWH (which can be used with once daily dosing postpartum) because they have become accustomed to its administration, and they appreciate the convenience of not having to attend clinics to have their international normalized ratio (INR) checked. Before discontinuing treatment the ongoing risk of thrombosis should be assessed including a review of personal and family history of VTE and any thrombophilia testing.

Breast-feeding

Neither heparin (unfractionated or LMWH) nor warfarin is contraindicated in breast-feeding. There is little published data on whether LMWHs are secreted in breast milk, but neither unfractionated heparin nor LMWH are orally active and no effect would be anticipated in the fetus.

The new oral anticoagulants such as dabigatran, rivaroxaban, edoxaban, and apixaban while widely licensed for use in the treatment and secondary prevention of VTE outside of pregnancy have not been investigated in pregnancy because animal studies suggest teratogenicity. Moreover, such small molecules may be transferred to the fetus. There is also lack of data of their safety during breast-feeding. Thus, they are not indicated during pregnancy or during breast-feeding[7,15,27].

Post-thrombotic Syndrome

The post-thrombotic syndrome (PTS) is a common complication following DVT[24]. It is found in over 60% of previous DVTs in pregnancy followed up over a median of 4.5 years. It is characterized by chronic persistent leg swelling, pain, a feeling of heaviness, dependent cyanosis, telangiectasis, chronic pigmentation, eczema, associated varicose veins and in some cases lipodermatosclerosis, and chronic ulceration. Symptoms are made worse by standing or walking and improve with rest and recumbency. The syndrome is more common where there is a recurrent DVT, with obesity, and where there has been inadequate anti-coagulation. In the past, it was recommended that graduated elastic compression stockings (class II) should be worn on the affected leg for 2 years after the acute event to reduce the risk of post-thrombotic syndrome. Graduated elastic compression stockings were thought to improve the microcirculation by assisting the calf muscle pump, reducing swelling and reflux, and reducing venous hypertension[4]. This recommendation is based upon studies in non-pregnant patients where such therapy reduces the incidence of PTS from 23% to 11% over 2 years but these data have been challenged recently by the results of the SOX clinical trial, which showed no benefit in reducing the risk of PTS[25]. Active management of PTS by using endovenous ballooning and stenting is currently an active research area.

Management of Massive, Life-threatening PE

Massive, life-threatening PE may be defined as embolus associated with hemodynamic compromise (a systolic blood pressure <90 mmHg or a drop in systolic blood pressure of ≥40 mmHg from baseline for a period >15 minutes), not otherwise explained by hypovolemia, sepsis, or new arrhythmia. This is an obstetric and medical emergency and hospitals should have in place guidelines for the management of non-hemorrhagic obstetric shock (see Figure 12.1). The

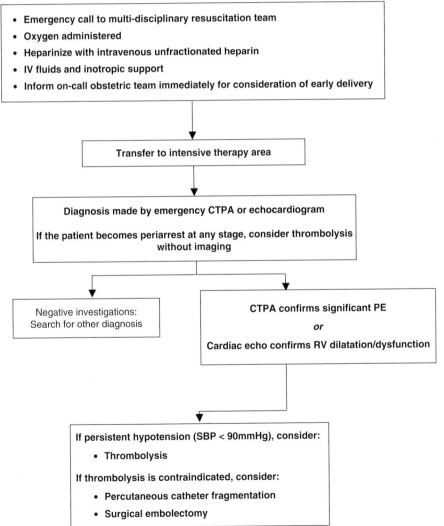

Figure 12.1 Symptoms and signs of VTE in pregnancy.

- Emergency call to multi-disciplinary resuscitation team
- Oxygen administered
- Heparinize with intravenous unfractionated heparin
- IV fluids and inotropic support
- Inform on-call obstetric team immediately for consideration of early delivery

Transfer to intensive therapy area

Diagnosis made by emergency CTPA or echocardiogram

If the patient becomes periarrest at any stage, consider thrombolysis without imaging

Negative investigations: Search for other diagnosis

CTPA confirms significant PE

or

Cardiac echo confirms RV dilatation/dysfunction

If persistent hypotension (SBP < 90mmHg), consider:
- Thrombolysis

If thrombolysis is contraindicated, consider:
- Percutaneous catheter fragmentation
- Surgical embolectomy

collapsed, shocked pregnant woman needs to be assessed by a multidisciplinary resuscitation team of experienced clinicians including senior obstetricians, hematologists, cardiothoracic surgeons, and interventional radiologists, who should decide on an individual basis whether a woman receives intravenous unfractionated heparin, thrombolytic therapy, or thoracotomy and surgical embolectomy[7].

Oxygen should be administered and the circulation supported using intravenous fluids and inotropic agents if required. Intravenous unfractionated heparin is the traditional method of heparin administration in acute VTE and remains the preferred treatment in massive PE because of its rapid effect and extensive experience of its use in this situation. The diagnosis should be established using either portable echocardiogram or CTPA performed within 1 hour of presentation.

In massive life-threatening PE with hemodynamic compromise, there is a case for considering catheter-directed or systemic thrombolytic therapy as anticoagulant therapy will not reduce the obstruction of the pulmonary circulation. After thrombolytic therapy has been given, an infusion of unfractionated heparin can be given. There are now a large number of published case reports on the use of thrombolytic therapy in pregnancy, streptokinase being the agent most frequently employed. Streptokinase does not cross the placenta; this is also thought to be true for other thrombolytics. The maternal bleeding complication rate is approximately 6%, which is consistent with that in non-pregnant patients receiving thrombolytic therapy. Most bleeding events occur around catheter and puncture sites and, in pregnant women, from the genital tract. If the patient is not suitable for thrombolysis or is moribund, a discussion with the cardiothoracic surgeons with a view to urgent thoracotomy or extracorporeal life support should be had [7,28,29].

Case Studies

Case Study 1
A 39-year-old primigravida who had a BMI of 31 was pregnant after her third round of IVF. An early scan showed a twin pregnancy. She developed hyperemesis in the eleventh week of pregnancy and was unable to keep any fluids down and so was admitted for intravenous fluids and antiemetics and was given thromboprophylaxis with 5000 units of dalteparin. The hyperemesis settled on conservative management and she was discharged home after 3 days. However, 2 days later she developed pain in the left calf and returned for review. On examination, there was no evidence of swelling or redness in the calf. She was sent for a Duplex ultrasound scan, which showed a popliteal thrombus extending into the calf.

She was anticoagulated with 1 mg/kg dalteparin twice daily and the calf pain settled within 48 hours. She disliked giving herself subcutaneous injections and so after 2 weeks was switched to dalteparin 1.5 mg/kg once daily. The rest of the pregnancy proceeded well. However, at 32 weeks her blood pressure started to rise and she developed swelling and proteinuria. Repeat Doppler ultrasound scanning showed some minor residual clot following dissolution of most of the previous clot. It was decided in view of her multiple problems that she should undergo an elective cesarean section. The last dose of therapeutic dalteparin was given 24 hours before delivery and she had an uncomplicated delivery with little bleeding. Six hours postpartum she had a dose of dalteparin 5000 units and was started back on full dose dalteparin the following morning. She was offered the option of switching to warfarin for 6 weeks but decided to continue with dalteparin for this time. She had no significant post-thrombotic syndrome 1 year later.

Comment: IVF pregnancies are associated with an increased risk of VTE, which endures for the entire pregnancy. She had multiple risk factors for VTE, which included IVF pregnancy, her age, increased BMI, multiple pregnancy, and hyperemesis.

This case also illustrates that many DVTs do not present with significant signs, for she had no swelling or change in color in her leg.

Case Study 2
A 28-year-old primip developed spontaneous left iliac vein thrombosis at 39 weeks' gestation. Pregnancy until then had been uncomplicated, and there were no other obvious acquired risk factors. Her father had an extensive DVT during immobilization of the leg in a plaster cast, after a traumatic ankle fracture.

On examination, there was marked erythema and gross tender swelling of the entire left leg, with a calf girth 6 cm greater than the right. Ultrasound confirmed extensive occlusive thrombus in the iliofemoral veins and she was commenced on therapeutic doses of low-molecular-weight heparin (LMWH). As she was near term, consideration was given to an inferior vena caval filter. However, delivery was not thought imminent and the cervix was unfavorable, so a decision was made to review the following day. After the first day of full anticoagulation her leg was less tense and painful and she was better able to mobilize. Daily review showed continued subsidence of the pain and swelling and a filter was avoided.

A week after presentation, labor was induced, 24 hours following her injection of LMWH. As labor was prolonged, she was commenced on an intravenous infusion of unfractionated heparin, aiming for an aPTT within the given therapeutic range for the laboratory. When finally the cervix was 4 cm dilated, the infusion was discontinued and there was no excess blood loss at delivery. She was given a prophylactic dose of LMWH at 4 hours after delivery and recommenced on therapeutic LMWH the next morning. Warfarin was introduced at 1 week postpartum, overlapping with the LMWH until an INR >2 was sustained for more than 24 hours. She was discharged with a below-knee, class 2 compression stocking on the left leg (although the benefit in reducing post-thrombotic syndrome is unclear) and reassured of the safety of breast-feeding with heparin and warfarin.

At 3 months postpartum, there was minimal residual swelling of the lower leg and the warfarin was discontinued.

References

1. Bates SM, Ginsberg JS. How we manage venous thromboembolism during pregnancy. *Blood* 2002; 100: 3470–3478.

2. Bates SM, Greer IA, Pabinger I *et al*. Venous thromboembolism, thrombophilia, antithrombotic therapy, and pregnancy: American College of Chest Physicians Evidence-Based Clinical Practice Guidelines (8th Edition). *Chest* 2008; **133**: 844S–886S.

3. Sultan AA Grainge M West J *et al*. Impact of risk factors on the timing of first postpartum venous thromboembolism: a population-based cohort study from England. *Blood* 2014; **124**(18): 2872–2880.

4. Kamel H, Navi BB, Sriram N, *et al*. Risk of a thrombotic event after the 6-week postpartum period. *New England Journal of Medicine* 2014; **370**: 1307–1315.

5. Knight M, Kenyon S, Brocklehurst P *et al*. on behalf of MBRRACE-UK. *Saving Lives, Improving Mothers' Care – Lessons learned to inform future maternity care from the UK and Ireland Confidential Enquiries into Maternal Deaths and Morbidity 2009–12*. Oxford: National Perinatal Epidemiology Unit, University of Oxford; 2014.

6. Lewis G, ed. *The Confidential Enquiry into Maternal and Child Health – Saving Mothers' Lives: Reviewing Maternal Deaths to Make Motherhood Safer 2003–2005*. The seventh report on Confidential Enquiries into Maternal Deaths in the United Kingdom. London: CEMACH; 2007.

7. Royal College of Obstetricians and Gynecologists (RCOG). *Thromboembolic Disease in Pregnancy and the Puerperium: Acute Management. Green-Top Guideline No. 37b*. London: Royal College of Obstetricians and Gynecologists; 2015 (https://www.rcog.org.uk/ globalassets/ documents/ guidelines/ gtg-37b.pdf).

8. British Thoracic Society Standards of Care Committee Pulmonary Embolism Guideline Development Group. British Thoracic Society guidelines for the management of suspected acute pulmonary embolism. *Thorax* 2003; **58**: 470–484.

9. Scarsbrook AF, Evans AL, Owen AR, Gleeson FV. Diagnosis of suspected venous thromboembolic disease in pregnancy. *Clinical Radiology* 2006; **61**: 1–12.

10. Royal College of Obstetricians and Gynecologists (RCOG). *Reducing the Risk of Thrombosis and Embolism During Pregnancy and the Puerperium. Green-Top Guideline No. 37a*. London: Royal College of Obstetricians and Gynecologists; 2015 (https://www.rcog.org.uk/globalassets/documents/guidelines/gtg-37a.pdf).

11. Jacobsen AF, Skjeldestad FE, Sandset PM. Ante- and postnatal risk factors of venous thrombosis: a hospital-based case-control study. *Journal of Thrombosis and Hemostasis* 2008; **6**: 905–912.

12. Lindqvist P, Dahlbäck B, Marŝál K. Thrombotic risk during pregnancy: a population study. *Obstetrics and Gynecology* 1999; **94**: 595–599.

13. James AH, Jamison MG, Brancazio LR, Myers ER. Venous thromboembolism during pregnancy and the postpartum period: incidence, risk factors, and mortality. *American Journal of Obstetrics and Gynecology* 2006; **194**: 1311–1315.

14. Knight M on behalf of UKOSS. Antenatal pulmonary embolism: risk factors, management and outcomes. *BJOG: An International Journal of Obstetrics and Gynecology* 2008; **115**: 453–461.

15. Greer IA. Pregnancy complicated by venous thrombosis. *New England Journal of Medicine* 2015; **73**: 540–547.

16. Dentali F, Douketis JD, Gianni M *et al*. Meta-analysis: anticoagulant prophylaxis to prevent

symptomatic venous thromboembolism in hospitalized medical patients. *Annals of Internal Medicine* 2007; **146**(4): 278–288.

17. Cutts BA, Dasgupta D, Hunt BJ. New directions in the diagnosis and treatment of pulmonary embolism in pregnancy. *American Journal of Obstetrics and Gynecology* 2013; **208**(2): 102–108.

18. Cutts BA, Tran HA, Merriman E *et al.* The utility of the Wells clinical prediction model and ventilation-perfusion scanning for pulmonary embolism diagnosis in pregnancy. *Blood Coagulation and Fibrinolysis* 2014; **25**(4): 375–378.

19. Cook JV, Kyriou J. Radiation from CT and perfusion scanning in pregnancy. *BMJ* 2005; **331**: 350.

20. Hurwitz LM, Yoshizumi TT, Goodman PC *et al.* Radiation dose savings for adult pulmonary embolus 64-MDCT using bismuth breast shields, lower peak kilovoltage, and automatic tube current modulation. *AJR American Journal of Roentgenology* 2009; **192**: 244–253.

21. The Task Force for the Diagnosis and Management of Acute Pulmonary Embolism of the European Society of Cardiology. Guidelines on the diagnosis and management of acute pulmonary embolism. *European Heart Journal* 2008; **29**: 2276–2315.

22. Robertson L, Wu O, Langhorne P, *et al.* Thrombophilia in pregnancy: a systematic review. *British Journal of Haematology* 2006; **132**: 171–196.

23. Greer IA, Nelson-Piercy C. Low-molecular-weight heparins for thromboprophylaxis and treatment of venous thromboembolism in pregnancy: a systematic review of safety and efficacy. *Blood* 2005; **106**: 401–407.

24. McColl D, Ellison J, Greer IA, *et al.* Prevalence of the post thrombotic syndrome in young women with previous venous thromboembolism. *British Journal of Haematology* 2000; **108**: 272–274.

25. Kahn SR, Shapiro S, Wells PS *et al.*; SOX Trial Investigators. Compression stockings to prevent post-thrombotic syndrome: a randomised placebo-controlled trial. *Lancet* 2014; **383**(9920): 880–888.

26. Greer I, Hunt BJ. Low molecular weight heparin in pregnancy: current issues. *British Journal of Haematology* 2005; **128**: 593–560.

27. Tang AW, Greer IA. A systematic review on the use of new anticoagulants in pregnancy. *Obstetric Medicine* 2013; **6**: 64–71.

28. Colombier S, Niclauss L. Successful surgical pulmonary embolectomy for massive perinatal embolism after emergency cesarean section. *Annals of Vascular Surgery* 2015; **29**(7): 1452.e1–4. doi: 10.1016/j.avsg.2015.04.066.

29. Bataillard A, Hebrard A, Gaide-Chevronnay L *et al.* Extracorporeal life support for massive pulmonary embolism during pregnancy. *Perfusion* 2015; **31**(2): 169–171.

Chapter 13

Thromboprophylaxis in Pregnancy

Anna Lawin-O'Brien and Catherine Nelson-Piercy

Introduction and Epidemiology

Venous thromboembolism (VTE) has been the leading direct cause of maternal death in the UK for decades[1].

Although the CEMACH report (2007) and CMACE report (2011) showed a significant reduction in the maternal mortality rate from pulmonary embolism (PE) – falling from 1.56 per 100 000 maternities (95% CI 1.43–2.63) in 2003–05 (33 deaths) to 0.70 per 100 000 maternities (95% CI 0.49–1.25) in 2006–08 (16 deaths) [2,3], the most recent UK maternal mortality report (MBRRACE 2014) showed an increase to 1.26 (95% CI 0.85–1.8) in 2009–11 and 1.08 (95% CI 0.71–1.59) in 2010–12[4]. Between 2003–05 and 2006–08, there was a reduction in maternal deaths from antenatal VTE (from 11 to 3) and postnatal VTE after vaginal delivery (from 8 to 2)[1,2]. The incidence of PE in pregnancy was calculated as 1.3 per 10 000 maternities according to the UK Obstetric Surveillance System (UKOSS) study[4]; this accounts for 5–10 maternal deaths every year, many of which may be preventable [1].

The recent enquiries into maternal death[2,3] as well as the UKOSS study[5] identified risk factors in the majority of women with fatal and non-fatal PE: CEMACH 2003–05 (79%), CMACE 2006–08 (89%), and UKOSS (70%)[2,3,5]. All reports have repeatedly highlighted the need to identify those risk factors, ideally prior to pregnancy or as early as possible in the first trimester. In addition to the physiologically increased VTE risk in pregnancy, risk factors can be continuous or transient, pregnancy related, or pregnancy independent[2,3]. The Royal College of Obstetricians and Gynecologists (RCOG) published the first Green-Top Guideline on risk stratification and prevention of VTE in pregnancy in 2004[6] and have since updated these guidelines twice (2009, 2015) [1,7]. The absolute risk of VTE in pregnancy and puerperium is small but significant (overall incidence of VTE is approximately 1–2 per 1000 births)[8–11] and increases with gestation[11,12]. The relative risk of antenatal VTE is increased four- to sixfold[8,9] and the relative risk postpartum is fivefold higher compared to antepartum[13,14].

The CEMACH enquiry from 2007 reported two-thirds of fatal antenatal PE occurring in the first trimester[2]. Antenatal deaths are as frequently reported as postnatal deaths[15] but pregnancy lasts longer than the puerperium. Despite good evidence for the increased risk of VTE from early pregnancy onwards there remains a higher threshold for initiating preventive thromboprophylaxis in the first trimester[16]. The risk is higher in the third trimester[13] but the time of highest risk per day for VTE remains the postpartum period with a 22-fold increase in risk compared with baseline non-pregnant, non-postpartum state[13,14,16,17]. The mode and complexity of delivery contribute significantly to the postpartum thromboembolic risk with women after vaginal delivery facing half the risk of those delivered by cesarean section[1].

The guideline on "Reducing the risk of venous thromboembolism" by the National Institute for Health and Clinical Excellence (NICE) estimates that low-molecular-weight heparin (LMWH) reduces VTE in 60% of medical and 70% of surgical patients [18]. In the obstetric population evidence suggests a relative risk reduction of VTE of over 80% with LMWH prophylaxis[19]. Good evidence for efficacy and safety of pharmacological thromboprophylaxis throughout pregnancy and growing knowledge about risk factors for VTE allow improved risk stratification and better preventive strategies[16,19,20]. Current guidelines support clinicians to initiate and continue thromboprophylaxis if appropriate from the first trimester to the puerperium[1].

Pathogenesis and Risk Factor Assessment

Pregnancy itself puts women at higher risk of VTE, with a four- to sixfold increase compared to an age-matched non-pregnant female population[6,8,9]. This is primarily related to the procoagulant changes occurring from early pregnancy to promote hemostasis post-delivery [10]. Other components of Virchow's triad[21] are also present, namely increased venous stasis and vascular trauma, the latter particularly around the time of delivery. Superimposed on the pregnancy background risk are a range of additional risk factors (see Tables 13.1 and 13.2), which may either predate the pregnancy or develop during the pregnancy or puerperium and can be persistent or transient. In order to stratify risk the current recommendation includes a documented assessment of risk factors for VTE for all women in early pregnancy or pre-pregnancy ideally (Table 13.3)[1]. This assessment should be repeated in case of hospital admission, development of any medical or obstetric complications, and again intrapartum and postpartum (Table 13.4)[1].

Previous VTE and Thrombophilia

Any previous VTE increases the risk for pregnancy-related VTE by 2–12%[10,13,22], and antenatal and postnatal prophylaxis is recommended. The exception is a single VTE related to major surgery, where thromboprophylaxis can be withheld until 28 weeks of pregnancy[1]. A large retrospective study calculated an odds ratio of 24.8 (95% CI 17.1–36) for previous VTE [24]; further studies show recurrence rates following a single previous DVT or PE of 5.8% for antenatal and 8.3% for postnatal VTE[28]. Even in the absence of objective clinical documentation of VTE but a good history of the past event and treatment, antenatal thromboprophylaxis should be started[1]. Testing for heritable thrombophilia here is not indicated as the recommended management will not change[1]. However, women with an unprovoked VTE should be offered testing for antiphospholipid antibodies[1].

Women with thrombophilia carry a higher risk of pregnancy-related VTE. Thrombophilias may either be heritable (antithrombin [AT] deficiency, protein C deficiency, protein S deficiency, factor V Leiden, or prothrombin gene variant) or acquired (antiphospholipid syndrome, including lupus anticoagulant and anticardiolipin antibodies). Up to 50% of women who develop VTE during pregnancy or the postpartum period have an underlying thrombophilia[15]. The relative risk of VTE in pregnancy varies depending on the thrombophilia, but can be as high as tenfold with antithrombin deficiency. The risk is further increased in those women with a personal, rather than a family, history of thromboembolism. Deficiencies of natural anticoagulants are associated with a higher recurrence

risk: protein C deficiency 12–17%, protein S deficiency 22–26%, and AT deficiency 32–51%. The risk of recurrence is lower in those women with heterogeneous factor V Leiden or prothrombin variant[29–31]. Testing for thrombophilia is recommended in women with recurrent, atypical, or unprovoked VTEs or a family history of thromboembolism[1,25].

Other Risk Factors

Additional risk factors of particular importance are obesity, increasing maternal age, and immobility. Obesity was found in 60% of women dying of PE in the UK between 2003 and 2008[2,3]. The risk of thromboembolism from obesity (body mass index [BMI] of 30 or higher) rises with increasing BMI[5,26,27] and is higher for PE (adjusted OR [aOR] 14.9, 95% CI 3.0–74.8) than for DVT (aOR 4.4, 95% CI 1.6–11.9)[26]. The data on age as a risk factor for VTE in pregnancy remain conflicting with studies suggesting a modestly increased relative risk for women over 35 years [11,12,32], or an up to 50% increased risk for the oldest age group (35–44 years) compared to women aged 25–34 years[13]. The recent RCOG guideline[1] recommends age over 35 years as a risk factor for antenatal or postnatal VTE. Moreover, general immobility, hospital admission, or long distance travel (more than 4 hours and not exclusively by air) are recognized risk factors for antenatal or postnatal VTE[33–35].

Many comorbidities have been identified as risk factors for VTE, such as active inflammatory bowel disease[36], urinary tract infection[36], systemic lupus erythematosus (SLE)[32], heart disease, or pre-eclampsia (PET)[12]. Current evidence does not allow an accurate estimation of cumulative VTE risk from combining the different risk factors[1], hence a pragmatic approach to women with risk factors is proposed by the RCOG[1]. Thromboprophylaxis from early pregnancy is recommended in the presence of four or more risk factors antenatally, from 28 weeks with three risk factors and postnatally with two risk factors or more[1].

Management

The management strategy for thromboprophylaxis during pregnancy and the postpartum period is based on risk stratification according to current RCOG guidelines as detailed in Table 13.3[1]. All women should have an assessment of risk factors for VTE, ideally pre-pregnancy or in early pregnancy as well as intrapartum and postpartum (Tables 13.4 and 13.5). This risk assessment should be repeated in the

Table 13.1 Risk factors for VTE in pregnancy and postpartum

Pre-existing risk factors

Previous VTE

Heritable thrombophilia

Antithrombin deficiency
Protein C deficiency

Protein S deficiency

Factor V Leiden
Prothrombin 20210

Acquired thrombophilia

Antiphospholipid antibodies

Persistent lupus anticoagulant and/or

persistent moderate/high titer

anticardiolipin antibodies and/or β2-

glycoprotein 1 antibodies

Medical comorbidities

e.g. cancer; heart failure; active SLE, inflammatory

polyarthropathy/IBD; nephrotic syndrome; T1 DM with

nephropathy; sickle cell disease; current intravenous drug user

Age >35 years

Obesity (BMI ≥30 kg/m^2) either prepregnancy or in early pregnancy

Parity ≥3

Smoking

Gross varicose veins (symptomatic or above knee or with associated phlebitis, edema/skin changes)

Paraplegia

Obstetric risk factors

Multiple pregnancy

Current pre-eclampsia

Cesarean section

Prolonged labor (>24 hours)

Mid-cavity or rotational operative delivery

Stillbirth

Preterm birth

Postpartum hemorrhage (>1 L/requiring transfusion)

New onset/transient risk factors

Any surgical procedure in pregnancy or puerperium except

immediate repair of the perineum, e.g. appendicectomy,

postpartum sterilization

Bone fracture

Hyperemesis, dehydration

Ovarian hyperstimulation syndrome (first trimester only)

Assisted reproductive technology (ART), in vitro fertilization (IVF)

Admission or immobility (≥3 days' bed rest)

Current systemic infection (requiring intravenous antibiotics or admission to hospital)

Long-distance travel (>4 hours)

From RCOG[1].
All of the above are accepted VTE risk factors. The degree of increased VTE risk associated with them varies, as indicated in Table 13.2.

Table 13.2 Quoted adjusted odds ratios for individual risk factors

Risk factor for VTE	aOR	95% CI
Previous VTE[25]	24.8	17.1–36
Age >35[9]	1.3	1.0–1.7
BMI >30[23]	5.3	2.1–13.5
Smoking[25]	2.7	1.5–4.9
Parity ≥3[9]	2.4	1.8–3.1
Hyperemesis	2.51	
Immobility[26]	7.7	3.2–19
Heart disease[23,27]	7.1	6.2–8.3
Pre-eclampsia[26]	3.1	1.8–5.3
+Fetal growth restriction	5.8	2.1–16
ART[26]	4.3	2.0–9.4
Twins[26]	2.6	1.1–6.2
APH[26]	2.3	1.8–2.8
PPH[26]	4.1	2.3–7.3
Cesarean section[9]	3.6	3.0–4.3
Varicose veins	2.4	1.04–5.4
Transfusion[15]	7.6	6.2–9.4

Adapted from RCOG[1].
ART, assisted reproductive technology; APH, antepartum hemorrhage; PPH, postpartum hemorrhage.

Table 13.3 Risk factors for VTE and management

Risk factors	Management
≥4 Risk factors	LMWH prophylaxis from 1st trimester and 6 weeks postnatally
3 Risk factors	LMWH prophylaxis from 28 weeks and 6 weeks postnatally
2 Risk factors	LMWH prophylaxis if admitted to hospital and 10 days postpartum

According to RCOG[1].

event of admission to hospital or development of any further medical problems. The estimated risk of VTE should be discussed with the woman and a written individualized plan for her thromboprophylaxis should be documented[1]. Antenatal thromboprophylaxis, if required, can be prescribed if the woman is already pregnant. If the woman is not yet pregnant, the prescription can still be given, so LMWH can be started as soon as a pregnancy test is positive. This is particularly important for women in the very-high- and high-risk groups, as the pregnancy-related increase in VTE risk starts from the beginning of the first trimester[37]. The recommendations should be detailed in a letter copied to both the GP and patient, so prophylaxis can be started without the woman needing to come back to the hospital clinic first.

A woman with a previous history of VTE is high risk; LMWH must be prescribed throughout the antenatal period and until 6 weeks postnatally and a referral should be made to the Trust-nominated expert in thrombosis in pregnancy[1].

Women at intermediate risk should be prescribed LMWH antenatally and for at least 10 days postnatally, while considering extending thromboprophylaxis if risk factors persist or with more than three risk factors [1]. Women with four or more current risk factors (Table 13.3) should be considered for prophylactic LMWH throughout antenatal period and 6 weeks

postnatally[1]. Women with three current risk factors (Table 13.3) (other than previous VTE or thrombophilia) should be considered for prophylactic LMWH from 28 weeks and 6 weeks postnatally[1]. Women with two current risk factors (Table 13.3) should be considered for prophylactic LMWH for at least 10 days postpartum[1].

It is particularly important to identify those women with a previous VTE and/or known thrombophilia. If there is a past history of VTE, then details of presentation, means of diagnosis, drug treatment, and length of course should be determined. If deemed appropriate, women with a previous VTE should be screened for both heritable and acquired thrombophilia prior to pregnancy, as interpretation of some of the tests (especially protein S) is unreliable in pregnancy. The specific thrombophilia (Table 13.6) and other risk factors (Table 13.2) should be considered, as well as any family history of VTE in a first-degree relative.

Women with a history of VTE in association with a high-risk thrombophilia such as antithrombin deficiency (AT)[30,37] or antiphospholipid syndrome (APS) [32,38,39] (who may be on long-term anticoagulation) should be offered thromboprophylaxis with a higher dose LMWH (either 50%, 75%, or full treatment dose) antenatally and 6 weeks postpartum or until returned to oral anticoagulation[1]. These high-risk women should be managed together with a hematologist with expertise in thrombosis in pregnancy and consideration given to antenatal anti-Xa monitoring and the potential for antithrombin replacement at initiation of labor or prior to cesarean section[30,40]. If anti-Xa levels are measured, a test that does not use exogenous antithrombin should be used and 4-hour peak level of 0.5–1.0 iu/mL aimed for [30]. Other heritable thrombophilias carry a lower VTE risk and can be managed with standard doses of LMWH [1]. Women with previous recurrent VTE, with no diagnosis of thrombophilia, should also be managed together with a hematologist with expertise in thrombosis in pregnancy. They may require higher doses of LMWH [39,41].

Table 13.4 Antenatal assessment of risk factors for VTE according to RCOG[1]

Risk factors	Management
≥4 risk factors	LMWH prophylaxis from 1st trimester and 6 weeks postnatally
3 risk factors	LMWH prophylaxis from 28 weeks and 6 weeks postnatally
2 risk factors	LMWH prophylaxis if admitted to hospital and 10 days postpartum.

High risk

- Any previous VTE (except a single event related to major surgery)

Intermediate risk

- Known high-risk thrombophilia
- Hospital admission
- Single previous VTE related to major surgery
- High-risk thrombophilia + no VTE
- Medical comorbidities (cancer, heart failure, active SLE, inflammatory bowel disease, inflammatory polyarthropathy, nephrotic syndrome, T1 DM +nephropathy, SCD, current IDU)
- Myeloproliferative disorders (essential thrombocythemia, polycythemia vera)
- Any surgical procedure (e.g. appendicectomy)

Other risk factors

- Obesity (BMI >30 kg/m^2, pre-pregnancy/in early pregnancy)
- Age >35 years
- Parity ≥3
- Gross varicose veins
- Immobility: paraplegia, PGP
- Smoker
- Family history of unprovoked/estrogen provoked VTE in 1st degree relative
- Low-risk thrombophilia
- Multiple pregnancy
- IVF/ART

Transient risk factors

- Dehydration, hyperemesis, current systemic infection, long-distance travel

Women on long-term warfarin or other oral anticoagulants should be counseled regarding teratogenicity pre-pregnancy and advised to stop their oral anticoagulant therapy and change to LMWH as soon as an intrauterine pregnancy is confirmed, ideally before the sixth week of pregnancy[1]. Women not on warfarin or other oral anticoagulants should be advised to start LMWH as soon as they have a positive pregnancy test[1].

Table 13.5 Postnatal assessment of risk factors for VTE according to RCOG[1]

High risk
- Any previous VTE
- Anyone requiring antenatal LMWH
- High-risk thrombophilia
- Low-risk thrombophilia + family history

Intermediate risk
- Cesarean section in labor
- BMI ≥40 kg/m^2
- Readmission or prolonged admission (≥3 days) in the puerperium
- Any surgical procedure in the puerperium except immediate repair of the perineum
- Medical comorbidities; e.g. cancer, heart failure, active SLE, IBD or inflammatory polyarthropathy; nephrotic syndrome, type I DM with nephropathy, sickle cell disease, current IVDU

General risk factors
- Obesity (BMI >30 kg/m^2, either pre-pregnancy or in early pregnancy)
- Age >35 years
- Parity ≥3
- Elective cesarean section
- Gross varicose veins
- Immobility: paraplegia, PGP, long-distance travel
- Smoker
- Family history VTE
- Low-risk thrombophilia
- Current PET
- Multiple pregnancy
- Preterm delivery (<37 weeks)
- Stillbirth in this pregnancy
- Prolonged labor (>24 hr)
- Mid-cavity rotational or operative delivery
- PPH >1 L or blood transfusion

The VTE risk may change for a woman as pregnancy progresses, e.g. with hospital admission, development of infections, or pre-eclampsia, influencing the risk. The risk factor assessment should be repeated if there is any change in circumstances, and LMWH initiated as appropriate. An additional risk factor may only exist temporarily, e.g. hyperemesis gravidarum, and the original regimen can be returned to once the condition has resolved.

Plans for peri-delivery anticoagulation should be discussed and documented early, including recommended timing of regional anesthesia (discussed further in Chapter 15).

The level of VTE risk should be reassessed postnatally, as it may be increased depending on the mode of delivery and any associated complications. Women on long-term warfarin are usually managed with high-dose prophylactic LMWH for the first week postnatally and then converted back to warfarin from day 4–6 postpartum.

Table 13.6 Recommendation for thromboprophylaxis for women with previous VTE/thrombophilia

Risk	Thrombophilia	Management
Very high	Previous VTE on long-term oral anticoagulant therapy	Antenatal high-dose LMWH & 6 weeks' postnatal LMWH or until switched back to oral anticoagulant therapy
	Antithrombin deficiency	Require specialist management by experts in hemostasis and pregnancy
	Antiphospholipid syndrome with previous VTE	
High	Any previous VTE (except a single VTE related to major surgery)	Antenatal and 6 weeks' postnatal prophylactic LMWH
Intermediate	Asymptomatic high-risk thrombophilia: homozygous factor V Leiden/compound heterozygote protein C or S deficiency	Refer to local expert &consider antenatal LMWH. Postnatal prophylactic LMWH for 6 weeks
	Single previous VTE associated with major surgery without thrombophilia, family history, or other risk factors	Consider antenatal LMWH (not routinely recommended) Recommend LMWH from 28 weeks of gestation & 6 weeks' postnatal prophylactic LMWH
Low	Asymptomatic low-risk thrombophilia (prothrombin gene mutation or factor V Leiden)	Recommend 10 days' postnatal prophylactic LMWH if other risk factor postpartum or 6 weeks' if significant family history

According to RCOG[1].

Non-pharmacological and Pharmacological Measures for Thromboprophylaxis in Pregnancy

Non-pharmacological

Non-pharmacological measures include appropriate hydration, early mobilization, anti-embolism stockings (AES, formerly known as TEDS), and intermittent pneumatic compression. No randomized controlled trials (RCTs) have been carried out in pregnancy to study the efficacy of AES and recommendations are extrapolated from studies of non-pregnant populations [41]. The RCOG advises the use of correctly applied AES (providing graduated compression of 14–15 mmHg) for hospitalized women with contraindication to LMWH, for high-risk women post-CS, or for women traveling for more than 4 hours[1].

Pharmacological

Aspirin

Aspirin inhibits the enzyme cyclo-oxygenase in platelets, thus reducing thromboxane production and platelet aggregation. There are no RCT data on the use of aspirin as a thromboprophylactic agent in pregnancy. Current literature suggests that benefit of aspirin in VTE prevention in pregnancy is uncertain and significantly less than that of LMWH. Hence aspirin is not recommended for thromboprophylaxis in pregnancy[1].

Heparin

Neither unfractionated (UFH) nor low-molecular-weight (LMWH) heparin crosses the placenta and there are no adverse effects on the fetus. LMWH is the anticoagulant of choice in the UK for prophylaxis and treatment of VTE both ante- and postnatally.

LMWH is as effective and safer than UFH for VTE prophylaxis in pregnancy and provides a number of advantages over UFH: predictable and reliable pharmacokinetics and a longer half-life allowing once daily administration as well as providing good antithrombotic effect with a lower risk of bleeding. LMWH is composed of shorter molecules than UFH and the ratio of anti-Xa (antithrombotic) to anti-IIa activity (anticoagulant) is increased. This enables an increased antithrombotic-benefit to bleeding risk ratio [15]. LMWH also has less of an effect on platelet aggregation, function, and activation, and binds platelet factor 4 less well, hence reducing the risk of both early and late heparin-induced thrombocytopenia (HIT)[42]. LMWH in prophylactic doses is not associated with a reduction in bone density over and

Table 13.7 Thromboprophylactic doses of LMWH

Weight	Enoxaparin (mg daily)	Dalteparin (units daily)	Tinzaparin (units daily)
<50 kg	20	2500	3500
50–90 kg	40	5000	4500
91–130 kg	60[a]	7500	7000[a]
131–170 kg	80[a]	10 000	9000[a]
>170 kg	0.6 mg/kg/d[a]	75 units/kg/d	75 units/kg/d[a]
High prophylactic dose for 50–90 kg	40 mg 12 hrly	5000 units/12 hrly	4500 units/12 hrly

[a] May be given in two divided doses.
According to RCOG[1].

above what is expected in normal pregnancy[42]. Doses are based on booking weight or most recent weight (see Table 13.7), and should be reduced with known renal impairment. Monitoring of platelets with LMWH is only recommended when UFH has been given before, and monitoring of factor anti-Xa is usually not required with LMWH in thromboprophylactic doses. LMWH is safe with breast-feeding[1,43].

Unfractionated heparin has the benefit of a shorter half-life and quicker reversibility compared to LMWH and is therefore useful to manage very high-risk women peripartum, with increased risk of hemorrhage or possible requirement of anesthesia [1,42]. The recommended time interval between a prophylactic dose of UFH and insertion of regional anesthesia is 4 hours compared to 12 hours after LMWH[1]. Monitoring of platelet count is recommended every 2–3 days until UFH is stopped if used after surgery as UFH is associated with an increased risk of HIT[1,42].

In women at risk of both VTE and bleeding a careful balance between risks and benefits of LMWH must be applied and a multidisciplinary team approach including hematologists is recommended[44].

In case of heparin intolerance or HIT alternative treatment with heparinoids is recommended in conjunction with hematologists[1]. Danaparoid is appropriate for prophylaxis or treatment of VTE in pregnancy; however, its long half-life of 24 hours has to be especially accounted for when used antenatally. Safety data are overall limited but no adverse outcome has been attributed to danaparoid and it appears safe in breast-feeding[45].

A further alternative for heparin intolerant women is the synthetic pentasaccharide fondaparinux, which works through inhibition of factor Xa via antithrombin[1]. Data on safety of its use in pregnancy are limited but reassuring[46,47]. Dosing recommendations in and outside pregnancy are the same and fondaparinux has a long half-life of 18 hours[46]. Fondaparinux does not cross the placenta, very small amounts of anti-factor Xa activity were found in neonatal plasma, and oral absorption through breast milk appears unlikely[46,48]. New oral anticoagulants (NOACs) such as dabigatran, rivaroxaban, or apixaban act through inhibition of thrombin or factor Xa. As there are no data on their use in pregnancy, they should be avoided[25].

Warfarin

Warfarin crosses the placenta and is teratogenic, with a risk of causing "warfarin embryopathy" (chrondrodysplasia punctata, nasal hypoplasia, heart defects, and short proximal limbs) in approximately 5% of fetuses exposed in the first trimester[49, 50]. Warfarin is also associated with an increased rate of miscarriage, stillbirth, neonatal neurological problems, and a significant risk of fetal and maternal hemorrhage[51, 52].

Because of these effects, warfarin is generally not recommended for thromboprophylaxis in pregnancy. An exception is those women requiring full anticoagulation with warfarin for metal prosthetic heart valves (particularly of the older type and those in the mitral position), whose thrombotic risk is extremely high, and in whom valve thrombosis carries a high mortality (see Chapter 14).

For women needing long-term anticoagulation warfarin can be reintroduced 4–6 days postpartum. This needs close monitoring, INR testing, and follow-up in an anticoagulation clinic. However, further self-administration of LMWH can be avoided and warfarin is safe in breast-feeding.

In very high-risk women appropriate thromboprophylaxis may be difficult, and the risk/benefit balance for the particular individual has to be considered. This would include those with a known thrombophilia and VTE or cerebral arterial thrombosis in APS despite full dose LMWH. A compromise option here is to use LMWH for the highest risk periods of warfarin side effects, namely, the first trimester and after 36 weeks' gestation, and convert back to warfarin for the second and early third trimesters. This obviously requires very close supervision and thorough discussion with the woman.

Current Research and Future Direction

- Interaction and accumulation of risk factors for VTE in the antenatal and postpartum periods.
- Reduction and avoidance of risk factors for VTE in pregnancy.
- VTE risk for women undergoing surgical management of miscarriage and surgical termination of pregnancy.
- Thromboprophylaxis regimes for different heritable thrombophilias.

Summary

- Venous thromboembolism is the leading direct cause of maternal mortality in the UK, and many cases are potentially preventable.
- Pregnancy itself is a risk factor for VTE, and additional risk factors include previous VTE, thrombophilia, cesarean section, and obesity.
- Risk factors for VTE should be identified pre-pregnancy, at least early in pregnancy, and reassessed throughout pregnancy and the puerperium, as level of risk may change.
- Thromboprophylaxis should be started according to current guidance, in the first trimester if indicated, throughout pregnancy and in the puerperium.

Case Study 1

A 38-year-old primiparous woman booked for antenatal care. This was a spontaneous conception and her BMI was 36. She had no personal or family history of venous thromboembolism. She was risk assessed by her midwife at booking and her VTE score was 2.

Her antenatal care was uneventful until 33 weeks when she was admitted with hypertension (blood pressure 148/96 mmHg – booking blood pressure 116/66 mmHg) and proteinuria (protein:creatinine ratio 160 g/mol) and a diagnosis of pre-eclampsia was made. Dalteparin 7500 units daily was commenced as her weight was 93 kg, and she was now admitted.

At 35 weeks her platelet count dropped from 156 x 10^9/L on admission to 80 x 10^9/L and she was requiring maximum doses of two antihypertensive drugs to control her blood pressure. A decision was taken that she required delivery and an induction of labor was planned.

She had her last dose of dalteparin at 6pm the day before planned induction. However after 24 hours of Propess (vaginal prostaglandin), she was not in labor so another dose of 7500 units of dalteparin was given (having first confirmed that her platelet count remained above 50 x 10^9/L). Once she was in established labor, further doses were withheld and an epidural was sited for pain relief. An interval of 16 hours had elapsed since the last dose of dalteparin before siting the epidural and her coagulation screen was normal and platelet count 85 x 10^9/L. She went on to have a spontaneous vaginal delivery of a baby boy. The epidural was removed after delivery and she received her first postpartum dose of dalteparin 7500 units 4 hours later. She was advised to continue the dalteparin for 6 weeks after the baby was born.

Case Study 2

A 28-year-old multiparous woman underwent an elective cesarean section because she had a previous cesarean section. Her antenatal care was uneventful and she was VTE risk assessed with a score of 0 antenatally and 1 postpartum. She was discharged on day 3 but readmitted on day 6 postpartum with suspected endometritis (fever, uterine tenderness, heavy lochia). She was commenced on intravenous antibiotics and dalteparin 5000 units once daily as she was now at increased risk of VTE. This was continued until her discharge from hospital 3 days later as she had improved clinically and was mobile.

Comment: it is important to risk assess all pregnant and postpartum women at every admission and especially postpartum, when the absolute risk of VTE is elevated.

References

1. Royal College of Obstetricians and Gynecologists. *Reducing the Risk of Thrombosis and Embolism during Pregnancy and Puerperium. Green-Top Guideline No. 37a*. London: Royal College of Obstetricians and Gynecologists; 2015.

2. Lewis G, ed. *The Confidential Enquiry into Maternal and Child Health (CEMACH) – Saving Mothers' Lives: Reviewing Maternal Deaths to Make Motherhood Safer – 2003–2005*. The Seventh Report on Confidential Enquiries into Maternal Deaths in the United Kingdom. London: CEMACH; 2007.

3. Center for Maternal and Child Enquiries (CMACE). Saving Mothers' Lives: Reviewing maternal deaths to make motherhood safer: 2006–08. The Eighth Report of the Confidential Enquiries into Maternal Deaths in the United Kingdom. *BJOG: An International Journal of Obstetrics and Gynecology* 2011; **118** (Suppl 1): 1–203.

4. MBRRACE. *Saving Lives, Improving Mothers' Care – Lessons learned to inform future maternity care from the UK and Ireland Confidential Enquiries into Maternal Deaths and Morbidity 2009–12*. Oxford: National Perinatal Epidemiology Unit, University of Oxford; 2014.

5. Knight M; UKOSS. Antenatal pulmonary embolism: risk factors, management and outcomes. *BJOG: An International Journal of Obstetrics and Gynecology* 2008; **115**: 453–461.

6. Royal College of Obstetricians and Gynecologists. *Thromboprophylaxis during Pregnancy, Labor and After Normal Vaginal Delivery. Green-Top Guideline no. 37*. London: Royal College of Obstetricians and Gynecologists; 2004.

7. Royal College of Obstetricians and Gynecologists. *Reducing the risk of Thrombosis and Embolism during Pregnancy and Puerperium. Green-Top Guideline No. 37a*. London: Royal College of Obstetricians and Gynecologists; 2009.

8. Heit JA, Kobbervig CE, James AH *et al.* Trends in the incidence of venous thromboembolism during pregnancy or postpartum: a 30-year population-based study. *Annals of Internal Medicine* 2005; **143**: 697–706.

9. Jacobsen AF, Skjeldestad FE, Sandset PM. Ante- and postnatal risk factors of venous thrombosis: a hospital-based case–control study. *Journal of Thrombosis and Hemostasis* 2008; **6**: 905–912.

10. James AH. Prevention and management of venous thrombo-embolism in pregnancy. *American Journal of Medicine* 2007; **120**: S26–34.

11. Lindqvist P, Dahlbäck B, Maršál K. Thrombotic risk during pregnancy: a population study. *BJOG: An International Journal of Obstetrics and Gynecology* 1999; **94**: 595–599.

12. Kane EV, Calderwood C, Dobbie R *et al.* A population-based study of venous thrombosis in pregnancy in Scotland 1980–2005. *European Journal of Obstetrics & Gynecology and Reproductive Biology* 2013; **169**: 223–229.

13. Sultan AA, West J, Tata LJ *et al.* Risk of first venous thromboembolism in and around pregnancy: a population-based cohort study. *British Journal of Haematology* 2012; **156**: 366–373.

14. Pomp ER, Lenselink AM, Rosendaal FR, Doggen CJ. Pregnancy, the postpartum period and prothrombotic defects: risk of venous thrombosis in the MEGA study. *Journal of Thrombosis and Haemostasis* 2008; **6**: 632–637.

15. Nelson SM, Greer IA. Thrombophilia and the risk for venous thromboembolism during pregnancy, delivery, and puerperium. *Obstetric Gynecologic Clinics of North America* 2006; **33**: 413–427.

16. Bates SM, Greer IA, Middeldorp S *et al.*; American College of Chest Physicians. VTE, thrombophilia, antithrombotic therapy, and pregnancy: Antithrombotic Therapy and Prevention of Thrombosis, 9th ed: American College of Chest Physicians Evidence-Based Clinical Practice Guidelines. *Chest* 2012;**141** (2 Suppl): e691S–736S.

17. Jackson E, Curtis KM, Gaffield ME. Risk of venous thromboembolism during the postpartum period: a systematic review. *Obstetrics and Gynecology* 2011; **117**: 691–703.

18. National Institute for Health and Clinical Excellence. *Venous Thromboembolism: Reducing the Risk. Reducing the risk of Venous Thromboembolism (Deep Vein Thrombosis and Pulmonary Embolism) in Patients Admitted to Hospital. NICE Clinical Guideline 92*. London: NICE; 2010.

19. Lindqvist PG, Bremme K, Hellgren M. Swedish Society of Obstetrics and Gynecology (SFOG) Working Group on Hemostatic Disorders (Hem-ARG). Efficacy of obstetric thromboprophylaxis and long-term risk of recurrence of venous thromboembolism. *Acta Obstetricia et Gynecologica Scandinavica* 2011; **90**: 648–653.

20. Hunt BJ, Gattens M, Khamashta M, Nelson-Piercy C, Almeida A. Thromboprophylaxis with unmonitored intermediate-dose low molecular weight heparin in pregnancies with a previous arterial or venous thrombotic event. *Blood Coagulation and Fibrinolysis* 2003; **14**: 735–739.

21. Virchow R. *Thrombose und Embolie. Gefässentzündung und septische Infektion: Gesammelte Abhandlungen zur wissenschaftlichen Medicin* [in German]. Frankfurt am Main: Von Meidinger & Sohn. 1856: 219–732.

22. McColl MD, Walker ID, Greer IA. The role of inherited thrombophilia in venous thromboembolism associated with pregnancy. *British Journal of Obstetrics and Gynaecology* 1999; **106**: 756–766.

147

23. James AH, Jamison MG, Brancazio LR, Myers ER. Venous thromboembolism during pregnancy and the postpartum period: incidence, risk factors, and mortality. *American Journal of Obstetrics and Gynecology* 2006; **194**: 1311–1315.

24. Jamison MG, Brancazio LR, Myers ER. Venous thromboembolism during pregnancy and the postpartum period: incidence, risk factors, and mortality. *American Journal of Obstetrics and Gynecology* 2006; **194**: 1311–1315.

25. Nelson-Piercy C. *Handbook of Obstetric Medicine*, 5th edn. Florida: CRC Press, Taylor & Francis Group; 2015: 49–60.

26. Larsen TB, Sorensen HT, Gislum M, Johnsen SP. Maternal smoking, obesity, and risk of venous thromboembolism during pregnancy and the puerperium: a population-based nested case-control study. *Thrombosis Research* 2007; **120**: 505–509.

27. Simpson EL, Lawrenson RA, Nightingale AL, Farmer RD. Venous thromboembolism in pregnancy and the puerperium: incidence and additional risk factors from a London perinatal database. *BJOG: An International Journal of Obstetrics and Gynecology* 2001; **108**: 56–60.

28. De Stefano V, Martinelli I, Rossi E *et al*. The risk of recurrent venous thromboembolism in pregnancy and puerperium without antithrombotic prophylaxis. *British Journal of Haematology* 2006; **135**: 386–391.

29. Baglin T, Gray E, Greaves M *et al*. British Committee for Standards in Hematology. Clinical guidelines for testing for heritable thrombophilia. *British Journal of Haematology* 2010; **149**: 209–220.

30. Bramham K, Retter A, Robinson SE. How I treat heterozygous hereditary antithrombin deficiency in pregnancy. *Thrombosis and Haemostasis* 2013; **110**: 550–559.

31. Rogenhofer N, Bohlmann MK, Beuter-Winkler P *et al*. Prevention, management and extent of adverse pregnancy outcomes in women with hereditary antithrombin deficiency. *Annals of Hematology* 2014; **93**: 385–392.

32. Liu S, Rouleau J, Joseph KS *et al*. Maternal Health Study Group of the Canadian Perinatal Surveillance System. Epidemiology of pregnancy-associated venous thromboembolism: a population-based study in Canada. *Journal of Obstetrics and Gynecology Canada* 2009; **31**: 611–620.

33. National Collaborating Center for Women's and Children's Health. *Antenatal Care: Routine Care for the Healthy Pregnant Woman*. London: RCOG Press; 2008.

34. Royal College of Obstetricians and Gynecologists. *Air Travel and Pregnancy. Scientific Impact Paper No. 1*. London: RCOG; 2013.

35. Hezelgrave NL, Whitty CJ, Shennan AH, Chappell LC. Advising on travel during pregnancy. *BMJ* 2011; **342**: d2506.

36. Sultan AA, Tata LJ, West J *et al*. Risk factors for first venous thromboembolism around pregnancy: a population-based cohort study from the United Kingdom. *Blood* 2013; **121**: 3953–3961.

37. James AH, Tapson VF, Goldhaber SZ. Thrombosis during pregnancy and the postpartum period. *American Journal of Obstetrics and Gynecology* 2005; **193**: 216–219.

38. Stone S, Hunt BJ, Khamashta MA, Bewley SJ, Nelson-Piercy C. Primary antiphospholipid syndrome in pregnancy: an analysis of outcome in a cohort of 33 women treated with a rigorous protocol. *Journal of Thrombosis and Haemostasis* 2005; **3**: 243–245.

39. Casele H, Grobman WA. Cost-effectiveness of thromboprophylaxis with intermittent pneumatic compression at Cesarean delivery. *Obstetrics and Gynecology* 2006; **108**: 535–540.

40. Rogenhofer N, Bohlmann MK, Beuter-Winkler P *et al*. Prevention, management and extent of adverse pregnancy outcomes in women with hereditary antithrombin deficiency. *Annals of Hematology* 2014; **93**: 385–392.

41. Bates SM, Greer IA, Pabinger I *et al*. Venous thromboembolism, thrombophilia, antithrombotic therapy, and pregnancy. American College of Chest Physicians Evidence-Based Clinical Practice Guidelines (8th edn). *Chest* 2008; **133**: 844S–886S.

42. Clark NP, Delate T, Witt DM, Parker S, McDuffie R. A descriptive evaluation of unfractionated heparin use during pregnancy. *Journal of Thrombosis and Thrombolysis* 2009; **27**: 267–273.

43. Andersen AS, Berthelsen JG, Bergholt T. Venous thrombo-embolism in pregnancy: prophylaxis and treatment with low molecular weight heparin. *Acta Obstetricia et Gynecologica Scandinavica* 2010; **89**: 15–21.

44. Greer IA, Nelson-Piercy C. Low-molecular-weight heparins for thromboprophylaxis and treatment of venous thromboembolism in pregnancy: a systematic review of safety and efficacy. *Blood* 2005; **106**: 401–407.

45. Lindhoff-Last E, Bauersachs R. Heparin-induced thrombocytopenia-alternative anticoagulation in pregnancy and lactation. *Seminars in Thrombosis and Hemostasis* 2002; **28**: 439–446.

46. Gerhardt A, Zotz RB, Stockschleder M, Scharf RE. Fondaparinux is an effective alternative anticoagulant in pregnant women with high risk of venous thromboembolism and intolerance to low-molecular-weight heparins and heparinoids. *Thrombosis and Haemostasis* 2007; **97**: 496–497.

47. Bomke B, Hoffmann T, Dücker C, Scharf RE. P01-09 Successful prevention or treatment of venous

thromboembolism (VTE) with fondaparinux in pregnant women with allergic skin reactions to low-molecular-weight heparins (LMWHs) and danaparoid. *Hämostaseologie* 2010; **30** (Suppl): A35.

48. Lagrange F, Vergnes C, Brun JL, *et al.* Absence of placental transfer of pentasaccharide (Fondaparinux, Arixtra®) in the dually perfused human cotyledon in vitro. *Thrombosis and Haemostasis* 2002; **87**: 831–835.

49. Holzgreve W, Carey JC, Hall BD. Warfarin-induced fetal abnormalities. *Lancet* 1976; **ii**: 914–5.

50. Born D, Martinez EE, Almeida PA *et al.* Risk of warfarin during pregnancy with mechanical valve prostheses. *Obstetrics and Gynecology* 2002; **99**: 35–40.

51. Sbarouni E, Oakley CM. Outcome of pregnancy in women with valve prostheses. *British Heart Journal* 1994; **71**: 196–201.

52. Born D, Martinez EE, Almeida PA. Pregnancy in patients with prosthetic heart valves: the effects of anticoagulation on mother, fetus, and neonate. *American Heart Journal* 1992; **124**: 413–417.

Chapter 14

Management of Prosthetic Heart Valves in Pregnancy

Claire McLintock

Introduction

There are few management decisions in obstetric hematology that present such a major challenge as the choice of anticoagulation during pregnancy for women with mechanical prosthetic heart valves. Oral anticoagulants such as warfarin and coumadin are the most effective agents for prevention of maternal thromboembolism, but freely cross the placenta, are teratogenic, and also cause late fetal loss in as many as 1 in 10 pregnancies. Alternative anticoagulants, unfractionated heparin (UFH) and low-molecular-weight heparin (LMWH), do not cross the placenta but while these agents do not cause embryopathy or fetopathy they are likely to be less effective at preventing maternal valve thrombosis that can result in valve failure, systemic thromboembolism, or even maternal death. Therein lies the challenge: a choice between the most effective anticoagulant to protect a woman's own health but one with the highest risk of adverse outcome for her baby or an anticoagulant that is associated with higher maternal risk but is safer for her baby. Clinicians must help women make the best choice based on the available information about maternal and fetal risks with different types of anticoagulant. The safest option for the woman is to avoid pregnancy altogether but for the many women who choose to have a pregnancy, clear guidance and support can help them avoid the most dangerous choice, that of no anticoagulation at all.

This chapter presents the data relating to maternal and fetal outcomes in pregnancy in women with mechanical heart valves, to help clinicians and women make the most informed choice in this challenging clinical situation.

Indication for Valve Replacement

The most common indications for replacement of a native heart valve are congenital valvular disease and rheumatic heart disease. While the incidence of congenital valvular disease is relatively stable at 0.8% of births, there is marked variation in the rates of rheumatic fever and rheumatic heart disease (RHD) across different countries. Rheumatic fever is more common in resource-poor countries but it is also relatively prevalent in certain groups in affluent countries with high rates in Aboriginal and Torres Strait Islanders in Australia, in Maori and Pacific Island people in New Zealand, and in people living in the Pacific Islands[1].

Valve Type: Bioprosthetic or Mechanical?

For patients who require heart valve replacement the alternatives include bioprosthetic valves – either homograft (human tissue) or heterograft (porcine or bovine tissue) – or mechanical valves, e.g. Starr–Edwards valves, Björk–Shirley valves, Medtronic-Hall valves, St Jude's valves and On-X valves. The major advantage of bioprosthetic valves for young women of childbearing age is that, in the absence of other risk factors, anticoagulant therapy is not required. However, structural valve deterioration and the need for redo valve surgery is a significant issue and while the rate of structural valve deterioration is more rapid in younger patients, it is not further accelerated by pregnancy[2]. In contrast, structural valve failure is extremely uncommon with mechanical heart valves but the risks of valve thrombosis and systemic thromboembolism mean that patients must take long-term oral anticoagulant therapy with vitamin K antagonists (VKA). The requirement for effective ongoing anticoagulation creates the dilemma for women with mechanical heart valves during pregnancy. It is recommended that clinicians take this into account when considering which type of valve to use in young women who require valve replacement [3] and discuss options with the patient.

Valve-related factors
- Ball-cage type valves, i.e. Starr–Edwards valve
- Valve in mitral position
- ≥2 valve replacements

Clinical risk factors
- Previous thromboembolism
- Atrial fibrillation
- Dilated left atrium
- Heart failure

Prevention of Thromboembolism

The risks of valve thrombosis and need for anticoagulation in patients with mechanical prosthetic valves (MPHV) became clear soon after the first operations were carried out. Valve thrombosis can cause valve obstruction and failure as well as systemic embolization leading to cerebrovascular accidents (CVA) with permanent or transient disability but also myocardial infarction or other arterial embolization. In non-pregnant patients with MPHV the annual rate of major systemic embolization in those taking no anticoagulation is in the order of 4% and is reduced to around 1% in patients taking VKA such as warfarin or acenocoumarol. The direct oral anticoagulant (DOAC) dabigatran is not as effective as warfarin at prevention of thromboembolism in patients with MPHV, and this and the other DOACs, rivaroxaban, edoxaban, and apixaban, are not licensed for use in this setting and should not be used[4]. Risk factors for thromboembolism are shown in Table 14.1.

Anticoagulation for Mechanical Prosthetic Heart Valves during Pregnancy

The prothrombotic changes of pregnancy are likely to further increase the risk of thromboembolism in women with MPHV reinforcing the need to continue therapeutic anticoagulation to prevent thromboembolic complications (TEC) that may result in major morbidity and even the death of the mother. The paucity of randomized clinical trial data means that published guidelines or recommendations relating to anticoagulant regimens are mainly based on expert opinion. Interpretation of existing data by different groups of experts has led to variation in recommendations for anticoagulation during pregnancy in women with MPHV (Table 14.2). The European[5] and American guidelines[6] recommend

that all women continue VKA in the second and third trimesters, with options in the first trimester related to the dose of VKA. In contrast, the American College of Chest Physicians offers a number of alternatives[7]. While it is accepted that VKA provide the most effective protection against TEC[8] these drugs cross the placenta and are associated with fetal complications, i.e. warfarin embryopathy and warfarin fetopathy, including miscarriage and stillbirth. This makes them unacceptable to many women. As will be discussed later, while it is likely that there is a relationship between the dose of VKA and development of warfarin fetopathy, a dose relationship has not been demonstrated for the risk of classic warfarin embryopathy. Women's concerns with the adverse fetal effects of VKA led a move to explore alternative anticoagulants. Heparins, including low-molecular-weight heparin, do not cross the placenta and are not teratogenic. Despite concerns about clinical efficacy, many centers offer anticoagulant regimens with therapeutic dose LMWH during pregnancy to women who are unwilling to take VKA. There are increasing calls to ensure that women's preferences are considered when making decisions on management of anticoagulation, and a discussion of the risks and benefits of different therapeutic approaches is critical in this clinical setting[7,8].

Key points for discussion to enable development of an optimal treatment plan that reflects the woman's preferences and values include:

1. The efficacy of VKA, such as warfarin, in prevention of TEC.
2. Potential fetal complications with VKA, such as fetal loss and neurological and ocular abnormalities, and the influence of dose of VKA.
3. The efficacy of anticoagulation with therapeutic dose LMWH.
4. The most appropriate monitoring for LMWH, including whether peak *and* trough anti-Xa levels should be measured and the target therapeutic range.
5. The place of low-dose aspirin.

Once a joint treatment plan has been decided, close clinical follow-up is essential as poor compliance with anticoagulation and monitoring is associated with worse maternal and fetal outcomes. Close monitoring for obstetric complications such as antepartum hemorrhage and preterm labor is essential and a careful peri-delivery plan must be made to minimize the risks of major bleeding at the time of birth and in the postpartum period.

Table 14.2 Summary of recommendations for anticoagulation during pregnancy in women with mechanical prosthetic heart valves

	1st trimester	2nd & 3rd trimesters
European Society of Cardiology 2011[5]	**Warfarin[a] dose <5 mg/day** Continue VKA or switch to therapeutic dose UFH or LMWH[b] may be considered between 6 and 12 weeks **Warfarin[a] dose >5 mg/day** Switch to therapeutic dose UFH or LMWH[b] should be considered between 6 and 12 weeks Continuation of VKA may be considered between 6 and 12 weeks	**All women** **(irrespective of warfarin dose)** VKA recommended for all women until 36th week
American Heart Association 2014[6]	**Warfarin dose ≤5 mg/day** Continue warfarin or Dose-adjusted LMWH ≥2 times daily[b] or Dose-adjusted continuous infusion UFH (aPTT ≥2× control) **Warfarin dose >5 mg/day** Dose-adjusted LMWH ≥ 2 times daily[b] or Dose-adjusted continuous infusion UFH (aPTT ≥2× control)	**All women** **(irrespective of warfarin dose)** Warfarin to goal INR + low-dose aspirin 75–100 mg daily) continued until planned vaginal delivery – switch to dose-adjusted continuous infusion UFH (aPTT ≥2× control)
American College of Chest Physicians 2012[7]	All options can be considered in any trimester: 1. Adjusted dose twice daily LMWH throughout pregnancy (to achieve manufacturer's peak anti-Xa 4 hours post-dose) or 2. Adjusted dose sc UFH twice daily throughout pregnancy (mid-interval aPTT at least twice control or anti-Xa heparin level 0.35–0.70 IU/mL) or 3. Dose-adjusted UFH or LMWH (as above) until 13th week then substitution by VKA until close to delivery when UFH or LMWH is resumed or 4. VKA with replacement of sc UFH or LMWH (as above) close to delivery for women at high risk of thromboembolism	

[a] Equivalent doses of phenprocoumon 3 mg/day and acenocoumarol 2 mg/day.
[b] Peak anti-Xa levels only recommended 4–6 hours (target range 0.8–1.2 IU/mL).
VKA, vitamin K antagonists; UFH, unfractionated heparin; LMWH, low-molecular-weight heparin; sc, subcutaneous; aPTT, activated partial thromboplastin time.

Vitamin K Antagonists

Prevention of Thromboembolism

The anticoagulant effects of the VKA such as warfarin, acenocoumarol, and phenprocoumon are the result of direct inhibition of the enzyme vitamin K epoxide reductase, which is essential for the post-translational modification that activates the vitamin K-dependent clotting factors II, VII, IX, and X[9]. While VKA are the most effective anticoagulants for preventing valve thrombosis and its complications, they do not eliminate the risk. Thromboembolic complications are reported in almost 4% of women with MPHV taking VKA during pregnancy (Table 14.3). The risk of thrombosis may in part be due to non-compliance with VKA as some studies report that women[10,11] discontinued this medication prior to pregnancy; however, TEC also occur in women who have therapeutic levels of coagulation on VKA[11,12].

Adverse Fetal Effects of Warfarin

Warfarin Embryopathy

Warfarin freely crosses the placenta. The first published case of warfarin embryopathy was reported in the infant of a woman with a Starr–Edwards mitral valve for RHD who was taking long-term warfarin. The infant had severe nasal hypoplasia and blindness due to bilateral optic atrophy[13]. Subsequent case reports described epiphyseal stippling in addition to the nasal hypoplasia in exposed infants and authors noted similarities between the clinical features in warfarin-exposed infants and infants with a rare inherited condition, chondrodysplasia punctata[13]. The seminal review by Hall and co-workers[14] suggested that "warfarin embryopathy" should only be diagnosed where women had been exposed to coumarin derivatives in the first trimester of pregnancy and whose infants had "characteristic nasal hypoplasia" or "stippled epiphyses." Their review reported

Table 14.3 Pregnancy outcomes and maternal thromboembolic complications in women with mechanical heart valves treated with VKA including warfarin

Study	Pregnancies (N)	All fetal loss n (% all pregnancies)	Spontaneous abortion n (% all pregnancies)	Stillbirth n (% ongoing pregnancies)	Live births n (%)	Early neonatal death n (% live births)	Warfarin embryopathy n (% all pregnancies[a])	Thromboembolic complications[b] N (%)
Arnaout[30]	18	9 (50.0)	7 (38.9)	2 (11.1)	9 (50)	1 (11.1)	0	1 (5.5)
Basude[31]	22	17 (77.3)	17 (77.3)	0	5 (22.7)	0	0	0
Chan[29]	792	196 (24.7)	196 (24.7)	47 (7.9)	549 (69.3)	23 (4.2)	35 (4.4)	31
Cotrufo[24]	71	28 (39.4)	23 (32.4)	5 (10.4)	43 (60.6)	0	3 (4.2)	0
Lee[27]	8	4 (50.0)	4 (50.0)	0	4 (50.0)	0	0	2 (25.0)
Mazibuko[11]	57	18 (31.6)	12 (21.1)	6 (13.3)	39 (68.4)	2 (4.9)	4 (7.5)	4 (7.0)
McLintock[a][10]	3	0	0	0	3 (100)	1 (33.3)	1 (33.3)	0
Meschengieser [32]	61	15 (24.6)	12 (19.7)	3 (6.1)	46 (75.4)	0	0	2 (3.3)
Nassar[33]	30	13 (42.3)	11 (44.0)	2 (14.3)	12 (40.0)	0	0	0
Soma-Pillay[25]	62	23 (37.1)	14 (22.6)	9 (14.5)	38 (61.3)	0	5 [12]	0
Suri[12]	45	13 (28.9)	9 (20.0)	4 (12.1)	31 (68.9)	1 (2.2)	0	3 (6.7)
All	1169	336 (28.7)	305 (26.1)	31 (9.1)	779 (66.6)	5 (3.6)	48 (4.2)	44 (3.8)

Therapeutic abortions were carried out in five women[33].

[a] Only pregnancies where women were exposed to warfarin.

[b] Transient ischemic attack, cerebrovascular accident, valve thrombosis.

warfarin embryopathy in 4% of infants (16 of 418), with exposure during gestational weeks six to nine being critical to development of embryopathy.

The precise mechanism of warfarin embryopathy is unclear but it seems likely that it is the result of inhibition of vitamin K-dependent osteocalcins, which play a critical role in calcification that occurs during embryogenesis[15], rather than inhibition of vitamin K-dependent clotting proteins, which are not produced by the fetal liver until later in gestation. Development of the nasal septum begins at the sixth week of gestation and there is a period of rapid growth of the nasal septum between gestational weeks six and nine[16]. Studies of chondrodysplasia punctata, a clinical and genetically heterogeneous group of skeletal dysplasias characterized by epiphyseal stippling and underdevelopment of the nasal cartilage, have provided insights into the potential role of warfarin in embryonic development. A clinically mild X-linked recessive form of chondrodysplasia punctata (CPDX) due to mutations in the vitamin K-dependent arylsulfatase E gene is phenotypically very similar to warfarin embryopathy, and the inhibition of this enzyme by warfarin is the subject of ongoing study[17].

A more recent review of 63 published cases of warfarin-related abnormalities described skeletal anomalies in 81% of cases (n=51) with midfacial hypoplasia described in 47 infants and epiphyseal calcific stippling of long bones, vertebrae, calcanei, or phalanges in 32 infants[18]. Breathing and feeding problems were present in 24 of 47 infants who had severe midfacial hypoplasia. The period of exposure to warfarin common to infants who developed embryopathy was between 6 and 9 weeks' gestation. Long-term follow-up information was available on 20 of 46 children who survived the neonatal period, with abnormalities persisting in about half of the children with midline hypoplasia and spinal deformities.

Warfarin Fetopathy

Other adverse effects of VKA include late fetal loss and stillbirth, which are reported in as many as 1 in 10 women who take VKA in pregnancy[19]. In addition, microcephaly, cerebral atrophy, hydrocephalus, optic atrophy, and intracranial hemorrhage are among the central nervous system abnormalities described in 1% of live-born infants exposed to warfarin during pregnancy. Long-term

neurological problems, such as developmental delay and low IQ, in infants who appear normal after in utero exposure to warfarin, have been reported in some small studies[20] but have not been confirmed in larger studies[21]. These effects seem likely to be due to warfarin-induced bleeding. Vitamin K_1 is present in low or undetectable levels in the term newborn, and limited amounts of vitamin K cross the placenta so that the fetus is likely to be essentially vitamin K naïve[22]. It can be anticipated that the dose of warfarin required to produce a therapeutic INR in the mother will significantly over anticoagulate the vitamin K-deficient fetus and lead to higher bleeding rates.

The Relationship between Dose of Vitamin K Antagonist and Fetal Complications

Warfarin Fetopathy

In 1999, Vitale and co-workers[23] first suggested the possibility of a dose-dependent effect of warfarin on development of fetal complications. Their retrospective study of 58 pregnancies in 43 women with MPHV reported fetal loss in 12% of pregnancies to women taking "low-dose" warfarin (≤5 mg) compared to 76% in women taking more than 5 mg warfarin (Table 14.4). A subsequent study[24] published by authors from the same center, which appears to include an overlapping cohort and uses different gestational cut-offs for spontaneous miscarriage and stillbirth, again reports higher rates of fetal loss in women taking more than 5 mg warfarin compared to those taking ≤5 mg (Table 14.3). A dose-dependent increase in stillbirth (fetal loss after 24 weeks' gestation) was also described in a cohort of South African women (n=56) taking warfarin in pregnancy[25]. Stillbirth was reported in 3.6% (1/28) of women taking <5 mg warfarin, in 14% (3/21) of women taking between 5.1 and 7.5 mg warfarin, and in 38.5% (5/13) of women taking >7.5 mg warfarin. In contrast, the European-based registry of pregnancy outcomes in women with MPHV[26], which demonstrated higher rates of miscarriage and later fetal death in women taking VKA compared to heparin (28.6% versus 9.2% and 7.1% versus 0.7%, respectively), did not show a difference in rates of fetal loss between women taking high-dose versus low-dose warfarin or other VKA. In

Table 14.4 Comparison of fetal complications with warfarin dose in women with mechanical prosthetic heart valves from two Italian cohorts

	Vitale[23]		Cotrufo[24]	
	≤5 mg	>5 mg	≤5 mg	>5 mg
Pregnancies (N)	33	25	38	33
All fetal loss (n)	4 (12%)	19 (76%)	2 (5.3%)	26 (78.8%)
Spontaneous abortion	4	18	2	21
Stillbirth	0	1	0	5
Warfarin embryopathy	0	2	1	2
Other fetal anomalies (VSD)	0	1	0	1
Live births	29 (87.9%)	6 (24%)	36 (94.7%)	7 (21.2%)
Valve thrombosis	1	1	None reported	None reported

Definitions of fetal loss: Vitale and co-workers[23] – spontaneous abortion = fetal loss prior to 28 weeks' gestation, stillbirth = fetal loss after >28 weeks' gestation; Cotrufo and co-workers[24] – spontaneous abortion = fetal loss prior to 20 weeks' gestation, stillbirth = fetal loss after >20 weeks' gestation.
VSD, ventricular septal defect.

a Korean cohort[27] of women with MPHV, all women were taking less than 5 mg warfarin during pregnancy and four had spontaneous miscarriage.

Warfarin Embryopathy

To date, a dose-dependent relationship in classical warfarin embryopathy has not been described. The initial publication[23] from the Italian group reported typical features of warfarin embryopathy (nasal hypoplasia, depressed nasal bridge, cartilage maldevelopment, and bifid spine) in two fetuses that spontaneously aborted in the sixth month of pregnancy in women taking 6.5 mg and 7.5 mg warfarin (Table 14.3). In the later paper[24], again there were two spontaneously aborted fetuses with features of warfarin embryopathy in the group of women taking more than 5 mg of warfarin but it also reported nasal hypoplasia in a live-born term infant whose mother took ≤5 mg warfarin during pregnancy. A live-born term infant in the high-dose warfarin group had a very small VSD detected on echocardiography that was surgically repaired in the first year of life.

The prospective cohort study[25] of South African women reported warfarin embryopathy in 5 of 41 (12.2%) pregnancies where there was drug exposure during the first trimester. Warfarin embryopathy was reported in infants of two women taking ≤5 mg warfarin and in three infants whose mothers took >5 mg warfarin. A separate South African study reported warfarin embryopathy in 4 of 56 (7.1%) warfarin-exposed pregnancies: two

women were taking 7.5 mg warfarin and two were taking ≤5 mg warfarin[11].

One group's approach to minimize the risk of adverse fetal outcomes in women with MPHV involves carrying out preoperative anticoagulation tests to identify those able to maintain an INR in a target range of 1.5–2.5 with warfarin doses <5 mg, before offering them a third generation St Jude's aortic valve[28]. Of 17 women who followed this approach, 16 subsequently became pregnant and continued with the same dose of warfarin with the same target INR. There were no maternal thromboembolic complications and all women had healthy babies born at term. However, the authors themselves acknowledge that the study results should be viewed with caution and that further studies are needed to validate such an approach given the small sample size and the lack of safety and efficacy data on using lower target INRs for patients with MPHV.

A number of key publications continue to confuse the data about the effect of dose and development of complications with warfarin and other VKA in pregnancy. The American Heart Association states that "the risk of embryopathy is dose dependent" while the "risk of embryopathy is >8% with a dosage of warfarin >5 mg per day" compared with a risk of "<3% with a warfarin dosage of 5 mg per day"[6]. Ensuring clarity is critical if women and clinicians are to receive the best information on which to make an informed decision.

A summary of maternal and fetal complications reported in a systematic review and subsequent published studies[10–12,24,25,27,29–33], where women with MPHV took warfarin or other VKA, is outlined in Table 14.3.

Alternatives to Vitamin K Antagonists

Unfractionated Heparin and Antiplatelet Agents

Concerns about the adverse fetal outcomes with VKA prompted consideration of alternative anticoagulants for pregnant women with MPHV. Unfractionated heparin (UFH) and antiplatelet agents such as aspirin were used initially. Antiplatelet agents avoided the risk of congenital anomalies but thromboembolic complications were reported in around 25% of pregnancies where women took antiplatelet agents alone [29]. Although warfarin embryopathy was not reported in women (n=317) who substituted UFH for warfarin prior to 6 weeks' gestation, continuing until 12 completed weeks of gestation, thromboembolic complications occurred in around 10% of pregnancies, while the women were on UFH. Whereas therapeutic levels of anticoagulation are unlikely to have been achieved in all regimens, thromboembolic complications were reported in studies where dose-adjusted UFH was given[12,32,34]. In 21 pregnancies where UFH was used throughout, thromboembolic complications were reported in 33%[29] with dose-adjustment done in only two studies, although no target range for monitoring of the activated partial thromboplastin time (aPTT) was provided. High rates of thromboembolism with UFH prompted clinicians to use low-molecular-weight heparin (LMWH), with its more predictable anticoagulant effect, as an alternative anticoagulant for pregnant women unwilling to take warfarin during pregnancy.

Maternal and Fetal Outcomes in Women Receiving LMWH during Pregnancy

Various regimens for therapeutic dose LMWH have been used during pregnancy in women with MPHV; some use LMWH throughout pregnancy and others give it during the first trimester only and recommend warfarin at other times. The first published studies reporting TEC in women with MPHV were often single case studies or small case series where inadequate doses of LMWH were given and anti-Xa levels were not uniformly carried out. Fewer events were reported in those centers where full therapeutic doses of LMWH were given and regular anti-Xa levels were measured[35,36]. A summary of maternal and fetal outcomes from seven centers that used dose-adjusted therapeutic LMWH during pregnancy in women with MPHV who were unwilling to take VKA is presented in Table 14.5[10,31,37–41]. Low-dose aspirin was recommended as an adjunct to LMWH in five centers[10,31,37,40,41]. Peak anti-Xa levels were measured in all centers but only one of these routinely measured trough anti-Xa levels[10]. Eleven thromboembolic events were reported in 104 (10.6%) pregnancies with five episodes of valve thrombosis – one resulting in a maternal death, three transient ischemic attacks, and two cerebrovascular accidents leading to permanent disability (Table 14.5). Active treatment failure (thromboembolism occurring in a woman taking her prescribed dose of LMWH and with anti-Xa levels recorded in the target therapeutic range) occurred in five women (4.8%). Subtherapeutic doses of LMWH had been prescribed initially to two of these women but they were taking therapeutic doses at the time of the event. In the remaining six cases women were either noncompliant with LMWH (n=3) or had subtherapeutic anti-Xa levels (n=3).

The HiP-CAT (heparin in pregnancy cardiac valve thromboprophylaxis) study is the only randomized study comparing outcomes in women treated with LMWH or warfarin. It was halted early because of the deaths of two women in the LMWH arm. In this study, anti-Xa levels directed adjustment of the LMWH dose to maintain the peak anti-Xa levels below 1.2 IU/mL and levels were <0.7 IU/mL in both women who died[42]. The drug manufacturer released a black box warning against the use of enoxaparin for anticoagulation in patients with mechanical heart valves but this has subsequently been modified to state that enoxaparin "has not been adequately studied for long-term use in this patient population" and that "inadequate anticoagulation" may complicate the evaluation of cases of prosthetic heart valve thrombosis in pregnant women who may be at "higher risk for thromboembolism."[43]

Anti-Xa: Peak and Trough Levels?

The appropriate time to determine the peak anticoagulant effect of LMWH given twice daily is 3–4 hours post-dose[44]. Most centers reporting outcomes in

Table 14.5 Details of maternal and fetal outcomes in women anticoagulated with dose-adjusted therapeutic level low-molecular-weight heparin (LMWH) throughout pregnancy

Study	Pregnancies (women)	LMWH	Anti-Xa monitoring (target range)	Maternal TEC n (%)	Late loss (>20/40) n (%)[b]	Live births n (%)[b]
Abildgaard[37]	12(11)	Dalteparin	Peak[a] (0.7–1.2)	2 (16.7)	0	12/12 (100)
Basude[c][31]	4(4)	Enoxaparin	Peak (1.0–1.2)	2(50)	0	3/3 (100)
Chitsike[38]	15(15)	Enoxaparin	Peak (1.0–1.2)	0	–	–
Goland[39]	8(8)	Enoxaparin	Peak (0.8–1.2)	0	0	8/8 (100)
McLintock[c][10]	34(23)	Enoxaparin	Trough (0.4–0.7)	5 (14.7)	1(3)	22/23 (95)
			Peak (1.0–1.2)			
Quinn[40]	8(7)	Dalteparin	Peak (1.0–1.2)	1 (12.5)	1[13]	7/8 (88)
Yinon[41]	23(17)	Enoxaparin/ Dalteparin	Peak (1.0–1.2)	1 (4.3)	2(10)	19/21 (91)
Total	104			11 (10.6)	4 (3.8)	71/75 (94.7)

Starting dose: enoxaparin 1 mg/kg twice daily; dalteparin 100 IU/kg twice daily.
[a] Measured 4–6 hours post-dose.
[b] Live birth rate excluding spontaneous abortions and terminations of pregnancy.
[c] Includes only women from cohort taking LMWH throughout pregnancy; fetal outcomes not reported in paper.
TEC, thromboembolic complications including valve thrombosis, cerebrovascular accident, transient ischemic attacks.

women with MPHV on dose-adjusted therapeutic dose LMWH measure only peak anti-Xa levels, with slight variations in the target therapeutic range (Table 14.5). Two groups [19,45] advocate measurement of trough as well as peak anti-Xa levels in this group of women, to ensure that a baseline level of anticoagulation is maintained, especially given that the increased renal clearance of LMWH in pregnancy[46], due to the increased glomerular filtration rate, may lead to a reduced anticoagulant effect. Goland and co-workers[39] demonstrated that adjusting the dose of LMWH to maintain peak anti-Xa levels in a therapeutic range of 0.7–1.2 IU/mL resulted in trough anti-Xa levels of <0.6 IU/mL in up to 80% of women. Targeting trough anti-Xa levels of ≥0.6 IU/mL was rarely associated with excessive peak levels and was not associated with bleeding. They have recommended that this should be the target trough level. At National Women's Health in Auckland, New Zealand, we have also increased the target therapeutic range for trough anti-Xa levels to 0.6–0.7 IU/mL in an attempt to minimize the risk of thrombotic complications and aim for peak anti-Xa levels of 1.0–1.4 IU/mL.

Addition of Aspirin

Low-dose aspirin (100–150 mg) is recommended in addition to warfarin, as the significant reduction in the risk of major thromboembolism more than offsets the slight increase in bleeding[47].

Management of the Labor and Birth

Management of women during labor and birth requires careful clinical monitoring. Labor and birth must be planned given the bleeding risks if on therapeutic levels of anticoagulation. The mode of birth should be determined by maternal and obstetric indications but induction of labor with vaginal birth is preferable to elective cesarean section as in the postpartum period women can restart therapeutic dose anticoagulation more quickly.

The need to minimize time off anticoagulation in these women at high risk of thromboembolism requires early reinstitution of anticoagulation postpartum, which increases the risk of primary and secondary postpartum hemorrhage. One study reported primary PPH rates of 12% and secondary postpartum hemorrhage, or other major bleeding requiring transfusion, readmission or return to theater, occurred in one in five women[10]. Continuation of intravenous

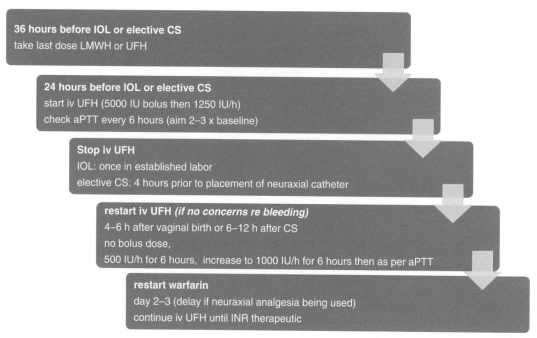

36 hours before IOL or elective CS
take last dose LMWH or UFH

24 hours before IOL or elective CS
start iv UFH (5000 IU bolus then 1250 IU/h)
check aPTT every 6 hours (aim 2–3 x baseline)

Stop iv UFH
IOL: once in established labor
elective CS: 4 hours prior to placement of neuraxial catheter

restart iv UFH *(if no concerns re bleeding)*
4–6 h after vaginal birth or 6–12 h after CS
no bolus dose,
500 IU/h for 6 hours, increase to 1000 IU/h for 6 hours then as per aPTT

restart warfarin
day 2–3 (delay if neuraxial analgesia being used)
continue iv UFH until INR therapeutic

Figure 14.1 Suggested regimen for peripartum anticoagulation in women with mechanical prosthetic heart valves on subcutaneous low-molecular-weight heparin (LMWH) or unfractionated heparin (UFH). IOL, induction of labor; CS, cesarean section; iv, intravenous; aPTT, activated partial thromboplastin time.

UFH instead of LMWH postpartum while waiting for VKA to become therapeutic allows more flexible control of anticoagulation if bleeding occurs, but does require women to remain in hospital for longer.

Management of Women on VKA

Oral anticoagulants should be stopped at around 34–35 weeks' gestation (or earlier if there is the risk of preterm birth), to allow normalization of the anticoagulant effect in the infant, to reduce the risk of bleeding. Cessation of VKA will generally lead to normalization of the INR in the mother within 3–4 days even without active reversal. The fetus will be over-anticoagulated as it is effectively vitamin K deficient with low levels of clotting factors, so reversal of anticoagulation after discontinuation of VKA will take longer. Options for anticoagulation after discontinuation of VKA until preparation for birth include either therapeutic dose LMWH, dose-adjusted subcutaneous UFH, or dose-adjusted UFH given by intravenous infusion. Women would require admission to hospital for intravenous UFH but can be managed as outpatients for the other two options. Heparin does not anticoagulate the fetus, but the mother is at risk of hemorrhage if she delivers on therapeutic anticoagulation with UFH or LMWH.

A suggested approach to management of anticoagulation in women at around the time of labor and birth is outlined in Figure 14.1.

Rapid Reversal of Anticoagulation

Onset of labor is unpredictable, and women may go into preterm labor or require urgent delivery for maternal or fetal complications. In women taking LMWH, the activated partial thromboplastin time will not provide an accurate indication of the degree of anticoagulation and risk of bleeding. Most laboratories do not provide urgent testing of anti-Xa levels. Protamine administration may partially reverse the anticoagulant effect of therapeutic dose LMWH[48] and should be given to women who have taken a dose within 24 h. Fresh frozen plasma has no role in reversal of UFH or LMWH.

Reversal of Vitamin K Antagonists

Rapid and effective reversal of the anticoagulant effect of VKA can be achieved using prothrombin complex concentrates (PCC). Fresh frozen plasma (FFP) can also be used but is not recommended due to the superior efficacy of PCC[49]. Vitamin K 1–2 mg should also be given but it is not fully effective for around 6 hours. Importantly, these maneuvers will not reverse the anticoagulant effect of VKA on the fetus. The nature of the emergency is likely to dictate the mode of birth but, as infants born to mothers taking oral anticoagulants will be over-anticoagulated, delivery should be as atraumatic as possible; fetal scalp electrodes, rotational forceps, and ventouse are contraindicated. A cord blood INR should be taken at birth, before reversal with PCC or FFP using adult protocols adjusted for infant weight.

Valve Thrombosis

Development of valve thrombosis is associated with a major risk of valve failure and systemic thromboembolism. Women with valve thrombosis may be asymptomatic or can present with symptoms of

heart failure (shortness of breath, dyspnea, orthopnea, or paroxysmal nocturnal dyspnea) or embolism including cerebrovascular accidents, with permanent or transient limb weakness, dysarthria, dysphasia, visual loss, or acute myocardial infarction. Women who develop any symptoms of concern require an urgent echocardiogram to assess the valve. Treatment of valve thrombosis is controversial[50] and will depend on the clinical presentation. Approaches include administration of more intensive anticoagulation often with intravenous UFH and warfarin, or thrombolysis or urgent cardiac surgery with valve replacement[6].

The woman's compliance with the anticoagulation regimen should be determined. If she has clearly been non-compliant then a discussion of ways to improve

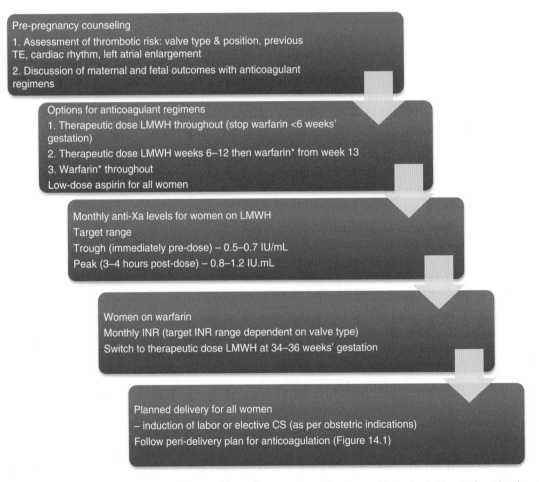

Figure 14.2 Approach to management of anticoagulation during pregnancy in women with mechanical heart valves.*Or other vitamin K antagonist. TE, thromboembolism; LMWH, low-molecular-weight heparin; CS, cesarean section.

her compliance is essential but often the anticoagulant regimen will need to be changed. Women who have complications due to valve thrombosis despite therapeutic anti-Xa levels or who are unable to comply with a regimen of twice daily LMWH injections should be counseled to switch to warfarin.

Other Considerations

Both warfarin and LMWH are safe in breast-feeding [51,52].

Women with MPHV as a result of rheumatic heart disease should receive benzathine penicillin by intramuscular injection every 28 days to prevent recurrent attacks of rheumatic fever. It is recommended that this be continued until the age of 30 years, or longer for individuals living or working with children in a high group A streptococcus environment[53].

The risk of congenital heart disease (CHD) in the infants of women who have CHD is around 3–5%[54], so these women require fetal cardiac echocardiogram

during pregnancy and the infant should have a clinical review by a pediatrician in the newborn period.

Routine antibiotic prophylaxis solely to prevent infective endocarditis is no longer recommended for vaginal birth or for cesarean section in women with MPHV[6,55].

Summary

Management of anticoagulation in pregnancy in women with MPHV is complex and requires care from a dedicated multidisciplinary team. Women must be counseled that they are at risk of thromboembolic complications irrespective of the anticoagulant regimen they choose but the clinician has a duty to provide the most objective discussion of the available evidence on outcomes. A suggested approach to management is outlined in Figure 14.2. Support for women during pregnancy to ensure optimal compliance with therapy and testing is paramount to attain best results for the woman and her unborn child.

Case Studies

Case Study 1

A primigravid woman, recently arrived from the Pacific Islands, was admitted at 22+4 weeks' gestation with history of increasing shortness of breath, paroxysmal nocturnal dyspnea, and orthopnea. She was found to be in heart failure secondary to severe mitral regurgitation due to rheumatic heart disease although she had no known history of previous rheumatic fever. She was unresponsive to medical therapy and required emergency cardiac bypass surgery carried out at 23+4 weeks' gestation. Valve repair was not possible and she had On-X mitral valve replacement and tricuspid annuloplasty. The surgery was uncomplicated and there were no fetal concerns during bypass. The pregnancy continued and the woman was counseled about the requirement for ongoing anticoagulation given the MPHV and the pros and cons of warfarin and LMWH discussed. She opted to take LMWH and started enoxaparin 60 mg (1 mg/kg) twice daily with 100 mg aspirin. The first anti-Xa trough level was 0.3 IU/mL with a 4-hour peak of 0.7 IU/mL and the enoxaparin dose was increased to 80 mg twice daily. Repeat anti-Xa trough and peak levels were 0.4 IU/mL and 0.8 IU/mL, respectively, and the dose was increased again to 90 mg twice daily. At 29 weeks' gestation, the trough and peak anti-Xa levels were 0.6 IU/mL and 0.9 IU/mL, respectively, and subsequent anti-Xa levels remained in this therapeutic range. Her pregnancy continued with no maternal cardiac or obstetric complications. An induction of labor was planned at 38+2 weeks' gestation with a careful plan for peri-delivery anticoagulation using the approach outlined in Figure 14.1. An epidural was sited when she was in active labor, 6 hours after the IV UFH infusion had been discontinued. She progressed to 9 cm but ultimately required an emergency CS for obstructed labor. The CS was uncomplicated, estimated blood loss 600 mL, and 6 hours postpartum IV UFH was reintroduced following the unit protocol. Warfarin was introduced after the epidural was removed and after 3 days on IV UFH her INR was 2.1 and heparin was discontinued. She had no postpartum complications. Contraception was discussed and the woman opted to have a Jadelle progesterone-releasing implant. She wishes to have more children in future and will attend our clinic for pre-pregnancy counseling.

Case Study 2

A 33-year-old woman (G5P1) presented for care in her second ongoing pregnancy to our unit. In 1989, at the age of 8, she had required mitral and aortic valve replacement (27 mm Medtronic–Hall mitral valve and 21 mm Medtronic–Hall aortic valve) with tricuspid annuloplasty (28 mm Carpentier ring) for severe rheumatic heart disease. She had a history of two thromboembolic events due to non-compliance with warfarin; the first was a TIA in 1993 and the second CVA occurred in 2003 leaving her with permanent mild left-sided weakness. In 2008, she presented to our unit at 15 weeks' gestation in her first ongoing pregnancy, prior to which she had two uncomplicated first trimester miscarriages. After discussion with the patient, it was decided to continue warfarin given her high risk of thromboembolism. Although she claimed to be compliant with warfarin she did not have regular INR testing but was therapeutic on the few occasions when the INR was measured. She was switched to LMWH at 35 weeks' gestation, then followed our unit protocol for induction of labor transitioning to iv UFH and went on to have an uncomplicated vaginal birth with a 500 mL estimated blood loss at delivery. Her baby was small for gestational age on the 7th centile by customized birth weight centiles (for age, weight, parity, gestation, and ethnicity). Warfarin was restarted postpartum. Five years later she presented at 10 weeks' gestation. She was only taking warfarin every 3–4 days and her INRs, when measured, were subtherapeutic. She did not want to take warfarin in pregnancy and we reluctantly prescribed therapeutic dose enoxaparin (1 mg/kg bd) and aspirin. A scan for nuchal translucency at 11 weeks showed a missed miscarriage, and she had an uncomplicated dilatation and curettage (D&C) done with bridging with IV UFH.

In early 2015, she presented to our unit at 17 weeks' gestation. Against our advice the patient refused to take warfarin and opted for therapeutic dose enoxaparin with low-dose aspirin. However, it became clear that she was not compliant with this medication and after further discussion at 20 weeks' gestation she agreed to take warfarin and continued this having INRs measured regularly, which were in the therapeutic range.

Echocardiograms done in pregnancy showed increasing gradient across the mechanical aortic valve thought to represent pannus. At 30 weeks' gestation, she presented in threatened preterm labor as a result of a urinary tract infection. Fetal fibronectin test was positive suggesting that she was at a high risk of preterm birth. At this stage she was switched to therapeutic dose enoxaparin and aspirin and was compliant with injections and monitoring with anti-Xa levels, which were in the therapeutic range. She was discharged and had one further episode of threatened preterm labor so remained on enoxaparin. At 37+5 she had a planned induction of labor, switching to IV UFH as per unit protocol. Because of staffing issues there was a delay in transferring her to a labor and birthing unit for an artificial rupture of membranes so she was off IV UFH for around 18 hours. In the first stage of labor she developed an acute dyspnea due to pulmonary edema and went for an emergency CS under general anesthetic. A transesophageal echo done during surgery showed a small mobile thrombus on the aortic valve. She was transferred to the cardiovascular intensive care unit post-CS and anticoagulation with IV UFH was reintroduced 6 hours post-CS with the dose of UFH increased over 18 hours to the therapeutic range. She had no postoperative bleeding complications but developed postpartum sepsis due to CS wound infection. Redo valve surgery was carried out 2 weeks postpartum. At operation, the aortic valve showed significant pannus extending into the left ventricular outflow tract underneath the valve. Pannus was noted in the mechanical mitral valve but it was surgically removed and was not replaced. The woman had a Jadelle placed for contraception. At the time of follow-up the clinical team are aware that the patient has had very few INRs done since discharge and these were not in the therapeutic range.

References

1. McLintock C. Still casting its long shadow: rheumatic heart disease in Australia and New Zealand. *International Medical Journal* 2012; **42**(9): 963–966.

2. Sadler L, McCowan L, White H *et al.* Pregnancy outcomes and cardiac complications in women with mechanical, bioprosthetic and homograft valves. *BJOG: An International Journal of Obstetrics and Gynecology* 2000; **107**(2): 245–253.

3. Elkayam U, Bitar F. Valvular heart disease and pregnancy. *Journal of the American College of Cardiology* 2005; **46**(3): 403–410.

4. Eikelboom JW, Connolly SJ, Brueckmann M *et al.* Dabigatran versus warfarin in patients with mechanical heart valves. *New England Journal of Medicine* 2013; **369**(13): 1206–14.

5. European Society of Gynecology; Association for European Pediatric Cardiology; German Society for Gender Medicine; Regitz-Zagrosek V, Blomstrom Lundqvist C, Borghi C *et al.* ESC Guidelines on the management of cardiovascular diseases during pregnancy: the Task Force on the Management of Cardiovascular Diseases during Pregnancy of the European Society of Cardiology (ESC). *European Heart Journal* 2011; **32**(24): 3147–3197.

6. Nishimura RA, Otto CM, Bonow RO *et al.* 2014 AHA/ACC guideline for the management of patients with valvular heart disease: a report of the American College of Cardiology/American Heart Association Task Force on Practice Guidelines. *Journal of the American College of Cardiology* 2014; **63**(22): e57–185.

7. Bates SM, Greer IA, Middeldorp S *et al.* VTE, thrombophilia, antithrombotic therapy, and pregnancy: Antithrombotic Therapy and Prevention of Thrombosis, 9th ed: American College of Chest Physicians Evidence-Based Clinical Practice Guidelines. *Chest.* 2012; **141**(2 Suppl): e691S–736S.

8. McLintock C. Anticoagulant choices in pregnant women with mechanical heart valves: balancing maternal and fetal risks – the difference the dose makes. *Thrombosis Research* 2013; **131** (Suppl 1): S8–10.

9. Schelleman H, Limdi NA, Kimmel SE. Ethnic differences in warfarin maintenance dose requirement and its relationship with genetics. *Pharmacogenomics* 2008; **9**(9): 1331–1346.

10. McLintock C, McCowan LM, North RA. Maternal complications and pregnancy outcome in women with mechanical prosthetic heart valves treated with enoxaparin. *BJOG: An International Journal of Obstetrics and Gynecology* 2009; **116**(12): 1585–1592.

11. Mazibuko B, Ramnarain H, Moodley J. An audit of pregnant women with prosthetic heart valves at a tertiary hospital in South Africa: a five-year experience. *Cardiovascular Journal of Africa* 2012; **23**(4): 216–221.

12. Suri V, Keepanasseril A, Aggarwal N *et al.* Mechanical valve prosthesis and anticoagulation regimens in pregnancy: a tertiary center experience. *European Journal of Obstetrics & Gynecology and Reproductive Biology* 2011; **159**(2): 320–323.

13. Becker MH, Genieser NB, Finegold M, Miranda D, Spackman T. Chondrodysplasis punctata: is maternal warfarin therapy a factor? *American Journal of Diseases of Childhood* 1975; **129**(3): 356–359.

14. Hall JG, Pauli RM, Wilson KM. Maternal and fetal sequelae of anticoagulation during pregnancy. *American Journal of Medicine* 1980; **68**(1): 122–140.

15. Howe AM, Lipson AH, de Silva M, Ouvrier R, Webster WS. Severe cervical dysplasia and nasal cartilage calcification following prenatal warfarin exposure. *American Journal of Medical Genetics* 1997; **71**(4): 391–396.

16. Howe AM, Hawkins JK, Webster WS. The growth of the nasal septum in the 6–9 week period of foetal development – Warfarin embryopathy offers a new insight into prenatal facial development. *Australian Dental Journal* 2004; **49**(4): 171–176.

17. Franco B, Meroni G, Parenti G *et al.* A cluster of sulfatase genes on Xp22.3: mutations in chondrodysplasia punctata (CDPX) and implications for warfarin embryopathy. *Cell* 1995; **81**(1): 15–25.

18. van Driel D, Wesseling J, Sauer PJ *et al.* Teratogen update: fetal effects after in utero exposure to coumarins: overview of cases, follow-up findings, and pathogenesis. *Teratology* 2002; **66**(3): 127–140.

19. McLintock C. Thromboembolism in pregnancy: challenges and controversies in the prevention of pregnancy-associated venous thromboembolism and management of anticoagulation in women with mechanical prosthetic heart valves. *Best Practice & Research Clinical Obstetrics & Gynaecology* 2014; **28**(4): 519–536.

20. Wong V, Cheng CH, Chan KC. Fetal and neonatal outcome of exposure to anticoagulants during pregnancy. *American Journal of Medical Genetics* 1993; **45**(1): 17–21.

21. Van Driel D, Wesseling J, Rosendaal FR *et al.* Growth until puberty after in utero exposure to coumarins. *American Journal of Medical Genetics* 2000; **95**(5): 438–443.

22. Greer FR. Vitamin K the basics – what's new? *Early Human Development* 2010; **86** (Suppl 1): 43–47.

23. Vitale N, De Feo M, Cotrufo M. Anticoagulation for prosthetic heart valves during pregnancy: the importance of warfarin daily dose. *European Journal of Cardiothoracic Surgery* 2002; **22**(4): 656; author reply 7.

24. Cotrufo M, De Feo M, De Santo LS *et al.* Risk of warfarin during pregnancy with mechanical valve prostheses. *Obstetrics and Gynecology* 2002; **99**(1): 35–40.

25. Soma-Pillay P, Nene Z, Mathivha TM, Macdonald AP. The effect of warfarin dosage on maternal and fetal outcomes in pregnant women with prosthetic heart valves. *Obstetric Medicine* 2011; **4**: 24–27.

26. van Hagen IM, Roos-Hesselink JW, Ruys TP *et al.* Pregnancy in women with a mechanical heart valve: data of the European Society of Cardiology Registry of Pregnancy and Cardiac Disease (ROPAC). *Circulation* 2015; **132**(2): 132–142.

27. Lee JH, Park NH, Keum DY, Choi SY, Kwon KY, Cho CH. Low molecular weight heparin treatment in pregnant women with a mechanical heart valve prosthesis. *Journal of Korean Medical Science* 2007; **22**(2): 258–261.

28. De Santo LS, Romano G, Della Corte A *et al.* Mechanical aortic valve replacement in young women planning on pregnancy: maternal and fetal

outcomes under low oral anticoagulation, a pilot observational study on a comprehensive pre-operative counseling protocol. *Journal of the American College of Cardiology* 2012; **59**(12): 1110–1115.

29. Chan WS, Anand S, Ginsberg JS. Anticoagulation of pregnant women with mechanical heart valves: a systematic review of the literature. *Archives of Internal Medicine* 2000; **160**(2): 191–196.

30. Arnaout MS, Kazma H, Khalil A *et al.* Is there a safe anticoagulation protocol for pregnant women with prosthetic valves? *Clinical and Experimental Obstetrics & Gynecology* 1998; **25**(3): 101–104.

31. Basude S, Hein C, Curtis SL, Clark A, Trinder J. Low-molecular-weight heparin or warfarin for anticoagulation in pregnant women with mechanical heart valves: what are the risks? A retrospective observational study. *BJOG: An International Journal of Obstetrics and Gynecology* 2012; **119**(8): 1008–1013; discussion 12–3.

32. Meschengieser SS, Fondevila CG, Santarelli MT, Lazzari MA. Anticoagulation in pregnant women with mechanical heart valve prostheses. *Heart* 1999; **82**(1): 23–26.

33. Nassar AH, Hobeika EM, Abd Essamad HM *et al.* Pregnancy outcome in women with prosthetic heart valves. *American Journal of Obstetrics and Gynecology* 2004; **191**(3): 1009–1013.

34. Kawamata K, Neki R, Yamanaka K *et al.* Risks and pregnancy outcome in women with prosthetic mechanical heart valve replacement. *Circulation Journal* 2007; **71**(2): 211–213.

35. McLintock C. Anticoagulant therapy in pregnant women with mechanical prosthetic valves: no easy option. *Thrombosis Research* 2011; **127** (Suppl 3): S56–60.

36. Oran B, Lee-Parritz A, Ansell J. Low molecular weight heparin for the prophylaxis of thromboembolism in women with prosthetic mechanical heart valves during pregnancy. *Thrombosis and Haemostasis* 2004; **92**(4): 747–751.

37. Abildgaard U, Sandset PM, Hammerstrom J, Gjestvang FT, Tveit A. Management of pregnant women with mechanical heart valve prosthesis: thromboprophylaxis with low molecular weight heparin. *Thrombosis Research* 2009; **124**(3): 262–267.

38. Chitsike RS, Jacobson BF, Manga P *et al.* A prospective trial showing the safety of adjusted-dose enoxaparin for thromboprophylaxis of pregnant women with mechanical prosthetic heart valves. *Clinical and Applied Thrombosis/Hemostasis* 2011; **17**(4): 313–319.

39. Goland S, Schwartzenberg S, Fan J *et al.* Monitoring of anti-Xa in pregnant patients with mechanical prosthetic valves receiving low-molecular-weight heparin: peak or trough levels? *Journal of Cardiovascular Pharmacology and Therapeutics* 2014; **19**(5): 451–456.

40. Quinn J, Von Klemperer K, Brooks R *et al.* Use of high intensity adjusted dose low molecular weight heparin in women with mechanical heart valves during pregnancy: a single-center experience. *Hematologica* 2009; **94**(11): 1608–1612.

41. Yinon Y, Siu SC, Warshafsky C *et al.* Use of low molecular weight heparin in pregnant women with mechanical heart valves. *American Journal of Cardiology* 2009; **104**(9): 1259–1263.

42. Aventis Pharma. Heparin in pregnancy: cardiac valve thromboprophylaxis. Data on file; 1999.

43. Sanofi. Product monograph for Lovenox; 2015.

44. Gouin-Thibault I, Pautas E, Siguret V. Safety profile of different low-molecular weight heparins used at therapeutic dose. *Drug Safety* 2005; **28**(4): 333–349.

45. Elkayam U, Goland S. The search for a safe and effective anticoagulation regimen in pregnant women with mechanical prosthetic heart valves. *Journal of the American College of Cardiology* 2012; **59**(12): 1116–1118.

46. Barbour LA, Oja JL, Schultz LK. A prospective trial that demonstrates that dalteparin requirements increase in pregnancy to maintain therapeutic levels of anticoagulation. *American Journal of Obstetrics and Gynecology* 2004; **191**(3): 1024–1029.

47. Turpie AG, Gent M, Laupacis A *et al.* A comparison of aspirin with placebo in patients treated with warfarin after heart-valve replacement *New England Journal of Medicine* 1993; **329**(8): 524–529.

48. Massonnet-Castel S, Pelissier E, Bara L *et al.* Partial reversal of low molecular weight heparin (PK 10169) anti-Xa activity by protamine sulfate: in vitro and in vivo study during cardiac surgery with extracorporeal circulation. *Hemostasis* 1986; **16**(2): 139–146.

49. Tran HA, Chunilal SD, Harper PL *et al.* An update of consensus guidelines for warfarin reversal. *Medical Journal of Australia* 2013; **198**(4): 198–199.

50. Casais P, Rolandi F. Prosthetic valve thrombosis in pregnancy: a promising treatment for a rare and mostly preventable complication. *Circulation* 2013; **128**(5): 481–482.

51. Orme ML, Lewis PJ, de Swiet M *et al.* May mothers given warfarin breast-feed their infants? *BMJ* 1977; **1**(6076): 1564–1565.

52. Richter C, Sitzmann J, Lang P *et al.* Excretion of low molecular weight heparin in human milk. *British Journal of Clinical Pharmacology* 2001; **52**(6): 708–710.

53. NZ Heart Foundation. New Zealand Guidelines for Rheumatic Fever: Diagnosis, management and secondary prevention of acute rheumatic fever and rheumatic heart disease; 2014 (Update). Heart Foundation of New Zealand.

54. Swan L. Congenital heart disease in pregnancy. *Best Practice & Research Clinical Obstetrics & Gynaecology* 2014; **28**(4): 495–506.

55. UK National Institute for Health and Clinical Excellence (NICE). *Prophylaxis Against Infective Endocarditis: Antimicrobial Prophylaxis Against Infective Endocarditis in Adults and Children Undergoing Interventional Procedures.* London: NICE; 2008.

Chapter 15

Management of Anticoagulants at Delivery

Christina Oppenheimer, Paul Sharpe, and Andrew Ling

Introduction

This chapter will address:

1. Practical obstetric and anesthetic management of women on prophylactic heparin and therapeutic anticoagulation in the peripartum period.
2. Dilemmas for obstetricians, anesthetists, and hematologists.
3. Use of novel anticoagulants and how this can affect obstetric and anesthetic planning.
4. Issues surrounding use of thrombolytic agents in pregnancy and unusual but complex situations such as cardiopulmonary bypass in pregnancy.

Increasing use of prophylactic anticoagulants in pregnancy, both for venous thromboprophylaxis and to modify fetal risk (as in antiphospholipid syndrome), means that more women are now reaching the peripartum period on anticoagulants, usually a low-molecular-weight heparin (LMWH). Therapeutic doses are used for treatment of acute venous thromboembolic events, prevention of thromboembolism in women with cardiac disease (including mechanical heart valves), acute cardiac events, and cardiomyopathy. It is also used for those on long-term anticoagulation outside of pregnancy for a variety of other indications. This situation necessitates careful assessment of risks, close multidisciplinary discussion and planning, and expert management by the medical and midwifery teams during labor or cesarean section (CS). Careful discussion of risks and therapeutic decisions with the patient and her partner are also essential.

Anesthesia using central neuraxial blockade (CNB), that is subarachnoid (spinal) blocks and epidural (extradural) blocks, makes up the overwhelming majority of all anesthesia provided for obstetric indications in the UK. In 2009, the Royal College of Anesthetists conducted the Third National Audit Project to ascertain the number of CNB procedures carried out in the UK and their relative complications[1]. Forty-five percent of around 700 000 CNBs carried out were for the obstetric population, with only one vertebral canal hematoma

that did not fully recover. Though none of the discussed obstetric morbidity cases were in anticoagulated women, the results remain reassuring that CNB is a safe technique, providing due diligence is paid to individual patient risk factors. Though it remains safer than general anesthesia, the rare complications of CNB, such as temporary or permanent nerve damage, can be life changing for an otherwise fit and healthy woman.

The exact risk of CNB complications in anticoagulated women is not known but it is logical to suggest it would be higher than in the general obstetric population. Even though the relative risk of complications when performing CNB in an anticoagulated woman may increase significantly, the absolute number of vertebral canal hematomas would still likely be extremely low. Proceeding with CNB in an anticoagulated woman, for labor analgesia or operative procedure, is not absolutely contraindicated but there must be perceived higher risk in doing nothing or attempting general anesthesia. Clearly, these patients should be informed of all the risks and the consent process extremely thorough.

Thromboprophylaxis

The use of a variety of anticoagulants in obstetric practice has been increasing steadily over the last 20 years, bringing with it increasing awareness of the need for attention to thromboprophylaxis, but also the need to adapt and plan for the risks associated with this. The Royal College of Obstetric and Gynecology (RCOG) guidance on thromboprophylaxis[2] and the recent MBRRACE-UK Report[3] have both significantly raised awareness of the importance of risk assessment for venous thromboembolism. This has increased the use of low-molecular-weight heparins in particular (see Chapter 13). The recent and rapid rise in prevalence of obesity in women of childbearing age also brings many more women into a high-risk category necessitating use of general as well as pharmacological antithrombotic measures.

Antiplatelet Agents

Following the publication of the CLASP trial in 1994[4] and then the work on antiphospholipid syndrome in recurrent miscarriage by Regan and colleagues, low-dose aspirin therapy in pregnancy increased. More recently NICE guidance[5] has also contributed to this rise. There has also been a gradual increase in numbers of women on long-term aspirin for medical conditions, such as previous stroke, that has led to development of guidelines for aspirin use around the time of delivery.

The use of low-dose aspirin (75 mg) up to the time of labor and delivery is not contraindicated on either obstetric or anesthetic grounds. At this dose, there is no increased risk of bleeding either at vaginal or cesarean delivery, nor is there evidence of any increase in the risk of vertebral canal hematoma after spinal or epidural block insertion. However, if aspirin use is combined with either heparin or warfarin in the postpartum period, there may be an additive effect and particular care should be taken with timing of dose administration and epidural catheter removal. There is no contraindication to breast-feeding on low-dose aspirin, in particular there is no evidence of risk of Reye's syndrome at this dose.

The safety in pregnancy of other antiplatelet agents such as clopidogrel or ticlopidine at usual therapeutic doses has not been established and they are rarely used. Both the indication for use and a clear plan of management should be available to those directly caring for the patient to minimize risk at the time of delivery. Decisions about when to discontinue these drugs around the time of delivery should be made on an individual case basis with consultation between responsible obstetrician, physician, and anesthetist.

Non-steroidal anti-inflammatory drugs are largely contraindicated in pregnancy. If used for other maternal indications they should be avoided around the time of delivery to minimize risk to the fetus.

Low-Molecular-Weight Heparins (LMWH)

Most of the women requiring prophylactic doses of anticoagulant will be given one of the low-molecular-weight heparins, usually once daily. Those with a particularly high risk of recurrent venous thromboembolism (VTE), high-risk mechanical heart valves, and the morbidly obese[2] may be on twice daily dosing.

While increasing numbers of women being prescribed LMWH for thromboprophylaxis leads to increased experience for staff in managing such pregnancies, it also necessitates sufficient knowledge for safe practice. This would take into account the half-life, increased clearance in pregnancy, and different therapeutic index of different heparins[6]. Underpinning all of the clinical management described below must be:

1. collaboration;
2. clear local guidelines;
3. knowledge and education of medical and midwifery staff;
4. written information for patients; and
5. individual care plans based on a woman's particular risk factors.

Obstetric Aspects

Labor and Delivery

In the presence of increased risk of venous thromboembolism, the optimum management is to aim for a spontaneous onset of labor, as these are generally shorter and have a lower risk of operative delivery. Clearly, this advantage needs to be weighed against other obstetric and medical risks if present.

A standard approach is to omit the LMWH at the onset of labor and ensure general antithrombotic measures, including:

1. adequate hydration, with early recourse to intravenous fluids if necessary;
2. mobilization, with passive movements or massage if mobility restricted by epidural; and
3. wearing of graduated compression stockings.

If a woman has no additional complications, other than a need for LMWH thromboprophylaxis, there is no contraindication to delivering in a midwifery-led setting, provided at least 8 hours has elapsed since the last dose by delivery. If women in this situation request a home confinement, this should be discussed on an individual basis.

Induction of Labor

If an induction of labor is planned, the LMWH should be omitted at the start of the process. We suggest that women who take evening doses omit their dose the day before induction and those who take a morning dose omit their dose on the day of induction. If an omission of more than 48 hours is thought to be contraindicated, intermittent dosing with unfractionated heparin (UFH)

5000 units subcutaneously can be considered at 6-hourly intervals until artificial rupture of the membranes (ARM) is possible; although this is rarely needed. UFH has a half-life of about 3 hours, so that an anticoagulant effect at a level suitable for regional anesthetic blockade is possible around that point. With LMWH this delay needs to be 8–12 hours depending on dose (see Table 15.2). Attention should be paid to general antithrombotic measures including compression stockings, hydration, and mobility.

A prolonged induction process is more likely in primigravida and those with an unfavorable cervix at the start of the induction. Thus, where possible, careful assessment should be made to try to delay induction until the cervix is more favorable. If this is not possible there will then be the dual additional risk of a prolonged period where the woman is covered by general antithrombotic measures only and an increased risk of instrumental delivery or CS inherent in an induced labor.

Practical Issues

At prophylactic doses of LMWH or UFH there is no contraindication to intramuscular analgesics or Syntometrine at delivery. The LMWH should be recommended 3–6 hours after delivery, once hemostasis is ensured and the timing to be determined in conjunction with removal of any epidural catheter if present, as described below.

It should also be emphasized that for standard prophylactic doses of LMWH there is no increase in the risk of intra- or postpartum bleeding, and no increased risk of paravaginal hematoma or prolonged lochia. There is no contraindication to pudendal or perineal block for analgesia. Also, there is no risk of excess surgical bleeding at CS. However, it is good practice to ensure adequate and timely use of uterotonics and early suturing of any tear or episiotomy.

Breast-feeding

There should be a clear plan of the length of time to continue the LMWH postpartum. The woman should be assured that there is no contraindication to breast-feeding since although the LMWH will be present in breast milk, it will be broken down in the gastric acid before absorption can occur.

Anesthetic Aspects

One of the major anesthetic concerns about the use of heparins in the peripartum period is the risk of vertebral

Table 15.1 Estimated incidence for vertebral canal hematoma in spinal and epidural anesthesia

	Epidural	Spinal
Without heparin		
Atraumatic	1/220 000	1/320 000
Traumatic	1/20 000	1/29 000
Heparin given after procedure		
Atraumatic	1/70 000	1/100 000
Traumatic	1/2000	1/2900
UFH more than 1 hr after puncture	1/100 000	1/150 000
UFH less than 1 hr after puncture	1/8700	1/13 000

canal hematoma and its severe sequelae after CNB. This was first raised as a significant issue in publications from the USA[7] and subsequently much study and debate leading to some standardization and guidance [8,9]. Over 40 cases of vertebral canal hematoma were reported in the American literature from 1997 to 1998, from a 5-year observation period. Women were given enoxaparin, a commonly used LMWH, mostly following epidural, spinal, or lumbar puncture needle insertion. However, subsequent European reports included only two cases with vertebral canal hematoma. Incidence has been estimated at 1 in over 2 million in a European study, but about 1 in 15 000 in American studies. Numerous factors have been implicated including timing of LMWH (in relation to needle insertion or epidural catheter removal) and dosing schedules. Other studies have suggested that technical difficulties with needle, particularly epidural catheter, insertion, multiple insertion attempts or blood-stained tap[10] may also be associated with increased risk of hematoma (Table 15.1).

Choosing the Central Neuraxial Block

Single shot subarachnoid anesthesia (spinal block) remains a popular choice among obstetric anesthetists to provide suitable operative conditions for elective CS. This is primarily because of the superior nature of the block quality but also due to the more rapid speed of onset, when compared with epidural anesthesia. Because there is no catheter to be removed, this technique facilitates the use of a single anticoagulant agent in the postoperative period (Figure 15.1).

The use of an epidural catheter in isolation, for example to provide more controlled onset of anesthesia in patients with cardiovascular instability, is less

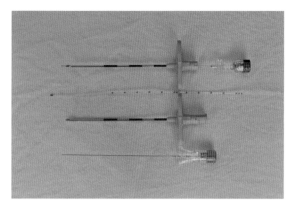

Figure 15.1 From bottom to top: A typical 25 G atraumatic spinal needle, a typical epidural needle, a typical epidural catheter, and an example of a needle-through-needle CSE.

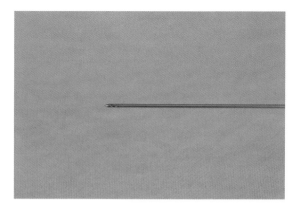

Figure 15.2 Close up of an atraumatic spinal needle.

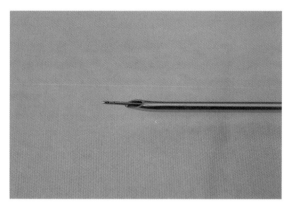

Figure 15.3 A close up of a needle-through-needle CSE.

common in the elective setting. The time from drug administration to achieving surgical anesthesia with this method can take around an hour. This has led to the introduction of the combined spinal-epidural (CSE) as a very useful tool with a flexible approach (Figure 15.2). The epidural space is located with a 16 or 18 gauge Tuohy needle using a loss of resistance technique. A non-cutting spinal needle, of smaller gauge such as 25, is then introduced through the Tuohy needle to pierce the dura and enter the subarachnoid space. Once this thinner spinal needle has been removed the epidural catheter can then be threaded through the Tuohy needle into the epidural space. This technique has provided great flexibility. Administration of reduced doses of local anesthetic into the subarachnoid space, with further doses administered via the epidural catheter, allows excellent control over the cardiovascular system. The presence of an epidural catheter also allows the anesthetist to provide additional doses of anesthetic in cases of inadequate anesthesia or prolonged operative delivery (Figure 15.3).

Thromboprophylaxis for Elective Operative Procedures

If a LMWH is given as a sole agent it is preferable to wait a minimum of 2 hours after completing the subarachnoid injection and 4 hours after removal of the Tuohy needle at epidural insertion.

When the epidural is used as part of a CSE in elective surgery there will then be an epidural catheter present at the end of surgery. This presents the operative team with two options in women requiring thromboprophylaxis:

1. administration of a single anticoagulant, most commonly a LMWH; or
2. a combination approach.

The epidural catheter should be left in place until the drug levels have reached a safe trough (see Table 15.2). A combination of unfractionated heparin followed by LMWH allows the epidural catheter to be removed in a highly monitored environment in the recovery area and also permits more controlled reversal of heparin effects if required in cases of massive postpartum hemorrhage. When UFH is given at the end of CS, local data suggest that coagulation profiles are equal to preoperative values at 4 hours post-operation, providing there has been no significant peripartum bleed.

Labor Analgesia

Despite difficulties with timings of anticoagulant drugs, it is likely that a "safe window" will be available to administer epidural analgesia once labor starts, but it is essential that all members of the multidisciplinary team have a clear plan to appropriately manage anticoagulant dosing from that point. For prophylactic dosing, there is current guidance on timings for insertion of epidural blockade. This should be utilized regularly as part of antenatal planning and agreed between obstetric, anesthetic, and hematology teams. The demonstrated increase in clearance of LMWH in the pregnant woman allows a slightly different regime from surgical patients in general. A scheme allowing neuraxial analgesia 8–10 hours following the administration of 2500 units and 12 hours following a dose of 5000 units of dalteparin, for example, would be appropriate (see Table 15.2). The ability to predict an appropriate time is harder when higher doses of LMWH have been used, or in situations where a woman presents on full anticoagulant therapy but several hours after her last dose. An assessment based on previous anti-Xa levels (if available) and on a risk–benefit analysis for each patient and situation is then needed.

If anticoagulation is to commence after delivery, an adequate gap should be left after the removal of the epidural catheter before the heparin or other anticoagulant is administered, usually 4 hours for LMWH.

Full Anticoagulation

Women who are fully anticoagulated at the time of labor and delivery include those with significant risks of morbidity: a recent venous thromboembolic event; those normally on long-term warfarin for a variety of conditions; cardiac disease including mechanical valves; ischemic heart disease and cardiomyopathy, and symptomatic homozygous or combination heritable thrombophilias[11–13].

The management of women with a need for therapeutic levels of anticoagulation in the peripartum period involves balancing the need for continuing anticoagulation to prevent the risk of thrombosis associated with the underlying condition against the risks of excessive bleeding and difficulties with analgesia and anesthesia. This requires a careful and individualized approach and thorough forward planning by a multidisciplinary team (obstetrician, midwife, anesthetist, and hematologist), in full consultation with the patient (Table 15.3). This is particularly important for the small number of women in whom the usually recommended temporary peripartum reduction in level of anticoagulation may be considered unsafe.

Table 15.2 Guidance for relative timings of anticoagulants and epidural or spinal block

A. **Subcutaneous prophylactic dose unfractionated heparin**

Catheter placement or removal >2–4 hours after injection
Delay next dose until >2 hours after catheter insertion or >4 hours after removal

B. **Intravenous infusion of unfractionated heparin**

Catheter placement >4 hours after stopping infusion, when aPPT back to baseline
Restart infusion >2 hours after catheter insertion or >4 hours after removal

C. **Low-molecular-weight heparin**

Spinal or epidural catheter insertion:

>8 hours after last injection – low dose
>12 hours after last injection – intermediate dose
>24 hours after last injection – full anticoagulation

Removal epidural catheter:

12 hours after any dose
Delay next dose until >2 hours after catheter insertion or subarachnoid injection or >4 hours after catheter removal

D. **Fondaparinux**

Perform spinal or epidural:

>36 hours after injection of low dose (≤2.5 mg/day)

Relatively contraindicated during therapeutic dosing, consider anti-Xa activity

Delay next dose after spinal or epidural until:

>6 hours after procedure for low-dose regime (≤2.5 mg per day)
>12 hours after procedure for therapeutic dose regime

Table 15.3 Recommended thromboprophylactic and anti-hemorrhagic measures

General measures:	Optimize anticoagulation antenatally Formulate intrapartum care plan Multidisciplinary intrapartum care Senior staff involvement in care throughout Aim for vaginal delivery whenever possible
Specific thromboprophylactic measures:	Mobilize during labor Maintain hydration Graduated compression stockings throughout labor and postpartum
Specific anti-hemorrhagic measures:	Minimize maternal soft tissue trauma (e.g. difficult instrumental delivery, perineal trauma) Active third stage with intravenous oxytocics Prompt management of complications (e.g. retained placenta, perineal trauma)

Table 15.4 Treatment of severe heparin overdosage

Protamine sulfate regime	(1) Heparin infusion:
	25–50 mg after stopping heparin infusion
	(1 mg of protamine sulfate neutralizes 80–100 units of heparin)
	(2) Heparin bolus
	1.00–1.5 mg/100 IU heparin can be given if 30 minutes have elapsed
	0.5–0.7 mg/100 IU heparin can be given if 30–60 minutes have elapsed
	0.25–0.375 mg IU heparin can be given if 2 hours have elapsed
	(3) Subcutaneous heparin injection:
	1–1.5 mg/100 IU heparin: 25–50 mg can be given by slow IV injection and the remainder by slow IV infusion over 8–16 hours (or the expected duration of absorption of heparin), or 2 hourly divided doses
	(4) Heparin during extracorporeal circulation:
	1.5 mg per 100 IU heparin. Sequential aPTTs may be needed to calculate correct dosage
Dose in renal/hepatic impairment	For hepatic impairment, seek further advice
	No dose adjustment necessary for renal hepatic impairment
Note	Excessive protamine doses may have an anticoagulant effect

Obstetric and General Aspects

If it has been necessary to use warfarin during the pregnancy, this should be stopped by 34–36 weeks' gestation to allow correction of the fetal coagulopathy (which takes longer than in the mother) and minimize the risk of intracranial hemorrhage at delivery. The most common practice is to replace it with a therapeutic dose of LMWH, monitored with anti-Xa levels as well as clinically. The anti-Xa level is checked at 3–5 days following the first dose and if in the desired therapeutic range does not usually need repeating.

If vaginal delivery is intended, planned induction of labor (once the cervix is sufficiently favorable) should be considered. This allows more accurate timing of events and minimizes the risk of delivery while fully anticoagulated.

The LMWH should be omitted on the morning of induction. If prophylaxis needs to be continued for the day of labor, 5000 IU of UFH can be given subcutaneously 8 hourly. If treatment doses are necessary, an infusion of UFH at 1200 u/hour should be started. Activated partial thromboplastin time (aPTT) should be checked at 4 hours after the infusion was commenced, aiming for the therapeutic range as determined by the local laboratory. It should be noted that the aPTT is less reliable in pregnancy due to increased levels of factor VIII and heparin-binding proteins.

This regime has been shown to be useful when stopped 1–6 hours (typically 4) pre-labor, with minimal obstetric or anesthetic complication[14]. However, if this interruption prior to labor is not appropriate, the UFH infusion should be stopped when cervical dilatation reaches 5 cm in primipara, or an appropriate pre-planned dilatation (depending on previous labor experience) in multipara. It should also be stopped if unscheduled blood loss is noted or urgent CS is required[15].

When a woman is fully anticoagulated with UFH, protamine sulfate, the regime for its use, and four units of cross-matched red cells should be immediately available. An example of a protamine sulfate regime is described in Table 15.4.

Graduated compression stockings should be worn throughout induction and labor and throughout the in-patient stay. Mobility should be encouraged and hydration ensured.

After delivery, the third stage of labor should be actively managed by oxytocin bolus 10 units intravenously followed by an infusion of 40 units over 4 hours. Perineal tears or episiotomies should be repaired immediately with careful attention to hemostasis and heparin restarted as soon as hemostasis has been secured.

A high index of suspicion must always be maintained when caring for fully anticoagulated women with regard to hemorrhagic complications during pregnancy. The incidence of antepartum hemorrhage and abruption is not increased, but it is more likely to be significant should it occur. A careful plan for investigation and management of unexplained abdominal pain (that may be abruption) and of unscheduled bleeding must be available in the notes.

Other issues that must be considered are the relative contraindication to performing pudendal block, the potential maternal risks during an instrumental delivery (if labor occurs spontaneously and without the lapse of time since last dose of heparin), and the importance of meticulous exclusion of postpartum hematomata.

If the woman is anticoagulated with warfarin when labor starts, the international normalized ratio (INR) must be checked urgently. If the INR is greater than 3 or a CS is required, then normalization of the INR should be targeted with vitamin K, and if more urgent, prothrombin complex as well. In this instance, a cord blood clotting screen must be taken after delivery as intravenous vitamin K may be required for the neonate. Early involvement of a neonatologist is essential.

Anesthetic Considerations

Analgesia and anesthesia in this group of women is a major challenge and early involvement of a senior anesthetist is essential in planning intrapartum care. A review by Loo *et al.* documented an overall incidence of 0.2–0.3/100 000 spinal hematomas following obstetric epidural analgesia (in all women), with coagulation abnormalities being identified as a major risk factor[16]. It is vanishingly rare for epidural labor analgesia to be performed in the fully anticoagulated woman when other options for analgesia are available.

Analgesia for Labor

The role of a consistent intrapartum care provider, particularly midwifery, is of high importance. One-to-one care from a single carer has been shown to reduce analgesia requirements and will also reduce the many anxieties associated with labor in such a situation[15]. Other guidance, such as decision-making concerning the need for continuity of anticoagulation or a window to reduce risk of hemorrhage, may alter the range of analgesics available[17].

Pharmacological intervention includes inhaled analgesia in the form of Entonox, or administration of systemic opioids. In a fully anticoagulated woman intramuscular injection is contraindicated, so intravenous bolus or patient-controlled intravenous administration of opioid analgesia is a suitable option.

Traditional opioid therapy used by most delivery suites across the UK was intermittent bolus administration of intramuscular drugs such as pethidine. The desire to match the pharmacokinetics of opioids to the time course of the cyclical pain associated with labor has led to the investigation of shorter acting opioids administered in small repeated doses. Patient-controlled analgesia pumps deliver a small pre-set dose of opioid to the woman in labor via an intravenous cannula.

Fentanyl is a synthetic phenylpiperidine derivative and is a highly selective μ-opiate peptide (MOP) receptor agonist. When given by the intravenous route the dose is effective within 2 to 5 minutes. Fentanyl is highly lipid soluble and therefore the drug in the plasma rapidly redistributes to fat-rich areas. This accounts for the short duration of fentanyl in clinical practice. If large doses are given, such as may occur in a prolonged labor, then the reservoir for redistribution becomes full. The duration of action then becomes exaggerated from each subsequent dose, behaving more like morphine. In practice, it can be difficult for the laboring woman to coincide the analgesic action with the peak of each contraction. For these reasons, fentanyl is not an ideal analgesic for labor.

Remifentanil is another synthetic opioid of the anilidopiperidine group also with action at the MOP receptor. It has an ultra-short duration of action due to unique metabolism by plasma esterases. This metabolic pathway cannot be saturated. It has a peak onset of 1 to 3 minutes, thus making the timing relative to contractions easier to manage. Remifentanil can be given by bolus dose, or a combination of background infusion with supplemental bolus doses. The pharmacokinetic profile of remifentanil means that of all the opioids available it should most closely match the time profile of a contraction. In a recent survey of opioid use in labor remifentanil is now the most commonly used opioid in the UK for women laboring with a live fetus. The recommended dose varies across studies and while the presence of a background infusion seems to increase analgesia, it is often at the expense of increased adverse events. The narrow therapeutic window means respiratory depression, and indeed apnea, is a significant risk. The degree of monitoring required is often well in excess of that which can be offered on a delivery suite.

Anesthesia for Operative Delivery

General anesthesia is associated with significant morbidity and even mortality during pregnancy[3]. The risk of failing to intubate and protect the trachea is increased by a factor of ten during pregnancy. This must be considered in a risk–benefit assessment for every woman presenting for delivery.

Procedures that require surgical anesthesia in this group leave the anesthetist with the unenviable task of providing the patient the *least risky* of two modes of anesthesia at inherently increased risk. In this situation, general anesthesia will almost always be chosen. If certain maternal risk factors combine that significantly decrease the likelihood of the anesthetist to successfully intubate, oxygenate, and ventilate the patient, then it may be considered safer to continue with a CNB. In this rare scenario, steps should be taken to minimize the complications of CNB: minimize number of attempts (most experienced person performing procedure), use of the single shot spinal technique instead of catheters, use of atraumatic needles, and where appropriate or possible, reversal of anticoagulation.

Communicating increasing amounts of risk that cannot be easily quantified is far from straightforward, particularly when trying to weigh one against another. To compound the problem, this is frequently required to be presented to women in emergency situations. Categorizing relative risk of CNBs in the obstetric population with abnormalities of coagulation (including drugs and diseases) has been suggested as a useful tool by a working party of UK experts and provides some concise guidance for use in the acute clinical setting[18].

General advice regarding timing of CNBs for anesthesia relative to anticoagulant dose remains the same as for analgesia (see Table 15.2) although the use of a single shot spinal anesthetic with a fine gauge needle may be considered earlier than standard guidance.

The anesthetist must be aware of the increased risk of bleeding at CS in those women taking higher doses of LMWH. The introduction of cell salvage machines in obstetric practice to collect autologous blood may help in the management of these patients.

Problems with Blood Patches

Accidental puncture of the dura mater occurs in 0.5 to 2.0% of all epidural procedures. Seventy percent of these women will develop a post-dural puncture headache. If this headache is severe it is often treated with an epidural blood patch. Maternal blood is withdrawn aseptically from a suitable vein and introduced via a Tuohy needle into the epidural space. As this requires further passage of a Tuohy needle, the same time delay should be introduced after LMWH administration to avoid bleeding risk.

If the woman is fully anticoagulated in the post-delivery period, a blood patch should not be performed. If headache is severe, then a hiatus in anticoagulant therapy may be considered; a risk–benefit decision must be made regarding the possible progression of

Table 15.5 The cauda equina syndrome

Low back pain
Bilateral, occasionally unilateral, sciatica
Perineal numbness (saddle numbness)
Bladder dysfunction
Bowel dysfunction
Variable lower limb weakness and sensory loss

low intracranial pressure leading to morbidity (e.g. nerve palsy due to brainstem pressure at the foramen magnum) versus the inherent dangers of discontinuing anticoagulation. Focal neurological symptoms warrant urgent imaging with MRI.

Decisions to blood patch an anticoagulated woman must be taken at a senior level but headache alone is unlikely to warrant blood patching in this group. Review of the literature suggests that continuing on prophylactic doses of LMWHs does not affect the ability of the epidural blood patch to treat the headache effectively.

Cauda Equina Syndrome

The cauda equina is formed from the terminal nerve roots of the spinal cord, after the spinal cord has formally terminated around the L2 lumbar disk space. Compression of the cauda equina presents in a common pattern. Table 15.5 shows the symptoms and signs classically displayed by patients with a cauda equina syndrome. Patients on anticoagulant therapy who have had regional analgesia or anesthesia should be carefully monitored in the post-delivery period. Imaging of a potential lesion is usually undertaken with MRI scanning. Cauda equina syndrome is a medical emergency and in the case of hematoma, requires urgent surgical opinion to schedule evacuation of the clot. Any delay is likely to increase the risk of residual neurological dysfunction.

Thrombolysis and Bypass

It has been traditional to consider pregnancy and puerperium as an absolute contraindication for use of thrombolytic agents. However, in situations in which they are liable to be used, the life of the mother is likely to be at high risk. Examples of these include cardiac compromise following massive central pulmonary embolus (PE) or acute myocardial infarction. In this situation, the balance of risks needs careful consideration but if thrombolysis is likely to be life saving it should not be delayed. Should major hemorrhage occur, it can be managed with a combination of surgical and hematological techniques. Clearly, for massive central PE, targeted injection via catheter is the ideal (if appropriate staff are available), but there are reports of successful thrombolysis without this [19]. Life-saving treatment should not be delayed or withheld for theoretical risk that cannot be substantiated. Senior and experienced decision-making is essential; for example, if a CS is required as part of resuscitation in a woman collapsed from PE or myocardial infarction, the timing and management of thrombolytic agents would need to be discussed carefully but swiftly.

The risk–benefit balance when cardiopulmonary bypass is contemplated in pregnancy is different. Clearly, the seriousness of the situation giving rise to the need for bypass is usually associated with cardiac surgery. This combined with prolonged and significant anticoagulation means that to facilitate optimization of both maternal condition for anesthesia and surgery and postoperative recovery, emptying of the uterus prior to bypass is advisable. There are case reports of successful prolongation of pregnancy in this situation, but also numerous reports published and unpublished of significant retroplacental bleeding, inability to maintain maternal blood pressure or oxygenation, and difficulty in maintaining good perioperative conditions associated with attempting to continue pregnancy. Clearly, in a viable fetus these risks are unacceptable and delivery should be expedited. Prior to this, serious consideration should be given to medical or surgical termination.

New Oral and Parenteral Anticoagulants

Recent developments in both prophylactic and therapeutic anticoagulation have occurred with the development of agents that target different points in the coagulation pathways. This has provided alternatives in situations where side effects, lack of effectiveness, or problems with compliance necessitate review. There is as yet little experience in using these agents in pregnancy and the puerperium, although there are case reports and series describing the use of the parenteral anticoagulants following development of heparin-induced thrombocytopenia (HIT) or cutaneous allergy to heparins[20–25]. Parenteral agents given subcutaneously include danaparoid, a low-molecular-weight heparinoid (heparan derivative), which does not cross the placenta, and fondaparinux, a synthetic polysaccharide based on the active moiety of heparin. Experience with fondaparinux during pregnancy is growing but data regarding placental passage are mixed. The long half life of these drugs requires careful attention at delivery. Fondaparinux has been recommended by the Pregnancy and Thrombosis Working Group[26] as a reasonable alternative to heparins in both pregnancy and the puerperium and during breastfeeding.

Newer oral agents are direct factor Xa and thrombin inhibitors and include rivaroxiban, apixaban, edoxaban, betrixaban, and dabigatran.

Reproductive toxicity has been shown in animal studies but in most of these studies plasma levels have been considerably higher than clinically necessary. Experience in humans is limited and current recommendations advise against their use in pregnancy and breastfeeding[27].

Near Patient Testing and Anticoagulation

The basic principles of thromboelastography (TEG®) are described in Chapter 2. Other near patient tests include rotational thromboelastometry (ROTEM®) and platelet function analysis (PFA-100®). These near patient tests have become useful additions to standard laboratory coagulation testing and their availability to clinicians in areas such as delivery suite is increasing. Although laboratory coagulation tests remain the gold standard, point-of-care tests can offer useful information in a fraction of the time. These tests have dramatically improved management of obstetric hemorrhage, particularly where cause of the coagulopathy is uncertain.

One particular difficulty in interpreting both laboratory and near patient testing of parturients is that reference ranges were derived from samples of healthy non-pregnant adults. It is well established that pregnancy leads to a hypercoagulable state, but individual coagulation study tests vary widely during normal pregnancy. Small studies on parturients using point-of-care tests, such as TEG and ROTEM, have demonstrated a hypercoagulable state[28,29] while testing using the PFA-100 has not shown significant differences to normal population values[30].

TEG and ROTEM may be helpful in the ongoing management of a bleeding anticoagulated parturient as they can:

• confirm poor clot formation;

- help to diagnose coagulopathy contributed to by:
  1. heparins
  2. aspirin
  3. relatively reduced fibrinogen (compared with the normal parturient);
- guide the choice of clotting products.

For patients with exposure to heparin, the heparinase cup (TEG) and the hep-tem S® reagent (ROTEM) should be used, alongside standard assays. For diagnosis of relative fibrinogen deficit, the fib-tem® assay (ROTEM) should be used alongside standard assay.

Although near patient testing may aid both diagnosis and treatment, it is not a replacement for laboratory coagulation studies, which remain central to management in this patient group.

Summary

Management of women with any degree of anticoagulation in the peripartum period is often challenging. However, attention to detail, careful planning and documentation, departmental education, and involving appropriate disciplines as well as the patient should allow optimal management to be achieved.

Case Studies

Case Study 1

This case involved severe cutaneous allergy secondary to LMWH. A 32-year-old woman was diagnosed with multiple small emboli in her left lung at 34 weeks' gestation in her third ongoing pregnancy. She had a BMI of 27 at booking but no other significant risk factors for venous thromboembolism. Previous pregnancies had been uncomplicated and she had delivered healthy, normally grown babies by spontaneous labor with vaginal deliveries at term, the last being 3 years previously.

Investigation for increasing shortness of breath over 2 weeks revealed not only multiple emboli on a ventilation–perfusion scan, but also a proximal DVT, which had given few symptoms.

Dalteparin was started in a twice daily regimen with dose as per guidelines. At review 7 days later she had obvious red itchy areas of reaction around the last three days' injection sites. A similar reaction occurred with enoxaparin.

At 2 weeks after diagnosis therapeutic doses were still needed, but at 36 weeks the patient was concerned about bleeding at delivery. After discussion of risks and benefits, fondaparinux 2.5 mg BD was started. Documented planning included analgesia if labor occurred within 24 hours of last injection (due to long half-life), careful attention to surgical and obstetric aspects of prevention and management of bleeding (early suturing, active management third stage), and use of blood products and tranexamic acid.

At 39 weeks symptoms were resolving but the patient remained increasingly concerned and requested delivery. This was agreed if the cervix was favorable.

ARM was performed 18 hours after the last dose of fondaparinux. Syntocinon was started immediately so that time off anticoagulation was minimized. Labor and delivery were uncomplicated.

Had she required epidural analgesia, fondaparinux was to be restarted 6 hours after catheter removal, with close attention to hydration and mobilization.

As the patient wished to breast-feed it was planned to restart fondaparinux and consider a single daily dose after 2 weeks (when she would be 7 weeks post diagnosis).

This case illustrates the importance of careful planning, weighing up risks at each decision, and involving the patient in care planning and assessing options. This is particularly so in the light of Montgomery vs Lanarkshire Health Board (https://www.supremecourt.uk/cases/).

Case Study 2

This case highlights dose of prophylactic heparin required for a woman with high BMI. A 37-year-old woman presented in antenatal clinic at 13 weeks in her fourth pregnancy. Her dating scan had shown dichorionic twins (spontaneous conception). Her BMI at booking was 46 and she smoked 25 cigarettes per day. Her first three children had been born at term, but she had gestational diabetes in the previous pregnancy. This had resulted in induction of labor at 39 weeks and a baby weighing 4.6 kg. This led to shoulder dystocia at delivery, requiring internal maneuvers.

She was assessed as having four risk factors for venous thromboembolism and was started on dalteparin 5000 units BD.

She again developed gestational diabetes, requiring metformin, and had severe symphysis pubis dysfunction from 26 weeks with reduced mobility. Her dose of dalteparin was therefore increased to 7500 units BD. An assessment in the obstetric anesthetic clinic was undertaken to plan with regard to safe timing of CNB and to highlight any potential concerns with airway management should the need for general anesthesia arise. It was agreed at a multidisciplinary team meeting that a cesarean section should be performed at 38 weeks.

The patient was admitted in established labor with ruptured membranes at 34 weeks, 2 hours after her last dose of dalteparin. Ten minutes later she was fully dilated and began to push, the anesthetic team having been requested urgently. The first twin was delivered uneventfully. On examination, a cord prolapse was diagnosed and position of the second twin was unclear due to obesity. Ultrasound scan revealed the second twin was a transverse lie.

An attempt was made to perform external cephalic version, with the patient using Entonox analgesia, to facilitate breech extraction. Unfortunately, fetal bradycardia and maternal distress necessitated cesarean section under general anesthesia for the second twin. Though the fetal heart rate normalized in theater, it was considered too soon after the dalteparin for spinal anesthesia to be attempted.

The procedure was uneventful from a surgical point of view, but inability to maintain maternal oxygen saturation occurred in recovery and she was transferred to critical care for advanced respiratory and airway support.

This case demonstrates that while thromboprophylaxis is important, the risks versus benefits of anticoagulation are dynamic and can vary rapidly during delivery. It is vital that decision-making is a shared process between specialties and a clear strategy agreed. The risks of general anesthesia in this group are significant.

References

1. Cook TM, Counsell D, Wildsmith JAW; on behalf of the Royal College of Anesthetists Third National Audit Project. Major complications of central neuraxial block: report on the Third National Audit Project of the Royal College of Anesthetists. *British Journal of Anesthesia* 2009; **102**: 179–190

2. Royal College of Obstetricians and Gynecologists. *Thrombosis and Embolism during Pregnancy and the Puerperium: Reducing the Risk. Green-Top Guideline 37a*. London: Royal College of Obstetricians and Gynecologists; 2015. https://www.rcog.org.uk/globalas sets/documents/guidelines/gtg-37a.pdf

3. Knight M *et al.* (eds.) on behalf of MBRRACE. *Saving Lives, Improving Care*. Oxford:NPEU, University of Oxford; 2015. https://www.npeu.ox.ac.uk/downloads/ files/mbrrace-uk/reports/MBRRACE-UK%20Maternal %20Report%202015.pdf

4. CLASP (Collaborative Low dose Aspirin Study in Pregnancy) Collaborative Group. CLASP: a randomised trial of low-dose aspirin for the prevention and treatment of pre-eclampsia among 9364 pregnant women. *Lancet* 1994; **343**: 619–629.

5. NICE. Hypertension in Pregnancy: diagnosis and management. Sections 1.1.1.2.1–2 NICE Guidelines CG107; 2010. https://www.nice.org.uk/guidance/cg107/ chapter/guidance

6. James AH, Abel DE, Braucazio LR. Anticoagulants in pregnancy. *Obstetrical and Gynecological Survey* 2005; **61**: 59–61.

7. Wysowski DK, Talarico L, Bacsanyi J, Botstein P. Spinal and epidural hematoma and low molecular weight heparin. *New England Journal of Medicine* 1998; **338**: 1774–1775.

8. Scottish Intercollegiate Guidelines Network. Section 7: Spinal and epidural blocks; Section 9: Pregnancy and puerperium. In *Prophylaxis of Venous Thromboembolism*. Publication No. 62. Edinburgh: SIGN; 2002: 24–26; 30–35.

9. Horlocker TT, Wedel DJ, Benzon H *et al.* Regional anesthesia in the anticoagulated patient: Defining the risks (The Second ASRA Consensus Conference on Neuraxial Anesthesia and Anticoagulation). *Regional Anesthesia and Pain Medicine* 2003; **23**: 172–197.

10. Stafford-Smith M. Impaired hemostasis and regional anesthesia. *Canadian Journal of Anesthesia* 1996; **43**: R129–R141.

11. Royal College of Obstetricians and Gynecologists. *Thrombosis and Embolism during Pregnancy and the Puerperium: Acute Management. Green-Top Guideline 27b*. London: Royal College of Obstetricians and Gynecologists; 2015. https://www.rcog.org.uk/ globalassets/documents/guidelines/gtg-37b.pdf

12. Asghar F, Bowman P. A clinical approach to the management of thrombosis in obstetrics Part 2: diagnosis and management of venous thromboembolism. *The Obstetrician and Gynecologist* 2007; **9**: 3–8.

13. Gelson E, Johnson M, Gatzoulis M, Uebing A. Cardiac disease in pregnancy Part 2: acquired heart disease. *The Obstetrician and Gynecologist* 2007; **9**: 83–87.

14. Austin SK, Lambert J, Peebles D, Cohen H. Managing peri-delivery anticoagulation in women on therapeutic dose low molecular weight heparin: a role for unfractionated heparin? *Journal of Thrombosis and Hemostasis* 2007; **5** (Supp 1): P-S-622.

15. Akkad A, Oppenheimer C, Mushambi M, Pavord S. Intrapartum care for women on full anticoagulation. *International Journal of Obstetric Anesthesia* 2003; **12**: 188–192.

16. Loo CC, Dahlgren G, Irestedt L. Neurological complications of obstetric regional analgesia. *International Journal of Obstetric Anesthesia* 2000; **9**: 99–124.

17. Bates SM, Greer IA, Pabinger I, Sofer S, Hirsh J. Venous Thromboembolism, Thrombophilias, Anti-thrombotic therapy and Pregnancy. American College of Chest Physicians Evidence-Based Clinical Practice Guidelines (8th Edition). *Chest* 2008; 844S–886S.

18. Harrop-Griffiths *et al.* on behalf of the Association of Anesthetists of Great Britain and Ireland, Obstetric Anesthetists' Association and Regional Anesthesia UK. Regional anesthesia and patients with abnormalities of coagulation. *Anesthesia* 2013; **68**: 966–972.

19. Leonhardt G, Gaul C, Nietsch HH *et al.* Thrombolytic therapy in pregnancy. *Journal of Thrombosis and Thrombolysis* 2006; **21**: 271–276.

20. Ekbatani A, Asaro LR, Malinow AM. Anticoagulation with argatroban in a parturient with heparin-induced thrombocytopenia. *International Journal of Obstetric Anesthesia* 2010; **19**: 82–87.

21. Young SK, Al-Mondhiry HA, Vaida SJ, Ambrose A, Botti JJ. Successful use of argatroban during the third trimester of pregnancy: case report and review of the literature. *Pharmacotherapy* 2008; **28**: 1531–1536.

22. Tanimura K, Ebina Y, Sonoyama A, *et al.* Argatroban therapy for heparin-induced thrombocytopenia during pregnancy in a woman with hereditary antithrombin deficiency. *Journal of Obstetrics and Gynaecology Research* 2012; **38**: 749–752.

23. Huhle G, Geberth M, Hoffmann U, Heene DL, Harenberg J. Management of heparin-associated thrombocytopenia in pregnancy with subcutaneous r-hirudin. *Gynecologic and Obstetric Investigation* 2000; **49**: 67–69.

24. Tang AW, Greer I. A systematic review on the use of new anticoagulants in pregnancy. *Obstetric Medicine* 2013; **6**: 64–71.

25. Ciurzyński M, Jankowski K, Pietrzak B *et al.* Use of fondaparinux in a pregnant woman with pulmonary embolism and heparin-induced thrombocytopenia. *Medical Science Monitor* 2011; **17**: CS56–59.

26. Duhl AJ, Paidas MJ, Ural SH *et al.* Pregnancy and Thrombosis Working Group. Antithrombotic therapy and pregnancy: consensus report and recommendations for prevention and treatment of venous thromboembolism and adverse pregnancy outcomes. *American Journal of Obstetrics and Gynecology* 2007; **197**: 457.e1–21.

27. Cohen H, Arachchillage DR, Middeldorp S, Beyer-Westendorf J, Abdul-Kadir R. Management of direct oral anticoagulants in women of childbearing potential: guidance from the SSC of the ISTH. *Journal of Thrombosis and Haemostasis* 2016. doi: 10.1111/jth.13366

28. Macafee B, Campbell JP, Ashpole K, *et al.* Reference ranges for thromboelastography (TEG®) and traditional coagulation tests in term parturients undergoing cesarean section. *Anesthesia* 2012: **67**: 741–747.

29. Armstrong S, Fernando R, Ashpole K, Simons R, Columb M. Assessment of coagulation in the obstetric population using ROTEM® thromboelastometry. *International Journal of Obstetric Anesthesia* 2011; **20**: 293–298.

30. Beilin Y, Arnold I, Hossain S. Evaluation of the platelet function analyser (PFA-100®) vs. the thromboelastogram (TEG) in the parturient. *International Journal of Obstetric Anesthesia* 2006; **15**(1): 7–12.

Chapter

16

Antiphospholipid Syndrome

Sue Pavord, Bethan Myers, Savino Sciascia, and Beverley Hunt

Introduction

Antiphospholipid syndrome (APS) is an autoimmune disorder characterized by vascular thrombosis and/or obstetric morbidity in the presence of persistent antiphospholipid antibodies (aPL). There are a number of potential complications for pregnancy but with optimal management, good maternal health and a live birth rate of 80–90% can be achieved.

The syndrome produces a spectrum of disease, both in terms of clinical manifestations and the presence of other autoimmune conditions. Arterial, venous, or small vessel thrombosis may occur, there is an array of adverse obstetric outcomes, and a number of additional clinical features may be present, involving any organ. The disease is classified as primary (PAPS) when it occurs in the absence of any features of other autoimmune disease and secondary where other autoimmune disease is present (SAPS). Predominantly, this is systemic lupus erythematosus (SLE), but other connective

tissue diseases or inflammatory bowel conditions may be involved. The term "primary" is useful for research and classification purposes, but there are few differences in complications related to APS or in antibody specificity in the presence or absence of SLE. Surprisingly few patients with primary APS progress to SLE, and it seems that in secondary APS, the antibodies to aPL develop at a similar time to the antibodies of SLE.

An international consensus statement on classification criteria for definite APS was first published after a workshop in Sapporo, Japan, in 1998. These criteria have subsequently been updated[1] (Table 16.1). At least one clinical manifestation, such as vascular thrombosis or pregnancy morbidity, together with positive laboratory tests, including lupus anticoagulant (LAC), anticardiolipin antibodies (aCL), or beta2 glycoprotein 1 (β2GPI), detected at least twice 12 weeks apart, are necessary to fulfil the classification criteria.

Table 16.1 Summary of the revised classification criteria for the Antiphospholipid Syndrome (APS)[1]

APS is diagnosed if at least one clinical and one laboratory criteria are met (although not if there is less than 12 weeks or more than 5 years between the positive aPL test and the clinical manifestation).

Clinical criteria

1. Vascular thrombosis
   One or more clinical episodes of arterial, venous, or microvascular thrombosis occurring in any tissue or organ (superficial venous thrombosis is not included)
2. Pregnancy morbidity
   (a) One or more unexplained deaths of a morphologically normal fetus at, or beyond, 10 weeks' gestation *or*
   (b) One or more premature births of a morphologically normal neonate before 34 weeks' gestation because of eclampsia, severe pre-eclampsia or recognized features of placental insufficiency*.
   (c) Three or more unexplained consecutive spontaneous abortions before the 10th week of gestation, with maternal anatomic or hormonal abnormalities and paternal and maternal chromosomal causes excluded.

Laboratory criteria

1. LAC present on two or more occasions at least 12 weeks apart detected according to the guidelines of the International Society on Thrombosis and Haemostasis[1]
2. aCL of IgG and/or IgM isotype in serum or plasma, present in medium or high titer (i.e. >40 GPL or MPL, or >the 99th percentile), on two or more occasions, at least 12 weeks apart, measured by a standardized ELISA
3. Anti-β_2 GP-I antibody of IgG and/or IgM isotype in serum or plasma (in titer >the 99th percentile), present on two or more occasions, at least 12 weeks apart, measured by standardized ELISA

*Generally accepted features of placental insufficiency include: (i) abnormal or non-reassuring fetal surveillance test(s), e.g. a non-reactive non-stress test, suggestive of fetal hypoxemia, (ii) abnormal Doppler flow velocimetry waveform analysis suggestive of fetal hypoxemia, e.g. absent end-diastolic flow in the umbilical artery, (iii) oligohydramnios, e.g. an amniotic fluid index of 5 cm or less, or (iv) a postnatal birth weight less than the 10th percentile for the gestational age.

Prevalence

aPL, identified using standardized techniques, are detected in less than 1% of apparently normal individuals and in up to 3% of the elderly population without clinical manifestations of the APS. However, the prevalence is dramatically higher in patients with a first stroke (10–26%) and 10–40% in women with recurrent pregnancy loss (10–40%). The syndrome occurs most commonly in young to middle-aged adults, with a mean age of onset of 31 years. Women are more frequently affected, with a female to male ratio of 5:1, which is even higher in SAPS associated with SLE. There is no defined racial predominance for APS, although an increased incidence of SLE occurs in African Americans and the Hispanic population. Among patients with SLE, the prevalence of aPL is 15–35%[2,3], but only around half of these cases will have clinical features of APS.

Pathophysiology and Etiology

Different pathological mechanisms may be responsible for the varying clinical manifestations. Recurrence of complications often follows a similar pattern of disease and recurrent thrombosis usually occurs in the same vascular field, although this is not always the rule.

It was originally thought that aPL were directed against negatively charged phospholipid, but it is now clear that they target plasma proteins with affinity for these anionic phospholipids. There is concordance between the LAC, aCL, and anti-β2GPI antibodies; however, they are not identical and some LAC antibodies react with phospholipids other than cardiolipin and proteins other than β2GPI, whereas some aCL and anti-β2GPI antibodies have no LAC activity. In general, LAC positivity has been shown to confer the highest risk for thrombosis when compared to other aPL[4]. However, there is no association with particular vessel occlusion or clinical manifestations and antibody type. Results of a recent prospective multi-center study support the concept that triple positivity (LAC, aCL, and anti-β2GPI antibodies) is associated with a very high thrombotic risk, with 37% of 104 asymptomatic carriers developing a first thromboembolic event within 10 years[5].

Procoagulant Effects of APL

β2GPI is a multifunctional apolipoprotein, which contributes to the regulation of hemostasis as well as other physiological processes. Not surprisingly

Table 16.2 Procoagulant effects of β2GPI-dependent aPL

Up-regulation of the tissue factor pathway
Inhibition of the activated protein C pathway
Inhibition of antithrombin activity
Inhibition of fibrinolysis
Activation of endothelial cells
Enhanced expression of adhesion molecules by endothelial cells with increased binding of leukocytes
Activation and degranulation of neutrophils
Potentiation of platelet activation
Enhanced platelet aggregation
Displacement of annexin V from cell membranes
Activation of complement

therefore, β2GPI-dependent antibodies have been associated with a number of different biological effects (Table 16.2). These include direct cellular effects caused by bound β2GPI–antibody complexes, with affinity for both anionic phospholipid expressed on the surface of activated cells and heparin sulfate-containing structures on non-activated cells. The binding of β2GPI to anionic structures, through domain 5, induces the expression of new cryptic epitopes in domain 1 and may increase the antigenic density, two events that seem to be pivotal for the antibody binding. Studies show that dimerization of β2GPI by anti-β2GPI antibodies causes a conformational change in the molecule increasing its affinity for phospholipids by 100-fold. β2GPI can bind to the low-density lipoprotein receptor, ApoER2, on the surface of platelets and thus mediate platelet activation, with increased thromboxane synthesis and platelet aggregation. In vitro, endothelial cells and monocytes can also be activated by aPL and β2GPI binding, resulting in tissue factor expression. In addition, in vitro studies have shown some aPL cause interference with hemostatic factors such as IX, X, and XII, resistance to activated protein C, and a reduction in fibrinolysis from antiplasmin or anti-tissue-type plasminogen activator (tPA) activity. At this time, there is no clarity as to how aPL cause thrombosis, and it is the subject of much research.

Indeed, despite the persistent presence of aPL in the circulation, thrombotic events in patients with aPL occur only occasionally, suggesting that the presence of aPL is necessary but not sufficient for clot formation in vivo. In this regard, a two-hit hypothesis has been suggested: aPL (first hit) increases the risk of thrombotic events that occur in the presence of another thrombophilic condition (second hit). According to this model, the initiating "first hit" injury disrupts the endothelium, and a "second hit" potentiates thrombus formation[6].

Obstetric Morbidity

The pathophysiological mechanisms underlying fetal loss or morbidity appear to be multiple. Owing to the wide spectrum of manifestations and heterogeneous findings in placental tissue in these patients, it is unclear whether one or several aPL subgroups are responsible for the varying phenotypes and whether concurrent, aPL-independent genetic and environmental factors affecting the maternal–fetal interface influence the potential pathogenicity of these antibodies.

Early histological studies demonstrated decidual vasculopathy and placental thrombosis in those with second and third pregnancy morbidity and mortality due to placental dysfunction. Displacement of annexin V from trophoblasts contributes to a procoagulant state through acceleration of coagulation reactions. A mouse model has demonstrated activation of complement through the classical pathway, with consequent influx of inflammatory cells into tissues, mediating placental injury, and leading to fetal loss and growth restriction. In this model, heparin prevented pregnancy loss by blocking activation of complement, rather than primarily via an anticoagulant effect[7].

Direct trophoblastic damage by aPL, independent of mechanisms involving thrombosis and complement activation, has also been demonstrated recently. Interaction of aPL with β2GPI, exposed during trophoblast syncytium formation, has been shown to cause inhibition of the intercytotrophoblast fusion process, gonadotrophin secretion, and trophoblast invasiveness. This mechanism has been hypothesized to contribute to early pregnancy loss. There is evidence of a significant reduction in intradecidual endovascular trophoblast invasion on analysis of the products of conception (first trimester failure) from APS patients.

The factors that determine whether aPL induce a thrombotic or non-thrombotic disease phenotype in the placenta are not known. It is likely that interplay between patient background traits and distinct aPL subgroups determines disease manifestation.

Clinical Features

International consensus criteria for the classification of definite APS were initially published in 1999[8] and updated in 2006[1] (Table 16.1).

Thrombosis

Thrombosis is the most common presenting feature of APS[9] and may occur in both the venous and arterial circulation as well as the microvasculature. It can involve vascular beds that are infrequently affected by other prothrombotic states and is independent of atherosclerotic vascular disease.

Venous Thrombosis

Studies suggest that aPL are found in approximately 2% of patients presenting with acute venous thromboembolism. Often, the venous thrombosis occurs in an unusual site such as the cerebral, retinal, splanchnic, axillary, and subclavian veins, and APS can account for up to 70% of such presentations. Venous thromboembolism, especially deep venous thrombosis of the legs, has been shown to occur in around 30–50% of patients with APS during an average follow-up of less than 6 years[10]. Following a first episode, the risk for future venous thrombosis increases significantly. Other sites such as the retinal vein, portal vein, sagittal vein, and renal vein may be affected. Essentially anyone with a venous thrombosis at an unusual site must be tested for aPL.

Arterial Thrombosis

The most common site of arterial thrombosis is the central nervous system, with strokes and transient ischemic attacks accounting for 50% of the arterial events seen with APS. Myocardial infarction accounts for around 20% and it is increasingly being recognized that aPL is an important cause of MINOCA (myocardial infarction with non-obstructive coronary occlusion), i.e. thrombosis in a normal, not atheromatous, coronary artery. Other vascular beds may be involved including those of the lungs, retina, gastrointestinal tract, spleen, kidney, and extremities. In many cases the event appears unprovoked, with no other identifiable risk factors for arterial disease, such as smoking, diabetes, or hypertension.

Obstetric Complications

Complications during pregnancy, in addition to maternal thrombosis, include recurrent spontaneous abortions in the first trimester as well as adverse outcomes occurring late in pregnancy. However, APS is not a "full-house" syndrome, for there are women with aPL who have no problems at all in pregnancy.

Early Pregnancy Loss

Pregnancy loss is one of the leading problems in women's health issues. Approximately one-third of all conceptions and 15% of clinically recognized pregnancies (<6 weeks of gestation) fail to result in a live birth. Five percent of women experience two or more losses and 1–2% suffer with three or more. Up to half of the cases remain unexplained after gynecological, hormonal, and karyotypic analyses. Of the women who have recurrent pregnancy loss, defined as three or more first trimester miscarriages, 10% to 20% have detectable aPL[11]. These women potentially have a 90% risk of further fetal loss if left untreated[12]. The diagnostic criteria for APS suggest that evaluation should begin after the third consecutive early miscarriage, defined by less than 10 weeks' gestation (Table 16.1). However, in practice, evaluation after two early miscarriages is often initiated at the discretion of the physician.

Late Pregnancy Complications of aPL

Complications occurring late in pregnancy relate to ischemic placental dysfunction caused by aPL. The manifestations include pre-eclampsia, prematurity, fetal distress, intrauterine growth restriction, and fetal death. Preterm delivery may be associated with premature rupture of the membranes or pre-eclampsia. The median rate of gestational hypertension or pre-eclampsia is 30–50% in untreated women with previously diagnosed APS but falls to 10% with effective management. In contrast, aPL are not found in a significantly higher proportion of general obstetric patients presenting with pre-eclampsia[13]. HELLP syndrome (hemolysis, elevated liver enzymes, and low platelets) may occur, being associated with pre-eclampsia/eclampsia in most cases and may occur earlier than in women without APS, often in the second trimester.

Other Clinical Manifestations

In addition to thrombosis and obstetric morbidity, there are a number of additional clinical manifestations which are not included in the official definition of APS. These include abnormalities of skin (particularly livedo reticularis, which occurs in up to 10% of patients), minor cardiac valve abnormalities, central nervous system, kidneys and hematological disturbances such as thrombocytopenia, and a positive direct Coombs test with occasional cases of clinical hemolytic anemia.

Thrombocytopenia

A significant minority of patients with APS have thrombocytopenia (platelets $<100 \times 10^9/L$). The pathogenic antibodies are directed toward epitopes on platelet membrane glycoproteins and are distinct from antiphospholipid antibodies, and therefore this can be considered to be an associated autoimmune thrombocytopenia. Conversely, aPL are found in approximately 25% of patients with chronic autoimmune thrombocytopenia. They do not confer a different clinical phenotype initially, but the persistence of aPL in these patients has been found to be an important risk factor for subsequent development of APS[14].

CNS Effects

A variety of neurological manifestations may occur, mostly secondary to cerebrovascular infarcts. The clinical features depend upon the size and location of the vessels occluded and include multi-infarct dementia, psychomotor agitation and insomnia, movement disorders such as chorea, dystonia, oral dyskinesias and speech impairment, transverse myelitis, seizures, and optic neuritis. Migraine has been associated with APS by some authors.

Valve Defects

Up to 30% of patients with APS have minor valvular abnormalities, including thickening and vegetations, which usually do not cause hemodynamic disturbance requiring surgical intervention. It is unclear whether the etiology is primarily thrombotic or inflammatory. Non-bacterial thrombotic endocarditis (Libman–Sacks endocarditis) is a rare disorder characterized by sterile, thrombotic vegetations of the heart valves and can occur in APS. These thrombotic lesions carry significant embolic potential.

APS Nephropathy

Renal involvement in APS was first described in 1992. Clinical features can include hypertension, renal artery stenosis, renal vein thrombosis, and a thrombotic microangiopathy (TMA), which can present for the first time during pregnancy. APS TMA is histologically characterized by the presence of fibrous intimal hyperplasia, focal cortical atrophy, and arterial occlusions.

Catastrophic Antiphospholipid Syndrome (CAPS)

This term defines a severe accelerated form of APS that results in multiorgan failure from widespread thromboses. The pathogenesis appears dependent on a multi-hit phenomenon, with infection, trauma or surgery, drug administration, or warfarin withdrawal exacerbating an already procoagulable state. We have noted that pre-eclampsia in APS is associated with CAPS. In 50% of cases no triggering factor is identified and in some it may be relatively minor, such as a biopsy. Around one-quarter may have disseminated intravascular coagulation (DIC), contributing to "thrombotic storm" and end-organ damage. Severe thrombocytopenia commonly develops. Acute adult respiratory distress syndrome (ARDS) occurs in one-third of patients and death in around 50%, mainly from cardiac or respiratory failure, despite treatment with anticoagulation and plasma exchange.

Laboratory Evaluation

Limitations to laboratory testing include lack of international laboratory standardization for aPL, and the heterogeneous nature of the antibodies results in low specificity of the assays. Many healthy individuals can have aPL without thrombosis or obstetric morbidity; indeed aPL are found in some studies to be present in 3–5% of the normal population. aPL may be transient after infection or infarction, or they may be induced by certain drugs. The clinical importance of these antibodies is uncertain. To satisfy the APS laboratory classification criteria, a patient has to be persistently positive for either one of the assays – anticardiolipin antibody, lupus anticoagulant, or β2GPI antibody, for at least 12 weeks. Testing should occur away from the acute event.

Lupus Anticoagulant (LAC)

These antibodies are detected by their ability to prolong phospholipid-dependent coagulation reactions, not usually corrected by mixing patient and normal plasmas (although about 25% of antibodies may show some correction on mixing with normal plasma). As aPL showing LAC activity are heterogeneous, it is recommended that at least two methods are performed; aPTT and a direct anti-Xa assay such as the dilute Russell viper venom assay (dRVVT). It should be confirmed that the anticoagulant is directed against protein bound to negatively charged phospholipids.

The International Society for Thrombosis and Hemostasis has identified the following criteria for the confirmation of a LAC[15]:

1. Prolongation of a phospholipid-dependent clotting assay
2. Evidence of an inhibitor demonstrated by mixing studies
3. Confirmation of the phospholipid-dependent nature of the inhibitor (platelet or other phospholipid neutralization procedure)

Most LACs are directed against either β2GPI or prothrombin. Recently methods to distinguish those associated with anti β2GPI have been developed but while these are highly specific, their sensitivity is low. LAC has been shown to be the most relevant assay in relation to vascular events and obstetric morbidity. The odds ratios for thrombotic risk range from 5 to 16.

Anticardiolipin Antibodies

Anticardiolipin antibodies (ACL) are measured by ELISA, although, again, concordance among laboratories is poor and it is difficult to distinguish between the significant antibodies associated with β2GPI and those bound to other plasma proteins or directly bound to cardiolipin. The correlation between aCL titer and thrombotic risk is well established, with the IgG subtype having a stronger association than IgM or IgA[16]. The revised classification criteria for APS use an IgG aCL cut-off of 40 U. Low levels of aCL, although statistically abnormal, may not be associated with a significant risk of thrombosis and in a systematic review of the literature, Galli *et al.* observed no correlation with venous thrombosis and only a weak correlation with arterial thrombosis[4].

Anti-beta 2 Glycoprotein 1 Antibodies

Anti-β2GPI antibodies show better correlation with thrombosis than aCL but there is a high false-positive rate. Recently, new guidelines have been published for the performance of an anti-β2GPI antibody ELISA, which might improve standardization of the assay. However, the specificity remains low as there are non-pathogenic antibodies that bind β2GPI. Indeed, of the five domains of β2GPI involved, only those antibodies directed against domain 1 correlate with thromboembolic complications, with an odds ratio of around 18.

Other aPL

The clinical utility of aPL assays for autoantibodies to phospholipids other than cardiolipin and to phospholipid-binding proteins other than β2GPI, such as prothrombin, is now a question of debate. Antibodies to prothrombin can be detected by directly coating prothrombin on irradiated ELISA plates (aPT) or by using the phosphatidylserine/prothrombin complex as antigen (aPS/PT).

Principles of Management

Individual treatment strategies for the management of the antiphospholipid syndrome in pregnancy in part depend on the assessment of a number of different factors. These include:

- history of prior thrombosis;
- whether the thrombotic event was provoked or spontaneous;
- whether the thrombotic event was venous or arterial;
- history of obstetric morbidity alone;
- evidence of any organ damage;
- the presence of SLE or other autoimmune disease; and
- other maternal risk factors, such as obesity and maternal age.

Background

The first treatment used and studied for pregnant patients with APS was a combination of corticosteroids and low-dose aspirin. Low-dose aspirin is known to be safe in pregnancy, in the first and second trimesters, and also recognized to reduce risk of preeclampsia.

Corticosteroids were an obvious choice as an immunosuppressant to suppress the antibodies present. Small, early studies were encouraging. Subsequent studies comparing heparin and prednisolone concluded that low-dose heparin was preferable, since, although effective, steroids induced significant maternal morbidity, and more premature deliveries[17]. Heparin (either unfractionated or low molecular weight) is the standard anticoagulant in pregnancy for prophylaxis and treatment of VTE. With improved understanding of the mechanisms of action of heparins and the pathophysiology of APS, it is a logical drug of choice in this condition. In addition to anticoagulant activity, it has anti-inflammatory and anti-complement effects, both of which may be involved in APS pathogenesis. In vitro heparin also appears to enhance trophoblast development, apparently limiting aPL attack on trophoblasts. Two systematic reviews of small studies recommended a combination of aspirin and heparin to reduce fetal loss, concluding that this regime may reduce pregnancy loss by 54%[18,19]. Some authors, however, question the role of pharmacological treatment in improved live birth rate, as some studies showed no difference between treatment and placebo arms in low-risk patients. Problems in interpretation are due to the small size of studies, variable entry criteria, lack of placebo arms, and absence of blinding.

Pre-pregnancy Management

Pre-pregnancy counseling should be offered, taking all factors into consideration. Where necessary, recommendations should be made to improve general health and reduce risk before a pregnancy is undertaken, such as the need for weight loss, to wait at least 3 to 6 months following an acute thrombotic event, or until SLE has been quiescent for 3 months. There may be rare circumstances where pregnancy should be actively discouraged; for example, if pulmonary hypertension is present the risk of maternal death is estimated at greater than 35%.

During this review, a clear proposed plan for pregnancy management should be outlined, both verbally and in writing. The following issues need to be addressed:

- Review detailed medical and obstetric history.
- Document and confirm persistent aPL, assess renal function and presence of thrombocytopenia and/or anemia.
- Optimize the patient's clinical state and pharmacological treatment before pregnancy. Advise postponing pregnancy if a thrombotic event has occurred within the last 3 to 6 months, SLE has been active, or hypertension uncontrolled.
- Assess individual additional risk factors such as obesity and maternal age and give a clear indication to the patient regarding the degree of risk for both thrombosis and obstetric complications.
- Assess for the presence of anti-Ro or La antibodies, even if no evidence of SLE. These antibodies are associated with a 2% risk of complete heart block in the fetus and up to a 10%

risk of neonatal lupus. If a mother has previously had a child with complete heart block, the risk of it occurring in a future pregnancy is 25%. If found, fetal cardiology assessment should be offered and any pregnancy affected by complete heart block should be managed by a specialized center where there is a pediatric cardiologist to manage the neonate. Many units now offer hydroxychloroquine during pregnancy to mothers with anti-Ro antibodies as there is some evidence they reduce the risk of complete heart block[20].

- Provide contact information for prompt, early referral at the onset of pregnancy and ensure a clear understanding of the need to substitute heparin and low-dose aspirin for warfarin at the time of the first positive pregnancy test. Ideally, the woman should be provided with a supply of low-molecular-weight heparin (LMWH) and lessons in self-injection so should they get pregnant, they can switch quickly from warfarin.

Management of Thrombosis in Pregnancy

The immediate management of thrombosis in pregnancy should be the same in those with or without the antiphospholipid syndrome, i.e. the use of full dose LMWH, ideally a twice daily dose because the half-life of LMWH is reduced in pregnancy due to improved renal function (see Chapter 12 on VTE). It may, indeed, be the first indication of underlying APS. Samples should not be sent for thrombophilia testing at the time of an acute event for physiological anticoagulant levels will be affected by a fresh thrombosis, and during pregnancy levels of protein S in particular are very low. Moreover, laboratory results do not change initial management.

Management of Women with Antiphospholipid Antibodies and a Previous Thrombotic Event

These women may be on long-term anticoagulants, although this depends on the circumstances of the thrombotic event; if it was a single venous event with a clear temporary provoking factor, a limited duration of anticoagulation may have been given.

In the former case, a change from warfarin to heparin can be made once a pregnancy test is positive. This requires the woman to be well motivated to check carefully in order to ensure that the substitution occurs before 6 weeks' gestation, to minimize risk of teratogenicity of warfarin. In the UK, it is usual to recommend a pregnancy test on the first or second day of a missed period and then to switch to low-molecular-weight heparin (LMWH) either at intermediate or full therapeutic doses, depending on the extent of risk when all factors are taken into account. Low-dose aspirin, at 75 mg daily, is also given.

The patient requires regular, frequent review throughout the pregnancy. Scans to assess fetal growth should be performed throughout the second half (monthly or more often as indicated). Uterine artery Doppler flow measurements (between 20 and 24 weeks onwards) are a further useful tool to indicate that the mother may be at risk of complications of ischemic placental dysfunction. The absence of bilateral notching is a good prognostic sign for fetal outcome.

Postnatally, the patient may be re-established on their oral anticoagulation or continued on LMWH for at least 6 weeks.

Management of Women with Multiple Previous Venous Events or Venous Plus Arterial Events

This group of women will likely be on long-term warfarin and possibly at a higher INR range (3–4), and are at very high risk during pregnancy. In this group, pre-pregnancy counseling is particularly important, to assess the extent of risk on an individual basis, and this risk clearly conveyed to the patient and partner prior to embarking on pregnancy. Low-molecular-weight heparin should be substituted for warfarin before 6 weeks' gestation, in intermediate or full dose. Some groups monitor anti-Xa levels, although they are not clearly predictive of antithrombotic effect. Other management is as above, i.e. low-dose aspirin, fetal growth assessment by regular ultrasound scanning, and warfarin reintroduced postnatally.

Management of Women with APS and Pregnancy Morbidity

A Cochrane systematic review in 2005 assessed 13 trials published between 1991 and 1999 on recurrent pregnancy loss associated with aPL. They commented that the quality of the studies was poor, which limited useful conclusions.

Aspirin

In obstetric patients, low-dose aspirin has been used to improve pregnancy outcome in those with hypertension, pre-eclampsia, preterm birth, and intrauterine growth restriction. The Cochrane review and meta-analysis summarized the studies with aspirin [21]. Three trials with aspirin alone showed no significant reduction in pregnancy loss; two studies using unfractionated heparin and aspirin showed a significant improvement in fetal outcome compared with aspirin alone; but in a further randomized controlled trial, while high success rates were achieved with low-dose aspirin, the addition of LMWH did not provide further benefit[22]. This latter study has been criticized as the laboratory criteria for APS were not met.

These studies were done at a time when LMWH was just being introduced, and it is difficult to draw firm conclusions from this collection of data. Subsequently obstetric hematology groups have accumulated a large volume of experience with LMWH, and it is considered as effective as unfractionated heparin, but considerably safer and more convenient with a once daily dosing regimen. Heparin-induced thrombocytopenic thrombosis (HIT) has not been described with LMWH during pregnancy. While the risk of osteoporotic fracture is as high as 2% with unfractionated heparin, it is rarely described with LMWH and prophylactic dose LMWH and low-dose aspirin has become standard practice. Improved outcomes for women with previous late fetal loss or early delivery due to placental insufficiency have been confirmed and a recent meta-analysis supports the efficacy of this approach for recurrent pregnancy loss[23].

Ultrasonography

In patients with poor obstetric history, pre-eclampsia, or evidence of fetal growth restriction, fetal growth scans every 4 weeks from 20 weeks are recommended, in addition to pharmacological treatments. Studies have shown uterine artery Doppler to be valuable in predicting placental dysfunction, i.e. pre-eclampsia and intrauterine growth restriction, and the discovery of bilateral uterine artery notching can allow the obstetrician to monitor the pregnancy more closely. Multivariate analysis of data on 100 pregnancies demonstrated that a notched uterine artery at the second trimester was the only predictor for adverse pregnancy outcome. Uterine artery Doppler assessment should be performed with the fetal scan between 20 and 24 weeks. Le Thi Huong et al.[24] showed the predictive value of the umbilical artery Doppler ultrasound examination for late pregnancy outcome, together with clinical examination and laboratory tests in women with SLE and/or APS.

Other Treatment Modalities

A summary of pharmacological management of APS in pregnancy is provided in Table 16.3.

If there is continued pregnancy loss despite prophylactic dose heparin and low-dose aspirin, the following options should be considered:

(a) The addition of first trimester low-dose prednisolone (10 mg daily) to conventional treatment has been shown to be successful in a small cohort of women with refractory aPL-related first trimester pregnancy loss.
(b) There is retrospective evidence supporting the beneficial use of hydroxychloroquine in women with aPL during pregnancy. It may also be useful in APS cases who have additional indications for its use, such us polyarthralgia.
(c) Increasing the dose of heparin to therapeutic levels, although there are no trials that have demonstrated this is effective.

Table 16.3 Summary of pharmacological management of APS in pregnancy

Clinical feature	Management
APS with prior fetal death or recurrent pregnancy loss	Aspirin 75 mg od, LMWH prophylactic dosage Doppler ultrasound for fetal assessment
APS with prior venous or arterial thrombosis	Low-molecular-weight heparin at intermediate or therapeutic dosage, plus aspirin
Antiphospholipid antibodies without clinical features and healthy previous pregnancies	No treatment, or low-dose aspirin
Primigravida with isolated aPL	Low-dose aspirin and fetal monitoring
APS with recurrent thrombotic events	Intermediate or full therapeutic dose LMWH; consider warfarin

(d) There are anecdotal case reports of use of intravenous immunoglobulin in refractory cases with success, although several studies have not demonstrated its benefit[25]. It may also be useful in APS cases who have additional indications for its use, for example in autoimmune thrombocytopenia.

(e) Successful use of plasma exchange, to temporarily remove antibodies, has been reported in high-risk pregnancies where plasma exchange was administered.

Management of Thrombocytopenia Associated with APS in Pregnancy

This may be due to pre-eclampsia, HELLP syndrome, or worsening maternal idiopathic thrombocytopenic purpura (ITP). This should be managed in the same way as those complications occurring without APS (see Chapters 5, 22, and 23).

Management Dilemmas

1. Management of women who have isolated aPL, with no prior pregnancy loss or thromboembolic phenomena, does not generally merit antenatal pharmacological treatment, although low-dose aspirin is often used. The best predictor of maternal and fetal outcome in APS pregnancies is the previous obstetric history. Mothers with a previously normal obstetric history despite aPL can be reassured that any future pregnancy has a low risk of complications.

2. For women with previous cerebrovascular thrombotic events (who have a 5% risk of recurrence in pregnancy despite the use of LMWH) or patients who develop a new thrombotic event during pregnancy despite anticoagulation, consideration should be given for warfarin usage from the second trimester, or even all trimesters. The risks of warfarin to the fetus must be explained – including the teratogenic risk in the first trimester and the ongoing risk of fetal loss, hemorrhage, and subtle neurological changes, which have been described after its use in the second and third trimester. Such patients should have their INR checked twice weekly, maintaining tight control of the INR, ideally dosed by one experienced physician alone.

3. Where in vitro fertilization (IVF) or other assisted reproductive techniques are planned, LMWH should be substituted for warfarin at the time at which the assisted reproductive procedure is performed, i.e. at the time of egg transfer; if the woman is not on anticoagulation prior to IVF, then prophylactic LMWH and aspirin should be used.

4. For the rare seronegative APS, or SNAPS, where typical clinical features occur in the absence of measurable standard antibodies, expert clinical judgment is required to make this diagnosis and to determine need for treatment.

5. Management of women with SLE in pregnancy is one of the few indications for the use of glucocorticoids during pregnancy with APS. SLE may flare during pregnancy and increasing or starting small doses (usually starting at 5–10 mg a day) of prednisolone is appropriate. Hydroxychloroquine and azathioprine, standard drugs for the management of SLE, are safe in pregnancy and should be continued if the disease is stable. Stopping such medications may lead to a flare of SLE which could be harmful to mother and fetus.

6. Chorea gravidarum is a rare complication in pregnancy and may be associated with primary or secondary APS. It is thought to be due to development of antibodies against components of the basal ganglia, or rarely due to infarction of this area. If antibody driven, it is usually self-limiting and resolves following pregnancy, although may recur in subsequent pregnancies. When severe, a variety of treatments have been described, including low-dose haloperidol, steroids, anticoagulants, antiplatelet medication, or a combination of treatments[26].

7. A careful management of anticoagulant treatment in women who will receive epidural anesthesia or analgesia is also mandatory. Epidural anesthesia can be safely carried out 12 hours after the last dose of thromboprophylactic LMWH and it can be resumed 6–8 hours after the procedure, or when hemostasis is achieved. When LMWH is used in full doses, it must be stopped 24 hours before the procedure. Low-dose aspirin has not been associated with significant risk for spinal hematoma, and it can be safely maintained.

8. The incidence of thrombosis in the purely obstetric form of APS is uncertain. Recent evidence suggests that the risks of venous thromboembolism, inside and outside pregnancy,

and of cerebrovascular manifestations are higher in women with purely obstetric APS (especially those positive for LAC) than in women with recurrent pregnancy losses without APS[27].

Neonatal Disease

Neonatal APS has been described, although the existence of this syndrome has not been fully accepted. It is a rare occurrence, characterized by neonatal thrombosis thought to be due to the transplacental passage of maternal aPL[28]. Ischemic stroke is the main event described. In comparison to a high incidence of thrombotic and obstetric complications in women with APS, the aPL-associated thrombotic events in neonates are extremely rare. There is no benefit from routine screening for aPL in neonates born to mothers with APS.

Case Studies

Case Study 1

A 33-year-old public relations manager came to clinic for advice about becoming pregnant. She had been found to have an antiphospholipid antibody after being (unnecessarily) checked during investigations for infertility. She had a lupus anticoagulant, with a DRVVT of 1.6 correcting to 1.1 after platelet correction, a titer of IgM anticardiolipin antibodies of 44 (normal 0–6) MPL/L, and anti-beta-2 glycoprotein I antibodies showed an IgM of 120 (normal 0–25) MPL/L.

Advice was sought because she was planning to undergo IVF (in vitro fertilization).

The first action was to repeat the tests more than 12 weeks after the first, to ensure the antibodies are persisting. Testing for anti-Ro antibodies was also carried out because anti-Ro is associated with complete heart block in 2% of fetuses and neonatal lupus in 10%. Many mothers with anti-Ro have no symptoms of lupus, so it is an important screening test. If present there is limited evidence that giving the mother hydroxychloroquine 200 mg daily during pregnancy might reduce the risk of complete heart block. Mothers with anti-Ro should be referred to a fetal cardiology unit for ultrasound during the second trimester. As a rule of thumb, complete heart block does not develop after 30 weeks, so a normal scan at 28–29 weeks is very reassuring.

Although the antibodies were found to be persistent, it was explained to her that in fact antiphospholipid antibodies, although associated with risk of pregnancy loss, are not associated with infertility. Aspirin 75 mg was prescribed for the period of IVF treatment and prophylactic LMWH was started after egg reimplantation in the mother, although the evidence for this, in someone with only aPL antibodies and no symptoms, is not clear.

Case Study 2

A GP telephoned for advice about a 32-year-old woman (weight 108 kg) who had just had a positive pregnancy test. She had been on warfarin for 12 years, following an extensive spontaneous femoral DVT and laboratory confirmation of antiphospholipid syndrome, with a persistently positive lupus anticoagulant and IgG anticardiolipin antibody of 98 GPLU/mL. The GP had changed her warfarin to clexane 40 mg daily, but was advised to increase the clexane to therapeutic doses and arrangements were made to see her in the next clinic.

Anticardiolipin antibodies and lupus anticoagulant were repeated and confirmed to be positive. Of note is that the platelet count was 67×10^9/L; hemoglobin and white cell count were normal.

Unfortunately, she miscarried 3 weeks later. She received counseling about the risks in her next pregnancy and advised to undertake a weight loss program beforehand. Clinical assessment and review of her old records excluded comorbidities such as hypertension and diabetes. There was no evidence of previous thrombocytopenia.

At the onset of a further pregnancy, the warfarin was substituted with therapeutic low-molecular-weight heparin and she was given aspirin 75 mg daily. The platelet count was monitored every 3–4 weeks. When it fell to below 50×10^9/L, at 29 weeks' gestation, she was started on 20 mg prednisolone daily, to allow continued therapeutic anticoagulation. There was a good response to this and it was lowered to 10 mg daily without a drop in platelets. The aspirin was discontinued at term but the prednisolone and LMWH were continued into the postpartum period. She was re-established on warfarin at 1 week postpartum.

This case highlights the conflict between the thrombotic risk and the ITP which are both associated with APS.

References

1. Miyakis S, Lockshin MD, Atsumi T *et al*. International consensus statement on an update of the classification criteria for definite antiphospholipid syndrome (APS). *Journal of Thrombosis and Hemostasis* 2006; **4**: 295–306.

2. McMahon MA, Keogan M, O'Connell P, Kearns G. The prevalence of antiphospholipid antibody syndrome among systemic lupus erythematosus patients. *Irish Medical Journal* 2006; **99**: 296–298.

3. Noori, AS, Jassim NA, Gorial FI. Prevalence of antiphospholipid antibodies in sample of Iraqi patients with systemic lupus erythematosus: a cross sectional study. *American Journal of Clinical Medicine Research* 2013; **1**: 61–64.

4. Galli M, Luciani D, Bertolini G, Barbui T. Lupus anticoagulants are stronger risk factors for thrombosis than anticardiolipin antibodies in the antiphospholipid syndrome: a systematic review of the literature. *Blood* 2003; **101**: 1827–1832.

5. Pengo V, Ruffatti A, Legnani C *et al*. Incidence of a first thromboembolic event in asymptomatic carriers of high-risk antiphospholipid antibody profile: a multicenter prospective study. *Blood* 2011; **118**(17): 4714–4718.

6. Meroni PL, Borghi MO, Raschi E, Tedesco F. Pathogenesis of antiphospholipid syndrome: understanding the antibodies. *Nature Reviews Rheumatology* 2011; 7(6): 330–339.

7. Girardi G, Redecha P, Salmon JE. Heparin prevents antiphospholipid antibody-induced fetal loss by inhibiting complement activation. *Nature Medicine* 2004; **10**: 1222–1226.

8. Wilson WA, Gharavi AE, Koike T *et al*. International consensus statement on preliminary classification criteria for definite antiphospholipid syndrome: report of an international workshop. *Arthritis and Rheumatism* 1999; **42**: 1309–1311.

9. Cervera R, Piette JC, Font J *et al*. Euro-Phospholipids Project Group. Antiphospholipid syndrome: clinical and immunologic manifestations and patterns of disease expression in a cohort of 1,000 patients. *Arthritis and Rheumatism* 2002; **46**: 1019–1027.

10. Asherson RA, Khamashta MA, Ordi-Ros J *et al*. The "primary" antiphospholipid syndrome: major clinical and serological features. *Medicine (Baltimore)* 1989; **68**: 366–374.

11. Yetman DL, Kutteh WH. Antiphospholipid antibody panels and recurrent pregnancy loss: prevalence of anticardiolipin antibodies compared with other antiphospholipid antibodies. *Fertility and Sterility* 1996; **66**: 540–546.

12. Rai RS, Clifford K, Cohen H, Regan L. High prospective fetal loss rate in untreated pregnancies of women with recurrent miscarriage and antiphospholipid antibodies. *Human Reproduction* 1995; **10**: 3301–3304.

13. Dreyfus M, Hedelin G, Kutnahorsky R *et al*. Antiphospholipid antibodies and preeclampsia: a case-control study. *Obstetrics and Gynecology* 2001; **97**: 29–34.

14. Diz-Küçükkaya R, Hacihanefioglu A, Yenerel M *et al*. Antiphospholipid antibodies and antiphospholipid syndrome in patients presenting with immune thrombocytopenic purpura: a prospective cohort study. *Blood* 2001; **98**: 1760–1764.

15. Brandt JT, Triplett DA, Alving B, Scharrer I. Criteria for the diagnosis of lupus anticoagulants: an update. On behalf of the Subcommittee on Lupus Anticoagulant/Antiphospholipid Antibody of the Scientific and Standardization Committee of the ISTH. *Thrombosis and Hemostasis* 1995; **74**: 1185–1190.

16. Harris EN, Pierangeli SS. Revisiting the anticardiolipin test and its standardization. *Lupus* 2002; **11**: 269–275.

17. Cowchock FS, Reece EA, Balaban D *et al*. Repeated fetal losses associated with antiphospholipid antibodies: a collaborative randomised trial comparing prednisone with low-dose heparin treatment. *American Journal of Obstetrics and Gynecology* 2003; **101**: 1319–1332.

18. Rai R, Cohen H, Dave M, Regan L. Randomised controlled trial of aspirin and aspirin plus heparin in pregnant women with recurrent miscarriage associated with phospholipid antibodies. *British Medical Journal* 1997; **314**: 253–257.

19. Kutteh WH. Antiphospholipid antibody associated recurrent pregnancy loss: treatment with heparin and low-dose aspirin is superior to low dose aspirin alone. *American Journal of Obstetrics and Gynecology* 1996; **174**: 1584–1589.

20. Izmirly PM, Costedoat-Chalumeau N, Pisoni C *et al*. Maternal use of hydroxychloroquine is associated with a reduced risk of recurrent anti-SSA/Ro associated cardiac manifestations of neonatal lupus. *Circulation* 2012; **126**(1): 76–82.

21. Empson M, Lassere M, Craig J, Scott J. Prevention of recurrent miscarriage for women with antiphospholipid antibody or lupus anticoagulant. *Cochrane Database of Systematic Reviews* 2005; (**2**): 002859.

22. Farquharson RG, Quenby S, Greaves M. Antiphospholipid syndrome in pregnancy: a randomised controlled trial of treatment. *Obstetrics and Gynecology* 2002; **100**: 408–413.

23. Mak A, Cheung MWL, Cheak AA, Ho RC. Combination of heparin and aspirin is superior to aspirin alone in enhancing live births in patients with recurrent pregnancy loss and positive anti-phospholipid

antibodies: a meta-analysis of randomized controlled trials and meta-regression. *Rheumatology* 2010; **49**: 281–288.

24. Le Thi Huong D, Weschler B, Vauthier-Brouzes D *et al.* The second trimester Doppler ultrasound examination is the best predictor of late pregnancy outcome in systemic lupus erythematosis and/or the antiphospholipid syndrome. *Rheumatology* 2006; **45**: 332–338.

25. Triolo G, Ferrante A, Ciccia F *et al.* Randomised study of subcutaneous low molecular weight heparin plus aspirin versus intravenous immunoglobulin in the treatment of recurrent fetal loss. *Arthritis and Rheumatism* 2003; **48**: 728–731.

26. Cervera R, Asherson RA, Font J *et al.* Chorea in the antiphospholipid syndrome: Clinical, radiologic and immunologic characteristics of 50 patients from our clinics and recent literature. *Medicine* 1997; **76**(3): 203–212.

27. Gris JC, Bouvier S, Molinari N *et al.* Comparative incidence of a first thrombotic event in purely obstetric antiphospholipid syndrome with pregnancy loss: the NOH-APS observational study. *Blood* 2012; **119**(11): 2624–2632.

28. Boffa MC, Lachassine E. Infant perinatal thrombosis and antiphospholipid antibodies: a review. *Lupus* 2007; **16**: 634–641.

Inherited Thrombophilia and Pregnancy Loss

Luuk Scheres, Isobel Walker, and Saskia Middeldorp

Introduction

Pregnancy loss is psychologically and emotionally extremely difficult for a woman, her partner, and wider family. Couples who have experienced such an event have many questions including, what caused the pregnancy to fail, will it happen again, and what can be done to minimize the risk of a recurrence?

It has been postulated that in some cases, pregnancy failure may be, at least in part, due to inadequate placental circulation and that thrombophilia, by increasing the risk of fibrin deposition or thrombosis within the placental circulation, may increase the risk of pregnancy loss. This postulate has led to the hypothesis that, for women with a history of (recurrent) pregnancy loss with no identifiable cause other than an underlying thrombophilia, intervention with antithrombotic therapy, mainly heparin with or without aspirin, may improve the outcome in subsequent pregnancies.

Epidemiology

Epidemiology of Pregnancy Loss

Pregnancy loss is a common phenomenon; it has been estimated that around 15% of clinically recognized pregnancies are lost before 24 weeks of gestation. As very early pregnancy losses often go unnoticed the percentage of actual pregnancy losses is estimated at around 30–50%. The terminology describing pregnancy loss varies in the literature. The World Health Organization employs the following definition of miscarriage: "a pregnancy which fails to progress, resulting in the death and expulsion of an embryo or fetus weighing no more than 500 g (which corresponds to a gestational age of 20 weeks or less)." A pregnancy loss after the 20th week is referred to as stillbirth or fetal death. Early fetal loss is defined as loss of fetal heart activity before the 12th week of gestation and late pregnancy loss after the 12th week of gestation. At present, there is no global consensus on the definition of recurrent miscarriage. When defined as two or

Table 17.1 Incidence of pregnancy loss

Spontaneous abortion of fertilized ova	30–50%
Spontaneous loss of clinically recognized pregnancy before 24 weeks	15%
Two or more pregnancy losses	3%
Three or more pregnancy losses	1%

more pregnancy losses, 3% of all fertile couples are affected. When employing the definition of three or more pregnancy losses, 1% of couples is affected (Table 17.1). Additionally, some definitions add "consecutive" to the description of recurrent pregnancy loss. Among experts, there is an increasing tendency to apply the definition entailing two or more pregnancy losses and to disregard the consecutive criterion to describe recurrent pregnancy loss. It is important to keep these varying definitions in mind, as among the published studies, literature, and guidelines different definitions are used. In this chapter pregnancy loss is the preferential term and describes miscarriage, stillbirth, and fetal death, and recurrent pregnancy loss refers to two or more losses.

Epidemiology of Thrombophilia

The term thrombophilia is used to describe disorders, usually in the coagulation cascade, which predispose to venous thromboembolism. Thrombophilia can be subdivided into acquired and inherited thrombophilia. Among acquired thrombophilias, antiphospholipid syndrome is the most well known. Other causes of a prothrombotic state include the presence of malignancy, infection, and inflammation. Inherited thrombophilia, the main focus of this chapter, includes inherited deficiencies of the natural anticoagulants antithrombin, protein C, and protein S, and common mutations in the genes encoding clotting factor V (called factor V Leiden) and clotting factor II, the prothrombin G20210A mutation. Antithrombin, protein C, and protein S are natural inhibitors of

Table 17.2 The prevalence of inherited thrombophilia in European populations

Thrombophilia	Prevalence (%)
Factor V Leiden (heterozygous)	2–7
Factor V Leiden (homozygous)	0.02
Prothrombin G20210A (heterozygous)	2
Antithrombin deficiency	0.25–0.55
Protein C deficiency	0.20–0.33
Protein S deficiency	0.03–0.13

thrombin generation, and an inherited deficiency (e.g. loss of function that can be caused by numerous different mutations) results in a hypercoagulable state. The consequence of a factor V Leiden variant is resistance of activated clotting factor V to be inactivated by activated protein C. The prothrombin mutation leads to higher circulating factor II levels. Both of these gain of function mutations carry an increased thrombotic tendency. Around 10% of Caucasians have an identifiable form of inherited thrombophilia, often without having symptoms (Table 17.2).

Pathogenesis

Placentation

Placentation in Normal Pregnancy
Successful pregnancy requires trophoblast invasion into the maternal uterine spiral arteries, converting them into large dilated vessels, which lack a functioning contractile smooth muscle wall. Prior to this remodeling, the spiral arterioles are occluded by endovascular trophoblasts. It is postulated that this plugging protects the early intervillous spaces from maternal systemic arterial pressure and protects the developing intervillous trophoblasts from high oxygen tension and oxidative damage. Although the blood flowing through the spiral arteries and the placental intervillous spaces is maternal, the cells lining these spaces are embryonic trophoblasts. Thus, the hemostatic balance within the placenta may be disturbed as a result of hypercoagulability of the maternal blood or as a result of abnormality of cellular regulatory mechanisms of fetal origin operating at the fetomaternal interface. Since the fetal blood is separated from the trophoblasts by fetal endothelial cells, the fetal hemostatic balance is influenced only by components of fetal origin[1].

Placental Pathology in Pregnancy Loss
Thrombi in the spiral arteries or fibrin deposition in the intervillous spaces on the maternal side of the placenta may result in inadequate placental perfusion. Microthrombi are frequently found in the vessels of the placentas from women who have experienced pregnancy loss and placental infarction has been described in placentas of some, but not all, women who have a fetal loss and who have thrombophilia. However, placental thrombosis and infarction are not uncommon in cases of fetal loss in the absence of any identifiable thrombophilia and no placental lesion is specific for thrombophilia.

It is appealing to ascribe pregnancy loss in women with thrombophilia to a hypercoagulable state.

However, recent observations implicate a role of the immune system and inflammatory pathways in pregnancy loss[2]. As coagulation and inflammation are closely related processes, there might be a role for both in the complex pathophysiology of pregnancy failure. Most of the studies that have reported on the placental pathology in women with thrombophilia and a history of pregnancy loss have concentrated on women with antiphospholipid syndrome and there is limited information about the placental pathology in women with an underlying heritable thrombophilia. Furthermore, there are methodological problems with many of the published studies. Some studies have compared the placentas from women with thrombophilia and pregnancy loss with the placentas from non-thrombophilic women with normal gestations – others with placentas from non-thrombophilic women with pregnancy loss. Others have included no control group at all.

Thrombophilia and Pregnancy Loss

Pregnancy Loss
Many studies have reported an association between maternal inherited thrombophilia and pregnancy complications, including pregnancy loss. The strengths of these associations vary among the studies and for the different types of inherited thrombophilia. Corresponding odds ratios and 95% confidence intervals (CI) for the different types of inherited thrombophilia are shown in Table 17.3.

The majority of published studies have been too small and therefore inadequately powered to detect odds ratios of 2 or more for inherited thrombophilias which usually have prevalences of less than 5% in the general population. Meta-analyses support the

Table 17.3 Associations between types of inherited thrombophilia and pregnancy loss

Type of thrombophilia	Odds ratio (95% confidence interval)				
	1st or 2nd trimester pregnancy loss	1st trimester recurrent pregnancy loss	2nd trimester single pregnancy loss	3rd trimester pregnancy loss	Any gestational age pregnancy loss
Factor V Leiden mutation (homozygous)	**2.7** (1.3–5.6)	*	*	2.0 (0.4–9.7)	*
Factor V Leiden mutation (heterozygous)	**1.7** (1.1–2.6)	1.9* (1.0–3.6)	**4.1*** (1.9–8.8)	**2.1** (1.1–3.9)	**1.52*** (1.06–2.19)
Prothrombin G20210A mutation (heterozygous)	**2.5** (1.2–5.0)	**2.7** (1.4–5.3)	**8.6** (2.2–34.0)	**2.7** (1.3–5.5)	1.13 (0.64–2.01)
Antithrombin deficiency	0.9 (0.2–4.5)	NA	NA	7.6 (0.3–196.4)	NA
Protein C deficiency	2.3 (0.2–26.4)	NA	NA	3.1 (0.2–38.5)	NA
Protein S deficiency	3.5 (0.4–35.7)	NA	NA	**20.1** (3.7–109.2)	NA

Table adapted from de Jong et al.[3]. Data are derived from systematic reviews, when possible[4,5]. Terminology of pregnancy loss at various gestational ages may vary among included studies. Statistically significant odds ratios are indicated in bold. NA, not available.
* Homozygous and heterozygous carriers were grouped together; it is not possible to extract data for zygosity.

hypothesis that at least some inherited thrombophilias are associated with pregnancy loss, but where the data are robust with narrow confidence intervals (i.e. for factor V Leiden and prothrombin G20210A), the point estimates of the odds ratios are small, suggesting that the associations, if they truly exist, are weak. Moreover, even if an association exists, it may not be a causal association. A few studies have shown that, compared with heterozygotes carrying a single thrombophilic variant, homozygous patients or patients with combinations of thrombophilic variants have increased odds ratios for pregnancy loss. This apparent dose effect would support the hypothesis of causality but needs further evidence. Evidence that pregnancy outcome could be improved in thrombophilic women with a history of pregnancy loss by reducing the hypercoagulability with anticoagulant treatment would offer indirect support to the hypothesis that maternal thrombophilia may cause pregnancy loss.

Recurrent pregnancy loss is recognized to be a multi-causal disorder. There is an increasing risk of pregnancy loss as the number of previous losses increases. Many factors including chromosomal abnormalities, endocrine disorders, anatomical aberrations, and infections have been shown to cause pregnancy loss, but around 40% of cases of recurrent pregnancy losses are unexplained after gynecological, hormonal, immunological, microbiological, and karyotypic investigations. While inherited thrombophilias alone may not cause pregnancy loss, it is possible that carriership of a thrombophilic variant may contribute to a complex of factors, which together result in pregnancy loss.

It is generally assumed that the mechanism of pregnancy failure associated with maternal thrombophilia involves fibrin deposition or thrombosis secondary to hypercoagulability but, although it is biologically plausible that placental thrombosis may have a role in the causation of fetal loss after 10 weeks' gestation, it is not plausible that this mechanism would cause embryo loss (before 10 weeks) prior to development of the placental vasculature. The vast majority of recurrent pregnancy losses occur early in pregnancy. In women with antiphospholipid syndrome, a non-prothrombotic mechanism, in addition to hypercoagulability, has been postulated. Antiphospholipid antibodies have been shown to inhibit extravillous trophoblast differentiation and subsequent placentation. Studies of trophoblast differentiation and early placental development are lacking in inherited thrombophilias, but experiments in mice have shown that maternal protein C is activated following binding to thrombomodulin on the trophoblast surface. Activated protein C then binds to endothelial protein C receptors also on the trophoblast surface and with protein S as a cofactor down-regulates local coagulation activation. Tight regulation of thrombin generation is essential for the regulation of trophoblast cell growth and limits the production of fibrin degradation products, which trigger trophoblast apoptosis. It is therefore possible that, in early pregnancy in humans, some maternal inherited thrombophilias may exert an adverse effect on normal trophoblast development.

191

Fetal Thrombophilia

It has been suggested that fetal carriership of thrombophilic mutations may have adverse clinical consequences. In one case–control study a twofold increase in factor V Leiden carrier frequency was noted in abortuses compared with unselected pregnant women, but most studies have not shown a significant association between fetal carriership of the most prevalent inherited thrombophilias (factor V Leiden and prothrombin G20210A) and fetoplacental thrombosis. As up to 10% of the population is affected by a form of inherited thrombophilia, from an evolutionary perspective it is unlikely that fetal thrombophilia plays a substantial role in pregnancy loss. On the contrary, there are several hypotheses on carriership of inherited thrombophilia having subtle evolutionary benefits[6].

Very Early Pregnancy Loss: Embryo Loss

Most reports do not separate very early pregnancy losses (before 10 weeks' gestation) from later first trimester losses. In a cohort study of 491 patients with a history of adverse pregnancy outcome, maternal thrombophilia was associated with an increased risk of pregnancy loss after 10 weeks' gestation (odds ratio 1.76, 95% CI 1.05–2.94 for women with one thrombophilia and odds ratio 1.66, 95% CI 1.03–2.68 for women with more than one identifiable thrombophilia). Paradoxically, the presence of one or more maternal thrombophilia seemed to be protective of recurrent very early (less than 10 weeks' gestation) pregnancy loss (odds ratio 0.55, 95% CI 0.33–0.92 for one and odds ratio 0.48, 95% CI 0.29–0.78 for multiple thrombophilias)[7].

Management

General Considerations and Prognosis

General considerations for women with inherited thrombophilia and recurrent miscarriage are not different from general preconception counseling and include a healthy lifestyle and cessation of smoking and alcohol and/or drug use. Women with recurrent pregnancy loss may often undergo (ineffective) invasive and costly diagnostic tests and interventions. Counseling couples on the prognosis of recurrent pregnancy loss may reduce their burden and decrease the number of unnecessary medical procedures. In a large cohort study of women with two or more unexplained consecutive pregnancy losses, 69.3% had a live birth in their subsequent pregnancy [8]. However, in this study the follow-up duration was

not specified. In another large cohort study, live birth rates were 66.7 and 71.1% after 5 and 15 years, respectively, for women with three or more consecutive unexplained pregnancy losses before the 22th week of pregnancy[9]. Studies evaluating live birth rates for patients with inherited thrombophilia and recurrent pregnancy loss are mostly observational and often concern women with a factor V Leiden or prothrombin mutation. The reported live birth rates in these studies vary greatly but on average, without antithrombotic treatment, live birth rates have been estimated at around 70% for patients with inherited thrombophilia and recurrent pregnancy loss[3]. Hence, the prognosis for future pregnancies in women with inherited thrombophilia who have a history of recurrent pregnancy loss may be better than generally expected[10].

Lack of Evidence

Observational studies on the effect of interventions to prevent pregnancy loss are frequently flawed. The subjects included are often poorly selected and form a heterogeneous group lacking stratification for important factors such as maternal age, past obstetric history, and stage of gestation. Some studies have compared pregnancy outcome in patients subjected to a new intervention with the outcome in their own previous pregnancies, which by definition was poor. This strategy ignores the fact that many of these women would have had a successful pregnancy outcome by its natural course (see section "General Considerations and Prognosis"), whereas the success is ascribed to the intervention. Reports of studies in which the pregnancy outcome in women with a history of pregnancy loss subjected to some experimental intervention is compared with pregnancy outcome in historical controls who were either untreated or treated differently are subject not only to the phenomenon of "regression to mean" in the treated patient group but also to problems with ascertaining the control information.

Summary of High-Level Evidence

A recent Cochrane review[11] concluded that there is only a limited number of randomized controlled studies on the efficacy and safety of aspirin and heparin in women with a history of at least two unexplained miscarriages with or without inherited thrombophilia. Of the included studies at low risk of bias, only one was placebo-controlled. In studies at low risk of bias, there was no beneficial effect of antithrombotic therapy. It was concluded that the effect of anticoagulants in women with inherited thrombophilia and otherwise unexplained recurrent miscarriages needs to be further investigated. At present, no landmark randomized controlled trials have been performed to show a definite beneficial effect of antithrombotic therapy in women with inherited thrombophilia and recurrent pregnancy loss.

Aspirin to Prevent Pregnancy Loss in Thrombophilia

To this date, no randomized controlled trials investigating the effectiveness of aspirin in women with inherited thrombophilia and recurrent pregnancy loss have been performed. Therefore, at present there is no role for aspirin in preventing pregnancy loss in women with inherited thrombophilia.

Heparin, with or without Aspirin, to Prevent Pregnancy Loss in Thrombophilia

Investigators in the Thrombophilia in Pregnancy Prophylaxis Study (TIPPS) trial[12] randomized 292 women with either acquired or inherited thrombophilia at increased risk of placenta-mediated pregnancy complications or/and venous thromboembolism to the low-molecular-weight heparin dalteparin 5000 IU or no treatment. No differences in live births were observed between the two groups (91.8% in the dalteparin group vs. 93% in the no treatment group, risk difference 1.2%, 95% CI −4.9–7.3). In the HABENOX trial[13], 207 women (of whom 51 [24%] had thrombophilia) were randomized to either enoxaparin 40 mg plus placebo, enoxaparin 40 mg plus 100 mg aspirin, or aspirin alone. The observed live birth rates were 71% in the enoxaparin arm (relative risk [RR] 1.17, 95% CI 0.92–1.48), 65% for enoxaparin plus aspirin (RR 1.08, 95% CI 0.83–1.39), and 61% in the aspirin alone arm (reference group). In the Scottish Pregnancy Intervention (SPIN) study[14], enoxaparin 40 mg with aspirin 75 mg was compared to no treatment, and in the ALIFE (Anticoagulants for Living Fetuses in Women with Recurrent Miscarriage and Inherited Thrombophilia) study[15], treatment with aspirin 80 mg, aspirin 80 mg plus nadroparin 2850 units, and placebo were compared in women with unexplained recurrent miscarriage. A number of the women included in these studies had inherited thrombophilia. For the subgroup of women with inherited thrombophilia in the ALIFE study, there was a non-significant increase in the chance of live birth for both the nadroparin with aspirin (69.2%, RR for live birth 1.31, 95% CI 0.74–2.33) and aspirin alone (64.7%, RR for live birth 1.22, 95% CI 0.69–2.16) treatment arms as compared to placebo

(52.9%, reference group). In summary, it remains uncertain whether LMWH, with or without aspirin, increases live birth rates among women with inherited thrombophilia and recurrent pregnancy loss.

To Treat or Not to Treat

From an evidence-based standpoint there is insufficient evidence on which to base antithrombotic intervention in women with a history of pregnancy loss with no other identified abnormality apart from inherited thrombophilia. This is the position adopted by many authors and guideline committees, by the British Committee for Standards in Hematology[16], and by the American College of Chest Physicians[17]. In support of this position it has to be reiterated that the use of antithrombotic drugs during pregnancy is not without risk for the mother and, in general, empirical intervention during pregnancy should be discouraged. Furthermore, LMWH carries the burden of daily subcutaneous injections, leads to a high incidence of type IV delayed skin reactions and bruises, and is very costly. Based on extrapolation from the limited evidence of benefit from intervention with heparin and low-dose aspirin in women with antiphospholipid syndrome and recurrent pregnancy loss, and the relative safety of prophylactic doses of LMWH in pregnancy, an increasing number of clinicians are willing to prescribe antithrombotic agents to women with inherited thrombophilia and a history of two or more otherwise unexplained pregnancy losses or one unexplained late intrauterine fetal death. We strongly advocate the position that more research is needed and that it is unethical to prescribe non-evidence-based, burdensome interventions to pregnant women, and to provide false hope in a situation where the prognosis is generally good.

Diagnosis

Thrombophilia Testing

What Test?

Currently, not only is there a lack of consensus about which individuals (if any) merit thrombophilia testing, but there is also no universal agreement regarding which tests should be included in the "thrombophilia screen." Most diagnostic laboratories would include functional assays of antithrombin and protein C, and an immunological assay of free protein S along with tests to detect factor V Leiden and the prothrombin G20210A mutation. A few centers still include an assay of homocysteine in the panel of tests they offer for women with a history of pregnancy loss, although homocysteine testing has been largely abandoned in the field of venous thromboembolism. There is no additional benefit in testing factor VIII levels as there is no association between factor VIII levels and pregnancy loss.

Who to Test?

Routine testing for thrombophilias in unselected populations is not recommended. There are important issues relevant to the clinical utility and cost-effectiveness of testing that must be addressed in considering who should be tested. Positive tests are not sensitive predictors of poor pregnancy outcome in women with no history of pregnancy complications. There are a number of published guidelines which suggest that women with a history of recurrent pregnancy loss and women with a history of unexplained late pregnancy loss be tested for antiphospholipid syndrome, i.e. lupus anticoagulant activity and elevated anti-cardiolipin antibodies or beta2-glycoprotein antibodies. At present, screening women with pregnancy loss or recurrent miscarriage for inherited thrombophilia is not indicated, unless in the context of subsequent participation in a randomized intervention trial. In case of a positive family history of venous thromboembolism, screening for inherited thrombophilia can be considered, as a positive test may have the result of offering thrombosis prophylaxis in the postpartum period[17].

Pitfalls

If testing for inherited thrombophilia is pursued, clinicians should be aware that there are numerous potential pitfalls in the interpretation of "thrombophilia screens" particularly in pregnant or recently pregnant women. Antithrombin activity falls slightly toward the end of a normal pregnancy, but usually levels remain within the reference range for non-pregnant women. Protein C activity is unaffected by gestation, although an elevation of protein C activity occurs in the early puerperium. Even in non-pregnant women there is considerable overlap of protein S levels between "normals" and women with inherited protein S deficiency. The levels of both free and total protein S are reduced by 60–70% in uncomplicated pregnancy. A diagnosis of possible protein S deficiency made on a sample collected during pregnancy or the puerperium requires confirmation when the woman is no longer pregnant, puerperal, or using hormonal contraception. Pregnancy is also

associated with a progressive increase in resistance to activated protein C (APC) due to the physiological rise in clotting factor VIII levels and fall in protein S levels. Using the original APC resistance test, around 40% of pregnant women in their third trimester have an APC sensitivity ratio below the general population reference range. Testing for factor V Leiden therefore requires genetic testing, or alternatively, the use of a modified APC resistance test with predilution of the test sample in factor V deficient plasma. Thrombophilia test results should always be interpreted by staff experienced in the reporting of thrombophilia tests and in the light of clear clinical information about each particular patient.

Dilemmas

Women who have suffered pregnancy loss have many questions and will seek information about the possible cause, the likelihood of recurrence, and the possibility of intervention to try to reduce the chances of further pregnancy loss. At present, however, there is a lack of solid evidence on which to base advice about the appropriateness or otherwise of testing these women for inherited thrombophilias or on the management of those who may be found to have an inherited thrombophilia.

Further Research

To fill the great knowledge gaps, international collaborative networks are required. Proper evaluation of interventions in women with a history of pregnancy loss requires randomized, preferentially double-blind, controlled trials to ensure that the treated and control groups are similar with respect to all of the important determinants of pregnancy outcome. Randomized controlled trials are difficult to complete because many women do not wish to run the chance of being randomized to the control group on one hand, or wish to avoid medication during pregnancy on the other hand. Nevertheless, in the past few years quite a few of those trials have been completed in women with unexplained recurrent pregnancy loss, which has contributed greatly to the evidence of absence of effect of antithrombotic therapy in this population[11,18,19]. For women with inherited thrombophilia, at least one randomized double-blind study is in progress. An example is the ALIFE2 trial (NTR 3361; www.trialregister.nl), which started recruiting early in 2013 and is still ongoing. In this trial women with inherited thrombophilia and two or more pregnancy losses are randomized to treatment with LMWH with standard pregnancy surveillance or to standard surveillance only[20]. It has to be hoped that studies like this will provide more solid evidence on which to base information and advice for women with a history of unexplained late pregnancy loss or recurrent early loss and inherited thrombophilia.

To our regret, in the meantime many clinicians choose to treat patients on an individual and pragmatic basis with prophylactic daily doses of LMWH (e.g. enoxaparin 40 mg daily or dalteparin 5000 units daily) throughout pregnancy and the puerperium. Some also advocate the addition of low-dose aspirin (<150 mg) daily. The pros and cons of intervention should be discussed with the patient and the lack of proof of efficacy and risks of antithrombotic therapy made clear. Ideally, this discussion should take place during preconception counseling.

Conclusion and Recommendations

There is convincing evidence supporting a weak association between inherited thrombophilia and recurrent pregnancy loss. However, at this moment there is insufficient evidence supporting the use of (low-molecular-weight) heparin, with or without aspirin, for women with inherited thrombophilia and recurrent pregnancy loss. There should be international collaborations to fill the huge evidence gaps, rather than prescribing expensive, burdensome medication of which the efficacy is unclear and that is potentially harmful.

Summary

- Many studies have examined the association between inherited thrombophilia and pregnancy loss, but the results are frequently contradictory, populations heterogeneous, and the absolute risk (if any) small.
- Women with a history of pregnancy loss merit increased surveillance in subsequent pregnancies.
- Currently, there is a lack of evidence on which to base antithrombotic intervention in women with a history of pregnancy loss and an inherited thrombophilia.

Case Studies

Case Study 1

A 38-year-old woman was referred to the outpatient clinic because of a prothrombin 20210A mutation and a history of three early pregnancy losses. The patient and her husband moved to the Netherlands years ago. They were convinced that LMWH and aspirin should be prescribed in the next pregnancy to decrease the chance of pregnancy loss, as this was suggested by the obstetrician in the patient's country of origin. The patient had been pregnant four times. The first pregnancy resulted in a loss of pregnancy around the 6th week of pregnancy. During the second pregnancy, she developed pre-eclampsia in the 34th week of gestation. At 35 weeks, delivery was induced and she delivered a healthy son of 2800 g. Her last two pregnancies ended in spontaneous early pregnancy loss. She was in otherwise good health and there was neither a personal history of venous thromboembolism, nor one in the family. She had a normal body mass index and blood pressure. Thrombophilia screening showed no laboratory criteria for antiphospholipid syndrome, the antithrombin, protein C and protein S levels were within normal ranges, and there was no activated protein C resistance (suggestive of absence of a factor V Leiden mutation). A heterozygous prothrombin 20210A mutation was present. The patient was counseled and offered to participate in the ALIFE2 trial. Outside study settings the patient would be prescribed aspirin only based on her history of pre-eclampsia. This case report has been published previously[21].

Case Study 2

A 29-year-old woman was referred to our outpatient clinic for evaluation of recurrent pregnancy loss. She had experienced two spontaneous pregnancy losses at 7 and 13 weeks of gestational age, respectively. Her medical history was otherwise unremarkable and besides folic acid supplements she was not using medication. The patient had one maternal aunt with a history of a single episode of venous thrombosis of the leg. The patients' body mass index and blood pressure were within normal ranges. Laboratory analyses revealed a heterozygous factor V Leiden mutation as well as a heterozygous prothrombin mutation. All other thrombophilia test results, including antiphospholipid antibodies screening, did not reveal abnormalities. We counseled her for the ALIFE2 study, in which she wanted to participate. The patient would not have been prescribed antepartum aspirin or heparin (including low-molecular-weight heparin) outside of study context. The presence of double heterozygous thrombophilia and a second-degree family history of venous thrombosis does not necessitate postpartum thrombosis prophylaxis. However, high level evidence on the risk of venous thromboembolism in combined thrombophilia mutations is scarce. After thoroughly discussing the options with the patient, she opted for postpartum prophylaxis (by means of low-molecular-weight heparin) with the aim to reduce the risk of thrombosis.

References

1. Pijnenborg R, Vercruysse L, Brosens I. Deep placentation. *Best Practice & Research Clinical Obstetrics & Gynaecology* 2011; **25**(3): 273–285.

2. Redecha P, Franzke C, Ruf W, Mackman N, Girardi G. Neutrophil activation by the tissue factor/Factor VIIa/PAR2 axis mediates fetal death in a mouse model of antiphospholipid syndrome. *Journal of Clinical Investigation* 2008; **118**(10): 3453–3461.

3. De Jong PG, Goddijn M, Middeldorp S. Antithrombotic therapy for pregnancy loss. *Human Reproduction Update* 2013; **19**(6): 656–673.

4. Robertson L, Wu O, Langhorne P et al. Thrombophilia in pregnancy: A systematic review. *British Journal of Haematology* 2006; **132**: 171–196.

5. Rodger MA, Walker MC, Smith GN et al. Is thrombophilia associated with placenta-mediated pregnancy complications? A prospective cohort study. *Journal of Thrombosis and Haemostasis* 2014; **12**: 469–478.

6. Van Mens TE, Levi M, Middeldorp S. Evolution of factor V Leiden. *Thrombosis and Haemostasis* 2013; **110**(1): 23–30.

7. Roqué H, Paidas MJ, Funai EF, Kuczynski E, Lockwood CJ. Maternal thrombophilias are not associated with early pregnancy loss. *Thrombosis and Haemostasis* 2004; **91**: 290–295.

8. Sugiura-Ogasawara M, Ozaki Y, Kitaori T, Suzumori N, Obayashi S, Suzuki S. Live birth rate according to maternal age and previous number of recurrent miscarriages. *American Journal of Reproductive Immunology* 2009; **62**(5): 314–319.

9. Lund M, Kamper-Jørgensen M, Nielsen HS et al. Prognosis for live birth in women with recurrent miscarriage. *Obstetrics and Gynecology* 2012; **119**(1): 37–43.

10. de Jong PG, Kaandorp SP, Kool RO et al. Time to live birth in women with recurrent miscarriage and inherited thrombophilia. Abstracts of the XXV Congress of the International Society on Thrombosis and Hemostasis, June 20–25. *Journal of Thrombosis and Hemostasis* 2015; **13**: 1–1090

11. De Jong PG, Kaandorp S, Di Nisio M, Goddijn M, Middeldorp S. Aspirin and/or heparin for women with unexplained recurrent miscarriage with or without inherited thrombophilia. *Cochrane Database of Systematic Reviews* 2014; (7): CD004734.

12. Rodger MA, Hague WM, Kingdom J et al. Antepartum dalteparin versus no antepartum dalteparin for the prevention of pregnancy complications in pregnant women with thrombophilia (TIPPS): A multinational open-label randomised trial. *Lancet* 2014; **384**(9955): 1673–1683.

13. Visser J, Ulander VM, Helmerhorst FM et al. Thromboprophylaxis for recurrent miscarriage in women with or without thrombophilia – HABENOX*: A randomised multicenter trial. *Thrombosis and Hemostasis* 2011; **105**(17): 295–301.

14. Clark P, Walker ID, Langhorne P et al. SPIN (Scottish Pregnancy Intervention) study: a multicenter, randomized controlled trial of low-molecular-weight heparin and low-dose aspirin in women with recurrent miscarriage. *Blood* 2010; **115**(21): 4162–4167.

15. Kaandorp SP, Goddijn M, van der Post JAM et al. Aspirin plus heparin or aspirin alone in women with recurrent miscarriage. *New England Journal of Medicine* 2010; **362**: 1586–1596.

16. Baglin T, Gray E, Greaves M et al. Clinical guidelines for testing for heritable thrombophilia. *British Journal of Haematology* 2010; **149**: 209–220.

17. Bates S, Greer IA, Middeldorp S et al. VTE, thrombophilia, antithrombotic therapy, and pregnancy: Thrombophilia, Antithrombotic Therapy, and Pregnancy Antithrombotic Therapy and Prevention of Thrombosis, 9th ed: American College of Chest Physicians Evidence-Based Clinical Practice Guidelines. *Chest* 2012; **141**.

18. Pasquier E, de Saint Martin L, Bohec C et al. Enoxaparin for prevention of unexplained recurrent miscarriage : a multicenter randomized double-blind placebo-controlled trial. *Blood* 2015; **125**(14): 2200–2205.

19. Schleussner E, Kamin G, Seliger G et al. Low-molecular-weight heparin for women with unexplained recurrent pregnancy loss. *Annals of Internal Medicine* 2015; **162**(9): 601.

20. De Jong PG, Quenby S, Bloemenkamp KW et al. ALIFE2 study: low-molecular-weight heparin for women with recurrent miscarriage and inherited thrombophilia – study protocol for a randomized controlled trial. *Trials* 2015; **16**(1): 208.

21. Middeldorp S. Anticoagulation in pregnancy complications. *Hematology* 2014; **1**: 393–399.

Management of Obstetric Hemorrhage: Obstetric Management

Annette Briley and Susan Bewley

Introduction and Epidemiology

Obstetric hemorrhage (OH) is the leading cause of maternal mortality worldwide. In the UK, mortality rates are relatively low, with 10 deaths per 100 000 maternities recorded in the latest Confidential Enquiry (Mothers and Babies: Reducing Risk through Audits and Confidential Enquiries across the UK – MBRRACE-UK) 2010–2012[1]. However, morbidity remains high, and timely recognition and management is of the utmost importance.

Antepartum hemorrhage (APH) is defined as bleeding from the genital tract after 24 weeks' gestation and affects approximately 3–4% of all pregnancies. The most common cause of APH is the presence of placenta previa, where the placenta is abnormally located in the lower uterine segment, covering or partially covering the internal os. As pregnancy progresses, especially as the lower segment forms or the cervix dilates, the woman is prone to episodes of bleeding that may be profuse. Another common cause of APH is placental abruption, when the placenta prematurely separates either partially or totally. It may be a single episode or recurrent, small or large, and the features may be typical and multiple (bleeding and pain, tender and woody Couvelaire uterus with stillbirth) or atypical and isolated (bleeding, premature labor, fetal growth restriction, abnormal CTG). However, the cause of many cases of APH is often unknown.

Primary postpartum hemorrhage (PPH) is the most common obstetric hemorrhage and is defined by the World Health Organization (WHO) as the loss of blood estimated to be >500 mL from the genital tract within 24 hours of delivery. After this, and until 6 weeks' postpartum, abnormal bleeding from the genital tract is defined as secondary PPH. Hemorrhage is considered severe when blood loss exceeds 1000 mL[2]. The major cause of postpartum hemorrhage is uterine atony, when the uterus fails to contract fully after delivery of the placenta. The incidence of PPH is variably reported, but is suggested as complicating at least 10% of deliveries worldwide. Globally, maternal deaths from hemorrhage have been estimated to have fallen from just over 71 000 annually in 1990 to just over 44 000 in 2013 [3]. Even with appropriate active management, around 3% of women will experience a PPH following vaginal delivery[4]. Recent studies in low-risk Australian women and all-risk women in southeast England suggested PPH was as high as 12%[5] or 34%[6]. Hemorrhage is the third leading cause of all maternal deaths worldwide, the majority occurring in the poorest countries[3]. Substandard care (defined as care which may have made a difference to the outcome) was highlighted as a factor in all 17 deaths from hemorrhage occurring in the UK and Ireland between 2009 and 2012 (rate 0.49/100 000 maternities)[1].

The Annual Scottish Confidential Audit of Severe Maternal Morbidity has found that the incidence of major PPH, i.e. >2500 mL, is high, is rising, and has more than doubled over its 10-year duration[7].

Table 18A.1 shows the estimated time to death for obstetric emergencies, highlighting APH and PPH in particular, and revealing obstetric hemorrhage as the most dangerous complication of pregnancy for the mother[8].

Table 18A.1 Estimated time to death for obstetric emergencies

Cause	Time to death
Postpartum hemorrhage	2 hours
Antepartum hemorrhage	12 hours
Uterine rupture	1 day
Eclampsia/severe PET	2 days
Obstructed labor	3 days
Infection	6 days

Prevention

Prevention of PPH occurs via the recognition of any risk factors present either antenatally or during the intrapartum period, and the subsequent implementation of preventive management/strategies.

Although there are a host of risk factors (see Table 18A.2), postpartum hemorrhage often occurs in women with no identifiable predictors and therefore clinicians must be prepared for this eventuality at each and every delivery[9].

The degree of risk will influence the management of these women from choice of place of birth to mode of delivery and postnatal care. Women at higher risk of hemorrhage should be advised to have their babies in, or alongside, an obstetric-led unit with an on-site blood bank. It is important to involve the woman and her family in

Table 18A.2 Risk factors for postpartum hemorrhage

	Factors	Risk (if known)
Pre-pregnancy	Maternal age >35 years	
	Nulliparity	× 3
	Grand multiparity (4 or more)	
	Asian ethnicity	× 2
	Obesity (BMI ≥35 kg/m²)	× 2
	Previous cesarean section	
	Previous retained placenta or PPH	× 3
	Existing uterine abnormalities (including uterine fibroids)	
	Factor VIII deficiency – hemophilia A carrier	
	Factor IX deficiency – hemophilia B carrier	
Pregnancy acquired	Overdistension of the uterus:	× 5
	• Multiple pregnancy	
	• Macrosomia	
	• Polyhydramnios	
	Anemia (maternal Hb <85 g/L)	
	Low-lying placenta	
	Placenta previa	× 15
	Abnormal placental implantation – accreta, increta, and percreta	
	APH in current pregnancy	
	Pre-eclampsia or pregnancy-induced hypertension	× 4
	Sepsis (including chorioamnionitis and/or endometritis)	
Delivery acquired	Cesarean section:	× 4
	• Elective	× 9
	• Emergency	
	Precipitate labor	
	Maternal pyrexia in labor	× 2
	Induction of labor	
	Oxytocin use	
	Prolonged 1st, 2nd, or 3rd stage	× 2
	Labor lasting >12 hours	
	Operative vaginal delivery	× 2
	Fetal macrosomia (baby weight >4 kg)	× 2
	Ruptured uterus	
Third stage	Tissue – retained placenta (causes 10% of PPH)	
	Tone – uterine atony (causes 70% of PPH)	
	Trauma – laceration to perineum, vagina, or cervix (causes 20% of PPH)	
	Thrombin – coagulopathies (causes 1% of PPH)	
	Infection	

Data from references [5], [8], and [12].

the multidisciplinary plan for her delivery, which must be well documented and reviewed as the pregnancy progresses and risk factors change. Planned management, particularly in cases of placenta percreta, has been recommended[10].

Ultrasound localization of the placenta should be reported and documented clearly in the handheld notes of all women, especially those who have had previous cesarean section[11]. Antenatal assessment of full blood count and treatment of anemia are essential.

The importance of communication with all members of the multidisciplinary team, and early involvement of senior medical and midwifery staff, have been highlighted in successive Confidential Enquiries to improve prognosis. Management has changed, with increasing use of fertility-conserving intrauterine balloon and a concomitant fall in peripartum hysterectomy. Interestingly, despite rising rates of PPH, use of blood transfusion has diminished over time and there have been falls in hysterectomy[7]. While the antenatal identification of women with risk factors for major hemorrhage has increased to over 90%, the proportion whose care followed an appropriate action plan fell to about 50%[7].

If a woman is at risk of PPH, there are preventive and anticipatory measures which can be implemented in the intrapartum period. Such interventions include giving oral ranitidine (150 mg), gaining intravenous access with two large-bore cannulas, and taking blood to send for a full blood count, group, and save.

Active management of the third stage of labor involves the administration of a uterotonic drug (oxytocin) with, or shortly following, delivery of the anterior shoulder of the baby. Active management is recommended for any woman at increased risk of PPH. This shortens the time between delivery of the baby and the placenta and membranes with no significant increase in retained placenta[13,14]. Immediate cord clamping is no longer recommended in view of the impact on the neonate[12,15,16]. Controlled cord traction may reduce the risk of retained placenta and subsequent need for medical intervention[17]. There have been no reported adverse effects of controlled cord traction[18–20].

Pathogenesis of PPH

The most common cause of PPH, accounting for approximately 70% of occurrences, is uterine atony. There are numerous reasons for the uterus failing to contract effectively, including exhaustion, sepsis, and retained products. Other causes of PPH include perineal trauma, uterine inversion, clotting disorders, pelvic hematomas, and cervical tears. An abnormally implanted placenta (placenta accreta, increta, or percreta) (see Figure 18A.1) can remain in situ and hence prevent the uterus from contracting properly. Placenta previa and accreta are becoming an increasing problem, attributed to abnormal adherence of the placenta in subsequent pregnancies following cesarean section[21].

If obstetric hemorrhage is not managed efficiently and effectively, this will lead to shock, hemostatic failure from disseminated intravascular coagulation (DIC), and ultimately death.

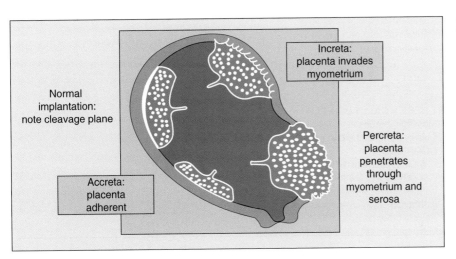

Figure 18A.1 Abnormal uteroplacental implantation.

Normal implantation: note cleavage plane

Increta: placenta invades myometrium

Accreta: placenta adherent

Percreta: placenta penetrates through myometrium and serosa

Diagnosis

Diagnosis of obstetric hemorrhage is typically by the visualization of blood loss from the genital tract. In the case of APH, bleeding can be concealed, and the only sign may be evidence of maternal compromise and/or fetal distress. With PPH, the volume of blood loss is usually estimated visually, although this is notoriously inaccurate and can be further compounded by clot formation in the uterus. In the acute situation before hemodilution, hemoglobin level will not represent the amount of blood lost. Fit, young women may appear to compensate and maintain vital signs until shortly before collapse. Clinician alertness and attention to symptoms and signs are vital. Some units attempt to measure blood loss by weighing blood-soaked items, for example sanitary pads and sheets. Modified Early Obstetric Warning Score (MEOWS) charts have been advocated to assess maternal compromise as they are supposed to provide a more accurate representation of maternal condition compared with visual estimation of blood loss and prevent delay in emergency management[22]. However, there is wide variation in the charts used and triggers for response, as well as barriers to their implementation[23,24].

Obstetric Management

In the case of APH, management will depend on the amount of bleeding, maternal compromise, and/or degree of fetal distress. A concealed APH large enough to cause intrauterine death is probably at least 1.5 L. DIC and PPH should both be assumed and anticipated.

Immediate Management of PPH

Once PPH has been diagnosed, action must be rapid. Figure 18A.2 is an effective tool in identifying what needs to be done and by whom, as often in the case of a PPH several actions need to be taken simultaneously.

HEAD
- Check airway
- Check breathing
- Administer O_2
- Lie flat
- Record time of relevant events

ARMS
- Check pulse and BP
- Establish LARGE BORE IV access x 2
- Check FBC, clotting and Xmatch 4–6 units
- Start FLUID RESUSCITATION
- 2 L crystalloid
- Drugs:
  - Ergometrine 0.5 mg IV (IM)
  - Syntocinon infusion (10 units/h)
  - Prostaglandin F2α 0.25 mg IM
  - Consider moving to theater if >2 doses required
  - Consider misoprostol 800 μg = micrograms

UTERUS
START HERE – CALL FOR HELP
- Massage uterus to stimulate contraction
- Deliver placenta if still in situ
- COORDINATE:
  - Assistant 1 at "HEAD"
  - Assistants 2 and 3 at "ARMS"
- Empty bladder – insert catheter
- If atony persists apply bimanual compression
- Review other causes; 4 Ts (Tone, Trauma, Tissue, Thrombin)
- Move to theater early if bleeding persists

Figure 18A.2 Management of PPH: organizing the team. Adapted from[4].

While constantly assessing maternal resuscitation requirements (pulse, blood pressure, respiration, temperature), the uterus should be massaged to stimulate a contraction, which may assist stemming of the bleeding should the cause be atony. This massaging action also helps expel retained products or blood clots. A full bladder could prevent the uterus from contracting properly by impeding on the space, and therefore catheterization is recommended. Table 18A.3 shows the standard drug management of PPH.

Table 18A.3 Drug management of PPH

Name of drug	How it works	Administration	Side effects
Oxytocin *Prevention*	Stimulates rhythmic upper uterine segment contractions	IM as part of Syntometrine (acts in 2–3 minutes, lasts up to 60 min) IV bolus 5 IU (acts in 1 min, has half-life of 3 min) IV 5 IU bolus can be repeated Infusion – 40 units/500 mL over 4 hours	Hypotension, due to vasodilatation, especially in cardiac patients • Administer slowly • In cardiac patients infuse 10 units over 30 min Antidiuretic hormone effect • Fluid overload – can lead to pulmonary edema • Hyponatremia
Ergometrine *Recognition*	Sustains uterine contraction via alpha receptors in the upper and lower uterine segment of the uterus Combined with oxytocin as Syntometrine Acts in 2–5 min, lasts up to 3 hours If atony persists give 0.5 mg IV		Potent agonist causes blood vessels to constrict Vomiting + + + most women WILL vomit Hypertension – ***do not give*** to women with pre-existing high BP, pre-eclampsia, or PIH or cardiac disease
Carboprost (Hemobate®) *Treatment*	This is a prostaglandin F2 alpha	*Not for IV administration* Intramyometrially into the fundus of the uterus to avoid blood vessels (but there are very large vessels in the uterus) Intramuscularly, 250 µg (microgram) every 15 min (maximum of 2 mg) In practice, most women are not given > 2 doses 85% of women respond to the first dose	Has predilection for smooth muscle of the bronchi and therefore ***caution is required with asthmatics*** Bronchospasm Significant intrapulmonary shunt Hypoxia
Microprostol (Cytotec®) *Treatment*	This is a prostaglandin E$_1$ analog It is thermostable and does not require refrigeration This drug is cheap and therefore useful in resource limited countries	Multiple routes of administration Orally, sublingually, rectally 800–1000 µg (effective within 3 min)	Shivering Pyrexia

Other uterotonics have been suggested with limited anecdotal evidence. These include:

- Carbetocin, not yet validated or proven cost effective[25].
- Dinoprostone; however, this is not suitable in hypovolemic situations.
- Gemeprost (cervogem).
- Sulproston – a prostaglandin E_2 widely used in France as a second-line drug after oxytocin (before ergometrine). Can cause coronary spasm, hypertension, pyrexia, nausea, and vomiting.
- Vasopressin® 5 IU in 19 mL normal saline given by subendothelial infiltration. Avoid intravenous administration as it causes severe hypertension.
- Tranexamic acid – a lysine derivative, which appears well tolerated. There is no evidence of increased thrombosis and this drug is probably underused: 1 g intravenously with, if necessary, repeat dose 4 hours later.
- Methotrexate – prevents DNA replication and may be useful in conservative management of placenta accreta.

Volume Maintenance in PPH

Initially, while blood is being cross-matched, volume replacement with crystalloid should be instituted. Close attention to fluid balance is required to avoid the perils of hypoxia–hypovolemia, on the one hand, and cardiopulmonary overload on the other. In massive hemorrhage, fluid replacement can be controlled with central venous and arterial lines and anesthetic and hematology input is vital both during the event and subsequently on high-dependency or intensive care units (see Chapter 18B).

Surgical Management of PPH

- **Manual removal of placenta.** This is an emergency procedure to separate the placenta manually that should be considered if it has not delivered within an hour of birth. Partial separation and delays can be associated with very heavy bleeding. Use of uterotonics via umbilical vein injection is not recommended[26].
- **Bimanual uterine compression.** This is an effective way of stemming bleeding by compressing the uterus with both hands (Figure 18A.3).
- **Examination under anesthesia (EUA) and evacuation of retained products of conception**

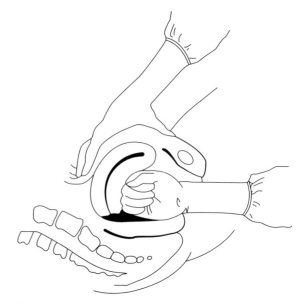

Figure 18A.3 Bimanual uterine compression.

(ERPC). This should be performed in theater with appropriate conditions, personnel, and instruments and in preparation for further procedures. It is important to explore the whole of the uterus, cervix, vagina, and perineum in a rigorous way, even if one cause is found or excluded. The aim of EUA is to assess the cause of bleeding and take action accordingly. The cause may be found, for example retained cotyledon, pelvic hematoma (common after a normal vaginal delivery and often requiring surgery), or cervical tears. ERPC for secondary PPH, especially if associated with sepsis, must be performed with great care as it can lead to perforation of the uterus.

- **Balloon tamponade** can be used, and is increasingly used to treat PPH[7]. This involves placing a balloon in the uterus and inflating it. Most commonly around 800–1000 mL is used to ensure the balloon does not fall out after a vaginal delivery, but less is required if only compressing the lower segment after elective cesarean; the balloon is then left in situ for 24 hours after which time it is gradually deflated. This is a cost-effective method. In an emergency, a condom could be filled with fluid and inserted into the uterus to apply pressure to stop the bleeding.
- **Packing with surgical gauze.** This is a traditional and effective way to stop surgical bleeding and

ooze from a raw or sutured surface, although the disadvantage is that a second procedure may be required for removal. Packs have to be placed under pressure, and can be left in the uterus, the vagina, or in the abdomen.

- **The B-Lynch brace suture**. This has steadily gained acceptance in recent years. The brace suture has not been evaluated in an RCT, but the case history evidence is compelling. It has been suggested that the B-Lynch brace suture may indent the uterus or cause necrotic uterus with potential long-term fertility consequences. Any speculated effect on fertility must be compared with hysterectomy, which would otherwise be the next surgical option. Prophylactic brace sutures can be advocated in Jehovah's Witnesses and in others who require cesarean section but refuse transfusion and are assessed as at increased risk of PPH (although risk assessment is difficult).
- **Internal iliac vessel ligation**. This is an old technique and less familiar to obstetricians nowadays, though more often used by gynecological oncologists. The principle of occluding the uterine blood supply has evolved into an interventional radiology technique of **uterine artery embolization** to stop bleeding. The collateral circulation is adequate to protect the uterus, but the equipment is not available in all units, and there is a risk to future fertility.

- **Hysterectomy**. Women may die if the decision to do a hysterectomy is either not made or made too late, but practitioners must be prepared to defend their decision-making in the legal process, as unnecessary loss of fertility is devastating. This must be the treatment of last resort, having attempted conservative measures first. The UKOSS study of hysterectomy showed a failure rate both for brace suture and interventional radiology embolization[27].

There is no evidence to guide the use of one surgical or medical management above others[12]. All women, and their companions, deserve a contemporaneous explanation, and a discussion afterwards about what happened, so that any questions can be answered. After a PPH, women can make a remarkable physical recovery. However, unrecognized or undocumented PPH may lead to dizziness, fainting, or collapse in the immediate postpartum period. All women with symptoms or a recognized PPH should be tested postpartum or on day 2–3 for hemoglobin levels in case iron supplements need to be prescribed. A prolonged recovery may be associated with fatigue, exhaustion, and interference with breast-feeding and bonding. Massive hemorrhage can be very traumatic, for women, their families, and for staff, and the need for explanation and reflection must not be underestimated, with increasing evidence of post-traumatic stress disorder associated with severe maternal morbidity[28]. Staff skills must be constantly updated.

Case Studies

Case Study 1

After a normal pregnancy and labor a woman had a spontaneous vaginal birth, followed by active management of the third stage and an estimated blood loss of 350 mL. Examination of the placenta and membranes showed the placenta was complete and the membranes ragged. After breast-feeding her infant and having 1 hour skin to skin she was transferred to the postnatal ward. Six hours later she complained of feeling unwell. She was pale, sweaty, tachycardic, and hypotensive. On examination her sanitary pad was blood-soaked and the uterus palpable above the umbilicus. Management to contract the uterus was commenced, as outlined in this chapter.

This case emphasizes the importance of postnatal observations, ensuring the membranes are complete and that the mother micturates within 4 hours of giving birth and regularly thereafter.

Case Study 2

A 41-year-old woman at 29 weeks in her fourth pregnancy was admitted feeling unwell, faint, and sweaty. She had been experiencing intermittent lower abdominal pains for 2 weeks. On examination, she was hypotensive, with a blood pressure of 85/45 mm Hg and tachycardia of 124 bpm. Initially vaginal blood loss was scant but soon became excessive, with an estimated loss of 1200 mL in the next 60 minutes. Hb was only 50 g/L, and emergency cesarean section was performed. The baby was taken to intensive care for resuscitation. Histology of the placenta showed massive retroplacental blood clot as well as bleeding and ischemic changes in the intervillous space.

This case demonstrates the hidden bleeding that occurs with placental abruption.

References

1. Knight M, Kenyon S, Brocklehurst P *et al.* (eds) on behalf of MBRRACE. *Saving Lives, Improving Mothers' Care – Lessons learned to inform future maternity care from the UK and Ireland Confidential Enquiries into Maternal Deaths and Morbidity 2009–12.* Oxford: National Perinatal Epidemiology Unit, University of Oxford; 2014.

2. World Health Organization. *WHO Recommendations for the Prevention and Treatment of Postpartum Hemorrhage.* Geneva: WHO; 2012.

3. Kassebaum NJ, Betozzi-Villa A, Coggeshall MS *et al.* Global, regional, and national levels and causes of maternal mortality during 1990–2013: a systematic analysis for the Global Burden of Disease Study 2013. *Lancet* 2014; **384**: 980–1004.

4. American Academy of Family Practitioners (AAFP). Advanced Life Support in Obstetrics. Syllabus Updates; 2008. www.aafp.org/online/en/home/cme /aafpcourses/clinicalcourses/also/syllabus.html#Parsy s0003 (accessed May 21 2008).

5. Ford JB, Roberts CL, Simpson JM, Vaughan J, Cameron CA. Increased postpartum hemorrhage rates in Australia. *International Journal of Gynecology and Obstetrics* 2007; **98**: 237–243.

6. Briley A, Seed PT, Tydeman G *et al.* Reporting errors, incidence and risk factors for postpartum hemorrhage and progression to severe PPH: a prospective observational study. *BJOG: An International Journal of Obstetrics and Gynecology* 2014; **121**(7): 876–888.

7. Scottish Confidential Audit of Severe Maternal Morbidity. Reducing Avoidable Harm. 10th Annual Report. http://www.healthcareimprovementscotland .org/our_work/reproductive,_maternal__child/repro ductive_health/scasmm.aspx (accessed June 12 2015).

8. Magann EF, Evans S, Chauhan SP *et al.* The length of the third stage of labor and risk of postpartum hemorrhage. *Obstetrics and Gynecology* 2005; **105**(2): 290–293.

9. Department of Health. *Why Mothers Die, 1997–1999. The Fifth Annual Report of the Confidential Enquiries into Maternal Deaths in the United Kingdom.* London: RCOG Press.

10. Lewis G. *The Confidential Enquiry into Maternal and Child Health (CEMACH). Why Mothers Die (2000– 2002).* London: CEMACH; 2005.

11. Magann EF, Evans S, Hutchinson M *et al.* Postpartum hemorrhage after cesarean delivery; an analysis of risk factors. *South Medical Journal* 2005; **98**: 681–685.

12. National Institute for Health and Clinical Excellence. NICE Intrapartum Guidelines. CG190; 2014.

http://www.nice.org.uk/guidance/cg190/evidence/ cg190-intrapartum-care-full-guideline3 (accessed June 12 2015).

13. Bais JM, Eskes M, Pel M, Bonsel GJ, Bleker OP. Postpartum hemorrhage in nulliparous women: incidence and risk factors in low and high risk women. A Dutch population-based cohort study on standard (> or = 500 ml) and severe (> or = 1000 ml) postpartum hemorrhage. *European Journal of Obstetrics & Gynecology and Reproduction Biology* 2004; **115**: 166–172.

14. Prendiville WJ, Elbourne D, McDonald S. Active versus expectant management of the third stage of labor. *Cochrane Database of Systematic Reviews* 2000 (**2**): CD00007.

15. Royal College of Obstetricians and Gynecologists. Clamping of the Umbilical Cord and Placental Transfusion. Scientific Impact Paper No. 14; 2015. https://www.rcog.org.uk/globalassets/documents/guide lines/scientific-impact-papers/sip-14.pdf (accessed June 12 2015).

16. World Health Organization. Delayed Umbilical Cord Clamping for Improved Maternal and Infant Health and Nutrition Outcomes; 2014. http://www.who.int/ nutrition/publications/guidelines/cord_clamping /en/ Accessed 12/06/2015

17. Hofmeyr GJ, Mshweshwe NT, Gülmezoglu AM. Controlled cord traction for the third stage of labor. *Cochrane Database of Systematic Reviews* 2015; (**1**): CD008020.

18. Khan GQ, John IS, Wani S *et al.* Controlled cord traction versus minimal intervention techniques in delivery of the placenta: a randomised controlled trial. *American Journal of Obstetrics and Gynecology* 1997; **177**: 770–774.

19. Zhao S, Xiaofeng S. Clinical study in curing postpartum hemorrhage in the third stage of labor. *Journal of Practical Obstetrics and Gynecology* 2003; **19**: 278–280.

20. Giacalone PL, Vignal J, Daures JP, *et al.* A randomised evaluation of two techniques of management of the third stage of labor in women at low risk of postpartum hemorrhage. *British Journal of Obstetrics and Gynecology* 2000; **107**: 396–400.

21. Royal College of Obstetricians and Gynecologists. *Placenta Previa, Placenta Previa Accreta and Vasa Previa: Diagnosis and Management. Green-Top Guideline No. 27.* London: Royal College of Obstetricians and Gynecologists; 2011. https://www .rcog.org.uk/en/guidelines-research-services/guide lines/gtg27/ (accessed June 12 2015).

22. Confidential Enquiries into Maternal and Child Health (CEMACH). *Saving Mothers' Lives: Reviewing Maternal Deaths to make Motherhood Safer: 2003–2005. The Seventh Report of the Confidential Enquiries into*

Maternal Deaths in the United Kingdom. London: RCOG Press; 2007.

23. Mackintosh N, Watson K, Rance S, Sandall J. Value of a modified early obstetric warning system (MEOWS) in managing maternal complications in the peripartum period: an ethnographic study. *BMJ Quality and Safety* 2014; **23**(1): 26–34.

24. Bick DE, Sandall J, Furuta M *et al.* A national cross sectional survey of heads of midwifery services of uptake, benefits and barriers to use of obstetric early warning systems (EWS) by midwives. *Midwifery* 2014; **30**(11): 1140–1146.

25. Su LL, Chng YS, Samuel M. Carbetocin for preventing postpartum hemorrhage. *Cochrane Database of Systematic Reviews* 2012; (**2**): CD005457.

26. Mori R, Nardin JM, Yamamoto N, Carroli G, Weeks A. Umbilical vein injection for the routine management of third stage of labor. *Cochrane Database of Systematic Reveiws* 2012; (**3**): CD006176.

27. Knight M, UKOSS. Peripartum hysterectomy in the UK: management and outcomes of the associated hemorrhage. *British Journal of Obstetrics and Gynecology: an International Journal of Obstetrics and Gynecology* 2007; **114**: 1380–1387.

28. Furuta M, Sandall J, Bick D. A systematic review of the relationship between severe maternal morbidity and post-traumatic stress disorder. *BMC Pregnancy and Childbirth* 2012; **12**: 125. http://doi: 10.1186/1471–2393-12–125.

Management of Obstetric Hemorrhage: Anesthetic Management

Catherine Collinson and Arlene Wise

Introduction

Obstetric hemorrhage is a common yet challenging emergency, which requires a prompt multidisciplinary response. Despite advances in obstetric care, hemorrhage remains the third most common cause of direct maternal death across the UK and Ireland according to the MBRRACE report (Mothers and Babies: Reducing Risk through Audits and Confidential Enquiries "Saving Lives, Improving Mothers' Care")[1]. The report identified areas where care could have been improved in each of the 17 maternal deaths that were attributable to hemorrhage. Death from obstetric hemorrhage is thought to be largely preventable. However, worldwide where many women deliver in resource-poor environments obstetric hemorrhage accounts for almost 25% of maternal mortality and can reach as high as 50% in some countries[1].

In resource-rich countries such as the UK, the rate of mortality from obstetric hemorrhage may be low but it does cause a significant burden of morbidity. The Scottish Confidential Audit of Severe Maternal Morbidity 2012 (SCASSM) reported that 80% of all maternal morbidity is related to hemorrhage[2].

Once a major hemorrhage has been declared, early senior anesthetic involvement is essential. The role of the anesthetist should be proactive, not reactive. Anesthetists have the practical skills (vascular access, invasive monitoring) and the clinical experience required to co-ordinate resuscitation efforts. They may also be required to provide anesthesia to facilitate surgery (or radiological procedures) to arrest the bleeding.

This chapter describes the approach to the anesthetic management of obstetric hemorrhage in the UK in consultant-led obstetric units. However, the same principles of management are applicable in other settings although the availability of equipment, drugs, and personnel may be different.

Antenatal Assessment

Anesthetists should play a role in the multidisciplinary antenatal management of women who:

- have an increased bleeding tendency
- are at risk of significant hemorrhage, i.e. placenta previa/accreta
- refuse blood products

These patients should be delivered in centers with facilities for blood transfusion, cell salvage, intensive care, and interventional radiology, and plans for their management should be made in advance. SCASMM 2012 reported that although 80–90% of women at high risk of obstetric hemorrhage were identified antenatally each year, an action plan was completed and followed for only 50–70% of these women[2].

Women who are anemic in pregnancy should be investigated and efforts made to optimize hemoglobin concentration using oral or intravenous iron, folic acid, and vitamin B_{12} as appropriate. If there are difficulties in cross-matching blood, e.g. pre-existing red cell antibodies, this should be flagged up antenatally and the need for blood pre-empted.

Recognition of Obstetric Hemorrhage

Many expert groups have recommended the use of track and trigger scoring systems (such as the Modified Early Warning Scores) for monitoring patients to facilitate early identification of those with ongoing hemorrhage. Scoring systems are never perfect and pregnant women will compensate well despite significant blood loss. Therefore, it should be borne in mind that physiological derangement, e.g. hypotension, may be a very late sign.

Careful repeated clinical assessment and a high index of suspicion for hemorrhage are important. This requires observations to be taken and recorded accurately, then acted upon in a timely fashion.

Communication

Early and clear communication among the multidisciplinary team (obstetricians, anesthetists, midwives, hematologists, laboratory and support staff) is vital. In most hospitals, this usually involves activating the major hemorrhage protocol. A team leader should be designated to facilitate a rapid and coordinated response with tasks allocated to specific team members: securing vascular access, communicating with the laboratory and other specialties, as well as clearly documenting events[3]. Consideration should be given to summoning extra and more senior help. Poor leadership featured in three deaths reviewed in the recent MBRRACE report[1].

Participation in multidisciplinary emergency drills such as PROMPT (PRactical Obstetric Multi-Professional Training) improves team working, situational awareness, and familiarity with the guidelines relevant to achieving a good outcome[4,5]. A major hemorrhage protocol must be available in all units and updated and rehearsed regularly.

Accurate and complete documentation of the sequence of events is also very important. Poor documentation is indefensible even if excellent care was provided. A person should be assigned the job of recording the drugs and fluids administered and of the personnel involved in the resuscitation.

Initial Resuscitation

Once obstetric hemorrhage has been identified, the multidisciplinary team must respond quickly in a co-ordinated manner. Early senior anesthetic involvement is essential. Rapid simultaneous evaluation (patient's airway, breathing, and circulation) and resuscitation should occur in accordance with the Resuscitation Council's guidelines[6]. High-concentration oxygen (10–15 L/min) should be administered via a non-rebreathing mask, and antenatally, women should be tilted to reduce aorto-caval compression. An emergency lifting sheet may be required to lift a bleeding patient from the floor or birthing pool onto a trolley to allow the resuscitation team safe and easy access to deliver care.

Goals of resuscitation are:

- restoration of circulating volume
- maintenance of adequate tissue perfusion
- prevention/treatment of coagulopathy

Access

- Intravenous (IV) access: two large bore (14 G/16 G) IV cannulae should be sited. Central venous catheterization may be needed but should not delay resuscitation.

- Intraosseous access, e.g. ARROW® EZ-IO® Intraosseous Vascular Access System: should be considered early if IV access is proving difficult.

Kit should be readily available and staff trained in its use; complications include local and/or systemic infection, hematoma, and extravasation (see Figure 18B.1).

Investigations

When significant hemorrhage is first diagnosed, blood should be taken and sent to the laboratory for a group and cross-match, full blood count, and coagulation screen (INR, aPTT, Clauss fibrinogen) in addition to baseline renal and liver function tests.

The clinical picture can change rapidly in major hemorrhage and as such "point-of-care" testing is invaluable by providing real time results that are used to guide resuscitation and blood replacement. These should be repeated at regular intervals in order to facilitate the logical use of blood products.

These include:

(a) HemoCue: gives an estimate of hemoglobin from a finger prick sample or drop of venous/arterial blood. Hemoglobin is a poor marker of acute blood loss, especially when fluid resuscitation has not yet commenced, but if low on initial testing, this suggests a significant volume of blood has been lost.

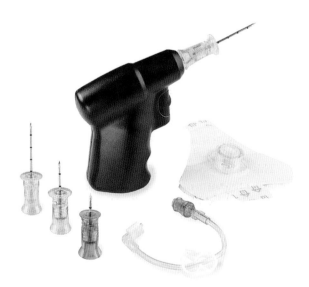

Figure 18B.1 ARROW® EZ-IO® Intraosseous Vascular Access System. Image courtesy of Teleflex Incorporated. © 2015 Teleflex Incorporated. All rights reserved.

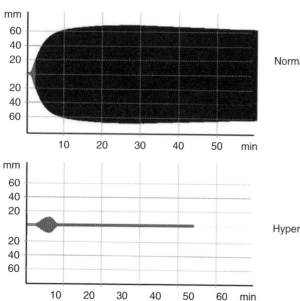

(b) Arterial blood gases (ABGs): provide information on oxygenation and ventilation, and lactate and base deficit are a useful monitor of tissue perfusion.

(c) Thromboelastograph, e.g. TEG or ROTEM: This technique uses whole blood and can provide information about hemostatic function within 5–10 minutes. A variety of reagents are added to assess different aspects of hemostasis: fibrinogen, platelets, and the effect of heparin. Institutions using thromboelastography should have protocols for the administration of blood components based on the results of the various assays (see Figure 18B.2). Although increasingly being used in obstetric practice, NICE (National Institute for Health and Care Excellence) supports the use of thromboelastography in cardiac surgery but found that there is currently insufficient evidence to recommend its routine use to monitor hemostasis during obstetric hemorrhage[7]. Standard formal coagulation tests do not reflect whole blood clotting function. In the vast majority of cases of major obstetric hemorrhage aPTT/PT will remain normal.

Monitoring

Non-invasive blood pressure, oxygen saturation, electrocardiogram (ECG), and temperature should be monitored. A urinary catheter should be inserted and hourly urine output measured. An arterial line permits continuous blood pressure monitoring and repeated blood sampling. Central venous pressure (CVP) monitoring may be required in cases of massive hemorrhage although not as a part of the initial resuscitation.

Choice of Fluid

There is no specific evidence about the correct choice of fluid (crystalloid vs. colloid) for initial resuscitation in obstetric bleeding but a systematic review of fluid choice in other critically unwell patients would suggest that isotonic crystalloids should be used in preference to colloids[8]. Hartmann's solution and Plasmalyte are physiologically balanced crystalloids; 0.9% saline can also be used but it may cause metabolic acidosis after several liters have been infused.

Colloids include gelatins, albumin, and starches. Gelatins (Geloplasma, Gelofusine) can interfere with blood grouping and cross-matching, and cause allergic reactions. Starches (Voluven) are no longer available in the UK due to concerns about risk of renal dysfunction and mortality in critically ill or septic patients.

Concern was raised in the SCASSM 2012 report about the excessive administration of clear fluid prior to blood transfusion. Consensus opinion suggests that a maximum of 3 L of crystalloid should be infused prior to consideration of blood transfusion[2]. O negative blood should be immediately available in all obstetric units and used if the patient is in extremis. If the clinical situation permits, it is preferable to await type-specific (20 minutes) or fully cross-matched (40 minutes) blood.

All fluids should be warmed. The RCOG guidelines state that every maternity unit should have access to a rapid infusion system, which can both pressurize and warm blood and fluids rapidly, e.g. Belmont Rapid Infuser[9] (see Figure 18B.3).

Ongoing Assessment

Response to Resuscitation
Clinical parameters, including level of consciousness, blood pressure, heart rate (both fetal and maternal), and urine output should be assessed in addition to

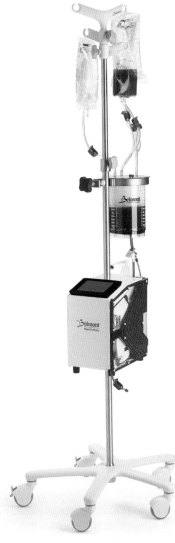

serial arterial blood gases. Blood pressure is generally maintained until 30% of the blood volume (1500–2000 mL) has been lost; tachycardia will usually represent uncorrected hypovolemia.

There is no place for permissive hypotension prior to delivery of the baby; however, this can be considered following delivery.

Volume of Blood Loss
Accurate assessment of blood loss is essential but notoriously difficult as visual estimation alone underestimates the volume of blood lost. In theater, surgical swabs are weighed and the volume of blood in the surgical suction measured. In the labor ward, bed linen, swabs, and pads should be weighed[10].

Blood loss should not just be considered as an absolute value but as a percentage of circulating blood volume. Estimated blood volume in late pregnancy is 100 mL/kg, although this may overestimate blood volume in obese women[9] (see Table 18B.1). Nine of the women who died from hemorrhage in the MBRRACE report weighed less than 60 kg, where blood loss of 1500 mL may be almost 30% of circulating blood volume, i.e. when cardiovascular decompensation is expected[1]. Major obstetric hemorrhage calls should therefore be activated when approximately 30% of circulating blood volume has been lost.

Pharmacological Hemorrhage Control
Uterine atony is the most common cause of obstetric hemorrhage so uterotonics should be given early.

(a) Oxytocin: Administration of a slow IV bolus (5 units) works within 2–3 minutes. However, due to its short half-life, an infusion, typically 40 IU in 500 mL of normal saline over 4 hours, should be given. Rapid IV administration can cause vasodilatation resulting in profound hypotension and tachycardia in hemodynamically unstable patients. Cardiac arrest has also been reported.

(b) Ergometrine: The recommended dose is 500 µg IM (intramuscular) or IV. Uterine contraction occurs within 5 minutes of an IM injection and 1 minute after an IV injection. Its effects last at least 1 hour. It is an extremely effective drug but is used as a second-line agent due to its side effects (nausea, vomiting, and hypertension).

Table 18B.1 Estimated blood volumes and proportionate losses according to body weight

Weight (kg)	Total blood volume (mL)	15% blood volume (mL)	30% blood volume (mL)	40% blood volume (mL)
50 kg	5000	750	1500	2000
55 kg	5500	825	1650	2200
60 kg	6000	900	1800	2400
65 kg	6500	975	1950	2600
70 kg	7000	1050	2100	2800

Table reproduced with kind permission from MBRRACE–UK[1].

(c) Carboprost (methyl prostaglandin F2): This potent smooth muscle constrictor should be administered only by intramuscular injection. It should be administered in 250-μg increments, which can be repeated at 15-minute intervals up to a maximum dose of 2 mg. The majority (85%) of patients will usually respond to the first or second dose, and in practice the full 2-mg dose will rarely be employed as ongoing severe hemorrhage usually necessitates further surgical/radiological intervention. It may cause significant bronchospasm and should be used with caution in asthmatics.

(d) Misoprostol: This is a prostaglandin E1 analog. It is supplied as 200-μg tablets, and 800 μg should be administered rectally or sublingually. Side effects include abdominal pain, diarrhea, pyrexia, and shivering which can be confused with signs of sepsis.

Anesthetic Considerations

Regional versus General Anesthesia

Regional anesthesia (RA) is generally the technique of choice in the obstetric population. It permits the mother to be awake at time of delivery and avoids general anesthesia (GA) in a group of patients whose anatomical and physiological changes make intubation and oxygenation more difficult.

However, RA is contraindicated in the presence of:

- coagulopathy: due to the increased risk of epidural hematoma;
- hemodynamic instability when sympathetic blockade can cause catastrophic cardiovascular collapse in a hypovolemic patient.

Therefore GA is indicated when blood loss exceeds 1000 mL and there is hemodynamic instability and/or

suspected or confirmed coagulopathy. The dose of induction agent should be altered according to the clinical scenario[1]. Consideration may be given to using an alternative agent with less depressant effects on the cardiovascular system, e.g. ketamine, if familiar with its use.

In an elective situation, where significant blood loss is anticipated, such as with anterior placenta previa, RA can still be considered, although patients should be warned of the potential need to convert to GA intraoperatively. Surgery may be prolonged so a combined spinal-epidural (CSE) technique rather than a single shot spinal may be useful to permit prolonged anesthesia. Baseline hemoglobin, vascular access, invasive monitoring, and cell salvage should be established prior to starting such cases. Sufficient blood should be cross-matched and immediately available[11].

Location of Anesthesia

If an unstable bleeding patient requires interventional radiology, transfer to the radiology department should be avoided. The interventional radiology team should come to the obstetric theater with a portable image intensifier where a carbon-fiber operating table should be used.

Blood and Blood Component Therapy (See Chapter 18C)

Transfusion Triggers/Strategies

There are limited data to inform a rational transfusion strategy in obstetric hemorrhage. However, it is vital not to wait for coagulation indices to deteriorate prior to consideration of transfusion of blood components.

The etiology and volume of bleeding predict the likelihood of impaired hemostasis. The most common causes of obstetric bleeding are uterine atony and genital tract trauma. This is generally not associated with coagulopathy so early empirical coagulation products are not indicated. Placental abruption or amniotic fluid embolism (AFE) are much more likely to cause hemostatic impairment; therefore, regular hemostatic monitoring with routine blood tests and/or thromboelastography should be used early to guide treatment. Fibrinogen falls most rapidly and is the best predictor of the progression into a major hemorrhage (fibrinogen <2 g/L)[12].

Current guidelines suggest the following transfusion triggers[13,14]:

- hemoglobin <80 g/L
- Platelets <75 × 10^9/L
- PT/ aPTT ratio of >1.5
- Fibrinogen <1.5–2 g/L

The 1:1:1 (red cells [RCC]:FFP:platelets) transfusion strategy used in military and major trauma settings has been considered in obstetrics when greater than 50% of the circulating blood volume has been lost. However, the large volumes may lead to circulatory overload; cryoprecipitate may be required as fresh frozen plasma (FFP) does not contain adequate replacement fibrinogen, which tends to fall at a faster rate than other coagulation factors.

Thrombocytopenia in PPH is unusual, unless in the context of placental abruption, severe pre-eclampsia, amniotic fluid embolism (AFE), and pre-existing thrombocytopenia (immune or inherited). A clean dedicated giving set should be used for all platelet transfusion.

Hemostatic Agents

Fibrinogen Concentrate, e.g. RiaSTAP/Hemocomplettan

Although unlicensed for use in obstetric hemorrhage in many countries, there is growing interest in the use of fibrinogen concentrate in the treatment of obstetric hemorrhage. It is easy to administer, immediately available, and it is thought to reduce blood product usage and fluid overload. Its production process includes viral inactivation, minimizing the risk of viral transmission compared to cryoprecipitate or FFP.

A number of RCTs are currently investigating whether fibrinogen concentrate has a role to play in PPH. The Fib-PPH study – Universal fibrinogen concentrate if PPH >1500 mL – demonstrated no role for fibrinogen concentrate in PPH. However, only 2% of the study population had fibrinogen less than 2 g/L, and the average was 4.5 g/L[15]. The OBS2 study – a weight-adjusted dose of fibrinogen concentrate given

if fibrinogen is low, based on ROTEM testing (FIBTEM A5 <15 mm), and found no improvement in outcome. Subgroup analysis, however, would suggest that there is no need for fibrinogen replacement if the Fibtem A5 is >12 mm or clauss fibrinogen is >2 g/L, the suggestion being that the raised fibrinogen is a buffer and is not actually required for hemostasis[16].

Tranexamic Acid

Tranexamic acid is an antifibrinolytic agent whose role in obstetric hemorrhage has been extrapolated from trauma and major surgery settings. The World Health Organization (WHO) suggest that it has a role to play in the treatment of bleeding caused by uterine atony or trauma if uterotonics have not been effective [17]. A small open-label study demonstrated a reduction in the volume of blood lost, the need for blood transfusion, and progression from moderate-to-severe PPH[18]. A recent international randomized controlled trial (the WOMAN study) has demonstrated that tranexamic acid is associated with a significant reduction in death due to bleeding and laparotomy to control bleeding with no evidence of any increased risk of thromboembolic events. When given soon after delivery, tranexamic acid reduces death due to bleeding by nearly one-third[19]. The dose of tranexamic acid is 1 g, which should be given as a slow IV bolus, and can be repeated at 30 minutes if bleeding is ongoing. In practice, if the thromboelastography trace shows signs of hyperfibrinolysis then tranexamic acid should be given.

Recombinant fVIIa

The role of recombinant fVIIa has diminished over the last 5 years due to a number of problems with its use, including a 5% rate of arterial thromboembolism. Although Lavigne-Lassalde *et al.* demonstrated a reduction in the need for second-line therapies with its use in PPH, the RCOG state that it should not be used in PPH unless as part of a clinical trial[20].

Complications from Massive Hemorrhage and Transfusion

Hypothermia

Patients develop hypothermia due to a number of factors: infusion of cold fluids, impairment of thermoregulatory heat-preserving mechanisms during anesthesia, and exposure for surgical access. Patients should be kept warm using forced air warming blankets, e.g. Bair hugger or under patient heating systems. All fluids should be warmed, preferably by a rapid infusion system. Patient temperature should be monitored to ensure these strategies are effective.

Acidosis

Inadequate tissue perfusion leads to metabolic acidosis due to the generation of lactic acid. Transfusion of blood products also contributes to the acidosis, as a result of the lower pH of stored blood and the fact that most blood products are anticoagulated with citrate, which is also an acid.

Electrolyte Imbalance

Massive transfusion and acidosis can lead to electrolyte imbalance, which can cause cardiac arrhythmias. Calcium concentration should be maintained above 0.9 mmol/L with slow intravenous boluses of 5–10 mL of calcium gluconate 10%. Hyperkalemia should be treated urgently: 5–20 mL of calcium gluconate 10% to stabilize the myocardium, and insulin and dextrose infusion to move the potassium intracellularly.

Coagulopathy

Most patients with major obstetric hemorrhage do not develop coagulopathy. However, if bleeding is not controlled a coagulopathy will develop. It has been demonstrated in trauma patients with massive bleeding that if they are allowed to become hypothermic and acidotic, their coagulopathy worsens and may become refractory to correction. This is known as the "lethal triad."

Certain types of hemorrhage are associated with certain types of coagulopathy:

- Placental abruption is characterized by a severe rapid-onset consumptive coagulopathy.
- AFE is associated with disseminated intravascular coagulation.

Transfusion-Related Acute Lung Injury (TRALI)

TRALI is characterized by the sudden onset of dyspnea, severe hypoxemia (SpO_2 <90% in room air), hypotension, and fever occurring 1–6 hours following the transfusion of blood products. It is very rare (1/5000 transfusions) but occurs most commonly following the transfusion of plasma components, e.g. FFP and platelets. The hypoxemia is unexplained by other cardiorespiratory disease with the clinical picture being similar to fluid overload (chest X-ray is consistent with bilateral pulmonary edema) but there is no improvement following treatment with diuretics. Treatment is entirely supportive and mortality is between 6 and 9%.

It has been suggested that TRALI is caused by two "hits": endothelial activation and neutrophil priming that occur as a result of the major hemorrhage, and a factor from the donated blood which causes endothelial damage and capillary leak.

Cell Salvage

Intraoperative cell salvage and auto transfusion is a technique for re-cycling intraoperative blood loss. It is well established in other surgical disciplines. Although the use of cell salvage in obstetrics has been endorsed by CEMACH, NICE, OAA, and AAGBI, the uptake has been slow due to concerns about amniotic fluid embolism[21–23]. The lack of availability of equipment and expertise in its use are also barriers to widespread adoption[24].

Salvaged blood compares favorably to donor blood in terms of red cell morphology and survival, potassium content, and 2,3-DPG levels. While it can be life saving, donor blood has additional risks including transfusion reactions, cross-matching errors, and infection. While salvaged blood has many advantages, it is important to note that it contains no coagulation factors or platelets.

Indications

Cell salvage is particularly appropriate for elective surgery where massive blood loss is anticipated, e.g. placenta previa/accreta and for mothers who refuse blood and/or blood products, e.g. Jehovah's Witnesses. Once skill has been acquired with the technique, the equipment can be rapidly set up in an emergency. While vaginal blood loss can be collected for cell salvage, the technique is best suited to an open abdomen[25].

Principles of Cell Salvage

Blood is collected from the surgical site or from surgical swabs (soak them in 0.9% saline and then aspirate this fluid) into a collecting reservoir. Cells are then separated by hemoconcentration and differential centrifugation, and washed in 0.9% saline. This process removes circulating fibrin, debris, plasma, micro-aggregates,

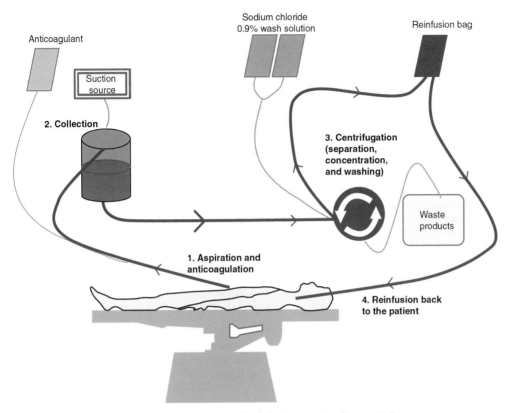

Figure 18B.4 Cell salvage machine. Image reproduced with kind permission of Danny McGee.

complement, platelets, free hemoglobin, circulating pro-coagulants, and most of the anticoagulant. At the end of the salvage process, the hematocrit of the salvaged blood is usually between 55 and 60% (see Figure 18B.4).

Potential Problems

AFE

The technique was initially thought to unsuitable for obstetric practice because of the risk of AFE. However, this is now known to be an immunological rather than embolic phenomenon. Nevertheless, some institutions have delayed initiating cell salvage until after delivery to minimize contamination of the salvaged blood with amniotic fluid. Practice is now changing such that blood collection commences at incision, as it has been shown that contamination with fetal squames is not significantly different between pre- and post-delivery collection so long as there a wash cycle and a leukocyte depletion filter is used[26]. Leukocyte depletion filters should routinely be used during re-infusion as these

remove any remaining fetal squames, white blood cells, and platelets from the salvaged blood. To date, no case of AFE has been reported in patients who received salvaged blood during cesarean section where a leukocyte filter was used.

Hypotension

A series of cases have been reported where sudden profound hypotension developed shortly after salvaged blood was re-transfused through a leukocyte depletion filter[27]. This is thought to be due to cytokine release. In this situation, the UK Cell Salvage Action Group would advocate stopping the transfusion, administering vasopressor, and removing the filter before continuing the transfusion[28]. If salvaged blood needs to be transfused rapidly, the filter may need to be removed to improve flow. Bags containing salvaged blood should never be pressurized because of the risk of air embolism.

Allo-immunization

Despite the use of several wash cycles and filters, it is not possible to separate the salvaged blood from fetal red blood cells. Transfusion of fetal cells (approximately 2–19 mL) into the maternal circulation therefore occurs [29]. Routine Kleihauer counts should be performed promptly in the postpartum period in all Rhesus negative mothers and anti-D treatment given as required.

Cost

Although the machines can be very expensive, most hospitals lease them from the manufacturer. The disposables cost approximately £140 per patient, equivalent to one unit of transfused blood. A systematic review of over 600 studies comparing various transfusion strategies to reduce allogenic blood transfusion found cell salvage was more cost-effective than all other strategies except acute normovolemic hemodilution[30].

SALVO

The recently completed UK-based randomized controlled trial into cell salvage in obstetrics (SALVO) has demonstrated a modest reduction in the need for donor blood transfusion when cell salvage was used routinely during cesarean section but this was not statistically significant. However, the increased rate of fetomaternal hemorrhage has raised concern about alloimmunization to Rhesus D and other red cell antigens[31]and the importance of adhering to anti-D prophylaxis.

Post Hemorrhage Care

Critical Care

The location for postoperative care depends on the volume of blood lost, the presence of ongoing coagulopathy, and whether any organ system requires support. The majority of patients will require high-dependency care that can usually be delivered in a maternity setting. A minority will require intensive care. The document "Providing equity of critical and maternity care for the critically ill pregnant or recently pregnant woman" calls for the standard of care to be high for both obstetric and critical care related needs irrespective of the setting in which this is delivered[32].

Critical care skills can be imported to labor ward via outreach or a critical care education program for midwives. Alternatively, obstetricians/midwives should provide specialist input to a patient in the intensive care unit.

Thromboprophylaxis

Once the bleeding has been controlled and the patient is stable, regular thromboprophylaxis should be commenced. If an epidural catheter or Bakri balloon remains in situ, the timing of thromboprophylaxis should be chosen carefully to facilitate its removal.

Debriefing and Counseling

Staff debriefing after a major hemorrhage can be a good opportunity to reinforce learning points and seek improvements for the future. This should be a blame-free forum, which takes place at the earliest possible opportunity.

Conclusion

Obstetric hemorrhage is a common yet challenging emergency responsible for significant maternal morbidity and mortality. A coordinated multidisciplinary response is required to identify, evaluate, and resuscitate the patient. General anesthesia is often the technique of choice. The use of blood and blood components should be guided by a combination of clinical assessment, point-of-care, and laboratory testing. Cell salvage can minimize the need for allogenic blood. Close observation of the patient will be required post bleed but this can be delivered in a maternity setting for the majority of patients.

Case Studies

Case Study 1
This case study describes the management of significant hemorrhage during an emergency cesarean section.
    The prior history was of a primigravida with a prolonged labor requiring augmentation with Syntocinon. An epidural was sited to provide labor analgesia.
    A trial of forceps in theater was unsuccessful, necessitating a full dilatation cesarean section. Post-delivery the uterus remained atonic despite uterotonics (Syntocinon, ergometrine, and carboprosthemabate) so a uterine tamponade (Bakri) balloon was inserted with good effect. Surgery was prolonged, so a further dose of local anesthetic was given via the epidural to maintain adequate anesthesia.

The patient required fluid resuscitation with 3000 mL of crystalloid and point-of-care testing was as follows – Hemocue: Hb 87, ROTEM: normal clotting profile – therefore no blood products were given. Additional IV access was secured and an arterial line was sited as blood loss reached 2 Lwith ongoing losses. Total blood loss was 2700 mL. A second dose of prophylactic antibiotics was administered.

Postoperatively, the patient received high-dependency care with regular observations and hourly urine output recorded on a track and trigger early warning chart. The epidural catheter was left in situ until the results of a full blood count, coagulation screen, and ROTEM were seen to be within safe limits for removal. The timing of thromboprophylaxis with low-molecular-weight heparin was chosen carefully so that the epidural catheter and uterine tamponade balloon could be removed when appropriate to do so.

This case illustrates the important peri- and postoperative considerations following unanticipated major obstetric hemorrhage.

Case Study 2

This case study describes the management of a patient undergoing elective cesarean section where major hemorrhage is anticipated.

The prior history is of a para 1 who underwent an elective cesarean section (CS) for breech presentation in a previous pregnancy. The 20-week gestation ultrasound scan showed an anterior placenta previa thought to be an accreta, which was confirmed on MRI imaging. Elective CS with interventional radiology was planned for 38 weeks' gestation.

Prophylactic internal iliac artery balloon catheters were inserted in the radiology suite and the patient then transferred to the operating theater. Two large-bore intravenous cannulae, an arterial line, and a central line were sited prior to induction of general anesthesia. Cell salvage commenced at the time of skin incision. After delivery, the placenta began to separate causing profuse bleeding despite inflation of the iliac artery balloons. In view of ongoing losses (5 L) a hysterectomy was performed.

Regular FBC, ABG, and ROTEM analysis guided transfusion: 2 units of RCC and subsequently 800 mL of salvaged blood were given. Two pools of FFP were given in response to a reduced amplitude FIBTEM trace at 10 minutes (A10, 5 mm) in the context of a slight reduction in EXTEM (Extrinsic Screening Test) trace at 10 minutes (A10, 41 mm) suggestive of fibrinogen deficiency. Platelet transfusion was not required. Total blood loss was 6 L.

The patient was transferred to the intensive care unit and after a period of observation, indicating hemodynamic stability and no signs of ongoing bleeding, she was extubated 4 hours later and transferred back to the labor ward for high-dependency care the next day.

This case illustrates the management of a morbidly adherent placenta where despite the use of additional monitoring, equipment, and multidisciplinary involvement, blood loss approached 100% of the patient's circulating volume.

References

1. Knight M, Kenyon S, Brocklehurst P *et al.* (eds) on behalf of MBRRACE. *Saving Lives, Improving Mothers' Care – Lessons learned to inform future maternity care from the UK and Ireland Confidential Enquiries into Maternal Deaths and Morbidity 2009–12*. Oxford: National Perinatal Epidemiology Unit, University of Oxford; 2014.

2. Healthcare Improvement Scotland. Scottish Confidential Audit Severe Maternal Morbidity 10th Annual Report; 2014. http://www.healthcareimprovementscotland.org/our_work/reproductive,_maternal_child/programme_resources/scasmm.aspx (accessed April 28 2015).

3. Association of Anesthetists of Great Britain and Ireland; Thomas D, Wee M, Clyburn P *et al.* Blood transfusion and the anesthetist: management of massive hemorrhage. *Anaesthesia* 2010; **65**(11): 1153–1161.

4. Draycott T, Winter C, Crofts J, Barnfield S. *Practical Obstetric Multi-professional Training (PROMPT) Trainer's Manual*. London: RCOG Press; 2008.

5. Crofts JF, Ellis D, Draycott TJ *et al.* Change in knowledge of midwives and obstetricians following obstetric emergency training: a randomised controlled trial of local hospital, simulation center and teamwork training. *BJOG: An International Journal of Obstetrics and Gynecology* 2007; **114**: 1534–1541.

6. https://www.resus.org.uk/pages/alsABCDE.htm (accessed April 28 2015).

7. National Institute for Health and Care Excellence. Detecting, Managing and Monitoring Hemostasis: Viscoelastometric Pointofcare Testing (ROTEM, TEG and Sonoclot Systems) Diagnostic Guidance 13: DG13; 2014. http://www.nice.org.uk/guidance/dg13 (Accessed July 13 2015).

8. Perel P, Roberts I. Colloids versus crystalloids for fluid resuscitation in critically ill patients. *Cochrane Database Systematics Reviews* 2007; **17**: CD000567.

9. RCOG. *Postpartum Hemorrhage, Prevention and Management. Green-Top Guideline No. 52*. London: Royal

College of Obstetricians and Gynecologists; 2015. https://www.rcog.org.uk/globalassets/documents/guidelines/gt52postpartumhemorrhage0411.pdf (accessed April 28 2015).

10. Lilley G, Burkett-St-Laurent D, Precious E et al. Measurement of blood loss during postpartum hemorrhage. *International Journal of Obstetric Anesthesia* 2015; **24**(1): 8–14.

11. RCOG. *Placenta Previa, Placenta Previa Accreta and Vasa Previa: Diagnosis and Management. Green-Top Guideline No. 27*. London: Royal College of Obstetricians and Gynecologists; 2015. https://www.rcog.org.uk/globalassets/documents/guidelines/gtg_27.pdf (accessed April 28 2015).

12. Charbit B, Mandelbrot L, Samain E et al. PPH Study Group. The decrease of fibrinogen is an early predictor of the severity of postpartum hemorrhage. *Journal of Thrombosis and Haemostasis* 2007; **5**(2): 266–273.

13. Stainsby D, MacLennan S, Thomas D, Isaac J, Hamilton PJ. Guidelines on the management of massive blood loss. *British Journal of Haematology* 2006; **135**: 634–641.

14. Allard S, Green L, Hunt BJ. How we manage the hematological aspects of major obstetric hemorrhage. *British Journal of Haematology* 2014; **164**(2): 177–188.

15. Wikkelsø AJ, Edwards HM, Afshari A et al. FIB-PPH trial group. Pre-emptive treatment with fibrinogen concentrate for postpartum hemorrhage: randomized controlled trial. *British Journal of Anaesthesia* 2015; **114**(4): 623–633.

16. Collins PW, Cannings-John R, Bruynseels D et al.; the OBS2 Study Team. Viscoelastometric-guided early fibrinogen concentrate replacement during postpartum haemorrhage: OBS2, a double-blind randomized controlled trial. *British Journal of Anaesthesia* 2017; aex181. doi:10.1093/bja/aex181 (accessed July 26 2017).

17. World Health Organization. *Recommendations for the Prevention and Treatment of Postpartum Hemorrhage*. Geneva: WHO; 2012. http://www.who.int/reproductivehealth/publications/maternal_perinatal_health/9789241548502/en/ (accessed April 28 2015).

18. Ducloy-Bouthors AS, Jude B, Duhamel A et al. High-dose tranexamic acid reduces blood loss in postpartum hemorrhage. *Critical Care* 2011; **15**(2): R117.

19. WOMAN Trial Collaborators. Effect of early tranexamic acid administration on mortality, hysterectomy, and other morbidities in women with post-partum haemorrhage (WOMAN): an international, randomised, double-blind, placebo-controlled trial. *Lancet* 2017; **389**: 2105–2116.

20. Lavigne-Lissalde G, Aya AG, Mercier FJ et al. Recombinant human FVIIa for reducing the need for invasive second-line therapies in severe refractory postpartum hemorrhage: a multicenter, randomized, open controlled trial. *Journal of Thrombosis and Haemostasis* 2015; **13**(4): 520–529.

21. UK National Institute for Health and Clinical Excellence. Intraoperative Blood Cell Salvage in Obstetrics. IP Guidance Number: IPG144; 2005. http://www.nice.org.uk/guidance (accessed April 28 2015).

22. Allam J, Cox M, Yentis SM. Cell salvage in obstetrics. *International Journal of Obstetric Anesthesia* 2008; **17**: 37–45.

23. Catling S, Thomas D. Intraoperative autologous blood transfusion. In Arulkumaran S, Karoshi M, Keith LG, Lalonde AB, B-Lynch C (eds) *A Comprehensive Textbook of Postpartum Hemorrhage*, 2nd edn. Sapiens Publishing.

24. Teig M, Harkness M, Catling S, Clark V. Survey of cell salvage use in obstetrics in the UK. Poster presentation OAA meeting Sheffield June 2007. *International Journal of Obstetric Anesthesia* 2007; **16** (Suppl 1): 30.

25. Teare KM, Sullivan IJ, Ralph CJ. Is cell salvaged vaginal blood loss suitable for re-infusion? *International Journal of Obstetric Anesthesia* 2015; **24**(2): 103–110.

26. Catling SJ, Williams S, Fielding A. Cell salvage in obstetrics: an evaluation of ability of cell salvage combined with leucocyte depletion filter to remove amniotic fluid from operative blood loss at cesarean section. *International Journal of Obstetric Anesthesia* 1999; **8**: 79–84.

27. Hussain S, Clyburn P. Cell salvage-induced hypotension and London buses. *Anesthesia* 2010; **65**(7): 661–663.

28. UK Cell Salvage Action Group. Intraoperative Cell Salvage in Obstetrics. http://transfusionguidelines.org.uk/transfusion-practice/uk-cell-salvage-action-group/technical-factsheets-and-frequently-asked-questions-faq (accessed April 28 2015).

29. Sullivan I, Faulds J, Ralph C. Contamination of salvaged maternal blood by amniotic fluid and fetal red cells during elective Cesarean section. *British Journal of Anesthesia* 2008; **101**: 225–229.

30. Davies L, Brown TJ, Haynes S et al. Cost effectiveness of cell salvage and alternative methods of minimizing perioperative allogeneic blood transfusion: a systematic review and economic model. *Health Technology Assessment* 2006; **10**: 1–228.

31. Khan K, Moore P, Wilson MJ et al. LB01: Cell Salvage during Caesarean Section: A Randomised Controlled Trial (The SALVO Trial). *American Journal of Obstetrics and Gynecology* 2017; **216**(1): S559 (Abstract).

32. The Maternal Critical Care Working Group. Providing Equity of Critical and Maternity Care for the Critically Ill Pregnant or Recently Pregnant Woman. https://www.rcoa.ac.uk/system/files/CSQ-ProvEqMatCritCare.pdf (accessed July 24 2017).

Management of Obstetric Hemorrhage: Hemostatic Management

Peter Collins and Rachel Collis

Introduction

Bleeding at the time of childbirth remains a common and demanding clinical emergency. Obstetric bleeding results mainly from physical causes which may be exacerbated by hemostatic impairment. The likelihood, severity, and timing of hemostatic impairment are dependent on the etiology of the bleed and most obstetric bleeds resolve without hemostatic interventions. There is limited evidence on appropriate intervention triggers and management strategies, with much of the literature and clinical guidelines relying on audit, interpretation of secondary outcomes, extrapolation from major trauma, and expert opinion[1,2]. National Institute for Health and Care Excellence (NICE) and World Health Organization (WHO) guidelines offer no advice on blood product use during PPH[3,4].

Hemostatic Changes Associated with PPH

There is increasing evidence that hemostatic impairment associated with bleeding in the pregnant population differs from that associated with trauma and the type and time of onset of coagulopathies depends on the underlying cause of bleeding (Table 18C.1)[5–7]. In the majority of cases, coagulation studies (PT/aPTT) remain normal despite large volumes of blood loss, which suggests adequate levels of coagulation factors [6,8,9]. When these were measured in 128 women with PPH they remained normal throughout despite severe bleeding[8]. In contrast, fibrinogen falls progressively as blood loss increases and reaches critically low levels earlier than other coagulation factors[9].

Table 18C.1 Coagulation abnormalities associated with various causes of postpartum hemorrhage

	Women with fibrinogen <2 g/L at 1000–2000 mL (%)	Women with PT or aPTT abnormal at 1000–2000 mL (%)	Women with platelets <75 at 1000–2000 mL (%)	Women requiring transfusion FFP (%)	Women requiring platelet transfusion (%)	Time of onset of coagulopathy	Bleeds >2000 mL (%)
Uterine atony (n=146)	2.2	1.4	0	14	2.4	Late	27
Genital tract and surgical trauma (n=126)	1.6	0	0.8	4	0.8	Late	13
Uterine rupture (n=3)	0	0	0	66	0	Late	100
Retained or adherent placenta (n=36)	6	6	3	8	3	Late	24
Placenta previa (n=8)	0	0	0	37.5	0	Late	50
Placental abruption (n=14)	38	0	0	42	21	Early (often before PPH recognized)	57
AFE (no data)						Early (often before PPH recognized)	

Data from Collins et al. 2014[6].
AFE, amniotic fluid embolus.

Changes Early during PPH

The type, severity, and rate of onset of coagulopathy vary with the etiology of the bleeding[5,10]. Uterine atony and surgical and genital tract trauma-induced bleeding (the cause of 80% of PPH) are usually associated with no significant coagulopathy with bleeds of 1000–2000 mL[6,8]. The fibrinogen level after 1000–2000 mL blood loss due to uterine atony, trauma, and retained or adherent placenta was, on average, 3.9 g/L, and PT and aPPT were normal in 98.4% and 98% of cases, respectively[7] (Table 18C.1). In placental abruption, the average fibrinogen was much lower at 2.2 g/L although the PT/aPTT ratios again remained normal[6]. In women in whom the diagnosis of PPH is delayed or underestimated, hemostatic abnormalities may be present at the time the bleeding is recognized.

Evolution of Hemostatic Failure

There is limited information on hemostatic changes during evolving PPH. A study measured serial coagulation factors during PPH and demonstrated remarkably little change in PT, fibrinogen, platelets, factor V, and factor II over time in both severe and non-severe cases. Factors V and II remained normal throughout the duration of the bleeds in almost all women. Only two women in this study had abruptions and so the findings may not apply in this situation[8]. If bleeding progresses, the majority of women will have a prolonged PT/aPTT after 5000 mL blood loss[9].

Dilutional Coagulopathy

Coagulopathies may develop secondary to infusion of crystalloid and colloid during resuscitation from dilution of coagulation factors[11]. If sufficiently large, volume replacement can lead to dilution of all coagulation factors and platelets.

Consumptive Coagulopathies

Consumption results from loss of blood and clots from the uterus and dysregulated activation of coagulation leading to a reduction in coagulation factors, especially fibrinogen and platelets[5,10,12]. Disseminated intravascular coagulation (DIC) is uncommon during PPH and very few cases fulfill internationally agreed criteria [5,6,10,13,14]. Consumptive coagulopathies are often localized to the placental bed (e.g. abruption) or related to coagulation factors being consumed in intrauterine clots (e.g. atony)[5]. DIC is associated with amniotic fluid embolism (AFE), some cases of severe pre-eclampsia/eclampsia, infected retained products, and some severe cases of abruption[15]. Whether localized or disseminated, consumption leads to critically low levels of coagulation factors, especially fibrinogen, earlier than would occur with dilution alone. Local activation of the fibrinolytic system at the time of delivery[16] contributes to a reduction in stable clot formation.

Thrombocytopenia

It is unusual for platelets to fall to clinically significant levels ($<75 \times 10^9$/L) due to atony or trauma [6,8] unless bleeds exceed 4000 mL or are associated with placental abruption or AFE[6,17]. Women may also develop clinically significant thrombocytopenia if platelets were low before labor, for example due to gestational thrombocytopenia, pre-eclampsia/eclampsia, or immune-mediated thrombocytopenia[17].

Role of Fibrinogen

There has been increasing interest in hypofibrinogenemia during PPH. Fibrinogen levels fall below the normal pregnancy range sooner than other coagulation factors[9] and, in some circumstances, may rapidly fall to <2 g/L[6,10]. There is strong evidence that a low Clauss fibrinogen is a good biomarker for progression from moderate to severe PPH[6,8,18–20].

In 128 women recruited at the time of a second-line uterotonic for resistant atony, a fibrinogen <2 g/L had a positive predictive value of 100% for progression to severe PPH while a level >4 g/L had a negative predictive value of 79%[8]. Another study reported a similar result, although all women with surgical bleeding or cesarean section were excluded[18]. A fibrinogen <2 g/L, taken on average 4 hours after the start of PPH, predicted progression to invasive procedures including iliac artery ligation, hysterectomy, and admission to level 3 intensive care[20]. In 346 women with any cause of PPH, recruited at around 1000–2000 mL blood loss, a fibrinogen <3 g/L, and especially <2 g/L, was associated with progression to larger bleeds, more prolonged bleeds, higher rates of RBC and FFP transfusion, and longer stays in high dependency (Figure18C.1)[6]. Fibrinogen is an independent predictor of successful arterial embolization: the mean (SD) fibrinogen level in the successful group was 2.89 (1.32) compared with 1.79 (0.9) in the unsuccessful group[21].

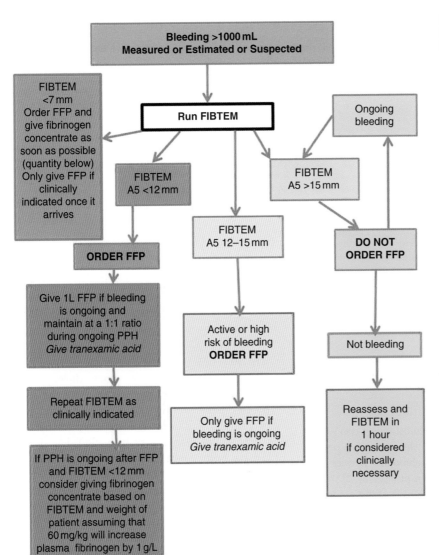

Figure 18C.1 Point-of-care FIBTEM algorithm used at The University Hospital of Wales 2015.

Combining studies in over 1700 women[6,8,18–20] demonstrates that a fibrinogen of less than 3 g/L and especially below 2 g/L, in the early phase of the PPH, is associated with progression, while a fibrinogen >4 g/L is not (Table 18C.2).

Monitoring Hemostasis during PPH

There are three strategies for assessing hemostasis during PPH: (i) clinical observation; (ii) laboratory-based PT/aPPT, Clauss fibrinogen, and platelet count; and (iii) point-of-care testing (POCT)[22]. All three may be used simultaneously. Coagulopathies may

evolve rapidly and repeated testing and observation of trends are more useful than single measurements.

Laboratory Coagulation Tests

Routine coagulation tests are widely available and have well-regulated quality control[5,22]. They are usually too slow to be clinically useful in acute and rapidly evolving bleeds and inevitably reflect past hemostatic status. The Clauss fibrinogen should always be measured as part of the routine coagulation screen because it falls early and may be reduced to a clinically significant level despite a normal PT/aPTT

219

Table 18C.2 Clauss fibrinogen as a biomarker for predicting progression of PPH

Paper	N	Entry criteria	Definition of progression	Fibrinogen level (g/L)	
				Non-progression	Progression
Charbit[8]	128	Second-line uterotonic after manual evacuation	Fall in Hb >40 g/L, ≥4 units RBC, need for invasive procedure[a]	Median (IQR) 4.4 (3.7–5.1)	Median (IQR) 3.3 (2.5–4.2)
Cortet[18]	738	Vaginal delivery >500 mL PPH	Fall in Hb >40 g/L, any RBC transfusion, need for invasive procedure, admission to ICU	Mean (SD) 4.2 (1.2)	Mean (SD) 3.4 (0.9)
		Excluding genital tract trauma, uterine rupture, accrete, and previa			
Gayat[20]	257	Admission to referral center for PPH[b]	Need for an invasive procedure	Median (IQR) 2.65 (2.08–3.46)[b]	Median (IQR) 1.8 (1.09–2.52)[b]
De Lloyd[19]	240	Any cause of PPH and time of first coagulation test	Need for ≥4 units RBC or PPH >2500 mL	Mean (SD) 4.4 (1.1)	Mean (SD) 3.1 (1.0)
Collins[6]	346	Any cause of PPH 1000–1500 mL	Need for ≥4 units RBC or PPH >2500 mL	Median (IQR) 3.9 (3.2–4.5)	Median (IQR) 2.8 (2.1–3.8)

[a] Most defined as progressing based on fall of Hb >40 g/L.
[b] Fibrinogen was taken on average 4 hours after the onset of bleeding on admission to a referral center, and this contributes to the lower fibrinogen levels in this cohort.

[5,22,23]. Derived fibrinogen (indirectly measured) may be misleading and should not be used[24].

Point-of-Care Tests of Hemostasis

POCT using viscoelastometric hemostatic assays (VHA) are becoming more common on delivery suites. A review of VHA, with the technology behind the devices and interpretation of results, has been published[22]. VHA normal ranges at the time of delivery differ from the non-pregnant normal range. The mean clot firmness/maximum amplitude are larger and clot/r time shorter and this should be taken into account during interpretation[22,25,26]. If fibrinolysis is severe and systemic, it can be detected by VHA although these systems are insensitive to local and less severe hyperfibrinolysis[27].

POCTs combined with a locally agreed treatment algorithm have been associated with decreased blood product use both outside and within the obstetric setting[7,22,28,29]. If POCTs are used, a quality control protocol should be agreed with the hematology laboratory. One expert group from the Association of Anaesthetists of Great Britain and Ireland has recommended the use of VHA for obstetric bleeding (http://www.aagbi.org/sites/default/files/obstetric_anesthetic_services_2013.pdf; accessed Jan 26 2015) although NICE state that there is currently insufficient evidence to recommend routine use of VHA for PPH (https://www.nice.org.uk/guidance/htdg13/chapter/1-executive-summary; accessed Feb 15 2015).

The ROTEM® FIBTEM assay can be used as a surrogate measure of fibrinogen during PPH [6,22,30,31]. This assay does not measure the same hemostatic parameter as Clauss fibrinogen but provides a similar indication of hemostatic competence and outcome[6]. Algorithms using ROTEM during PPH have been published (Figure 18C.2)[7,29]. To date, no validated algorithm for TEG® has been published[22,26]. POCT algorithms using ROTEM® are associated with reduced blood product usage without a detrimental effect on major PPH outcomes[7,29].

No studies have compared clinical outcomes when using coagulation screens and VHA during PPH, although it might be hypothesized that an earlier result would be beneficial. The major advantage of POCT is that the obstetric and anesthetic teams can rapidly identify whether bleeding has a purely obstetric cause with normal hemostasis or whether bleeding is exacerbated by abnormal hemostasis.

Treatment of Hemostatic Impairment

Blood Product Replacement

There are limited data to inform practice on the treatment of hemostatic impairment during PPH. It is not known whether hemostasis should be corrected to

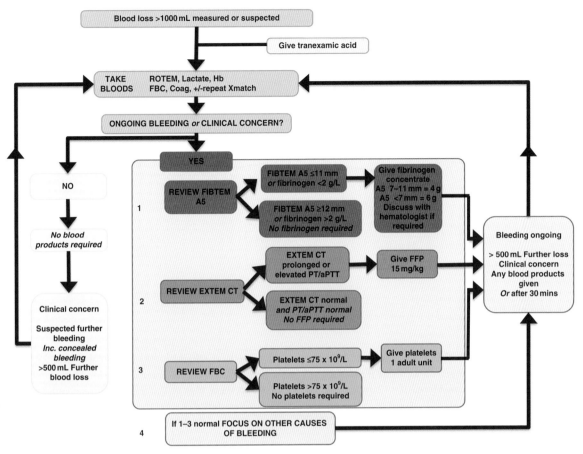

Figure 18C.2 Case 1 OBS1 outcomes.

normality for women at the time of delivery or to the non-pregnant healthy population. If bleeding has stopped, correction of abnormal hemostatic tests is not required but with ongoing bleeding, prompt correction is necessary. A suggested algorithm based on guidance from the Royal College of Obstetrics and Gynaecology Green-top Guideline published in 2016 is shown in Figure 18C.3[32].

The Role of Fibrinogen

Observational studies show that a fibrinogen level of 1–1.5 g/L is likely to be too low for adequate hemostasis during ongoing PPH. Fibrinogen below 3 g/L and especially below 2 g/L is associated with progression of bleeding, increased red blood cell and blood component requirement, and the need for invasive procedures. A fibrinogen >4 g/L is not associated with progression of bleeding[3,6,8,18–20]. A double-blind randomized controlled trial has shown that pre-emptive infusion of 2 g fibrinogen concentrate in women

with 500–1000 mL PPH has no benefit; however, in this study the fibrinogen level at the time of randomization was >4 g/L in almost all women and this is a likely explanation for the lack of a clinical effect[33].

Fibrinogen can be replaced by cryoprecipitate or fibrinogen concentrate, although fibrinogen concentrate is not licensed for this indication in some countries and cryoprecipitate is unavailable in others. Similar outcomes have been reported for cryoprecipitate and fibrinogen concentrate[34]. Two pools of cryoprecipitate increase the fibrinogen level by about 1 g/L in the average woman, although this will vary depending on consumption. Fibrinogen concentrate rapidly corrects severe hypofibrinogenemia during PPH and anecdotal studies report improved clinical hemostasis, but without adequate controls and appropriate study design, these reports are of limited value[23,34–36]. Increasing the fibrinogen level by 1 g/L requires about 60 mg/kg fibrinogen concentrate[35].

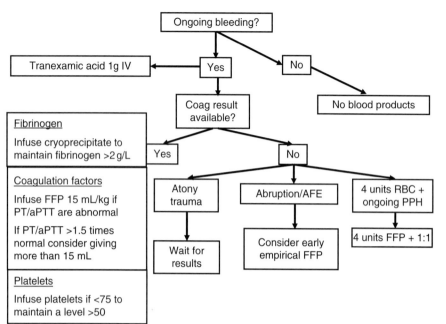

Figure 18C.3 Algorithm for hemostatic management of postpartum hemorrhage.

A description of service development showed that an infusion of 3 g fibrinogen concentrate if the FIBTEM A5 was <7 mm (and considered if <12 mm in severe bleeds) significantly reduced blood product usage, decreased transfusion-associated circulatory overload (TACO), and resulted in fewer bleeds requiring >5 units red cells compared with the use of shock packs (4 units red cells, 4 units FFP, and 1 pool of platelets)[29]. Three prospective randomized studies are investigating fibrinogen concentrate during PPH (NCT02155725, NCT01910675, and ISRCTN46295339).

A recently completed double-blind randomized controlled trial has shown that infusion of fibrinogen concentrate if the FIBTEM A5 was <16 mm did not improve outcomes. Further, if the Clauss fibrinogen at the time of the infusion was >2 g/L or the FIBTEM A5 was >12 mm, infusion of fibrinogen concentrate did not reduce blood product usage or bleed volume.

Based on available evidence, during ongoing PPH, cryoprecipitate or fibrinogen concentrate should be infused to maintain a fibrinogen level >2 g/L (FIBTEM A5 about 12 mm) even if PT/aPTT are normal[7]. There is no benefit of increasing the fibrinogen level above 4 g/L[33].

The Role of Fresh Frozen Plasma

Formulaic protocols such as 1:1, 3:2, or 6:4 RBC:FFP, based on data derived from massive trauma, have been advocated for PPH[1,37,38] (https://www.cmqcc.org/ob_hemorrhage; accessed Jan 27 2015). There is no evidence to show that this practice improves outcomes in PPH. One study describes the use of fixed ratio resuscitation of 3:2 and reports decreased red blood cell usage by 15% and increased FFP use by 60%. The study introduced many other practices to control PPH and so it is not possible to assess the impact of this transfusion policy[37,38]. The drawbacks of early FFP are that the majority of women will have normal coagulation at the time of administration[6,8,9] and its association with an increased risk of TACO[29] and transfusion-related acute lung injury (TRALI)[39]. TRALI is particularly associated with blood product use in women with pre-eclampsia[39]. Early FFP may result in women being infused with blood products with lower concentrations of fibrinogen and other coagulation factors (FVIII, VWF) than they have circulating because FFP has a fibrinogen level of around 2–2.5 g/L compared with an average fibrinogen of 4–4.5 g/L at the time of moderate/severe PPH[33,40].

There are limited data on the role of laboratory or POC coagulation tests to guide FFP replacement during PPH. An algorithm based on EXTEM and FIBTEM A5 has shown that it is safe to withhold FFP if the EXTEM is <100s and FIBTEM A5 above 12 mm (Clauss fibrinogen of about 2.2 g/L)[29]. Although this study was observational and not randomized, it is the first to suggest a potential intervention trigger in PPH.

Transfusion of Fresh Frozen Plasma

If bleeding has stopped no FFP is required. If POCTs are available, initial FFP transfusion can be guided by EXTEM and FIBTEM[7,29]. There are no published data to guide FFP transfusion based on TEG results.

If PT/aPTT results are available, most guidelines advocate FFP infusion to maintain a PT/aPTT ratio of less than 1.5× normal[1,2]. The Royal College of Obstetrics and Gynaecology[1] and the International Society on Thrombosis and Haemostasis[41] recommend transfusing FFP if the PT/aPTT is above the normal range (1.2× normal) to limit progression to 1.5× normal. If the PT/aPTT is >1.5× normal the volume of FFP required to correct hemostasis is likely to be greater than 15 mL/kg[42].

If results of hemostasis tests are not available and PPH is severe and ongoing, the only option is to use formulaic replacement. In the absence of high-quality evidence in PPH, guidelines recommend that if bleeding is ongoing after 4 units RBC have been transfused then 4 units of FFP should be infused and 1:1 RBC: FFP transfusion maintained until tests of hemostasis are available. It must be recognized, however, that this strategy will result in many women receiving FFP despite normal coagulation. FFP transfusion earlier than this could be considered for placental abruption or AFE and delayed presentations because early hemostatic impairment is more likely. In very severe bleeds, if 8 units of RBC and FFP have been transfused and tests of hemostasis are still not available then infusion of two pools of cryoprecipitate may be considered.

Transfusion of Platelets

There is wide consensus that platelets should be transfused at 75×10^9/L to maintain a level $>50 \times 10^9$/L during ongoing PPH[1,2]. Women who develop a platelet count $<75 \times 10^9$/L during PPH either have low platelets prior to labor, are bleeding secondary to placental abruption or AFE, or have bleeds >4000 mL[17]. A strategy of 1:1:1 RBC:FFP:platelet transfusion would, therefore, inevitably result in multiple platelet transfusions well above consensus levels, and we recommend against this practice. If women have received 8 units of RBC and no platelet count is available, infusion of one pool of platelets may be considered.

Other Hemostatic Agents

Tranexamic Acid

Tranexamic acid reduces bleeding and transfusion requirement in massive hemorrhage secondary to a number of non-obstetric causes[43]. Its role in obstetric bleeding has also now been demonstrated [44,45]. An open-label study of 144 women randomized to tranexamic acid or placebo after 800 mL blood loss reported a reduction in total blood loss, shorter period of bleeding, and fewer women progressing to severe PPH or blood transfusion[46]. A double-blind randomized control trial of tranexamic acid versus placebo at elective cesarean section reported reduced blood loss[47]. The double-blinded WOMAN study confirmed a reduction in death due to bleeding if tranexamic acid is given within 3 hours of PPH after 500 mL[48].

Recombinant Factor VIIa

rFVIIa has been used in life-threatening PPH or in an attempt to prevent hysterectomy, although this is an unlicensed indication and evidence is predominantly registry based[49,50]. The use of rFVIIa is associated with thrombotic complications[51]. A recent open-label study of 60 µg/kg rFVIIa versus placebo in PPH unresponsive to uterotonics demonstrated a reduction in invasive procedures from 93% to 52% (mainly because of fewer embolizations) although there was no difference in red cell or FFP usage or hysterectomy. There were two thrombotic events in the rFVIIa arm (not significantly different from placebo)[52]. The open-label design of this study means that the primary outcome may have been influenced by knowledge of whether rFVIIa had been given or not. NICE recommend that other coagulation factors should be normal before considering infusing rFVIIa[3]. The optimal dose of rFVIIa is unknown but restoration of normal thrombin generation is likely to be achieved with less than 90 µg/kg and lower doses may be less thrombotic. If two doses of rFVIIa have not arrested bleeding, further doses are unlikely to work. Our current policy is not to use rFVIIa for PPH.

Prothrombin Complex Concentrate (PCC)

PCC has been suggested during PPH (http://www.aagbi.org/sites/default/files/obstetric_anesthetic_servi

ces_2013.pdf; accessed Feb 15 2015). A study is currently investigating its role in combination with fibrinogen concentrate during PPH 2000–3000 mL (NCT01910675). PCCs are associated with thrombotic events in the non-obstetric population. A deficiency of FII, VII, IX, or X, either assayed directly[8] or assumed because of an abnormal PT/aPTT[9], is rare during PPH and so replacement of these coagulation factors will only occasionally be useful. We do not support the use of PCC outside a clinical trial.

Thromboprophylaxis

Women who have experienced PPH are at increased risk of venous thrombosis. Venous thromboprophylaxis should be started as soon as feasible once bleeding has been controlled, and continued according to local and national guidelines.

Conclusions

Hemostatic impairment is uncommon during PPH. The formulaic approach to management with shock packs does not take into account that in the majority of PPHs the mother's fibrinogen level will be greater than that in the FFP administered and therefore unmonitored usage will lead to dilution and possibly contribute to pulmonary complications. POC testing allows real time monitoring and a tailored approach to coagulopathy management. Monitored administration of fibrinogen concentrate has led to a fall in blood product usage but the results of trials are required before recommendations on its routine use can be made.

Case Studies

Case Study 1
A fit and well 18-year-old primigravida had a forceps delivery in theater under spinal block with a 700-mL measured blood loss. In the recovery room, she had a small bleed of 300 mL and then 60 minutes later was noted to be hypotensive and tachycardic and a further 1000 mL blood loss from uterine atony noted. Total measured blood loss was 2000 mL and was ongoing. The major hemorrhage protocol was activated and 4 units of RBC ordered. POC testing showed an Hb of 82 g/dL, a lactate of 3.5 mmol/L, and FIBTEM A5 of 22 mm. FFP was ordered but not delivered to the delivery suite. She returned to theater and had a small piece of residual placenta removed under the residual spinal block. Total blood loss was 3200 mL but despite 4 units of RBC and 2.5 L of clear fluids her FIBTEM remained at 19 mm then 14 mm, at which time the bleeding had completely settled. She made an uneventful recovery requiring no further blood and did not receive FFP.

Case Study 2
A multiparous woman with a previous history of placental abruption was admitted to the delivery suite complaining of abdominal pain. There was no overt bleeding but she was tachycardic and hypotensive. Fetal distress was noted on the cardiotocograph and a decision for immediate cesarean section under general anesthetic was made. The major hemorrhage protocol was activated and 4 units of RBC and FFP ordered. The A5 of 8 mm became available at the same time as the baby was delivered; a large retroplacental clot was noted, followed by a very rapid PPH of 2000 mL. The RBC arrived within 20 minutes of request but due to thawing, the FFP was delayed. Despite conventional uterotonics, ongoing bleeding was noted and a consultant hematologist issued 4 g of fibrinogen concentrate, which was given prior to the FFP arriving. Hemostasis improved and a repeat A5 was 11 mm. The total measured blood loss was 2800 mL and in total she received 4 units of RBC, 4 units of FFP, 1 g of tranexamic acid, and 4 g of fibrinogen concentrate. She made an uneventful recovery.

References

1. Mavrides E, Allard S, Chandraharan E *et al.* on behalf of the Royal College of Obstetricians and Gynecologists. Postpartum haemorrhage prevention and management. *BJOG: An International Journal of Obstetrics and Gynecology* 2016 http://onlinelibrary.wiley.com/doi/10.1111/1471-0528.14178/epdf (accessed Feb 21 Feb 2017).

2. Thomas D, Wee M, Clyburn P *et al.* Blood transfusion and the anesthetist: Management of massive hemorrhage. *Anesthesia* 2010; **65**: 1153–1161.

3. Kenyon S. Intrapartum Care: Care of Healthy Women and Their Babies During Childbirth. 2007. http://www.nice.org.uk/guidance/cg55/chapter/guidance

4. World Health Organization. WHO Guidelines for the Management of Postpartum Hemorrhage and Retained Placenta; 2009. http://apps.who.int/iris/bitstream/10665/75411/1/9789241548502_eng.pdf

5. Allard S, Green L, Hunt BJ. How we manage the hematological aspects of major obstetric hemorrhage. *British Journal of Haematology* 2014; **164**: 177–188.

6. Collins PW, Lilley G, Bruynseels D. Fibrin-based clot formation as an early and rapid biomarker for progression of postpartum hemorrhage: a prospective study. *Blood* 2014; **124**: 585–595.

7. Collis RE, Collins PW. Hemostatic management of obstetric hemorrhage. *Anesthesia* 2015; **70**: 78–86.

8. Charbit B, Mandelbrot L, Samain E *et al.* The decrease of fibrinogen is an early predictor of the severity of postpartum hemorrhage. *Journal of Thrombosis and Hemostasis* 2007; **5**: 266–273.

9. De Lloyd L, Bovington R, Kaye A *et al.* Standard hemostatic tests following major obstetric hemorrhage. *International Journal of Obstetric Anesthesia* 2011; **20**: 135–141.

10. Thachil J, Toh CH. Disseminated intravascular coagulation in obstetric disorders and its acute hematological management. *Blood Reviews* 2009; **23**: 167–176.

11. Hiippala ST, Myllyla GJ, Vahtera EM. Hemostatic factors and replacement of major blood loss with plasma-poor red cell concentrates. *Anesthesia and Analgesia* 1995; **81**: 360–365.

12. James AH, McLintock C, Lockhart E. Postpartum hemorrhage: When uterotonics and sutures fail. *American Journal of Hematology* 2012; **87**: S16–S22.

13. Levi M, Toh CH, Thachil J, Watson HG. Guidelines for the diagnosis and management of disseminated intravascular coagulation. *British Journal of Haematology* 2009; **145**: 24–33.

14. Wada H, Thachil J, Di Nisio M *et al.* Guidance for diagnosis and treatment of disseminated intravascular coagulation from harmonization of the recommendations from three guidelines. *Journal of Thrombosis and Haemostasis* 2013; **11**: 761–767.

15. Levi M. Pathogenesis and management of peripartum coagulopathic calamities (disseminated intravascular coagulation and amniotic fluid embolism). *Thrombosis Research* 2013; **131**: S32–S34.

16. Bonnar J, McNicol GP, Douglas AS. Coagulation and fibrinolytic mechanisms during and after normal childbirth. *BMJ* 1970; **2**: 200–203.

17. Jones R, de Lloyd L, Kealaher EJ *et al.* Platelet count and transfuion requirements during moderate or severe postpartum haemorrhage. *Anaesthesia* 2016; **71**: 648–656.

18. Cortet M, Deneux-Tharaux C, Dupont C *et al.* Association between fibrinogen level and severity of postpartum hemorrhage: Secondary analysis of a prospective trial. *British Journal of Anaesthesia* 2012; **108**: 984–989.

19. De Lloyd L, Collins PW, Kaye A, Collis RE. Early fibrinogen as a predictor of red cell requirements during postpartum hemorrhage. *International Journal of Obstetric Anesthesia* 2012; **21**: S13.

20. Gayat E, Resche-Rigon M, Morel O *et al.* Predictive factors of advanced interventional procedures in a multicenter severe postpartum hemorrhage study. *Intensive Care Medicine* 2011; **37**: 1816–1825.

21. Poujade O, Zappa M, Letendre I, *et al.* Predictive factors for failure of pelvic arterial embolization for postpartum hemorrhage. *International Journal of Gynecology and Obstetrics* 2012; **117**: 119–123.

22. Solomon C, Collis RE, Collins PW. Hemostatic monitoring during postpartum hemorrhage and implications for management. *British Journal of Anesthesia* 2012; **109**: 851–863.

23. Bell SF, Rayment R, Collins PW, Collis RE. The use of fibrinogen concentrate to correct hypofibrinogenemia rapidly during obstetric hemorrhage. *International Journal of Obstetric Anesthesia* 2010; **19**: 218–223.

24. Mackie IJ, Kitchen S, Machin SJ, Lowe GDO. Guidelines on fibrinogen assays. *British Journal of Haematology* 2003; **121**: 396–404.

25. De Lange NM, Lance MD, De Groot R, *et al.* Obstetric hemorrhage and coagulation: An update. Thromboelastography, thromboelastometry, and conventional coagulation tests in the diagnosis and prediction of postpartum hemorrhage. *Obstetrical and Gynecological Survey* 2012; **67**: 426–435.

26. Hill JS, Devenie G, Powell M. Point-of-care testing of coagulation and fibrinolytic status during postpartum hemorrhage: Developing a thrombelastography©-guided transfusion algorithm. *Anesthesia and Intensive Care* 2012; **40**: 1007–1015.

27. Raza I, Davenport R, Rourke C et al. The incidence and magnitude of fibrinolytic activation in trauma patients. *Journal of Thrombosis and Haemostasis* 2013; **11**: 307–314.

28. Afshari A, Wikkelso A, Brok J, Moller AM, Wetterslev J. Thrombelastography (TEG) or thromboelastometry (ROTEM) to monitor hemotherapy versus usual care in patients with massive transfusion. Cochrane Database of Systematic Reviews 2011; (**3**): CD007871.

29. Mallaiah S, Barclay P, Harrod I, Chevannes C, Bhalla A. Introduction of an algorithm for ROTEM-guided fibrinogen concentrate administration in major obstetric hemorrhage. *Anesthesia* 2015; **70**: 166–175.

30. Huissoud C, Carrabin N, Audibert F et al. Bedside assessment of fibrinogen level in postpartum hemorrhage by thrombelastometry. *BJOG: An International Journal of Obstetrics and Gynecology* 2009; **116**: 1097–1102.

31. Van Rheenen-Flach LE, Zweegman S, Boersma F et al. A prospective longitudinal study on rotation thromboelastometry in women with uncomplicated pregnancies and postpartum. *Australian and New Zealand Journal of Obstetrics and Gynaecology* 2013; **53**: 32–36.

32. Pavord S, Maybury H. How I treat postpartum hemorrhage. Blood 2015; **125**: 2759–2770.

33. Wikkelsoe AJ, Edwards HM, Afshari A et al. Pre-emptive treatment with fibrinogen concentrate for postpartum hemorrhage: randomized controlled trial. *British Journal of Anesthesia* 2015; **114**: 623–633.

34. Ahmed S, Harrity C, Johnson S et al. The efficacy of fibrinogen concentrate compared with cryoprecipitate in major obstetric hemorrhage – an observational study. *Transfusion Medicine* 2012; **22**: 344–349.

35. Gollop ND, Chilcott J, Benton A et al. National audit of the use of fibrinogen concentrate to correct hypofibrinogenemia. *Transfusion Medicine* 2012; **22**: 350–355.

36. Weinkove R, Rangarajan S. Fibrinogen concentrate for acquired hypofibrinogenemic states. *Transfusion Medicine* 2008; **18**: 151–157.

37. Shields LE, Smalarz K, Reffigee L et al. Comprehensive maternal hemorrhage protocols improve patient safety and reduce utilization of blood products. *American Journal of Obstetrics and Gynecology* 2011; **205**: 368.

38. Shields LE, Wiesner S, Fulton J, Pelletreau B. Comprehensive maternal hemorrhage protocols reduce the use of blood products and improve patient safety. *American Journal of Obstetrics and Gynecology* 2015; **212**: 272–280.

39. Teofili L, Bianchi M, Zanfini BA et al. Acute lung injury complicating blood transfusion in post-partum hemorrhage: Incidence and risk factors. *Mediterranean Journal of Hematology and Infectious Diseases* 2014; **6**: e2014.069.

40. Collins PW, Solomon C, Sutor K et al. Theoretical modelling of fibrinogen supplementation with therapeutic plasma, cryoprecipitate, or fibrinogen concentrate. *British Journal of Anaesthesia* 2014; **113**: 585–595.

41. Collins PW, Kadir R, Thachil J. Management of coagulopathy associated with postpartum haemorrhage: guidance from the SSC of ISTH. *Journal of Thrombosis and Haemostasis* 2016; **14**: 205–210.

42. Chowdhury P, Saayman AG, Paulus U, Findlay GP, Collins PW. Efficacy of standard dose and 30 ml/kg fresh frozen plasma in correcting laboratory parameters of hemostasis in critically ill patients. *British Journal of Haematology* 2004; **125**: 69–73.

43. CRASH-2 Collaborators. The importance of early treatment with tranexamic acid in bleeding trauma patients: An exploratory analysis of the CRASH-2 randomised controlled trial. *Lancet* 2011; **377**: 1096–1101.

44. Novikova N, Hofmeyr GL. Tranexamic acid for preventing postpartum hemorrhage. *Cochrane Database of Systematic Reviews* 2010; (**7**): CD007872.

45. Ferrer P, Roberts I, Sydenham E, Blackhall K, Shakur H. Anti-fibrinolytic agents in postpartum hemorrhage: A systematic review. *BMC Pregnancy Childbirth* 2009; **9**: 29.

46. Ducloy-Bouthors AS, Jude B, Duhamel A et al. High-dose tranexamic acid reduces blood loss in postpartum hemorrhage. *Critical Care* 2011; **15**: R117.

47. Gungorduk K, Yildirim G, Asicioglu O et al. Efficacy of intravenous tranexamic acid in reducing blood loss after elective cesarean section: A prospective, randomized, double-blind, placebo-controlled study. *American Journal of Perinatology* 2011; **28**: 233–239.

48. WOMAN Trial Collaborators. Effect of early tranexamic acid administration on mortality, hysterectomy, and other morbidities in women with post-partum haemorrhage (WOMAN): an international, randomised, double-blind, placebo-controlled trial. *Lancet* 2017; **389**: 2105–2116.

49. Alfirevic Z, Elbourne D, Pavord S et al. Use of recombinant activated factor vii in primary postpartum hemorrhage: The northern European registry 2000–2004. *Obstetrics and Gynecology* 2007; **110**: 1270–1278.

50. Franchini M, Franchi M, Bergamini V et al. The use of recombinant activated FVII in postpartum hemorrhage. *Clinical Obstetrics and Gynecology* 2010; **53**: 219–227.

51. Levi M, Levy JH, Andersen HF, Truloff D. Safety of recombinant activated factor VII in randomized clinical trials. *New England Journal of Medicine* 2010; **363**: 1791–1800.

52. Lavigne-Lissalde G. Recombinant human factor VIIa for reducing the need for invasive second line therapies in severe refractory postpartum hemorrhage: A multicenter, randomised open controlled study. *Journal of Thrombosis and Hemostasis* 2015; **13**: 520–529.

Management of Obstetric Hemorrhage: Radiological Management

Narayan Karunanithy and Athanasios Diamantopoulos

Background

Postpartum hemorrhage (PPH) is defined as estimated blood loss of >500 mL after vaginal delivery or >1000 mL after cesarean delivery. PPH accounts for 25% of maternal mortality and in some countries the rates are as high as 60%[1]. It is recognized that the morbidity and mortality associated with PPH are largely preventable[2]. While risk factors for developing PPH are known, the majority of cases of PPH (approximately two-thirds) occur in women with no known risk factors. The focus of management is hence on early identification and instigation of appropriate treatment[3].

In recent years, interventional radiology (IR) has established an important role in treating PPH in a minimally invasive manner, negating the need for the woman to undergo hysterectomy, which carries significant morbidity, and loss of fertility[4]. Further, women considered high risk of PPH could undergo certain prophylactic IR procedures at the time of delivery that reduces their risk of significant bleeding[4].

The aims of this chapter are to describe the relevant IR techniques and discuss patient selection, workup, and published guidelines on the role of interventional radiology in the management of PPH.

Etiology

Risk factors for PPH are summarized in Table 18D.1. Some of the causes may have been recognized prior to delivery. Abnormal placentation (placenta accreta and placenta previa) is diagnosed on antenatal ultrasound or magnetic resonance imaging[5]. Placenta accreta refers to a morbidly adherent placenta and dependent on the degree of invasion into and then through the myometrium is classified as acreta, increta, and percreta, respectively[6]. Placenta previa is defined as a low-lying placenta that wholly (major) or partially (minor/partial) covers the cervical os. Uterine atony remains the leading cause of PPH, accounting for approximately 80% of cases[3].

Apart from abnormal placentation and known coagulation defect, the other causes of PPH often only become apparent peripartum. Hence, although labor and childbirth are very much natural processes, contingency plans need to be put in place in every birth plan to manage significant PPH if it were to occur.

Management Algorithm of Postpartum Hemorrhage and the Role of Interventional Radiology

First-line management of PPH involves medical therapy with uterotonic agents like oxytocin, ergometrine, or a prostaglandin drug (misoprostol)[3]. Supportive measures initiated include fluid resuscitation (crystalloids and/or blood products) and correction of any coagulation defect. When there is persistent bleeding despite these supportive measures, uterine artery embolization (UAE) performed by interventional radiology is recommended[3]. When appropriate IR facility is unavailable or unsuitable, surgical intervention in the form of uterine compression suture or hysterectomy is performed. In cases where control of hemorrhage is required, such as in planned cesareans for pre-known or suspected placental abnormalities, and prior to either hysterectomy or uterine embolization, prophylactic balloon occlusion of the internal iliac or the anterior division of the internal iliac arteries is proposed.

Interventional Radiology: Technical Considerations

Treatment of Postpartum Hemorrhage

For interventional radiology procedures to be performed in a timely, safe, and effective manner, access to suitable imaging in the obstetric unit or in a

Table 18D.1 Risk factors for developing postpartum hemorrhage

Cause	Description
Early (<24 hours)	
Atonic uterus	Following prolonged labor
	Multiple pregnancies
	Obesity (BMI >35)
Abnormal placentation	Placenta previa
	Placenta accreta
	Placental abruption
Uterine & cervical injury	Instrumental vaginal delivery
	Surgical complications from cesarean section
	Episiotomies
Coagulation defects	Pre-eclampsia/gestational hypertension
Late (24 hours–12 weeks)	
Retained products of conception	
Infection	
Coagulation defects	

From ref. [3].

dedicated IR suite nearby is vital[3]. Interventional radiologists familiar with the vascular territory being treated and experienced in use of the various embolic materials are essential. Informed consent should be obtained if feasible following discussion with the patient and family.

Common femoral artery access is achieved either by palpation or under ultrasound guidance and a 5 Fr sheath (Johnson & Johnson, Fremont, CA, USA) inserted. It is the author's preference to gain access under ultrasound guidance, as it is safer and quicker considering the emergent situation and hypotension from blood loss causes reduction in the caliber of the arteries. An aortogram covering the pelvic vessels may be performed first using a 4/5 Fr pigtail catheter (Cook Medical, Bloomington, IN, USA) to localize a traumatic uterine/cervical injury if this is suspected. When a definite bleeding site is recognized, the feeding artery is selectively catheterized with a microcatheter (Progreat, Terumo Medical, Somerset, NJ, USA) and embolized with coils and/or Polyvinyl Alcohol particles (Cook Medical, Bloomington, IN, USA).

If, as is more often the case, a bleeding source is not identified, the anterior divisions of the respective internal iliac arteries are cannulated in turn. It is preferable to selectively catheterize the uterine arteries if time permits and it is technically feasible. The embolic agent of choice in these cases is absorbable gelatin sponge (Gelfoam, Pfizer Inc, New York,

NY, USA). Sometimes it may prove difficult to cannulate the internal iliac artery on the same side as that of the access common femoral artery. Under these circumstances, the contralateral common femoral artery access would allow straightforward access to the target internal iliac artery[7].

Prophylactic Balloon Occlusion

In patients with abnormal placentation and hence considered high risk during delivery, prophylactic balloon occlusion of both internal iliac arteries may help control/reduce postpartum hemorrhage[6]. The placement of the occlusion balloon catheters is ideally carried out prior to advanced labor. Via access from both common femoral arteries, occlusion balloon catheters (Boston Scientific, Hemel Hempstead, Herts, UK) are placed into the internal iliac arteries feeding the uterus. The catheters are connected to heparin infusion pumps to prevent surrounding thrombosis. The balloons can then be inflated to occlude the vessels if PPH occurs during delivery. Embolization can be performed through the balloon catheters if bleeding continues with absorbable gelatin sponge (Gelfoam, Pfizer Inc, New York, NY, USA). Even if the decision is to perform a hysterectomy, perioperative balloon occlusion +/– embolization may reduce blood loss and associated morbidity.

Outcomes

Transarterial embolization (TAE) to treat PPH was first described in 1979 and since then there have been a number of studies that have described its benefits. Reported clinical success rates range between 71 and 98%[8,9]. Absorbable gelatin sponge (Gelfoam, Pfizer Inc, New York, NY, USA) was the embolic agent of choice in all the studies. Factors that led to failure in achieving hemostasis were those most likely due to delayed instigation of IR treatment and included onset of disseminated intravascular coagulation (DIC), hemodynamic instability, and hemoglobin <8 g/dL.

Complications of TAE are relatively rare with an overall reported incidence of approximately 9%. Complications include transient fever, transient buttock ischemia, foot ischemia, iliac artery perforation, and abscess formation[9].

The role of prophylactic balloon occlusion in the management of abnormal placentation remains debatable. In small case-controlled series, mean estimated blood loss (2.1 L vs 2.8 L) and requirement of massive transfusions (31% vs 52%) has been shown to be lower with the use of prophylactic balloon occlusion[10]. The impact appears to be greater in cases of the more invasive placenta percreta[11].

Complications related to prophylactic balloon occlusion are estimated to be approximately 3% and include iliac artery thrombosis and transection[10].

Published Guidelines

Currently both WHO[1] and RCOG[3] recommend the use of arterial embolization to treat PPH following balloon tamponade and prior to surgery, if the necessary resources are available.

Summary

Transarterial embolization and prophylactic balloon occlusion are safe and effective methods in treating PPH. They can reduce transfusion requirement, preserve fertility, and thus have the potential to reduce maternal morbidity and mortality. Obstetric departments should incorporate early referral to IR and consideration of embolization into protocols for management of PPH.

Case Studies

Case Study 1

A 30-year-old woman presented with massive postpartum hemorrhage after forceps vaginal delivery, warranting transfer to the intensive care unit. Despite aggressive resuscitation, the patient showed evidence of hypotensive shock. A catheter angiogram performed of the right internal iliac artery (Figure 18D.1a) showed active extravasation from the inferior vesicle branch of the anterior division. Selective catheterization with a microcatheter (Fig 18D.1b) demonstrated the bleeding point more clearly. Coil embolization (Fig 18D.1c) was performed to effectively treat the hemorrhage source. A completion aortogram (Fig 18D.1d) showed complete embolization and no further bleeding source. The patient exhibited no further evidence of PPH and made a complete recovery.

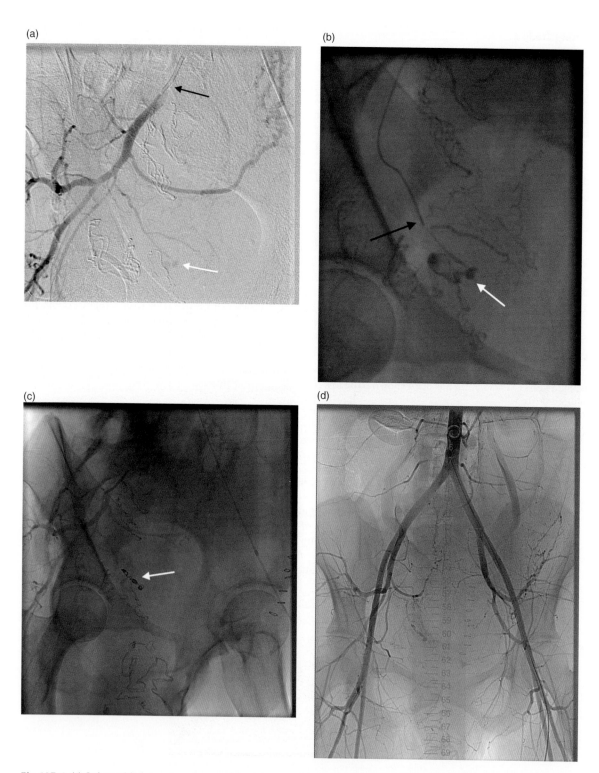

Fig 18D.1 (a) Catheter (black arrow) angiogram of the right internal iliac artery demonstrates active arterial extravasation from an inferior vesicle branch (white arrow). (b) Selective catheterization with a microcatheter (black arrow) shows the bleeding point (white arrow) more clearly. (c) Coil embolization (white arrow) has been performed, resulting in complete obliteration of the bleeding. (d) Completion aortogram confirms no further bleeding sources.

Case Study 2

A 39-year-old woman presented with massive postpartum hemorrhage 1 day after normal vaginal delivery, thought to be secondary to partial retained products. An aortogram (Figure 18D.2a) shows markedly hypertrophied left uterine artery. Selective catheterization (Figure 18D.2b) and embolization (Figure 18D.2c) was performed with gelfoam. There were no further episodes of PPH and the patient had an uneventful recovery.

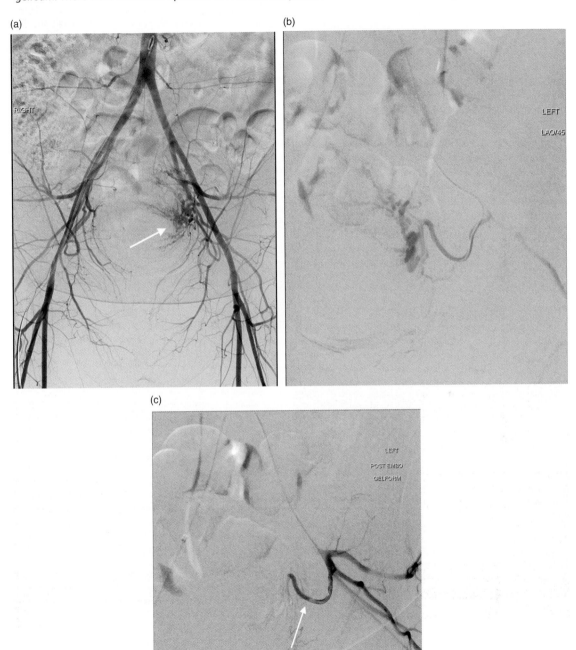

Fig 18D.2 (a) Aortogram shows markedly hypertrophied left uterine artery (arrow). (b) The left uterine artery has been selectively catheterized and embolization performed with injection of gelfoam to occlude flow. (c) Angiogram performed after gelfoam embolization confirms satisfactory occlusion of flow.

References

1. World Health Organization. *WHO Recommendations for the Prevention and Treatment of Postpartum Hemorrhage.* Geneva: WHO; 2012.

2. Healthcare Commission. *Investigation into 10 Maternal Deaths at, or Following Delivery at, Northwick Park Hospital, North West London Hospitals NHS Trust, Between April 2002 and April 2005.* London: Commission for Healthcare Audit and Inspection; 2006.

3. Royal College of Obstetricians and Gynecologists. *Postpartum Hemorrhage, Prevention and Management. Green-Top Guideline No. 52.* London: Royal College of Obstetricians and Gynecologists; 2011.

4. Royal College of Obstetricians and Gynecologists. *The Role of Emergency and Elective Interventional Radiology in Postpartum Hemorrhage (Good Practice No. 6).* London: RCOG; 2007.

5. Silver RM, Barbour KD. Placenta accreta spectrum: accreta, increta, and percreta. *Obstetrics and Gynecology Clinics of North America* 2015; **42**(2): 381–402.

6. Royal College of Obstetricians and Gynecologists. *Placenta Previa and Placenta Previa Accreta: Diagnosis and Management. Green-Top Guideline No. 27.* London: Royal College of Obstetricians and Gynecologists; 2005.

7. Gipson MG, Smith MT. Endovascular therapies for primary postpartum hemorrhage: techniques and outcomes. *Seminars in Interventional Radiology* 2013; **30**(4): 333–339.

8. Lee HY, Shin JH, Kim J *et al.* Primary postpartum hemorrhage: outcome of pelvic arterial embolization in 251 patients at a single institution. *Radiology* 2012; **264**(3): 903–909.

9. Kim YJ, Yoon CJ, Seong NJ *et al.* Failed pelvic arterial embolization for postpartum hemorrhage: clinical outcomes and predictive factors. *Journal of Vascular and Interventional Radiology* 2013; **24**(5): 703–709.

10. Ballas J, Hull AD, Senz C *et al.* Preoperative intravascular balloon catheters and surgical outcomes in pregnancies complicated by placenta accreta: a management paradox. *American Journal of Obstetrics and Gynecology* 2012; **207**(3): 216.e1–5.

11. Cali G, Forlani F, Giambanco L *et al.* Prophylactic use of intravascular balloon catheters in women with placenta accreta, increta and percreta. *European Journal of Obstetrics & Gynecology and Reproductive Biology* 2014; **179**: 36–41.

Chapter 19

Management of Inherited Disorders of Primary Hemostasis in Pregnancy

Sue Pavord and Carolyn Millar

Introduction

The process of primary hemostasis starts immediately following trauma or vessel injury and involves interaction between the vasculature, platelets, and von Willebrand factor (VWF) resulting in the formation of the primary platelet plug. This process is usually sufficient to control bleeding at sites of microvascular injury, such as within mucosal tissues like the genitourinary tract. The management of inherited disorders of primary hemostasis during pregnancy, delivery, and the postpartum period can pose particular challenges. Consideration should be given to the inheritance risk to the fetus and the bleeding risk to the mother, with appropriate multidisciplinary management plans to minimize complications for both. Good communication among the hematologists, obstetricians, anesthetists, neonatologists, and labor ward staff is required, as well as full information for the patient. Where possible this should begin prior to conception and be reviewed as pregnancy advances. Guidelines for management in pregnancy are provided by the Royal College of

Obstetricians and Gynaecologists in collaboration with the UK Hemophilia Center Doctors' Organization[1].

Von Willebrand Disease

von Willebrand disease (VWD) is the most common of the inherited bleeding disorders. It is characterized by a deficiency or defect of von Willebrand factor (VWF), a large multimeric glycoprotein responsible for platelet adhesion.

Von Willebrand Factor

VWF is synthesized by endothelial cells and megakaryocytes; it mediates the tethering of platelets at sites of injury and promotes platelet–platelet aggregation. VWF circulates in the plasma as a series of multimers, assembled from varying numbers of identical monomeric subunits. The size of the multimers influences VWF function; high-molecular-weight (HMW) multimers contain higher numbers of binding sites and are the most functionally active (Figure 19.1)

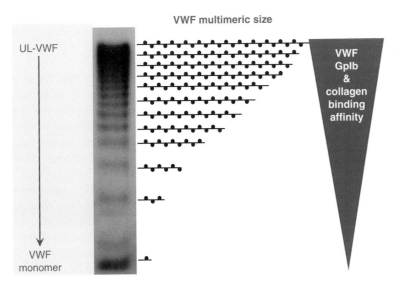

VWF multimeric size

UL-VWF

VWF GpIb & collagen binding affinity

VWF monomer

Figure 19.1 Relationship between VWF multimeric size and functional activity. UL-VWF, ultralarge von willebrand factor multimers; GP1b, glycoprotein 1b.

Genetic

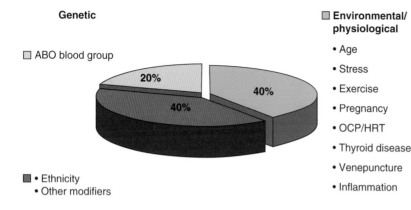

☐ ABO blood group

20%

40%

40%

■ • Ethnicity
  • Other modifiers

☐ **Environmental/
    physiological**

• Age

• Stress

• Exercise

• Pregnancy

• OCP/HRT

• Thyroid disease

• Venepuncture

• Inflammation

Figure 19.2 Factors affecting variation in VWF level.

In addition to its adhesive properties, VWF is a specific carrier molecule for factor VIII (FVIII); VWF protects FVIII from proteolytic degradation and localizes it to sites of vascular injury. Circulating levels of VWF in the plasma are determined by its synthesis in endothelial cells, secretion from its storage in Weibel Palade bodies, and clearance. A separate source of VWF is synthesized by megakaryocytes and stored in the alpha granules of platelets, from where it is released during platelet activation. The normal range of VWF is defined as 0.5–1.5 IU/mL, although VWF plasma levels vary widely in the population, ranging from 0.40 to 2.40 IU/mL[2]. Many factors contribute to this variation including ABO blood group (Figure 19.2). VWF levels are elevated at birth, falling to baseline by around 6 months of age.

Clinical Features of VWD

The bleeding disorder that results from deficiency of VWF varies in severity according to the degree of deficiency and the specific characteristics of the molecule. There may be features of both primary and secondary hemostatic defects to reflect the respective adhesive and carrier properties of VWF. Primary hemostatic defects result in a predominantly mucocutaneous pattern of bleeding such as menorrhagia, epistaxis, and excessive bleeding following trauma or surgery, while reduced levels of FVIII may result in prolonged or delayed bleeding following surgery. Both these effects can have serious implications for women in pregnancy.

Classification and Inheritance of VWD

VWD is classified according to whether the VWF defect is quantitative (types 1 and 3) or qualitative (type 2). Classification is focused on the facilitation of

diagnosis, treatment, and counseling of patients with VWD using laboratory tests which are widely available[3]. Table 19.1 summarizes how VWD classification is currently applied.

Although type 1 VWD, a partial quantitative deficiency of VWF, accounts for the majority of cases of VWD, this type can be the most challenging to diagnose given the subjective nature of bleeding histories, the many factors that may influence VWF levels, the lack of precision of some of the laboratory tests, and the frequency of bleeding symptoms in the normal population. To address this, attempts have been made in recent years to standardize the bleeding history by developing quantitative bleeding scoring systems. These can help ascertain the significance of bleeding symptoms and predict the likelihood of VWD, which is of particular value in type 1 VWD; the bleeding score has also been shown to have a good negative predictive value[4]. It is recommended that a bleeding assessment tool such as that developed by the Scientific and Standardization Committee of the International Society on Thrombosis and Hemostasis be used in the assessment of patients for primary hemostatic defects[5].

Quantitative deficiencies are characterized by concordant reductions in VWF level and functional activity. Patients with type 1 VWD have a VWF activity of less than 0.30 IU/mL, while it is now recommended that patients with an appropriate bleeding history and VWF activity of 0.3–0.5 IU/mL should be regarded as having primary hemostatic bleeding with reduced VWF as a risk factor (referred to as "low VWF"), rather than VWD[6]. This distinction is important for two reasons. First, significant bleeding symptoms may not only be attributable to VWF levels between 0.3 and 0.5 IU/mL, and investigations for an alternative explanation such as a primary platelet function defect should be completed. Second, the likelihood of there being a mutation in the

Table 19.1 Classification of von Willebrand disease

VWD subtype	Description	Comments	Inheritance pattern
1	Partial quantitative deficiency of VWF	Function: antigen ratio >0.6 All sizes multimers present or mildly abnormal Accounts for ~70% of all cases	AD with higher likelihood of *VWF* gene linkage when VWF levels <0.3 IU/mL
2 (except type 2N)	Qualitative VWF defects	Function: Ag <0.6 IU/mL	
2A	Decreased VWF-dependent platelet adhesion and a selective deficiency of HMW multimers	Loss of HMW multimers results in reduced platelet and collagen binding	Mostly AD
2B	Increased affinity for platelet glycoprotein Ib	RIPA +ve Variable loss of HMW multimers and thrombocytopenia; cases with normal platelet count and multimers have been reported	AD
2M	Decreased VWF-dependent platelet adhesion without a selective deficiency of HMW multimers	All multimer sizes present UL multimers may also be present Includes isolated defects of VWF collagen binding	AD
2N	Markedly decreased binding affinity for FVIII	Need to distinguish from mild hemophilia A	AR
3	Virtually complete deficiency of VWF	Most assays <0.03 IU/mL	AR, frequent null alleles

AD, autosomal dominant; AR, autosomal recessive; HMW, high molecular weight; RIPA, ristocetin-induced platelet agglutination; UL, unusually large.

VWF gene (*VWF*) is far greater when VWF levels are less than 0.3 IU/mL than when VWF levels are between 0.30 and 0.50 IU/mL[7,8]. This affects the predictability and pattern of inheritance: in cases where the reduction in VWF levels to less than 0.3 IU/mL results from a *VWF* mutation, inheritance is likely to be autosomal dominant and penetrant. On the other hand, "low VWF" levels between 0.3 and 0.5 IU/mL are more likely to result from a variety of factors that do not necessarily link to the *VWF* gene, and therefore the pattern of inheritance is more variable.

Type 2 VWD results from a variety of qualitative VWF defects as shown in Table 19.1, which usually demonstrate discordant reductions in VWF functional activity. The principal abnormality may be a selective loss in high-molecular-weight (HMW) multimers as seen in type 2A VWD, increased or reduced binding to platelet glycoprotein Ib-IX-V (GPI) in types 2B and 2M respectively, or reduced binding to FVIII (type 2N). Unlike type 1 VWD, type 2 variants are invariably linked to *VWF* and follow a more predictable laboratory and clinical phenotype. With the exception of type 2N VWD,

the inheritance of type 2 VWD is usually autosomal dominant.

Type 3 VWD is characterized by unmeasurable VWF levels and consequently, significantly lowered FVIII levels. Thus, in addition to clinical features of impaired primary hemostasis, the bleeding pattern resembles that of patients with hemophilia, with the potential for spontaneous joint and muscle bleeds. Inheritance follows an autosomal recessive pattern with patients being homozygous or compound heterozygous for the abnormal *VWF* gene. Importantly, the causative mutations in type 3 VWD do not usually cause type 1 VWD in heterozygous form, and type 3 VWD is therefore usually inherited from asymptomatic parents. The prevalence of type 3 VWD in the UK is around 1 per million, although it is more frequent in communities where consanguineous partnerships are common.

Laboratory Evaluation

Routine coagulation screening tests, including the prothrombin time (PT) and activated partial thromboplastin time (aPTT), do not detect VWD unless the factor VIII level is below normal, when the aPTT may be prolonged. Factor VIII (FVIII:C), VWF antigen (VWF:Ag), and measurements of VWF activity are the initial laboratory tests required to make a diagnosis of VWD and should be performed when VWD is suspected, along with a platelet count. VWF activity should be assessed by its ability to bind both platelets and collagen: a ratio of VWF activity to antigen of <0.6 should identify most cases of type 2 VWD[6]. The ristocetin cofactor assay (VWF:RCo) remains the gold standard for measuring the ability of VWF to bind to the platelet GPIb receptor and automated assays are being increasingly used. A diagnostic algorithm is shown in Figure 19.3. As a variety of environmental factors including physical activity and emotional stress may affect VWF levels, assays should be repeated and the diagnosis should be based on at least two sets of similar results. Further evaluation of type 2 VWD should include ristocetin-induced platelet agglutination (RIPA) to assess for the increased GPIb binding property that is characteristic of type 2B. Analysis of the size distribution and pattern of VWF multimers helps distinguish

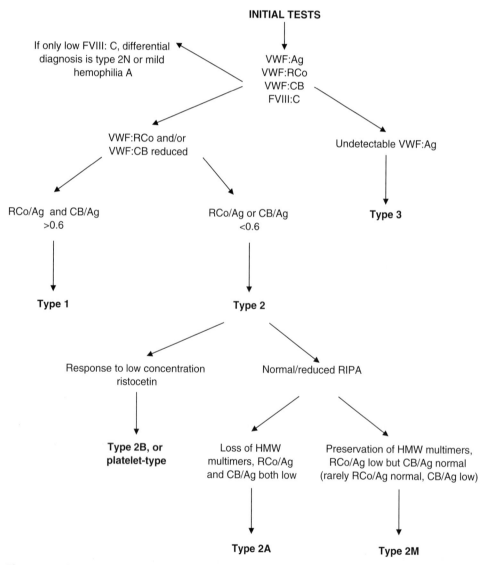

Figure 19.3 Diagnostic algorithm for VWD. VWF:Ag, von Willebrand factor antigen; RCo, ristocetin cofactor activity; CB, collagen binding activity; HMW, high molecular weight.

between types 2A and 2M, although information obtained from the collagen binding activity may serve as a useful surrogate where multimeric analysis is not available.

The Platelet Function Analyzer (PFA-200) simulates in vitro hemodynamic conditions for platelet adhesion and aggregation and has an overall sensitivity for detecting VWD of 90%: in type 2 (excluding 2N) and type 3 VWD the sensitivity is close to 100% although it is lower in type 1 VWD and results may be normal when VWF activity is 0.3–0.5 IU/mL.

Pregnancy can often prompt an individual to present with a historical diagnosis of VWD; in many cases this will be the first contact with healthcare systems for many years. Notwithstanding the physiological changes in VWF during pregnancy discussed below, it is important to consider recent improvements in the precision of laboratory assays and increased knowledge and understanding of the application of VWD classification when interpreting historical results, in particular in cases of mild quantitative deficiencies.

Hormonal Influences on VWF Levels in Pregnancy

Levels of maternal VWF start to rise from early in the first trimester, increasing progressively throughout pregnancy, and reaching two to three times baseline levels by the time of delivery[9,10]. FVIII levels also increase progressively throughout pregnancy: in some cases, the magnitude of rise is comparable to the rise in VWF while in others it may be less. These rises are often sufficient to correct the VWF deficiency in many patients with type 1 VWD, in whom normal levels are often reached by delivery. However, those with more severe VWF deficiency (e.g. less than 0.15 IU/mL) may fail to reach normal values and in patients with the qualitative abnormalities of VWF seen in type 2 disease, the condition may not improve and may even deteriorate. This is a particular challenge in type 2B where the rise in dysfunctional VWF may cause or exacerbate thrombocytopenia and worsen the bleeding tendency [11]. In patients with type 2N disease, FVIII levels tend to remain low because of impaired binding by the abnormal VWF and patients with type 3 disease show minimal or no rise in VWF.

VWF and FVIII levels start to fall soon after delivery, returning to baseline levels within a few weeks.

Obstetric Complications

Maternal Bleeding

Women with VWD have an increased risk of bleeding events and even death during childbirth[12]. Although the physiological rise in VWF and FVIII protects many women with type 1 VWD during delivery, they remain vulnerable in early pregnancy and in the postpartum period. Studies have found:

- One-third of women with VWD have bleeding during their first trimester.
- 15–30% of women with VWD have primary postpartum hemorrhage.
- Delayed postpartum bleeding occurs in 20–25% of women with VWD.
- There is a relatively high frequency of perineal hematoma, a normally rare complication of vaginal birth.
- The risk of receiving a blood transfusion is increased fivefold.
- Maternal mortality rate is ten times higher than that for women without the condition.

Pregnancy Outcomes

Women with VWD are no more likely to experience premature labor, placental abruption, fetal growth restriction, or intrauterine fetal death[11]. There is no convincing evidence to show increased risk of early miscarriage but this can be complicated by significant bleeding[12].

Pregnancy Management for Women with VWD

The safe management of women with VWD requires good communication between the hematologist, obstetricians, anesthetists, neonatologists, and labor ward staff. The patient should be fully informed of potential bleeding risks and the plan for management of pregnancy, delivery, and the postpartum period. This should begin prior to conception and should be reviewed as pregnancy advances (Table 19.2).

Antenatal Management

The physiological rise in levels of VWF and FVIII during pregnancy leads to most women with type 1 VWD achieving levels well above 0.50 IU/mL, the lower limit of the normal range outside of pregnancy. These women can be safely managed in standard obstetric units in collaboration with hemophilia

Table 19.2 Pre-pregnancy management of VWD

- Reassess severity of clinical bleeding tendency including previous responses to hemostatic challenges; use of a bleeding score may be helpful.
- Check baseline investigations and confirm accuracy of any historical diagnosis.
- Establish response to desmopressin.
- Obtain consent for use of plasma products after full counseling of risks.
- Where plasma-derived products have been received in the past, the presence of transfusion-transmitted infection should be excluded.
- Vaccinate against hepatitis A and B if not already immune.
- Check hemoglobin and serum ferritin and give oral supplements as necessary.
- All patients should receive counseling about risks of increased bleeding, particularly in the postpartum period and particularly for women with type 2 or 3 VWD.
- A management plan should be discussed with all patients.
- All patients should be offered genetic counseling as they are at risk of delivering an affected child.
- All patients should receive an explanation regarding evaluation of the infant after delivery.

Table 19.3 Antenatal management of VWD

- Check VWF antigen and activity and FVIII levels at booking, in the third trimester, and prior to any invasive procedure.
- In patients with type 2B VWD, the platelet count should also be monitored. Platelet transfusions, as well as VWF factor replacement, may sometimes be required for bleeding or surgical procedures.
- Aim for FVIII and VWF:RCo activity levels of ≥0.5 IU/mL to cover surgical procedures or spontaneous miscarriage.
- Treat with desmopressin in preference to blood-derived factor concentrates where possible, checking pre- and post-treatment VWF activity and FVIII levels.
- Distribute action plan for acute bleeding events to hematology and obstetric staff, and ensure patient is given an emergency number for contact.

center staff. Women with types 2 and 3 VWD, or moderate or severe type 1, or a history of severe bleeding, should be referred for prenatal care and delivery in a unit where there are specialists in high-risk obstetrics, as well as a Hemophilia Center. Laboratory, pharmacy, and blood bank support is also essential.

For all types of VWD, levels should be checked routinely at booking and in the third trimester. If an adequate rise is demonstrated, only a third trimester sample may be necessary for subsequent pregnancies, unless earlier interventions are required.

Prenatal diagnosis may be appropriate where there is a chance the fetus may have type 3 VWD. Given the likely normal VWF levels in parents of a child with type 3 VWD, this situation tends to arise in pregnancies subsequent to the diagnosis of an affected sibling.

VWF levels are always needed prior to invasive procedures such as chorionic villus sampling, amniocentesis, or cervical cerclage. Where levels of VWF activity or FVIII are <0.50 IU/mL, women should receive hemostatic support in the form of desmopressin where responsive, or VWF-containing concentrates (Table 19.3).

Desmopressin in Pregnancy

Desmopressin (DDAVP, 1-deamino-8-D-arginine vasopressin), a synthetic derivative of the antidiuretic

hormone vasopressin, stimulates release of endothelial stores of VWF. Intravenous, subcutaneous, and intranasal preparations are available that usually result in a three- to fivefold increase in both endogenous VWF and FVIII. To assess the response to desmopressin, VWF activity levels and FVIII should be measured before administration, at 30–60 mins and 4–6 hours, to determine peak levels and clearance rate, respectively.

Desmopressin is generally safe both in pregnancy and at delivery[13,14] but should be avoided in pre-eclampsia. Fluid intake should be restricted to 1 L for the following 24 hours, to prevent maternal hyponatremia. Repeated administration should be avoided in view of the sensitivity of the fetus to the effect of hyponatremia. The advantages of desmopressin are its low cost, unlimited availability, and most importantly, the avoidance of blood products. However, there are many situations where desmopressin may be contraindicated or ineffective and plasma products necessary (Table 19.4).

Coagulation Factor Replacement

There are several licensed plasma-derived high-purity and intermediate-purity VWF-containing concentrates available. Usually these also contain FVIII. The spectrum of multimeric size and ratio of VWF:RCo/FVIII activity differs between them, but this does not appear to cause a difference in efficacy[15]. These concentrates are available as lyophilized powders and, after reconstitution in water, can be administered by slow bolus intravenous injection. Therapeutic levels of FVIII and VWF:RCo >0.50 IU/mL should be maintained until hemostasis is secure. Situations where high-purity VWF concentrates are used that do not contain factor VIII and baseline FVIII:C levels are

Table 19.4 Situations where desmopressin may not be suitable

Patients with insufficient baseline levels	Patients with baseline VWF levels of less than 0.15 IU/mL may not achieve post-infusion levels which are sufficient to control or prevent bleeding.
Some subtypes of type 1, including Vicenza subtype	Some subtypes of type 1 VWD show decreased survival of endogenously produced VWF following desmopressin compared with normal survival of exogenously administered VWF.
Previous intolerance or severe adverse effects	During intravenous infusion, hypotension, headache, and facial flushing are common but generally mild. Blood pressure should be monitored during and after infusion.
Known cardiovascular disease, pre-eclampsia, or unstable blood pressure	There are anecdotal reports of myocardial and cerebral infarction and desmopressin should be avoided in patients known to have arterial disease or hypertension.
Tachyphylaxis after repeated doses	The response to desmopressin may diminish after repeated doses.
Type 2 VWD	Desmopressin is less likely to correct the functional defect in type 2 VWD.
Type 2B	The heightened and spontaneous binding of the abnormal VWF molecule to normal platelets may be aggravated by the rise in VWF levels after desmopressin, increasing platelet clearance from the circulation and exacerbating thrombocytopenia.
Type 2N	Desmopressin also causes release of factor VIII. However, due to the abnormal VWF:FVIII binding, the sustainability of response can be limited.
Type 3 VWD	These patients lack releasable stores of VWF and do not respond to desmopressin.

reduced require either co-infusion with factor VIII concentrate or administration of the initial dose around 12 hours prior to requirement of normalized FVIII levels.

Intrapartum Management

Although there are no large prospective studies that correlate VWF activity with the risk of bleeding at the time of childbirth, the opinion of experts is that VWF:RCo activity above 0.50 IU/mL and platelet count >50 × 10⁹/L should be achieved before and during vaginal delivery or cesarean section[1,6].

Neonates are at risk of intracranial hemorrhage and cephalhematomas during labor and delivery.

Table 19.5 Intrapartum management

- Allow spontaneous labor and normal vaginal delivery, if no other obstetric concerns, to minimize risk of intervention.
- Where VWF:RCo activity levels <0.50 IU/mL at the last check, the test should be repeated if time allows and a rapid turnaround is available.
- Where VWF:RCo <0.50 IU/mL, treat with desmopressin if previous documented response, otherwise VWF-containing concentrates. For dose calculation, aim for peak VWF:RCo level of 1.0 IU/mL. Treatment should be given at the onset of established labor and pre- and post-treatment VWF and FVIII levels should be obtained. Trough VWF:RCo level should be maintained above 0.5 IU/mL.
- Tranexamic acid 1 g intravenously may be helpful for low–normal VWF:RCo levels where VWF-containing concentrates are not thought necessary. It can also be given in conjunction with replacement factor concentrate but is not usually necessary.
- For fetuses at risk of having type 2 or 3 disease or moderate–severe type 1, avoid fetal blood sampling, fetal scalp monitoring, ventouse delivery, and mid-cavity or rotational forceps.
- Avoid aspirin and consider alternatives for NSAIDs. Intramuscular injections are suitable where FVIII:C >0.5 IU/mL.
- Active management of the third stage of labor and early suturing of episiotomy and lacerations.

The increase in FVIII and VWF, induced by the stress of labor, provides some protection for neonates with mild type 1 disease but in more severe types, trauma to the baby should be minimized by avoiding extracephalic version, invasive monitoring procedures, ventouse delivery, fetal blood sampling, scalp electrodes, and mid-cavity rotational forceps.

Analgesia

Where VWF activity is >0.50 IU/mL in patients with type 1 VWD, neuraxial anesthesia may be regarded as safe. However, in type 2 and 3 VWD, restoration of normal hemostasis cannot be reliably assumed even if VWF activity levels >0.50 IU/mL are achieved. Therefore, that unless normal global hemostasis can be demonstrated (PFA-200), it has been recommended that neuraxial anesthesia should be avoided in types 2 or 3 VWD irrespective of whether VWF activity has reached apparently normal levels, including following treatment[6].

Spinal anesthesia is preferred to epidural, as it requires a smaller needle and does not involve leaving a catheter in situ. However, if a catheter does remain, VWF levels should be rechecked at the time of catheter removal and further treatment should be given beforehand if necessary. Intramuscular injections are not contraindicated where FVIII level is normal. Prior to delivery, all women with VWD should have the opportunity to discuss analgesia with an anesthetist.

Postpartum Management (Table 19.6)

The pregnancy-induced increase in VWF and FVIII levels is usually maintained in the first 48 hours after delivery; however, levels may start to decline from day 3 following delivery[16]. In normal pregnancies, the median duration of bleeding after childbirth is 21 to 27 days, with delayed or secondary postpartum hemorrhage occurring in fewer than 1% of cases. In women with VWD this is much more common, affecting 20–25% of cases. In addition, there are multiple cases of postpartum hemorrhage that have occurred despite prophylaxis. The average time of presentation of postpartum hemorrhage in women with VWD is 10–20 days after delivery[17]. Women with VWD should be made aware of the risk of delayed bleeding and be encouraged to report excessive bleeding; for more severe cases, hemoglobin should be monitored and regular contact with the patient maintained for several weeks.

All patients with type 3 and most with type 2 disease, or severe type 1, require VWF concentrates, to maintain VWF:RCo and FVIII:C levels >0.50 IU/dL for at least 3 days after vaginal delivery and 5 days following cesarean section[1]. It is important to monitor both of these levels, as secondary hemostasis takes over from primary hemostasis as the predominant mechanism after the first 24–48 hours. If the bleeding risk is prolonged by complicated delivery and delayed recovery or development of sepsis, normal levels should be maintained for longer. Treatment may sometimes be required for several weeks. Close contact should be maintained with the patient after discharge (Table 19.6).

Tranexamic Acid

Patients with mild type 1 VWD can usually be safely managed in the postpartum period with oral tranexamic acid (TXA) alone. It may be given empirically or as treatment and can be a useful adjunct to VWF replacement therapy. The dose is 1 g tds and it is usually prescribed for up to 14 days, which can be continued for a longer period if needed. TXA is a lysine analog, which by saturating lysine binding sites on plasminogen prevents its interaction with fibrin, thereby inhibiting fibrinolysis. It has proven efficacy

Table 19.6 Postpartum management

Ensure careful surgical hemostasis and effective uterine contraction in all cases.

Repeat VWF activity levels and Hb prior to discharge.

Give oral tranexamic acid.

For patients with significantly low pre-pregnancy levels, consider desmopressin if known responder.

For all patients, ensure VWF activity levels are maintained at >0.50 IU/mL for at least 3 days following vaginal delivery or 5 days if cesarean section has been performed.

Factor VIII levels should also be monitored and maintained above 0.5 IU/mL. Additionally, care should be taken to avoid accumulation of FVIII with repeated doses of FVIII:VWF concentrate.

Risk assessment and prophylaxis for venous thromboembolism should be carried out in the normal way providing FVIII and VWF activity levels are being maintained.

Ensure regular contact with the patient after discharge and encourage them to report excessive or increasing blood loss.

Consider use of the combined oral contraceptive pill if excessive bleeding is ongoing despite prophylaxis.

in reducing blood loss, without increasing thrombotic risk. It is contraindicated in patients with hematuria and doses should be reduced in renal failure.

Tranexamic acid crosses the placenta but has been used to treat antenatal bleeding in a number of cases without reported adverse fetal effects. Recent guidelines from the UK Hemophilia Center Doctors' Organization have supported its use in pregnancy. Traces have been found in breast milk but this has not been associated with changes to fibrinolytic activity in the infant.

Thromboprophylaxis

Postpartum thromboprophylaxis should be considered in women with increased thrombotic risk factors (Chapter 13) provided VWF levels are within the normal range. However, caution must be exercised when VWF levels start to fall. Furthermore, patients receiving boluses of VWF-containing replacement concentrates have fluctuating levels, sometimes dropping below the desired therapeutic range. Prophylactic heparin during these times could have a significant effect on increased bleeding risk. Careful monitoring, dosing, and timing of replacement therapy is required to avoid low trough levels and also excessive accumulation of FVIII, which can occur after repeated treatments. Resulting thrombosis has been reported in these cases but most were perioperative without use of monitoring. Attention should be given to simple thromboprophylactic measures, including mobilization and hydration.

Transfusion-Transmitted Infections

The VWF-containing concentrates currently used are manufactured from thousands of pooled plasma donations. The processes now used for viral screening are very robust. In addition, at least two separate viral inactivation steps are incorporated into the manufacturing process of pooled plasma concentrates. These include dry heat treatment at 80°C for 72 hours, pasteurization at 60°C for 10 hours, or solvent detergent treatment with tri(n-butyl) phosphate and Tween-80 or Triton X. A third step of nanofiltration has been introduced for some products. No cases of infection with HIV, hepatitis B, or hepatitis C have occurred with products inactivated by the currently used processes. However, some viruses, such as parvovirus B19, are relatively resistant to these inactivation techniques. Parvovirus infection can have serious consequences in pregnancy, being associated with hydrops fetalis and intrauterine fetal death. Prion diseases such as variant Creutzfeldt–Jakob disease (vCJD), for which there is currently no available screening test, and as yet unidentified pathogens remain potential infective risks. Recombinant VWF concentrates are currently in development.

Neonatal Management

Type 1 VWD in which there is linkage to the *VWF* gene and most cases of type 2 VWD (with the exception of type 2N) are autosomal dominant conditions with a 50% chance of offspring being affected if either parent is affected. Milder forms of type 1 VWD are less likely to follow a clear inheritance pattern for the reasons explained earlier. The autosomal recessive inheritance of type 3 VWD results in a 25% risk if a previous sibling has been affected. The risk of perinatal intracranial hemorrhage appears low.

Diagnosis of VWD in neonates and infants may be complicated by the difficulty in obtaining a venous or cord sample that is not activated or contaminated and the prolonged physiological rise in VWF following delivery. Thus, in the absence of bleeding the diagnosis of VWD is often not attempted before at least 6 months of age. However, newborns at risk of moderate and severe VWD types should be tested using cord blood which should include a platelet count in cases of type 2B VWD; where known, *VWF* gene sequence analysis for the causative mutation can be performed. The neonate should be assessed to exclude intracranial hemorrhage. Intramuscular vitamin K should not be given until FVIII has been shown to be normal; it can be given orally if necessary (Table 19.7).

Table 19.7 Neonatal management

• If severe disease phenotype is anticipated, a cord sample should be tested for VWF activity and FVIII level and considered for *VWF* gene mutation testing where appropriate. The limitations of testing at this stage should be understood.

• Neonates with type 2B disease may require platelet transfusion if there is severe thrombocytopenia or bruising/bleeding manifestations.

• Intramuscular vitamin K should be avoided until FVIII results are known and given orally if necessary. Any heel prick tests should have pressure applied afterwards for 5 minutes.

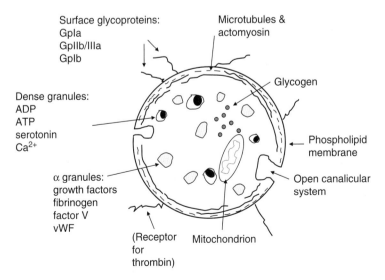

Figure 19.4 Diagram of a platelet showing range of platelet defects.

Inherited Disorders of Platelet Function

There are a number of inherited disorders of platelet function (Figure 19.4) and for most cases management requires assessment of maternal bleeding phenotype with consideration given to use of desmopressin to promote primary hemostasis, tranexamic acid, and pooled platelet concentrates to cover antenatal procedures and delivery. There may be a role in selected patients with disorders of platelet function to monitor during pregnancy using PFA-200 analysis and tailor hemostatic support accordingly[18]. Women with bleeding histories should continue tranexamic acid in the postpartum period until the lochia becomes clear. Where there is a neonatal risk of significant platelet dysfunction, traumatic delivery should be avoided, and if thrombocytopenia is a feature of the condition, a cord sample should be taken at birth.

Special mention is given to Glanzmann's thrombasthenia and Bernard–Soulier syndrome.

Glanzmann's Thrombasthenia

Glanzmann's thrombasthenia (GT) is a rare autosomal recessive disorder with a prevalence of around one per million although higher in areas where consanguinity is common. Platelets are normal in number, but their ability to aggregate is reduced due to loss of the surface receptor glycoprotein (GP) IIb-IIIa (α IIb β3 integrin). Pregnancy and delivery are rare in these patients but have been associated with a high risk of severe postpartum hemorrhage.

Recombinant activated factor VII (rFVIIa) is licensed for use in patients with this disorder. In pharmacological concentrations, rFVIIa is capable of binding to the surface of activated platelets and improving thrombin generation to enhance adhesion and aggregation of platelets lacking GPIIb-IIIa. The usual dose given is 90 μg/kg 2–3 hourly. Bleeding can also be successfully prevented by transfusion of platelets before and after delivery. However, platelet transfusion can stimulate isoantibody formation against platelet antigens, resulting in a decreased efficacy of subsequent transfusions and a risk of fetal/neonatal alloimmune thrombocytopenia. A single donor platelet preparation should be used in preference to pooled platelet transfusion to reduce this risk and where possible platelets should be HLA matched.

Delayed bleeding up to 2–3 weeks postpartum has been reported and in these circumstances, desmopressin and tranexamic acid are useful to reduce platelet transfusion requirements.

Bernard–Soulier Syndrome

The Bernard–Soulier syndrome (BSS) is a rare autosomal recessive bleeding disorder with similar prevalence to GT, characterized by impaired platelet agglutination with ristocetin as a result of a lack of the platelet glycoprotein GP Ib-IX-V complex. BSS patients also have thrombocytopenia with large circulating platelets. In some patients, the disease can go unrecognized until the third or fourth decade.

Four different features of BSS may contribute to the hemorrhagic diathesis: thrombocytopenia, abnormal platelet interaction with VWF, impaired platelet interaction with thrombin, and abnormal platelet coagulant activity. BSS is caused by genetic defects in the genes of GPIbα, GPIbβ, GPIX, or GPV. This variety of mutations could explain the heterogeneity of the syndrome; however, the clinical manifestation may even differ in consecutive pregnancies of the same patient.

The main complications encountered in reported cases have been antepartum hemorrhage, excessive intraoperative bleeding, immediate and delayed postpartum hemorrhage, and development of maternal antiplatelet antibodies leading to fetal intracranial hemorrhage and neonatal alloimmune thrombocytopenia.

Management

Management is similar to that for GT and includes the judicious and timely use of platelet transfusions to prevent bleeding while minimizing the risk of platelet refractoriness. Regional anesthesia should be avoided and postpartum tranexamic acid and desmopressin prescribed as necessary.

Neonatal Management of Glanzmann's Thrombasthenia and Bernard–Soulier Syndrome

Unless the father has the same condition or is a carrier, the fetus is heterozygous, with platelets carrying specific paternal antigens that are not present on the maternal platelets and thus are capable of causing maternal alloimmunization. Transplacental transfer of the maternal antiplatelet IgG antibodies can lead to severe alloimmune neonatal thrombocytopenia and a risk of intracranial hemorrhage in the fetus. Thus the management should follow that for fetal/neonatal alloimmune thrombocytopenia, with use of intravenous immunoglobulin and steroids and avoidance of intrauterine fetal blood sampling (see Chapter 10). In BSS, heterozygosity can also result in thrombocytopenia.

Monitoring for Maternal Alloimmunization

All women with severe GT or BSS should be monitored for the development of platelet-specific antibodies.

This involves testing for anti-HPA and anti-HLA alloantibodies at the start of pregnancy and regular testing during pregnancy as well as following any donor platelet transfusion.

Case Studies

Case Study 1

A 27-year-old woman presented at 28 weeks' gestation in her first pregnancy. She had a significant bleeding history and was known to have type 2B VWD, confirmed by factor assays and genetic mutation analysis (R1308C mutation). Her factor antigen and activity levels were checked at 28 and 34 weeks and showed no improvement above her known baseline levels.

Her intrapartum care plan was discussed and documented, and high-purity VWF/FVIII concentrate made available on the delivery suite. At 38 weeks there was spontaneous rupture of membranes. Two vials of factor concentrate were given (1000 IU FVIII:2400IU RCo/vial) and the baby was delivered 4 hours later by low-cavity lift out forceps. Unfortunately, the mother sustained a second degree tear, with estimated blood loss of 900 mL. The perineum and vaginal wall were sutured under general anesthesia with 1 g intravenous tranexamic acid.

RCo fell from 1.17 IU/mL after the pre-delivery treatment to 0.27 IU/mL the following morning, and treatment was given 12 hourly the next day followed by 24 hourly for a further 2 days and oral tranexamic acid for 14 days. Non-pharmacological thromboprophylactic measures were advised.

Her laboratory results highlight the relatively short half-life of VWF activity immediately following delivery (Figure 19.5) and the need for close monitoring. The thrombocytopenia of type 2B VWD is also demonstrated and in part corrected by the administration of exogenous (normal) VWF.

The cord sample was unsuccessful but at day 2 the neonatal levels showed FVIII 0.41 IU/mL, VWF Ag 0.40 IU/mL, RCo 0.08 IU/mL, and platelets 152×10^9/L. This is consistent with type 2 VWD. Had the cord sample been successful, it may well have shown a lower platelet count, due to a rise in the dysfunctional VWF molecule during birth.

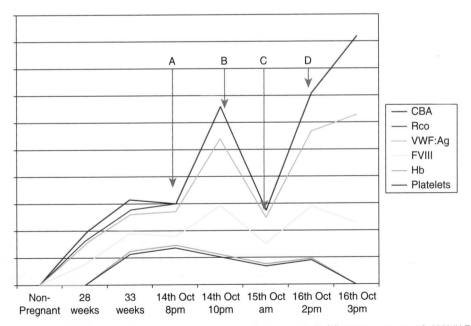

Figure 19.5 (A) Presentation with spontaneous rupture of membranes; (B) following treatment with 2000 IU FVIII and 4800 IU RCo; (C) 9 hours after delivery; (D) trough level, 24 hours following last treatment (level was unknown and further treatment was given empirically, as planned).

Case Study 2

A 32-year-old woman is referred at 20 weeks' gestation in her first pregnancy with a family history of von Willebrand disease. She informs you that the initial diagnosis was made in her mother following an episode of excessive bleeding after dental extractions. The patient recalls that she herself was tested in childhood although it was unclear whether a diagnosis of VWD had been made. On further questioning the patient reports a history of heavy menstrual blood loss since menarche for which she has tried a variety of medications including the combined oral contraceptive pill. She has been prescribed iron supplementation on multiple occasions. She recalls that both she and her siblings were troubled with nose bleeds in childhood. She has not undergone any invasive or surgical procedures.

Blood tests taken at 20 weeks' gestation showed normal VWF-related parameters and platelet count (Table 19.8). PFA-200 analysis demonstrated closure times to be prolonged: collagen/epinephrine 273 seconds (NR 105–165 seconds) and collagen/ADP 218 seconds (60–120 seconds). Hemoglobin was 116 g/L. A platelet function disorder was suspected; however, the increased platelet activation that may be associated with pregnancy precludes meaningful interpretation of platelet aggregation studies, which were therefore deferred. PFA-200 closure times remained abnormal when repeated at 32 and 36 weeks' gestation in the context of normal VWF levels and activity and platelet counts (Table 19.8). Following discussion with obstetric and anesthetic colleagues, plans were made for delivery: avoidance of spinal or epidural anesthesia, avoidance of NSAID analgesia, commencement of tranexamic acid 1 g tds at onset of labor and active management of the third stage of labor were agreed. Failure of progression of the second stage of labor resulted in delivery by cesarean section under general anesthesia. There was no excessive blood loss at the time of delivery; the patient was discharged 3 days later and advised to continue tranexamic acid for 10 days postpartum. She was provided with details of who to contact in the event of increasing or unexpected bleeding.

The neonate received intramuscular vitamin K and testing for bleeding diathesis was deferred with advice provided on what to do in the event of any bleeding symptoms.

Blood tests performed at follow-up in the hematology clinic 3 months later showed VWF:Ag 0.4 IU/mL, VWF:RCo 0.39 IU/mL (NR 0.5–1.5) (Table 19.8). PFA-200 closure times were significantly prolonged: collagen/epinephrine >300 seconds (NR 100–165 seconds) and collagen/ADP 276 seconds (60–120 seconds). Platelet aggregation studies were arranged which showed reduced aggregation at low concentrations of ADP, epinephrine, and arachidonic acid. Reduced granular storage and release of ATP were demonstrated on lumi-aggregometry.

A diagnosis of platelet function defect with low VWF was made. There were no bleeding symptoms in the infant, who underwent testing prior to tonsillectomy at the age of 3 years, which was normal. Subsequent review of family members previously diagnosed with VWD revealed similar platelet aggregometry patterns and revision of the original diagnosis.

Table 19.8 Laboratory resuts for Case Study 2

Time	Platelets (x10^9/L)	FVIII (IU/mL)	VWF:Ag (IU/mL)	VWF:RCo (IU/mL)	VWF:CB (IU/mL)	PFA-200 closure time
normal range	140–400	0.5–1.5	0.5–1.5	0.5–1.5	0.5–1.5	(Coll/Epi; Coll/ADP)
20/40	254	0.87	0.92	0.83	0.95	Prolonged ++
32/40	201	1.31	1.40	1.32	1.38	Prolonged +
36/40	189	1.53	1.69	1.76	1.73	prolonged+ +
12 weeks postpartum	270	0.62	0.40	0.39	0.45	Prolonged +++

References

1. Pavord S, Rayment R, Madan B *et al.* The Management of Inherited Bleeding Disorders in Pregnancy. RCOG Green-Top Guideline No. 71; 2017. http://onlinelibrary.wiley.com/doi/10.1111/1471-0528.14592/epdf

2. Abildgaard CF, Suzuki Z, Harrison J *et al.* Serial studies in von Willebrand's disease: variability versus "variants". *Blood* 1980; **56**(4): 712–716.

3. Sadler JE, Budde U, Eikenboom JC *et al.* Update on the pathophysiology and classification of von Willebrand disease: a report of the Subcommittee on von Willebrand Factor. *Journal of Thrombosis and Haemostasis* 2006; **4**(10): 2103–2114.

4. Rydz N, James PD. The evolution and value of bleeding assessment tools. *Journal of Thrombosis and Haemostasis* 2012; **10**(11): 2223–2229.

5. Rodeghiero F, Tosetto A, Abshire T *et al.* ISTH/SSC bleeding assessment tool: a standardized questionnaire and a proposal for a new bleeding score for inherited bleeding disorders. *Journal of Thrombosis and Haemostasis* 2010; **8**(9): 2063–2065.

6. Laffan MA, Lester W, O'Donnell JS *et al.* The diagnosis and management of von Willebrand disease: a United Kingdom Hemophilia Center Doctors Organization guideline approved by the British Committee for Standards in Hematology. *British Journal of Haematology* 2014; **167**(4): 453–465.

7. James PD, Paterson AD, Notley C *et al.* Genetic linkage and association analysis in type 1 von Willebrand disease: results from the Canadian type 1 VWD study. *Journal of Thrombosis and Haemostasis* 2006; **4**(4): 783–792.

8. Eikenboom J, Van Marion V, Putter H *et al.* Linkage analysis in families diagnosed with type 1 von Willebrand disease in the European study, molecular and clinical markers for the diagnosis and management of type 1 VWD. *Journal of Thrombosis and Haemostasis* 2006; **4**(4): 774–782.

9. Stirling Y, Woolf L, North WR *et al.* Hemostasis in normal pregnancy. *Thrombosis and Haemostasis* 1984; **52**(2): 176–182.

10. Sanchez-Luceros A, Meschengieser SS, Marchese C *et al.* Factor VIII and von Willebrand factor changes during normal pregnancy and puerperium. *Blood Coagulation and Fibrinolysis* 2003; **14**: 647–651.

11. Ranger A, Manning RA, Lyall H *et al.* Pregnancy in type 2B VWD: a case series. *Hemophilia* 2012; **18**(3): 406–412.

12. James AH, Jamison MG. Bleeding events and other complications during pregnancy and childbirth in women with von Willebrand disease. *Journal of Thrombosis and Haemostasis* 2007; **5**: 1165–1169.

13. Ray JG. DDAVP use during pregnancy: an analysis of its safety for mother and child. *Obstetrical & Gynecological Survey* 1998; **53**(7): 450–455.

14. Trigg DE, Stergiotou I, Peitsidis P *et al.* A systematic review: The use of desmopressin for treatment and prophylaxis of bleeding disorders in pregnancy. *Hemophilia* 2012; **18**(1): 25–33.

15. Mannucci PM, Tenconi PM, Castaman G, Rodeghiero F. Comparison of four virus-inactivated plasma concentrates for treatment of severe von Willebrand disease: a cross-over randomized trial. *Blood* 1992; **79**: 3130–3137.

16. Huq FY, Kulkarni A, Agbim EC *et al.* Changes in the levels of factor VIII and von Willebrand factor in the puerperium. *Hemophilia* 2012; **18**: 241–245.

17. Roqué H, Funai E, Lockwood CJ. von Willebrand disease and pregnancy. *The Journal of Maternal–Fetal Medicine* 2000; **9**: 257–266.

18. Lentaigne CE, Sodhi V, Usman N, McCarthy A, Millar CM. Hemostatic management of pregnant women with platelet function disorders: utility of PFA-100. *Journal of Thrombosis and Haemostasis* 2013; **11**: 1152.

Chapter 20

Management of Inherited Coagulopathies in Pregnancy

Sue Pavord

Hemophilia

Introduction

Hemophilia is characterized by a deficiency of factor VIII (hemophilia A) or factor IX (hemophilia B), both key components of the intrinsic pathway of the coagulation cascade. The gene is carried on the long arm of the X chromosome, so males are clinically affected and females are carriers. Female carriers may also have low factor levels due to skewed X chromosome inactivation, giving rise to an increased tendency to bleed. Thus management of pregnancy requires the assessment of bleeding risk for both mother and baby, with particular attention given to multidisciplinary planning and coordination of health care professionals at the time of and after delivery. Guidelines for management of inherited bleeding disorders in pregnancy are provided by the Royal College of Obstetricians and Gynaecologists in collaboration with the UK Hemophilia Centre Doctors' Organisation[1].

Disease Incidence

Hemophilia A and B occur with an incidence of around 1:5000 and 1:10 000 male births, respectively. The severity of the disease runs true in families and if the family history is known, the bleeding risk to male offspring can be largely predicted (Chapter 21). However, 40–50% of cases are sporadic and unexpected with no family history of the condition.

Clinical Features

The hallmark of the condition is hemarthrosis, resulting in progressive arthropathies requiring joint fusions or joint replacement to alleviate pain. The bleeding risk correlates with the level of coagulation factor (Table 20.1). Patients with severe hemophilia or those with recurrent joint bleeds require prophylaxis with factor concentrate to keep trough levels at or above 1 IU/mL and avoid spontaneous bleeds. Acute

Table 20.1 Severity of hemophilia according to factor level

Factor level (% of normal)	Severity of clinical condition	Bleeding risk
<1	Severe	Spontaneous joint and muscle bleeds
1–5	Moderate	Joint and muscle bleeds mainly after trauma. Occasional spontaneous bleeds
>5	Mild	Trauma/surgery-induced bleeding

bleeds require immediate treatment to minimize joint and soft tissue damage. After a period of training and assessment of competency, factor concentrate can be self-administered using home stocks, although many children on prophylaxis have difficulty with venous access and require insertion of portacaths, which are often complicated by recurrent infections.

Hormonal Influences on Levels in Pregnancy

Levels of factor VIII increase from 6 weeks' gestation, to 2–3 times baseline by term. Factor IX levels are relatively unaltered.

Obstetric Complications

Maternal Bleeding

Female carriers of hemophilia typically have half levels of factor VIII/IX. Unbalanced lyonization, where there is uneven X chromosome inactivation, may result in significantly lower levels and an associated bleeding risk. However, risk has also been shown to be increased in carriers with relatively normal factor levels of 0.4–0.6 IU/mL[2,3]. For most carriers of hemophilia A, the pregnancy-induced rise in factor VIII level alleviates any potential problems for childbirth, although they remain vulnerable in early pregnancy, and those with low baseline levels, for example <1.5 IU/mL, may not achieve normal levels by delivery. Women with low factor IX levels remain at risk of bleeding throughout pregnancy.

Pregnancy Outcomes

The incidence of miscarriage and placental insufficiency syndromes is not increased. The main risk is to the neonate at the time of delivery, as well as the maternal bleeding risk, particularly postpartum, for those mothers with low factor levels.

Neonatal Risk

The most significant potential complication for the neonate is intracranial hemorrhage (ICH), particularly following instrumental or traumatic birth. The risk is approximately 50 times greater than for the general population and affects around 4% of all hemophilia boys[4], although it is clearly highest in those with severe hemophilia or where the disease is unexpected and no preventive strategies, neonatal surveillance, or considered management plan are in place.

ICH is most often associated with extracranial hemorrhage (ECH) after trauma and any significant ECH in a newborn should raise the suspicion of underlying coagulopathy and ICH. Common complications are cephalhematomas and abnormal bleeding after injection or venepuncture. Other reported events are umbilical bleeding, hematuria, and retro-orbital bleeding.

Pre-pregnancy Management

All women with a family history of hemophilia should be assessed for carrier status, including pedigree profile and calculation of statistical risk, baseline factor levels, and genetic mutation analysis where possible. See Chapter 21.

Carriers should receive effective counseling regarding their risk of:

(a) bleeding, particularly in the postpartum period; and
(b) delivering an affected male.

These risks need to be determined and fully discussed with the patient, including options for prenatal diagnosis. Appropriate multidisciplinary management plans should be agreed to minimize complications for both mother and baby.

Table 20.2 Antenatal management of hemophilia carriers

Check factor levels at booking, 28 weeks' gestation, and if still abnormal, 34 weeks' gestation or prior to any invasive procedure. Aim for FVIII/FIX levels of ≥50 IU/dL to cover surgical procedures or spontaneous miscarriage.

For carriers with low factor VIII levels desmopressin may be used but recombinant factor concentrate is required to raise factor IX levels.

Antenatal Management (Table 20.2)

- All women should be offered prenatal diagnosis (Chapter 21) but women who do not wish for this should be encouraged to have the fetal sex determined by ultrasound when the anomaly scan is performed.
- Factor levels should be checked at booking and in the third trimester. Factor VIII levels usually rise in pregnancy but factor IX tends to remain constant. If an adequate rise in factor VIII is demonstrated, only a third trimester sample may be necessary for subsequent pregnancies, unless earlier interventions are required.
- Factor levels should also be checked prior to potentially hemorrhagic events such as invasive diagnostic procedures, spontaneous abortion, or termination of pregnancy. If levels are <0.5 IU/mL, women should receive prophylaxis.
- Desmopressin can be used to raise factor VIII levels by around three times but recombinant clotting factor concentrate is needed for factor IX-deficient women and may be required for those with factor VIII levels below 1.5 IU/mL, as the response to desmopressin may be insufficient. Pre- and post-treatment levels should be checked and therapeutic levels maintained for a suitable time period depending on the procedure.

Intrapartum Management (Table 20.3)

Although there are no large prospective studies that correlate FVIII or IX levels with the risk of maternal bleeding at the time of childbirth, the opinion of experts is that levels should be above 0.5 IU/mL. If treatment is required, the level should be brought to 1.0 IU/mL pre-delivery and maintained at >0.5 IU/mL for at least 3–5 days. Excessive treatment should be avoided due to the risk of thrombosis and thus careful titration and monitoring of levels is required. A continuous infusion of factor concentrate is sometimes easier to manage but must still be closely supervised.

Table 20.3 Intrapartum management of hemophilia carriers

If FVIII/IX levels <50 IU/dL at the last check, the test needs to be repeated on arrival in labor.

Recombinant factor concentrate is required to raise factor IX levels. Treatment should be given at the onset of established labor and pre- and post-treatment levels should be obtained.

Allow spontaneous labor and normal vaginal delivery, if no other obstetric concerns, to minimize risk of intervention.

Avoid prolonged second stage of labor, with early recourse to cesarean section if necessary, to reduce risk of trauma to the baby.

Avoid fetal blood sampling, fetal scalp monitoring, ventouse delivery, and mid-cavity forceps or forceps involving rotation of the head.

Active management of the third stage of labor and early suturing of episiotomy and lacerations for patients with low factor levels.

Regional anesthesia has been shown to be safe if the coagulation screen is normal and factor levels are >50 IU/dL but levels must be checked prior to removal of the catheter as they may fall rapidly in the postpartum period.

If maternal FVIII/IX levels <50 IU/dL caution with non-steroidal anti-inflammatory drugs and intramuscular injections.

Levels of >0.5 IU/mL may be required for a further 2–3 days.

Neonates are at risk of intracranial hemorrhage and cephalhematomas during labor and delivery. The second stage of labor should not be prolonged and early recourse to cesarean section may be required. Trauma should be minimized by avoiding extra cephalic version, ventouse delivery, fetal blood sampling, scalp electrodes, and rotational forceps. If a male baby is at risk of severe hemophilia, the mother should be offered a cesarean delivery, although there is no conclusive evidence of greater safety compared with an uncomplicated vaginal delivery.

The cut-off value for predicted factor VIII or IX, above which no birth restrictions are necessary, has not been defined although mild hemophilia is unlikely to be associated with severe bleeding at birth. Furthermore, the increase in FVIII, induced by the stress of labor, provides some protection for babies with mild hemophilia A. Female carriers have a small risk of extreme lyonization and low factor levels but this needs to be weighed up against the possibly greater risks of withholding instrumental delivery and invasive fetal monitoring. As factor IX levels are lower at birth and are not increased by the stress of delivery, female carriers of severe hemophilia B are theoretically at higher risk but bleeding has not yet been reported.

Analgesia

There is no consensus on the levels required for regional anesthesia but this is generally considered to be safe if FVIII/IX levels are >0.5 IU/mL[5,6]. Spinal is preferred over epidural but if a prolonged epidural catheter is required, levels should be checked at the time of catheter removal and repeat treatment given beforehand if necessary. Intramuscular injections and non-steroidal anti-inflammatory drugs are not contraindicated if factor levels are normal. All women with low factor levels should have the opportunity to meet with an anesthetist prior to delivery.

Postpartum

Postpartum blood loss should be assessed as factor levels start to fall rapidly after delivery. If factor concentrate is given to cover delivery, factor VIII/IX levels should not be allowed to fall below 0.5 IU/mL for at least 3 days, or 5 days if cesarean section has been performed[7].

Tranexamic acid may be used alone or in combination with factor concentrate to prevent excessive postpartum bleeding. It should be continued until the lochia is clear. Desmopressin may also be helpful in boosting FVIII levels in the postpartum period but is rarely required.

Neonatal Management

Affected babies may suffer bruising and bleeding at venepuncture and heel prick sites and even spontaneous organ or joint bleeding. To identify neonates at risk, a cord sample should be taken for coagulation factor assay and the result must be known before the patient leaves hospital. Female babies at risk of being carriers for severe hemophilia may also require a cord sample as very low levels may occur due to severely unbalanced lyonization. However, factors VIII and IX from the newborn do not reflect the true baseline level and may need repeating at 6 months of age, when adult values are reached.

Venepunctures and intramuscular injections, including vitamin K, should be avoided until the cord factor level is known. Vitamin K could be given orally if the results are delayed. Severely affected babies should receive ultrasound scan of the head to assess for signs of intracranial hemorrhage (ICH), particularly if delivery was traumatic or labor prolonged. This investigation is non-invasive but lacks sensitivity, particularly for subdural bleeds, which is the commonest site of ICH in the neonate.

The mean age for occurrence of ICH is 4.5 days[4], when the baby is likely to be at home. Hence parents and midwives should be informed of the early signs of ICH: poor feeding, listlessness, vomiting and seizures, so that treatment can be administered without delay. To date, there is no evidence for the benefit of prophylactic factor concentrate, about which the risk of inhibitor development is debated. However, it may be justified in selected cases, such as prematurity or traumatic delivery, where the risk of ICH is greater.

Factor XI Deficiency

Introduction

Factor XI is an important component of the intrinsic coagulation pathway, playing a key role in the amplification of initial thrombin production, via activation of factor IX. The additional amount of thrombin activates thrombin-activatable fibrinolysis inhibitor (TAFI), which consolidates the fibrin clot and protects it from degradation by fibrinolysis. Thus, deficiency of factor XI is manifest mostly by injury or surgery-related bleeding at sites which are prone to local fibrinolysis, such as the nose and genitourinary tract. Women with factor XI deficiency are at risk of menorrhagia and bleeding in relation to childbirth.

Disease Incidence

The inheritance of factor XI deficiency is autosomal. It is most common among Ashkenazi Jews, where the estimated heterozygosity rate is as high as 8%[8]. The incidence in the non-Jewish population is reported to be around 1:100 000 although this is likely to be an underestimate, as it may frequently remain undetected as routine coagulation assays may be normal in heterozygotes and there may be no bleeding history.

The predominant mutations in Ashkenazi Jews are a Glu117 stop codon in exon 5 designated type II and a Phe283Leu mutation in exon 9 designated type III. Homozygotes for type II and type III mutation have factor XI activities <0.1 IU/mL and 0.8–1.5 IU/mL, respectively, with compound heterozygotes for type II and III having factor XI levels between these values[9]. In non-Jewish populations, rapidly increasing numbers of mutations and polymorphisms have been reported, now reaching over 80. For the majority of these, the level of FXI antigen has not been reported.

Clinical Features

The bleeding tendency in FXI-deficient individuals is highly variable[10]. Factor XI activities <1.5 IU/mL have been designated as severe deficiency, although bleeding is not closely correlated with factor levels[11] as it is with hemophilia A and B. Neither does the abnormal genotype causing the condition seem to bear any relationship to bleeding tendency, which is inconsistent among family members. Indeed, in most patients spontaneous bleeding, as well as bleeding after hemostatic challenge, does not occur and phenotype may depend on other associated factors, such as coexistence of mild von Willebrand disease.

Hormonal Influences on Factor Levels

Factor XI levels usually remain constant in pregnancy but studies have shown inconsistencies in levels with increases or decreases as pregnancy advances[12].

Obstetric Complications

The main risk in pregnancy is of uterine hemorrhage during invasive procedures, miscarriage or postpartum. Patients with FXI levels <1.5 IU/mL have a 16–30% risk of peripartum bleeding[13] and this has been confirmed to almost exclusively affect those with a predetermined bleeding phenotype[12]. Thus, it is important to attempt to ascertain, by thorough history taking, which patients are at risk of bleeding, so that antenatal procedures, childbirth, and the postpartum period can be managed appropriately (Table 20.4).

Antenatal Management

As it is often not feasible to check levels in an acute situation, routine monitoring should be carried out at booking and in the third trimester. While low factor levels cause prolongation of the aPTT, test reagents vary in their sensitivity to factor XI levels and a normal aPTT does not exclude mild deficiency. This is particularly so in pregnancy where the increase in

Table 20.4 Pre-pregnancy management of women with factor XI deficiency

Assess clinical bleeding tendency and coexistence of confounding factors such as VWD or platelet dysfunction.

Offer prenatal diagnosis where there is a risk of severe deficiency and the mutation is known.

Discuss potential maternal bleeding risk and options for management.

Consent for use of blood products if necessary and ensure hepatitis A and B immunity.

Table 20.5 Antenatal management of women with factor XI deficiency

Check levels at booking, 28 and 34 weeks' gestation, and prior to invasive procedures.

Patients with severely low levels or a positive bleeding history should be given prophylaxis to cover invasive procedures.

Other patients can be managed expectantly with close observation and treatment available on standby should bleeding occur.

Table 20.6 Intrapartum management of women with factor XI deficiency

An on-demand policy can be advocated, including for those with severely low levels, during and after vaginal delivery.

Most patients undergoing cesarean section can be managed expectantly but those with severe deficiency should be given prophylaxis.

Measures should be taken to avoid unnecessary trauma to the baby during delivery.

The third stage of labor should be actively managed.

factor VIII may normalize the aPTT even when factor XI is reduced. Thus, a specific coagulation factor assay is required (Table 20.5).

Treatment Options to Cover Delivery and Antenatal Procedures

Most patients can be managed expectantly[14] but those with severely reduced levels or a positive bleeding history require prophylaxis for invasive antenatal procedures, miscarriage, and delivery.

Factor XI concentrate provides effective cover and has a mean half-life of 52 hours, so a single dose is usually sufficient. However, it is associated with a potential risk of transfusion-transmitted infections, common to all plasma products, as well as an increased risk of thrombosis due to coagulation activation[15]. The increased thrombotic risk may be further exaggerated in pregnancy where there is already activation of coagulation and increased thrombin generation.

Fresh frozen plasma contains variable amounts of factor XI and patients with severe deficiency are unlikely to achieve levels above 3 IU/mL. However, it is helpful for milder cases and involves less donor exposure than factor XI concentrate. A dose of 15–20 mL/kg is effective but the risk of fluid overload must be considered.

Monitoring of the response to FFP or factor XI concentrate is important and due to the thrombogenicity of the latter, levels should not be allowed to exceed 70 IU/mL. A recent study found inhibitor development, after transfusion of plasma-derived factor XI, in 33% of patients with severe factor XI deficiency due to homozygous type II mutation (which accounts for approximately 25% of Jewish patients with severe factor XI deficiency).

Recombinant factor VIIa (rFVIIa, NovoSeven®, Novo Nordisk Ltd, Bagsverd, Denmark) is a possible alternative to plasma-derived FXI replacement and avoids the risk of bacterial or viral infections, transfusion-related lung injury, and development of inhibitors to factor XI. It is as yet unlicensed for use in this setting and the optimal dose has not been ascertained. A suggested dose for minor procedures is 90 µg/kg administered intravenously before surgery and 4 hours later. For major surgery 2-hourly infusions are necessary due to the short half-life of the product.

Intrapartum Management

Around 70% of patients do not experience bleeding problems at delivery. This may be due to increased levels of coagulation factors, including factor VIII and fibrinogen, at term. Also the pregnancy-associated reduction in fibrinolytic activity, due to decreased levels of tissue plasminogen activator and urokinase and an increased level of plasminogen activator inhibitor-2, contributes to hemostasis. Thus, even for those with severe factor XI deficiency an on-demand policy can usually be adopted for vaginal delivery[16]. However, it is important that the patient is closely observed and that all relevant staff are aware of the management plan.

It may be that a similar policy can be adopted for patients with severe deficiency undergoing cesarean section but until further studies are done, these patients should probably receive prophylaxis with one of the agents described above (Table 20.6).

Regional Anesthesia

Epidural anesthesia should be avoided in patients with low factor XI levels. If the procedure is necessary, it should be covered with factor XI concentrate and an adequate response demonstrated. FFP is not recommended due to the variable levels of FXI. Recombinant factor VIIa may provide effective cover but further evaluation is required in this area.

Postpartum Management

The incidence of primary and secondary postpartum hemorrhage in patients with untreated factor XI deficiency has been reported to be 16% and 24%, respectively. Tranexamic acid is effective although its use with factor XI concentrate should be avoided. The standard dose is 1 g 6–8 hourly for 3–5 days, with the first dose being administered in labor.

Neonatal Management

Neonatal hemorrhage due to peripartum events is rare but nevertheless care should be taken during delivery to avoid unnecessary trauma to the baby, including avoidance of ventouse extraction, rotational forceps, and invasive monitoring techniques. Spontaneous bleeding or intracranial hemorrhage has not yet been reported in neonates but a cord blood sample should be taken to determine the potential for bleeding during high-risk procedures such as circumcision. Neonatal levels are approximately half those of adults and repeat testing after 6 months of age is required to provide an accurate baseline level.

Rare Coagulation Factor Deficiencies

The rare coagulation disorders include deficiencies of coagulation factors II, V, VII, X, V, and VIII, combined vitamin K-dependent factors, FXIII, and disorders of fibrinogen. The spectrum of bleeding manifestations in individuals with these disorders is variable but some may present with severe bleeds, including intracranial hemorrhage and hemarthroses. With the exception of dysfibrinogenemia, these disorders have autosomal recessive inheritance and their prevalence, in the severe form, varies between 1:500 000 and 1:2 000 000. Pregnancy in women with these disorders or couples at risk of having an affected child should be managed in an obstetric unit with close links to a hemophilia center.

Hormonal Influences on Factor Levels

Factors II, V, and XIII tend to remain constant throughout pregnancy or show a slight increase but there is a progressive rise in factors VII, X, and fibrinogen, particularly in the third trimester. This is beneficial to heterozygous women with mild or moderate factor deficiency but in homozygous women, with severe deficiency, levels remain low.

Pre-pregnancy Management

The clinical bleeding tendency and response to hemostatic challenges should be ascertained. Women should be counseled about their potential bleeding risk in relation to pregnancy, antenatal procedures, delivery, and the postpartum period. Consent for use of blood products should be obtained and immunity to hepatitis

A and B ensured. Genetic counseling should be given and prenatal diagnosis offered where possible.

Antenatal Management

Levels should be checked at booking and repeated at 28 and 34 weeks' gestation. Depending on the factor level and clinical bleeding tendency, prophylaxis may be required for antenatal procedures and delivery. There is little evidence to guide therapeutic decisions but in general, relatively low levels of factors II, V, VII, and X, of around 20 IU/dL, are sufficient for normal hemostasis[14,17]. Therefore, patients with partial deficiencies and no history of bleeding can be managed expectantly. Otherwise, replacement therapy should start at the onset of established labor and the factor half-life should be considered to determine the need for and timing of repeat doses. Pre- and post-treatment factor levels should be obtained and effective levels maintained for 3–5 days after delivery.

Treatment Options

Prothrombin complex concentrates can be used for patients with factor II or X deficiency. These are pooled plasma-derived products containing known quantities of factors II, IX, and X, with or without factor VII. The strength of the concentrate is expressed in terms of units of FIX but this is approximately equal to the units of prothrombin. Concomitant use of tranexamic acid should be avoided because of the risk of thrombosis.

FFP is the only available product for FV deficiency and may also be used for patients with prothrombin and FX deficiency. A virally inactivated product should be used. An initial dose of 15 mL/kg should be given, with repeat doses dictated by factor levels and clinical response. Women with factor V deficiency failing to respond to FFP may benefit from platelet transfusions, which provide a concentrated supply of platelet factor V.

Recombinant FVIIa is the treatment of choice for surgery or childbirth in women with FVII deficiency, at a dose of 20–25 µg/kg administered every 4–6 hours.

Tranexamic acid is useful in preventing postpartum bleeding, although it should not be used in conjunction with prothrombin complex concentrates.

Patients with combined vitamin K-dependent factors can be treated with daily vitamin K, although FFP may be needed in the event of bleeding.

251

Early Pregnancy Failure

Maternal FXIII plays a critical role in uterine hemostasis and maintenance of the placenta during gestation. The risk of miscarriage in women with severe factor XIII deficiency is around 50%, depending on the subtype. These women should receive prophylactic infusions of FXIII at 2–4 weekly intervals, aiming for a trough level of >0.2 IU/mL[18]. A systematic review found a median level of 0.35 IU/mL was obtained during labor and delivery[19]. Higher factor XIII levels may be needed for delivery[20].

Fibrinogen is important for implantation and patients with afibrinogenemia or hypofibrinogenemia have a high rate of early miscarriage occurring at 6–8 weeks' gestation. Regular infusions of fibrinogen concentrate, to maintain trough levels >0.6 g/L, should be started as soon as pregnancy is confirmed and continued throughout pregnancy and the peripartum period [21]. Fibrinogen consumption tends to increase as pregnancy advances. Repeated ultrasounds should be carried out to detect concealed placental bleeding and monitor fetal growth.

Dysfibrinogenemia has been associated with a high incidence of miscarriage and stillbirth[22] but clinical phenotypes vary and management should be individualized, depending on the fibrinogen level and the clinical presentation of the disorder in the family.

Thromboprophylaxis with low-molecular-weight heparin is required for those with personal or family history of thrombosis and fibrinogen replacement for bleeding phenotypes but many cases are asymptomatic without the need for specific treatment.

Thrombosis

The potential for thrombosis following factor replacement must be considered and attention given to simple thromboprophylactic measures such as adequate hydration, compression stockings, and early mobilization. Patients with afibrinogenemia or dysfibrinogenemia are at particular risk of thrombosis due to impaired regulation of thrombin generation. Loose platelet thrombi form and are susceptible to embolization, therefore careful consideration should be given to the balance of bleeding and thrombotic risk. For patients with afibrinogenemia or hypofibrinogenemia, a continual infusion of fibrinogen concentrate to maintain levels above 1.5 g/L during the peripartum period allows for fine control.

Neonatal Management

Perinatal trauma such as ventouse delivery, rotational forceps, and fetal blood sampling should be avoided. Severe and moderate deficiencies can be diagnosed on a cord blood sample. Severely affected babies require cranial ultrasound to detect any ICH.

Case Studies

Case Study 1

A known carrier for moderate hemophilia A was referred in her third pregnancy. Her baseline factor VIII level outside of pregnancy was 35%. Two previous pregnancies had been complicated by postpartum hemorrhage following spontaneous vaginal delivery, when her factor VIII levels were 46% and 42%, respectively. Estimated blood loss with the first was 800 mL and 1500 mL with the second, when she was given a 2 unit blood transfusion. On both occasions, she received DDAVP after delivery, with a rise in her factor VIII level to 86% and 81%, respectively.

She was counseled about the risks of bleeding at delivery and the 50% risk to a baby boy of inheriting moderate hemophilia and to a baby girl of being a carrier. She chose to wait until a scan at 14 weeks to determine the gender of the baby, rather than having maternal blood sampling for free fetal DNA as she would not have wanted a termination. Her factor VIII levels were measured at 28, 34, and 38 weeks but did not increment and at delivery her level was 44%.

A delivery plan was drawn up by the hematologist, obstetrician, and anesthetist and included measures to prevent bleeding in both the mother and baby, who was now confirmed to be male.

Allowing spontaneous delivery was thought to be preferable, with early recourse to cesarean section if labor was prolonged; she had two previous vaginal deliveries. Avoidance of ventouse, rotational forceps, fetal blood sampling, and fetal scalp electrodes was advised, as well as cross-matching blood on arrival and DDAVP and tranexamic acid given in established labor. If needed, spinal anesthesia was allowed and active management of the third stage of labor recommended. In view of her previous PPHs, a senior obstetrician was asked to be available, Bakri balloon prepared, and interventional radiologists notified in case embolization was necessary.

The DDAVP resulted in a rise in FVIII to 91% and delivery was uncomplicated with no excess bleeding. She was given intramuscular Syntometrine, the placenta was delivered by controlled cord traction, and a Syntocinon infusion was administered for 24 hours. A factor VIII level from the umbilical cord was 7% and vitamin K was given orally. The baby was referred to the hemophilia center for follow-up. At 1 day postpartum, she received a further dose of DDAVP as her factor level had fallen to 45% and tranexamic acid was continued orally. After both doses of DDAVP, she was asked to restrict fluid intake for 24 hours, to quenching thirst only.

This case illustrates the bleeding tendency in carriers even if the factor level is only just under the normal range (it compares with non-carriers who have a significant rise in FVIII at delivery) and the need for DDAVP to be given in established labor (rather than immediately after delivery), to raise factor VIII levels before delivery.

Case Study 2

A woman was referred at 14 weeks in her first pregnancy, with ultrasound confirmation of a male baby. She was an obligate carrier for severe hemophilia B, in that her father had the condition. She was advised of the 50% risk of her baby having severe hemophilia but declined offers for prenatal diagnosis, as she would not wish to terminate the pregnancy. She did agree to a third trimester amniocentesis to enable an unaffected baby to have a normal delivery without restrictions. However, the baby was found to have the same hemophilia genetic mutation and she opted for a cesarean section.

Her baseline FIX level was previously found to be 27% and this was confirmed by a repeat test. Therefore, for both the amniocentesis and delivery she was covered with FIX concentrate, with a post-treatment factor IX level of around 100%. After the cesarean, her factor IX levels were monitored and further concentrate given to maintain the level above 0.5 IU/mL for 5 days. Thereafter she was continued on oral tranexamic acid until the lochia was clear.

This case highlights the use of third trimester amniocentesis to inform choices for delivery.

References

1. Pavord S, Rayment R, Madan B *et al*. The management of inherited bleeding disorders in pregnancy. RCOG Green-Top Guideline No. 71. April 2017 http://onlineli brary.wiley.com/doi/10.1111/1471-0528.14592/epdf (accessed July 25 2017).

2. Plug I, Mauser-Bunschoten EP, Bröcker-Vriends AH *et al*. Bleeding in carriers of hemophilia. *Blood* 2006; **108**(1): 52–56.

3. Miesbach W, Alesci S, Geisen C, Oldenburg J. Association between phenotype and genotype in carriers of hemophilia A. *Hemophilia* 2011; **17**(2): 246–251.

4. Kulkarni R, Lusher JM. Intracranial and extracranial hemorrhages in newborns with hemophilia: a review of the literature. *Journal of Pediatric Hematology/Oncology* 1999; **21**: 289–295.

5. Kadir RA, Economides DL, Braithwaite J, Goldman E, Lee CA. The obstetric experience of carriers of hemophilia. *British Journal of Obstetrics and Gynecology* 1997; **104**: 803–810.

6. Letsky EA. Hemostasis and epidural anesthesia. *International Journal of Obstetric Anesthesia* 1991; **1**: 51–54.

7. Lee CA, Chi C, Pavord SR *et al*. UK Hemophilia Center Doctors' Organization. The obstetric and gynecological management of women with inherited bleeding disorders: review with guidelines produced by a taskforce of UK Hemophilia Center Doctors' organization. *Hemophilia* 2006; **12**: 301–336.

8. Asakai R, Chung DW, Davie EW, Seligsohn U. Factor XI deficiency in Ashkenazi Jews in Israel. *New England Journal of Medicine* 1991; **325**: 153–158.

9. Hancock JF, Wieland K, Pugh RE *et al*. A molecular genetic study of factor XI deficiency. *Blood* 1991; **77**: 1942–1948.

10. Bolton-Maggs PH, Patterson DA, Wensley RT, Tuddenham EG. Definition of the bleeding tendency in factor XI-deficient kindreds – a clinical and laboratory study. *Thrombosis and Haemostasis* 1995; **73**: 194–202.

11. Bolton-Maggs PH, Wan-Yin BY, McCraw AH, Slack J, Kernoff P. Inheritance and bleeding in factor XI deficiency. *British Journal of Haematology* 2008; **69**: 521–528.

12. Myers B, Pavord S, Kean L, Hill M, Dolan G. Pregnancy outcome in Factor XI deficiency: incidence of miscarriage, antenatal and postnatal hemorrhage in 33 women with Factor XI deficiency. *BJOG: an International Journal of Obstetrics and Gynecology* 2008; **114**: 643–646.

13. Kadir RA, Lee CA, Sabin CA, Pollard D, Economides DL. Pregnancy in women with von Willebrand's disease or factor XI deficiency. *British Journal of Obstetrics and Gynaecology* 1998; **105**: 314–321.

14. Bolton-Maggs PH, Perry DJ, Chalmers EA *et al*. The rare coagulation disorders – review with guidelines for management from the United Kingdom Hemophilia Center Doctors' Organization. *Hemophilia* 2004; **10**: 593–628.

15. Bolton-Maggs PH, Colvin BT, Satchi BT *et al.* Thrombogenic potential of factor XI concentrate. *Lancet* 1994; **344**: 748–749.

16. Salomon O, Steinberg DM, Tamarin I, Zivelin A, Seligsohn U. Plasma replacement therapy during labor is not mandatory for women with severe factor XI deficiency. *Blood Coagulation and Fibrinolysis* 2005; **16**: 37–41.

17. Kadir R, Chi C, Bolton-Maggs P. Pregnancy and rare bleeding disorders. *Hemophilia* 2009; **15**(5): 990–1005.

18. Mumford AD, Ackroyd S, Alikhan R, *et al.* and the BCSH Committee. Guideline for the diagnosis and management of the rare coagulation disorders. *British Journal of Haematology* 2014; **167**: 304–326.

19. Sharief LAT, Kadir RA. Congenital factor XIII deficiency in women: a systematic review of literature. *Hemophilia* 2013; **19**(6):e349–e357.

20. Asahina T, Kobayashi T, Takeuchi K *et al.* Blood coagulation factor XIII deficiency and successful deliveries: a review of the literature. *Obstetrical & Gynecological Survey* 2007; **62**: 255–260.

21. Kobayashi T, Kanayama N, Tokunaga N *et al.* Prenatal and peripartum management of congenital afibrinogenemia. *British Journal of Haematology* 2000; **109**: 364–366.

22. Haverkate F, Samama M. Familial dysfibrinogenemia and thrombophilia. Report on a study of the SSC Subcommittee on Fibrinogen. *Thrombosis and Hemostasis* 1995; **73**: 151–161.

Chapter 21

Genetic Counseling and Prenatal Diagnosis of Congenital Bleeding Disorders

Nicola Curry and Andrew Mumford

Introduction

Heritable bleeding disorders are a group of lifelong conditions of varying severity that confer increased bleeding risk to patients. Severe and moderate bleeding disorders are of particular importance during pregnancy as they increase the risk of fetal intracranial hemorrhage at the time of delivery[1]. Severe bleeding disorders may also be associated with significant morbidity later in life and may require intensive long-term treatment, which can be a considerable burden to affected families.

All families in which an unborn fetus is at risk of a heritable bleeding disorder should receive appropriate genetic counseling to convey the expected pattern of inheritance (see Table 21.1), the probability of having affected children, the anticipated disease severity, and the implications for pregnancy and delivery. Most affected families require no further management, as many heritable bleeding disorders are phenotypically mild. Prenatal diagnosis is generally reserved for the more severe bleeding disorders, such

as moderate and severe hemophilia A or B, type 3 VWD, and the rare bleeding disorders where both parents are known to be heterozygous carriers and the fetus is at risk of a severe factor deficiency[2]. This chapter focuses mainly on hemophilia, as the most common severe heritable bleeding disorder, but also includes management of rarer bleeding disorders.

Genetic Counseling

Genetic counseling refers to the process of communicating information to women and families to enable informed decision-making about the consequences of carrying a fetus with a heritable bleeding disorder. Successful genetic counseling should be supportive and requires careful two-way discussion between families and healthcare professionals who are familiar with management of bleeding disorders and with the techniques available for carrier testing and prenatal diagnosis. Since genetic counseling often raises complex ethical and moral issues, this process may require

Table 21.1 Inheritance patterns for heritable bleeding disorders

		Inheritance	
	X-linked	Autosomal dominant	Autosomal recessive
Hemophilia	Hemophilia A Hemophilia B		
von Willebrand disease		Type 1 VWD[a] Type 2A VWD[a] Type 2B VWD Type 2M VWD Platelet type VWD	Type 2N VWD Type 3 VWD
Rare coagulation bleeding disorders		Dysfibrinogenemia Factor XI deficiency	Factors II, V, VII, X, XIII deficiency Combined FV and VIII deficiency Combined FII, VII, IX, and X deficiency Fibrinogen deficiency Factor XI deficiency

[a] Denotes that most, but not all, forms follow autosomal dominant inheritance.

multiple face-to-face consultations supported by clear and objective written information. Genetic counseling may be provided by appropriately trained hemostasis clinicians or by clinical geneticists. However, families should be offered a choice of counselor since they may be more comfortable discussing complex issues, particularly termination of pregnancy, with a counselor who does not also regularly provide medical treatment to a member of their family. Ideally, genetic counseling should be initiated before pregnancy is planned[3].

Genetic counseling is a step-wise process and may require discussion about the following issues:

- family diagnosis of the bleeding disorder and its clinical severity;
- inheritance pattern of the disorder within the family to either exclude carriership or to identify "possible" and "obligate" carriers;
- penetrance of the bleeding disorder;
- pattern of transmission and consequences of the bleeding disorder in future offspring;
- benefits and hazards of carrier detection techniques; and
- options available for management of pregnancy, including prenatal diagnosis.

Genetic Counseling for Hemophilia

Hemophilia A and hemophilia B are X-linked disorders caused by absent or reduced synthesis of coagulation factors VIII (FVIII) or IX (FIX), respectively. The disorders are caused by mutations in the long arm of the X chromosome in the *F8* gene (Xq28) or the *F9* gene (Xq27). The X-linked inheritance means that hemophilia mostly affects males. In contrast female carriers of hemophilia do not typically experience abnormal bleeding, but may transmit hemophilia to males in the next generation (Figure 21.1). The two disorders represent the most common of the severe heritable coagulation disorders with a combined prevalence of around 1 in 10 000. Approximately 50–60% of males with hemophilia have a positive family history, which usually provides the opportunity for informed pre-pregnancy genetic counseling and prenatal diagnosis[4].

The analysis of an accurate family pedigree is essential to establish the probability of hemophilia carriership and transmission risk.

- Sons of female hemophilia carriers have a 50% chance of having hemophilia.

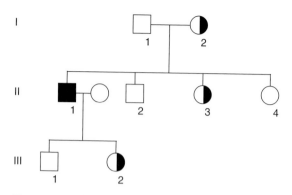

Figure 21.1 Pedigree of a family with hemophilia showing possible patterns of transmission of hemophilia over three generations. The offspring of a female hemophilia carrier (I.2) can include males with hemophilia (II.1), males without hemophilia (II.2), female hemophilia carriers (II.3), and females who are not hemophilia carriers (II.4). The offspring of males with hemophilia (II.1) can either be males without hemophilia (III.1) or female obligate hemophilia carriers (III.2).

- Daughters of female hemophilia carriers have a 50% chance of being carriers.
- Female hemophilia carriers may have partially reduced plasma FVIII or FIX activity.
- Sons of males with hemophilia will not have hemophilia unless there is also maternal hemophilia carriership.
- Daughters of males with hemophilia will always inherit hemophilia and will therefore be obligate hemophilia carriers.
- Approximately 40–50% of individuals newly diagnosed with hemophilia have no family history of hemophilia.
- Hemophilia is highly penetrant, meaning that the severity of the disease remains constant between generations.

Prediction of Hemophilia Carrier Status by Pedigree Analysis

For women from families with hemophilia, the probability that a pregnancy will yield a fetus that is a male with hemophilia can be estimated from the family pedigree using simple rules of Mendelian inheritance (Figure 21.2).

For families in which there is hemophilia in one individual but no antecedent history of hemophilia (sporadic hemophilia), calculating the risk of hemophilia in subsequent members of the same generation is more difficult (Figure 21.3). Sporadic hemophilia in males arises because of new mutations in the *F8* or *F9* genes occurring during gametogenesis in either the

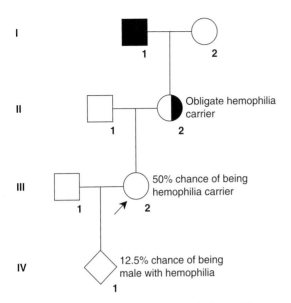

Figure 21.2 Example pedigree allowing calculation of the probability of carriership and transmission of hemophilia. The female proband (III.2 – arrowed) has a maternal grandfather (II.1) with hemophilia. Since I.1 is a male with hemophilia, the mother of the proband (II.2) is an obligate carrier of hemophilia. The proband III.2 therefore has a 50% chance of hemophilia carriership. Since the probability that a hemophilia carrier will carry a fetus that is a male with hemophilia at each pregnancy is 25%, the absolute probability that the unborn fetus IV.1 will be affected with hemophilia is 12.5%.

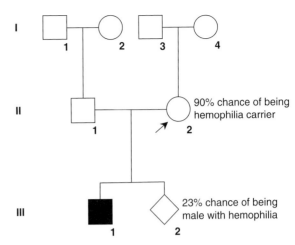

Figure 21.3 Example pedigree showing estimated probability of hemophilia carriership and transmission in a family with sporadic hemophilia. The female proband (II.2 – arrowed) already has a son who is affected with hemophilia (III.3) but has no other family history. The mutation responsible for hemophilia in III.3 is most likely to have occurred during spermatogenesis in individual I.3 and so the proband II.2 is likely to be a carrier of hemophilia. The estimated probability that II.2 is a carrier of hemophilia is approximately 90% and so the probability that each subsequent pregnancy will yield a male with hemophilia is approximately 23%.

mother or a maternal ancestor. However, spontaneous mutations occur more readily during spermatogenesis than oogenesis. Therefore, the causative mutation in a male with sporadic hemophilia is more likely to have arisen during spermatogenesis in the maternal grandfather than in oogenesis in the mother. It follows that mothers of males with sporadic hemophilia are likely to be constitutional hemophilia carriers. Observational population studies confirm this prediction and show that approximately 90% of mothers of males with sporadic hemophilia are carriers and therefore, have significant risk of transmitting hemophilia to future male offspring[5].

For women who have a history of hemophilia in antecedent male relatives, it may be possible to rule out carriership of the familial hemophilia mutation by analysis of the family pedigree alone. However, it is essential to recognize that there is a small probability of second hemophilia mutations arising through spontaneous mutagenesis. Therefore, women in whom carriership can be ruled out by pedigree analysis should be counseled that the risk of an affected male fetus is not zero, but instead is approximately the same as that of the background population. In pedigrees in which

there is any ambiguity over family relationships or paternity, it is good practice to offer laboratory carrier detection to all women by genetic testing, alongside testing of a confirmed affected male pedigree member.

Laboratory Detection of Hemophilia Carriership

Determining the probability of hemophilia carriership by pedigree analysis is essential for the genetic counseling process. However, all women who are potential hemophilia carriers should also be offered laboratory carriership detection. Two complementary approaches are available: coagulation factor activity assays and genetic testing.

Coagulation Factor Activity Assays

Female carriers of hemophilia may show reduced activities of coagulation factor VIII or IX to levels of 40–80% those of unaffected individuals[6]. However, there is wide variation in factor activity between carriers and there is significant overlap with women who are not hemophilia carriers. Therefore, measurement of coagulation factor activity may guide identification of hemophilia carriers but is insufficient for definitive diagnosis. The ratio of FVIII to von Willebrand factor antigen (VWF) may be helpful, as these two molecules normally circulate in the plasma with 1:1 stoichiometry. Thus, carrier status may be suspected if the ratio falls below 0.7, despite the absolute FVIII level being normal[7].

Genetic Detection of Carriership

Female hemophilia carriers are heterozygous for mutations in *F8* or *F9* and demonstration of a hemophilia-associated mutation in these genes is sufficient to diagnose carriership. It is good practice to confirm hemophilia carriership with genetic testing even in women identified as obligate carriers by pedigree analysis. Definitive exclusion of hemophilia carriership in potential carriers requires demonstration that the hemophilia mutation in the family is absent. In this circumstance, prior knowledge of the causative mutation in a male with hemophilia or an obligate female carrier from the family is essential. Diagnosis of hemophilia A or B mutations should follow national guidelines[8,9].

Testing the potential for transmission of hemophilia in asymptomatic women raises complex moral issues for the individual and families undergoing testing. The full implications of genetic testing should therefore be discussed during counseling and informed written consent is mandatory. Counseling should include specific discussion about the limitations of *F8* and *F9* genetic analysis. Parents should also be made aware that some forms of prenatal diagnosis, such as diagnostic CVS or amniocentesis, can only be offered if the familial genetic mutation is known, since testing for unknown mutations can be time consuming and without prior knowledge of the familial mutation rapid genetic diagnosis cannot be performed reliably[10].

Mutations Associated with Hemophilia

Although more than 1800 *F8* mutations have now been identified in individuals with hemophilia A, many defects are recurrent and have been recognized in multiple affected families. A major structural rearrangement of the *F8* gene resulting from an inversion involving intron 22 accounts for approximately 50% of cases of severe hemophilia A. Other recurrent mutations associated with severe hemophilia A include an inversion affecting intron 1, point mutations, nonsense mutations, deletions, or other major structural changes in *F8* that prevent expression of the gene. Mild hemophilia A and hemophilia B are usually associated with point mutations in *F8* and *F9*, respectively, although since mild hemophilia A and B are genetically heterogeneous, previously unreported mutations are common.

The mutation databases for hemophilia A (www .factorviii-db.org) and hemophilia B (www.factorix .org) contain bibliographic references and phenotypic data from previously reported families with hemophilia[11]. These resources are invaluable for confirming that a newly identified mutation in a hemophilia family is causative and in predicting the future clinical phenotype, including inhibitor risk, of affected males.

Both *F8* and *F9* databases are now housed within a central web portal at www.eahad-db.org, which also provides access to the VWF variant database: www .vwf.group.shef.ac.uk/.

Limitations and Hazards of Genetic Diagnosis of Carriership

Failure to Detect Causative Mutations

Approximately 5% of hemophilia mutations are not detected by inversion analysis or analysis of the coding sequence of *F8* or *F9*. Some mutations, such as large deletions, may be readily detected in males with standard Sanger sequencing techniques but this is not the case in heterozygous female carriers. When standard techniques fail, analysis using multiplex ligation-dependent probe amplification (MLPA) should be undertaken[12]. This technique is able to detect duplications and deletions by analyzing PCR copy number. For example, if a gene is duplicated so there are three copies, the final amount of PCR product produced by MLPA will be 1.5 times greater than normal (Figure 21.4). If MLPA fails to detect a mutation then detection of carriers may require techniques such as linkage analysis. This may not be informative in all families and, because of genetic recombination events, has lower diagnostic accuracy than direct mutation detection by sequencing.

False-Negative Carrier Detection Because of Somatic Mosaicism

An individual is a somatic mosaic for hemophilia when a spontaneous hemophilia mutation occurs in a somatic cell during early embryogenesis rather than during gametogenesis in one or other parent. This means that in an affected embryo, the hemophilia mutation is present in some cells, including germ

(a)

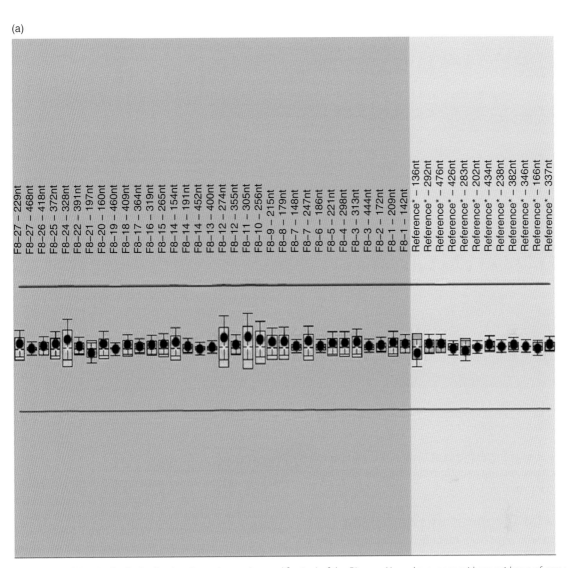

Figure 21.4 (a) MLPA (multiplex ligation-dependent probe amplification) of the *F8* gene. Normal sequence with no evidence of copy number variation (results lie between red and blue lines). (b) MLPA of *F8* gene showing heterozygous duplication of exons 1 to 10 (inclusive), detected in an obligate carrier of severe hemophilia A. Duplication is evident by the greater number of copies detected (blue dots).

cells, but not all cells. Those germ cells which contain the hemophilia mutation may then go on to form gametes, potentially resulting in transmission of the hemophilia mutation to subsequent generations.

Somatic mosaicism has been identified in a female proband in more than 10% of families with severe hemophilia and, in some cases, the hemophilia mutation was present in up to 25% of maternal cells[13]. In this circumstance, standard genetic testing of DNA obtained from peripheral blood cells may not identify a hemophilia mutation since the proportion of peripheral cells that contain the mutation is too low for

detection. This may result in mis-classification of somatic mosaic mothers as "not hemophilia carriers." Somatic mosaicism should be considered in all women who have a son with hemophilia but no other family history and who have been classified as "not a hemophilia carrier" by standard genetic testing. Estimates of the recurrence risk for non-carrier mothers due to mosaicism for X-linked disorders are variable, with reported values ranging from 3 to 10%. For families with sporadic hemophilia B, one study estimated that women have a risk of hemophilia B in a second fetus of <6%[14]. This very low probability

259

(b)

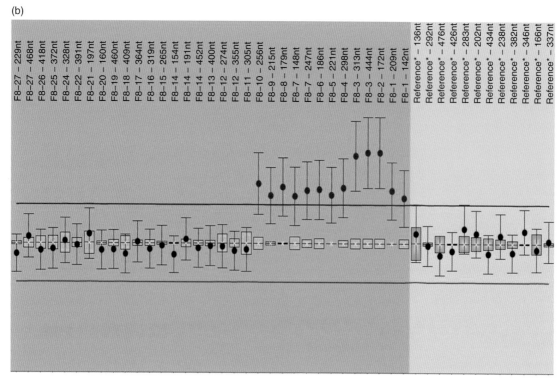

Figure 21.4 (cont.)

may be similar for all forms of hemophilia and should be discussed during genetic counseling for all potential carrier women.

Prenatal Diagnosis of Hemophilia

Women who have been identified as hemophilia carriers by pedigree analysis and laboratory investigation may be offered several different options for prenatal diagnosis. Involvement of healthcare professionals with expertise in fetal medicine is essential.

Prenatal diagnosis in hemophilia is currently offered to families for two different reasons:

1. For more accurate prediction of whether a fetus will be affected with hemophilia. This is achieved either by fetal sexing or by mutation detection to rule in or rule out an affected fetus. This option is typically performed in the third trimester when the absolute risk to the pregnancy by amniocentesis is low.

2. For early definitive diagnosis of hemophilia in a male fetus using first trimester prenatal genetic diagnosis to enable the option of termination of an affected pregnancy.

Prenatal Fetal Sexing

Fetal sexing is an important first step in the evaluation of the fetus of a pregnant hemophilia carrier since if a female fetus is identified, the probability of a significant bleeding disorder is very low and a restrictive delivery with hemostatic precautions is not necessary [15]. Fetal sexing may be performed by non-invasive (ultrasound or free fetal DNA [ffDNA] analysis) or invasive (chorionic villus sampling [CVS] or amniocentesis) techniques.

Non-invasive techniques

Non-invasive techniques are attractive to both parents and physicians since they present no direct risk to the pregnancy[16].

Fetal Ultrasound

Fetal ultrasound allows reliable sex determination (accuracy >99%) in most pregnancies from about 18–20 weeks' gestation. Earlier ultrasound can reliably determine fetal sex if performed in some specialist centers, but only from 13 weeks' gestation[17].

Free Fetal DNA Analysis

The ffDNA technique relies on the principle that identification of a genetic sequence associated with the Y chromosome indicates that a fetus is male. The most commonly used technique detects the *SRY* locus, although this is usually performed alongside analysis of the *DYS14* sequence to increase diagnostic accuracy[17]. This assay requires a maternal venous blood specimen of <20 mL and has >99% diagnostic accuracy at 8–12 weeks' gestation in expert centers [18]. A recent study that evaluated ffDNA testing in a cohort of 196 women that included hemophilia carriers showed 100% accuracy as early as 7 weeks' gestation[19]. If samples are taken very early in pregnancy, test failure may be more common due to lower levels of circulating ffDNA. It is advised that a dating ultrasound is used to confirm gestational age, to limit the need for a repeat test. Ideal timing for ffDNA is currently considered to be at 8–9 weeks' gestation[17].

Fetal sexing by ffDNA analysis has enabled female fetuses to be identified before 11–14 weeks. However, since the diagnostic accuracy for identifying a female fetus is less than that of identifying a male fetus, it is good practice to confirm gender by fetal ultrasound at 18 weeks' gestation.

Invasive techniques

The Royal College of Obstetricians and Gynecologists (RCOG) provide detailed evidence-based guidelines for chorionic villous sampling and amniocentesis[20].

Chorionic Villous Sampling

- First trimester prenatal genetic diagnosis allows definitive diagnosis of hemophilia in a fetus but still requires invasive testing using CVS.
- CVS is an important option for confirmed hemophilia carriers who are considering termination of a male fetus with hemophilia. The uptake of this approach is very low in most reported series of pregnancies in hemophilia carriers.
- CVS is available to those families where the hemophilia mutation is known. Genetic results can be expected within 3–5 working days of the procedure, thereby facilitating early termination, if appropriate.
- CVS for prenatal genetic diagnosis is performed at 11–13 weeks' gestation and carries a miscarriage

rate of approximately 1%. CVS has historically been associated with fetal limb reduction defects, particularly if performed before 10 weeks' gestation.
- Hemophilia carrier mothers with low coagulation factor levels may need hemostatic support before the CVS procedure (see Chapter 20).
- Placental cells obtained by CVS are first used to determine fetal sex. Detection of the hemophilia mutation present in the family is then performed only on cells from confirmed male fetuses.

Amniocentesis

Amniocentesis is an alternative technique for prenatal genetic diagnosis and can safely be performed from 15 weeks' gestation. This technique is therefore less suitable for women contemplating termination of pregnancy and is much less commonly used than CVS for diagnosis of hemophilia. Amniocentesis is associated with overall miscarriage rates of 0.5–1%. However, higher miscarriage rates and fetal talipes have been associated with amniocentesis performed before 15 weeks[21]. Cord blood sampling is unsuitable for prenatal diagnosis of hemophilia because of the risk of bleeding if the fetus is affected with hemophilia.

Third Trimester Amniocentesis

Amniocentesis performed at 34–36 weeks enables definitive genetic diagnosis in pregnancies where the fetus is at risk of a moderate or severe bleeding disorder. Late amniocentesis carries a risk of early rupture of membranes and premature labor of approximately 1% in experienced centers[20]. Consequently, women routinely receive steroid therapy prior to the procedure to improve fetal lung maturity. Late amniocentesis can only be performed where the causal hemophilia mutation is known and results can be expected within 3–5 working days. All mothers should be counseled about risks of early labor which could result in delivery before the genetic test result is known.

Third trimester amniocentesis allows hemostatic precautions and restrictive delivery to be applied only to male fetuses who are affected with hemophilia or to fetuses confirmed as having other severe bleeding conditions, such as type 3 VWD (see Chapter 19). In a recently reported case series of late amniocentesis in nine pregnancies in six women (four carriers of hemophilia A, one carrier of hemophilia B, and one at risk of a fetus with type 2B VWD), all women delivered successfully after 37 weeks' gestation[22]. Genetic analysis showed five unaffected fetuses, in which delivery using routine practice in local hospitals was possible, without restrictive pro-hemostatic precautions.

Preimplantation Genetic Diagnosis

Preimplantation genetic diagnosis (PGD) combines assisted reproductive technology with molecular genetics and cytogenetics to allow the identification of an abnormality of the embryo prior to implantation [23]. Preimplantation sexing with reimplantation of female or unaffected male embryos requires standard in vitro fertilization techniques, and then harvesting of cells from embryos at the 8-cell stage for analysis. Single-cell PCR enables detection of specific mutations in male embryos[24]. These approaches are technically feasible in hemophilia and have now been performed in small numbers of successful pregnancies. Preimplantation genetic diagnosis may be the preferred option for those women who do not wish to consider termination of an affected pregnancy. However, assisted reproductive technology is stressful and requires invasive transvaginal egg collection which in some carriers may require pro-hemostatic support. In the UK, PGD has limited availability through the National Health Service because of the high costs and approximately 30% success rate of each PGD cycle.

Future Techniques for Prenatal Diagnosis

Mutation Detection Using ffDNA or Fetal Cells in Maternal Blood

Detection of hemophilia mutations in ffDNA or in fetal cells in maternal blood in pregnancy potentially offers non-invasive prenatal diagnosis of hemophilia. This approach requires highly efficient purification of fetal material from maternal blood and may only be feasible in the third trimester when ffDNA and fetal cells are most abundant. Furthermore, detection of hemophilia mutations in ffDNA may be hampered by the presence of mutant alleles of maternal origin. One emerging approach is to quantify accurately the relative concentration of mutant compared to normal gene sequences in maternal blood using

sensitive techniques such as digital PCR. Early experience of this technique suggests that diagnosis may be achieved with high accuracy as early as 11 weeks' gestation[25].

Genetic Counseling for Other Severe Heritable Bleeding Disorders

Genetic counseling, carrier detection, and prenatal diagnosis should also be considered in families with other rare heritable bleeding disorders which may also present a bleeding risk to an affected fetus. Since most of the rare bleeding disorders show autosomal recessive inheritance, genetic counseling requires discussion about the transmission of homozygous or compound heterozygous mutations from both parents. Affected fetuses are usually sporadic and arise in families with no bleeding history in heterozygous "carrier" ancestors. For mothers who are known heterozygous "carriers" or who themselves are homozygous or compound heterozygous for a recessive bleeding disorder, accurate prediction of fetal bleeding risk may require partner testing. This is particularly important in consanguineous partnerships where the risk of transmission of homozygous recessive mutations is high.

Genetic counseling for the rare bleeding disorders should reflect that the relationship between plasma coagulation factor activity and bleeding risk in affected individuals is less predictable than in hemophilia and that some disorders show variable penetrance. Since the range of reported mutations in the rare bleeding disorders is less than for hemophilia, detection of previously undescribed mutations in affected families is common. Uncertainty about whether a candidate mutation is causal may hamper genetic carrier detection and prenatal diagnosis in some families.

Prenatal Diagnosis in Other Heritable Bleeding Disorders

Prenatal diagnosis can only be undertaken in those families where causal genetic mutations have been identified. Fetal sex testing plays no part in prenatal diagnosis of the rare bleeding disorders since these disorders are autosomally inherited. If the genetic cause is known, CVS, amniocentesis, and late amniocentesis can be performed as for hemophilia. Mothers may require factor concentrate therapy or other hemostatic measures such as tranexamic acid before invasive diagnostic procedures.

Case Studies

Case Study 1

A 26-year-old obligate carrier of severe hemophilia A attends the hemophilia center at 5 weeks' gestation. She has previously received genetic counseling and her carriership status has been confirmed by genetic testing. She and her partner have agreed that they would consider a termination if the fetus was an affected male. After a dating scan to confirm gestational age, a maternal blood sample was drawn at 8–9 weeks for ffDNA analysis to measure maternal FVIII activity and for blood group and antibody screen. Since ffDNA analysis typically requires 4–5 working days, testing at this time point enables fetal sex to be known by 10 weeks' gestation. For this reason, a preliminary date for a CVS was arranged at the time of blood sampling. The ffDNA test confirmed a male fetus and the mother went on to have CVS at 11 weeks' gestation for confirmatory fetal sexing by karyotype and then genetic testing of the *F8* gene. Since the familial hemophilia mutation was already known, the CVS genetic test result was available within 3–5 working days. In this case study, after detailed discussion and counseling, the family chose to proceed with termination of pregnancy using suction techniques, which are possible up to the end of the 12th week of gestation and are psychologically and physically less demanding than termination at a later gestation.

Case Study 2

A 14-month-old boy was referred to the hemophilia center for investigation of bruising and a prolonged aPTT. The boy had been born at term by spontaneous vaginal delivery, with no instrumentation. His development was normal and there was no history of bleeding, except an increased propensity to bruise. Coagulation testing revealed a diagnosis of severe hemophilia A (baseline FVIII level <0.01 IU/mL). Genetic testing of the *F8* gene using a Southern blotting technique confirmed the inversion 22 mutation in the boy but showed only normal *F8* in the mother. There was no family history of hemophilia. Therefore, the mother was informed that hemophilia in her son had arisen through a spontaneous mutation and that she was not a carrier.

Three years later, the mother delivered a second son through a normal vaginal delivery. Although the second son was initially asymptomatic, he presented at 14 months old with a knee hemarthrosis. Subsequent investigations confirmed that he also had severe hemophilia A caused by the inversion 22 mutation. Further detailed analysis of a genomic DNA sample from the mother using highly sensitive quantitative PCR confirmed that approximately 10% of her peripheral blood DNA harbored the inversion 22 mutation, indicating that she was a somatic mosaic for severe hemophilia.

This case highlights that women with a male child with apparently de novo hemophilia should be counseled very carefully if they are found not to be a carrier of the familial mutation by conventional genetic testing. Somatic mosaicism should be discussed with women in this scenario and should be evaluated using specialist genetic testing techniques.

References

1. Chi C, Kadir R. Inherited bleeding disorders in pregnancy. *Best Practice and Research Clinical Obstetrics and Gynecology* 2012; **26**: 103–117.

2. Kadir R, Chi C, Bolton-Maggs P. Pregnancy and rare bleeding disorders. *Hemophilia* 2009; **15**: 990–1005.

3. Ludlam CA, Pasi KJ, Bolton-Maggs P *et al.* A framework for genetic service provision for hemophilia and other inherited bleeding disorders. *Hemophilia* 2005; **11**: 145–163.

4. Miller R. Genetic Counseling for Hemophilia. World Federation of Hemophilia; 2002. www.wfh.org

5. Kasper CK, Lin JC. Prevalence of sporadic and familial hemophilia. *Hemophilia* 2007; **13**: 90–92.

6. Plug I, Mauser-Bunschoten EP, Broker-Vriends AH *et al.* Bleeding in carriers of hemophilia. *Blood* 2006; **108**: 52–56.

7. Shetty S, Ghosh K, Pathare A, Mohanty D. Carrier detection in hemophilia A families: comparison of conventional coagulation parameters with DNA polymorphism analysis – first report from India. *Hemophilia* 2001; **5**: 243–246.

8. Keeney S, Mitchell M, Goodeve A; on behalf of the UK Haemophilia Centre Doctors' Organisation (UKHCDO), the Haemophilia Genetics Laboratory Network and the Clinical Molecular Genetics Society. Practice Guidelines for the Molecular Diagnosis of Haemophilia A; 2010. http://www.acgs.uk.com/media/774613/haemophilia_a_bpg_revision_sept_2011_approved.pdf

9. Mitchell M, Keeney S, Goodeve A; on behalf of the UK Haemophilia Centre Doctors' Organisation (UKHCDO), the Haemophilia Genetics Laboratory Network and the Clinical Molecular Genetics Society. Practice Guidelines for the Molecular Diagnosis of Haemophilia B; 2010. http://www.acgs.uk.com/media/774631/haemophilia_b_bpg_revision_sept_2011_approved.pdf

10. Kessler L, Adams R, Mighion L et al. Prenatal diagnosis in hemophilia A: experience of the genetic diagnostic laboratory. *Hemophilia* 2014; **20**: e384–391.

11. Rallapalli PM, Kemball-Cook G, Tuddenham EG et al. An interactive mutation database for human coagulation factor IX provides novel insights into the phenotypes and genetics of hemophilia B. *Journal of Thrombosis and Haemostasis* 2013; **11**: 1329–1340.

12. Payne AB, Bean CJ, Hooper WC, Miller CH. Utility of multiplex ligation-dependent probe amplification (MLPA) for hemophilia mutation screening. *Journal of Thrombosis and Haemostasis* 2012; **10**: 1951–1954.

13. Leuger M, Oldenburg J Lavergne J-M et al. Somatic mosaicism in hemophilia A: a fairly common event. *American Journal of Human Genetics* 2001; **69**: 75–87.

14. Green PM, Saad S, Lewis CM, Gianelli F. Mutation rates in humans I: overall and sex-specific rates obtained from a population study of hemophilia B. *American Journal of Human Genetics* 1999; **65**: 1572–1579.

15. Lee C, Chi C, Pavord SR et al. The obstetric and gynecological management of women with inherited bleeding disorders – review of guidelines produced by a taskforce of UK Hemophilia Center Doctors' Organization. *Hemophilia* 2006; **12**: 301–336.

16. Lewis C, Hill M, Skirton H, Chitty LS. Non-invasive prenatal diagnosis for fetal sex determination: benefits and disadvantages from the service users' perspective. *European Journal of Human Genetics* 2012; **20**: 1127–1133.

17. Colmant C, Morin-Surroca M, Fuchs F et al. Non-invasive prenatal testing for fetal sex determination: is ultrasound still relevant? *European Journal of Obstetrics & Gynecology and Reproductive Biology* 2013; **171**: 197–204.

18. Avent N, Chitty LS. Non-invasive diagnosis of fetal sex; utilization of free fetal DNA in maternal plasma and ultrasound. *Prenatal Diagnosis* 2006; **26**: 598–603.

19. Bustamente-Aragones A, Rodriguez de Alba M, Gonzalez-Gonzalez C et al. Foetal sex determination in maternal blood from the seventh week of gestation and its role in diagnosing hemophilia in the foetuses of female carriers. *Hemophilia* 2008; **14**: 593–598.

20. RCOG. *Amniocentesis and Chorionic Villous Sampling. Green-Top Guideline No. 8.* London: Royal College of Obstetricians and Gynecologists; 2010. http://www.rcog.org.uk/

21. Alfirevic Z, Mujezinovic F, Sundberg K. Amniocentesis and chorionic villus sampling for prenatal diagnosis. *Cochrane Database of Systematic Reviews* 2003 (**3**): CD003252.

22. Cutler J, Chappell LC, Kyle P, Madan B. Third trimester amniocentesis for diagnosis of inherited bleeding disorders prior to delivery. *Hemophilia* 2013; **19**: 904–907.

23. Peyvandi F, Garagiola I, Mortarino M. Prenatal diagnosis and preimplantation genetic diagnosis: novel technologies and state of the art of PGD in different regions of the world. *Hemophilia* 2011; **17** (Suppl 1): 14–17.

24. Michelidis K, Tuddenham EG, Turner C et al. Live birth following the first mutation specific pre-implantation genetic diagnosis for hemophilia A. *Thrombosis and Hemostasis* 2006; **95**: 373–379.

25. Tsui NBY, Kadir RA, Chan KC et al. Noninvasive prenatal diagnosis of hemophilia by microfluidics digital PCR analysis of maternal plasma DNA. *Blood* 2011; **117**: 3684–3691.

Chapter 22

Pre-eclampsia

Eleftheria Lefkou and Beverley Hunt

Introduction

Ten million women develop pre-eclampsia each year around the world. Worldwide about 76 000 pregnant women die each year from pre-eclampsia and related hypertensive disorders. And, the number of babies who die from these disorders is thought to be in the order of 500 000 per annum[1]. In developing countries, a woman is seven times more likely to develop pre-eclampsia than a woman in a developed country. Ten to 25% of these cases will result in maternal death[2].

Pre-eclampsia, intrauterine growth restriction (IUGR), and placental abruption are complications of ischemic placental disease (IPD). While the clinical manifestations of IPD vary significantly, there are common underlying etiological and pathophysiological processes, as suggested by the shared medical, demographic and epidemiological risk factors, and the increased cross-recurrence risk. The underlying pathology for all three conditions may include endothelial activation, uteroplacental insufficiency, ischemia, and underperfusion, beginning from the stage of implantation, and indicated by placental histology, ultrasound indices, and several biological markers.

The three causes of IPD occur simultaneously in the same pregnancy more often than expected by chance, and any specific IPD condition in a prior pregnancy is a risk factor for that same or another IPD in a subsequent pregnancy. In terms of co-occurrence and recurrence risk, these conditions are more prevalent in preterm gestations than in term gestations and appear heavily influenced by the degree of severity.

This chapter will focus on providing a basic understanding of pre-eclampsia and its complications and will then go on to briefly describe IUGR and placental abruption followed by a more in depth consideration of pre-eclampsia.

Intrauterine Growth Restriction

Intrauterine growth restriction occurs when a fetus is unable to reach its predetermined growth potential, and affects an estimated 3–10% of pregnancies. Owing to the amount of information required to confer a diagnosis of IUGR (i.e. serial ultrasounds and Doppler studies), epidemiological studies frequently use small-for-gestational age (SGA) as a proxy for IUGR. Fetal abdominal circumference (AC) or estimated fetal weight (EFW) <10th centile can be used to diagnose an SGA fetus[3].

Placental insufficiency, as measured by structural abnormalities and histological findings, is the most frequent cause of IUGR, but fetal factors, including both chromosomal abnormalities and vertically transmitted congenital infections, as well as maternal factors also contribute to IUGR. Risk factors for IUGR include smoking during pregnancy, alcohol and/or drug abuse, low pre-pregnancy body mass index and nutritional status, poor weight gain during pregnancy, pre-gestational diabetes mellitus, gestational diabetes, celiac disease, sickle cell disease, chronic hypertension, and antiphospholipid syndrome (see Chapter 16). One of the strongest risk factors for IUGR in a current pregnancy is a previous IUGR-affected pregnancy. The risk factors are shown in Table 22.1.

Placental Abruption

Placental abruption, defined as complete or partial separation of the placenta from the uterus prior to delivery, is the least common of the three IPD conditions with an estimated prevalence of 0.5% or 1 in 200 deliveries. Risk factors for placental abruption include advanced maternal age, multiparity, multiple pregnancy, maternal trauma, cigarette, smoking, drug use during pregnancy, pre-eclampsia, chronic hypertension, antiphospholipid syndrome, and pre-gestational diabetes. The greatest risk factor for abruption is a prior placental abruption, with estimates ranging from 3- to 12-fold increased risk of a subsequent abruption.

Preterm placental abruption (<37 weeks) and term placental abruption (≥37 weeks) are believed to have

Table 22.1 Risk factors for pre-eclampsia (PET)

Nulliparity
High body mass index (BMI) (>35 at booking)
Multiple gestation (twins, triplet pregnancies)
Chronic hypertension
Diastolic pressure >89 mmHg at booking
Proteinuria at booking
Previous pregnancy with PET or IUGR child
Family history of PET (in mother or sisters)
Black race
Maternal age under 20 and possibly maternal age over 35 to 40
Diabetes mellitus or insulin resistance
Renal disease
Thrombophilias and hyperviscosity syndromes
Underlying maternal collagen vascular disease
Presence of antiphospholipid syndrome or antibodies
Increased circulating testosterone
Protein D deficiency in mother during pregnancy
Trisomy 13
High altitude
Mirror syndrome
Fetal (genetic) factors from donor eggs
Father of Hispanic origin
Parental specific genes

varied biological mechanisms. Risk factors and conditions associated with preterm abruption substantially differ from those associated with term abruption, thus implicating that these two diagnoses are truly distinct. IPD usually relates to preterm placental abruption.

Pre-eclampsia

Pre-eclampsia (PET) is a pregnancy-related multisystem syndrome, classically defined as the new onset of hypertension (blood pressure greater than 140/90 mmHg) after 20 weeks of gestation and proteinuria (or urinary excretion of protein ≥300 mg/24 hours) resolving after delivery. According to the Task Force Report on Hypertension in Pregnancy by The American College of Obstetricians and Gynecologists, the diagnosis of pre-eclampsia no longer requires the detection of high levels of protein in the urine (proteinuria)[4].

Recently the protein/creatinine ratio has been proposed as a more easily applicable screening test for suspected pre-eclampsia. A protein/creatinine (P/C) ratio <18 mg/mM can exclude proteinuria and a P/C >60 mg/mM correlates with severe proteinuria. Twenty-four-hour urine collection could be used for urinary protein:creatinine ratio values between 18 and 60 mg/mM in the detection of significant proteinuria[5].

PET is also termed toxemia, pregnancy-induced hypertension, and pre-eclamptic toxemia. Symptoms can occur any time after 20 weeks of gestation or even start in the first few days after delivery, and usually resolve within 2 weeks after delivery of the placenta. Early onset PET is when it develops before the 34th week of gestation and late-onset PET when it presents after the 34th week of pregnancy. Predisposing factors are shown in Table 22.1. It is not known why some women develop pre-eclampsia, while others with the same risk factors do not. Eclampsia occurs when PET is complicated by seizures.

Chronic hypertension is defined as a systolic pressure ≥140 mmHg and/or diastolic pressure ≥90 mmHg that antedates pregnancy, is present before the 20th week of pregnancy, or persists longer than 12 weeks' postpartum. PET with chronic hypertension is diagnosed when a pregnant woman has a history of chronic hypertension and then develops features suggestive of PET after the 20th week of pregnancy.

Gestational hypertension, or transient hypertension of pregnancy, refers to the situation that is characterized by elevated blood pressure (>140/90 mmHg) after the 20th week of gestation, but without proteinuria, that occurs uniquely during pregnancy and resolves after birth.

Epidemiology of Pre-eclampsia

Pre-eclampsia (PET), the commonest medical complication of pregnancy, affecting approximately 2–8% of all pregnancies, remains a major cause of maternal and fetal morbidity and mortality worldwide. It is estimated that 50 000 women die annually worldwide due to PET and eclampsia. In the United States, the incidence of PET is approximately 5–8% (with a 20% increase in the last decade), with 75% of cases being mild and 10% of cases due to early onset PET. According to the latest report from the Confidential Enquiry into Maternal and Child Health in the UK, the maternal mortality rate due to PET is at its lowest ever rate of 0.38 deaths per 100 0000 maternities[6]. The incidence of PET in the UK is reported as 2–8%, but mild PET is underreported and so the true incidence is potentially much higher.

PET is associated with intrauterine growth restriction (IUGR) in one-third of cases. Premature delivery to prevent the progression of PET is responsible for 15% of all preterm births. Infants of women with PET have a fivefold increase in mortality compared with infants of mothers without the disorder. The recurrence likelihood for PET is reported as 60% if it occurred before 34 weeks' gestation and 10–20% if it occurred near term. The key to appropriate management is early clinical recognition.

Diagnosis of PET

The diagnosis of PET is based on the maternal history, signs, and symptoms (Table 22.2). The current aim of antenatal care is to monitor for signs of PET at each clinic visit, with assessment of blood pressure, urinalysis, and the presence of edema. These visits occur more frequently in the third trimester of pregnancy, especially in women with risk factors. Most women with PET experience only mildly increased blood pressure and small amounts of proteinuria. Edema, especially in the face and hands, is a frequent sign of PET, but is not pathognomonic, for many women without PET also develop edema during pregnancy. Other forms of hypertensive disorders also occur in pregnancy and should be considered in the differential diagnosis of PET.

The maternal manifestations of PET can affect almost every organ, depending on severity. Possible complications of PET in the mother and in the fetus are listed in Table 22.3.

Current Concepts on the Pathogenesis of PET

Placental dysfunction is the central feature in the development of PET. In 1939 Ernest Page introduced the

Table 22.3 Complications of PET

(A) Maternal

Central nervous system
- Eclampsia
- Cerebral edema
- Cerebral hemorrhage
- Retinal edema
- Retinal blindness
- Cortical blindness

Liver
- HELLP syndrome
- Acute liver failure
- Hepatic rupture

Renal system
- Acute renal failure
- Renal cortical necrosis
- Renal tubular necrosis

Respiratory
- Pulmonary edema
- Laryngeal edema

Hemostatic system
- Thrombocytopenia
- DIC
- Microangiopathic hemolytic anemias

Cardiovascular system
- Risk factor for later cardiovascular disease

Labor
- Placental infarction
- Placental abruption
- Preterm delivery

(B) Fetal–Neonatal
- IUGR
- Prematurity
- Death
- Neurological complications
- Later cardiovascular disease

Table 22.2 Signs and symptoms of severe pre-eclampsia

Blood pressure greater than 160/110 mmHg

Impaired kidney function (serum creatinine concentration >110 µmol/L, urine protein greater than 5 g in a 24-hour urine collection), or low urine production (less than 500 mL in 24 hours)

Persistent severe headache

Papilledema and/or visual disturbances (blurred vision, diplopia, blind spots, flashes of light, or squiggly lines)

Hyperreflexia, brisk tendon reflexes (3+)

Pulmonary edema, shortness of breath

Nausea, vomiting

Abdominal pain, persistent new epigastric pain, or tenderness

Impaired functional liver tests (elevated alanine aminotransferase, aspartate aminotransferase)

Thrombocytopenia ($<100 \times 10^9$/L)

Microangiopathic hemolytic anemia

concept that PET may be due to the reduced perfusion of the placenta. The development of PET is hypothesized to be in two stages, according to a theory introduced by the Oxford Group in 1991, and supported and expanded by Roberts[7]. The first stage is reduced placental perfusion and the second the maternal response to this – maternal endothelial cell activation. Failure of endovascular trophoblast invasion is thought to lead to relative underperfusion of the placenta. Under conditions of hypoperfusion, the placenta probably releases factors into the circulation which then trigger maternal endothelial dysfunction.

Early in normal gestation, cytotrophoblast cells invade the decidua and myometrium. These cells also invade endovascularly, replacing first the endothelium

267

and then the media of the spiral arteries. This creates a system of flaccid, low-resistance, large-diameter, unresponsive arterioles that increase placental perfusion. The outcome is an increment in blood flow to the fetus and lack of adrenergic vasomotor control. The endothelial lining is replaced by the cytotrophoblast cells, which adapt to mimic an endothelial pattern of adhesion molecule expression.

In PET, this vascular phenotype is not expressed and the pattern of invasion is much more superficial. There is a restriction of trophoblast invasion into the spiral arteries, particularly those within the myometrium. These decidual vessels may later show atherosis, and superimposed thrombosis augments hypoperfusion. It seems plausible that, consequent to these changes, placental hypoperfusion causes a state of relative hypoxia.

Various factors have been postulated as the substance produced from the placenta that affects blood flow, arterial pressure, and maternal endothelial cell activation (ECA). These factors include oxidative stress, cytokines such as tumor necrosis factor α (TNF-α) and interleukin 6 (IL-6), insulin-like growth factors, nitric oxide (NO), heparin-binding endothelial growth factor-like growth factor, endothelin-1, arachidonic acid metabolites, angiotensin II type-1 receptor autoantibody (AT1-AA), and angiogenic factors.

Recently, the focus has been on angiogenic factors. It has been proposed that PET could be related to an imbalance between proangiogenic (such as vascular endothelial growth factor, VEGF) and antiangiogenic factors such as fms-like tyrosine kinase (sFlt-1) and soluble endoglin (sEng). sFlt-1 is an endogenous inhibitor of both VEGF and PGF and may regulate placental angiogenesis by preventing the interaction between circulating VEGF and PGF with their proangiogenic receptors. Levels of sFlt-1 in the plasma of women with PET are elevated compared with normal pregnancies. When sFlt-1 is exogenously administered via adenovirus-mediated gene transfer in pregnant rats and mice, there are increases in arterial blood pressure and proteinuria, as well as decreased levels of VEGF and PIGF, similar to those observed in PET[8,9]. Another observation was that VEGF infusion attenuates the increased blood pressure and renal dysfunction observed in pregnant rats overexpressing sFlt-1[10]. Also, uteroplacental ischemia has been shown to increase plasma and placental sFlt-1 and to decrease the levels of VEGF and PIGF in late gestation of rats and baboons[11]. Endoglin (Eng) is a component of the transforming growth factor (TGF)-beta receptor complex and a hypoxia inducible protein, and is related to cellular proliferation and NO signaling. Soluble Eng (sEng) has been shown to act as an anti-angiogenic factor, possibly via the inhibition of TGF-beta binding to cell-surface receptors[12]. In vitro work showed that sEng inhibits in vitro endothelial cell tube formation and that adenovirus-mediated increase of both sflt-1 and sEng in pregnant rats resulted in IUGR and in a syndrome resembling PET[13]. Recently, sEng levels have been proposed as a predictor of PET[14].

Whichever factor provokes maternal ECA, when the latter is established, it leads to up-regulation of a number of inflammatory molecules, including adhesion molecules. These procedures change the endothelium phenotype from antithrombotic to prothrombotic, with a decrease in the formation of the vasodilator and antiplatelet agents prostacyclin and nitric oxide, the production of endothelin, and finally the down-regulation of anticoagulant systems.

Redman's research group in Oxford proposed that the endothelial dysfunction seen in PET is part of a wider inflammatory response and that placental hypoperfusion is not necessarily the sole primary event. They argue that pregnancy normally elicits an inflammatory response[15]. This is evidenced by changes in granulocytes and monocytes such as increased intracellular production of reactive oxygen species and up-regulation of surface molecules such as CD11b and CD64, as well as release of L-selectin, which is related to granulocyte activation. During PET there is increased activation of platelets, neutrophils, and monocytes and an increase in the release of microparticles when compared with normal pregnancy. Perhaps these inflammatory changes are a response to the presence of fetal (or paternal) antigens. If so, then abnormalities of the normal immunomodulation seen at the fetoplacental interface could act to trigger PET. HLA-G is important in the prevention of recognition of the placenta as "non-self" and there is a reduction of expression of HLA-G in PET along with abnormal responsiveness of maternal lymphocytes toward fetal cells.

Microparticles are fragments of cell membranes released into the circulation as a result of cellular activation or apoptosis and can have a procoagulant effect. Microparticles in pregnancy are derived from a number of cells, but the predominant population is platelet derived. Vesicles prepared from syncytiotrophoblast microvillous membranes (STBM) have been shown to suppress the proliferation of endothelial cells in vitro. They also affected an in vitro model of endothelial cell-dependent arterial relaxation. The numbers of STBM

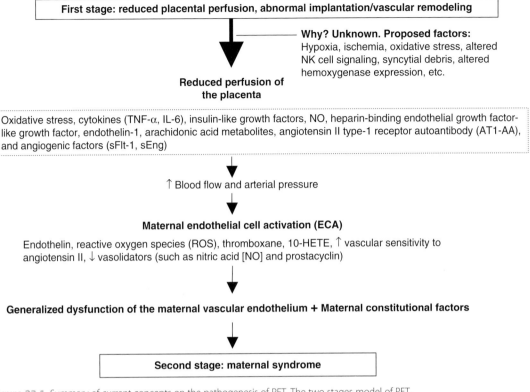

Figure 22.1 Summary of current concepts on the pathogenesis of PET. The two stages model of PET.

detected in the circulation of pre-eclamptic women have been shown to be significantly elevated compared with those with normal pregnancies[16].

A summary of the currently favored pathogenesis of PET is shown in Figure 22.1.

Relation between PET and IUGR

The consequences of placental dysfunction can be two-fold – IUGR and the maternal symptoms and signs of PET. What is not understood is why some women only have IUGR, while others have both IUGR and PET. It has been suggested that the maternal syndrome of PET may only occur in women with "constitutional factors" (genetics, environmental, dietary, behavior, etc.) that render the mother sensitive to the effects of reduced placental perfusion.

Constitutional factors that have been proposed to act as the inductors of the maternal syndrome of PET include several dietary factors, metabolic conditions such as diabetes, insulin resistance and uric acid, low melatonin levels, obesity, metabolic syndrome, folic acid and hyperhomocysteinemia, hyperlipidemia with elevated triglycerides, free fatty acids and low-density lipoprotein (LDL) cholesterol and reduced high-density lipoprotein (HDL), maternal vitamin D deficiency, and thrombophilia. The factors that cause ECA may contribute to the development or severity of PET.

Relation of PET with Later Medical Risk in Women and Their Babies

Despite PET and IUGR occurring only in pregnancy, they have been shown to have long-term consequences. Mothers who have had PET or have delivered a baby with IUGR experience a two- to eightfold increased risk of atherosclerotic cardiovascular disease (CAD) in later life[17]. It is unclear whether PET causes CAD or whether these two entities share the same causal origin. It has also been shown that the earlier PET presents in pregnancy, the more severe the later maternal CAD is. Women who developed PET before 37 weeks of gestation had an eightfold higher risk of cardiovascular death 14 years later than women with normal pregnancies.

There is a large body of epidemiological studies showing that the long-term consequences of FGR in the baby last well into adulthood. These individuals have a predisposition to develop a metabolic syndrome later in life, manifesting as obesity, hypertension, hypercholesterolemia, cardiovascular disease, and type 2 diabetes, in agreement with the theory of early origin of CAD, also known as "the Barker hypothesis"[18].

A recent study showed positive associations between maternal pre-pregnancy levels of triglycerides, cholesterol, low-density lipoprotein, and baseline systolic blood pressure and subsequent development of PET[19]. The authors concluded that the presence of cardiovascular risk factors prior to pregnancy is predisposing to PET. The prevalence of chronic hypertension is significantly higher among women with a history of PET (46.7%) as well as those with previous IUGR (8.9%)[20]. Women with PET and FGR with chronic hypertension on follow-up had increased carotid intimal-media thickness, suggesting a predisposition to atherosclerosis. Women with previous PET have significantly higher fasting glucose levels, waist circumference, body mass index, and higher prevalence of metabolic syndrome compared to normal women[21].

Recently it has been shown that early onset pre-eclampsia was associated with an increased risk of asthma in the offspring, but part of this association may be due to confounding by factors shared by siblings[22]. Interestingly data from the Childhood Autism Risks from Genetics and the Environment (CHARGE) study, a population-based, case–control investigation of autism spectrum disorder and developmental delay, showed that pre-eclampsia, particularly severe disease, is associated with the later development of both disorders[23].

New Modifications of Current Theories on the Pathogenesis of PET

As long as the initial causative factor for PET remains unrecognized, different theories continue to be generated, some of them challenging the currently accepted

origins of PET. It has been suggested that early-onset (before 34 weeks) and late-onset (after 34 weeks) PET are two different clinical entities with different pathogenesis, origins, etiology, severity, and clinical expression. Certainly, IUGR is more strongly associated with severe rather than with milder pregnancy-induced hypertension[24]. According to this theory, early PET is associated with reduced perfusion but PET at term may not, suggesting different genetic origins for early and late PET.

Huppetz has challenged the placental origins of PET and proposed that PET is a syndrome of early placental formation[25]. He suggested that an insult results in aberrant development and differentiation of the villous syncytiotrophoblast, causing impaired maintenance of the placental barrier. This subsequently leads to the release of necrotic and aponecrotic fragments culminating in a systemic inflammatory response of the mother. According to this theory IUGR is due, in contrast, to a failure of extravillous trophoblast invasion. This new concept clearly separates the origins of PET and IUGR, and proposes alterations in different trophoblast differentiation pathways as origins of both syndromes.

Genome-wide expression analysis in rodents showed that spontaneous differentiation of trophoblast stem cells is associated with the acquisition of an endothelial-cell-like thromboregulatory gene expression program[26]. This program is developmentally regulated and conserved between mice and humans. They further showed that trophoblast cells sense, via the expression of protease-activated receptors, the presence of activated coagulation factors. Engagement of these receptors results in cell-type specific changes. These observations define candidate fetal genes that are potential risk modifiers of PET and suggest that hemostasis can affect trophoblast physiology and thus affect placental function in the absence of frank thrombosis[27]. It is postulated that PET is not only due to a maternal cause, but also that fetal genes could contribute to the development of the disease[26]. Another study, by Salmon et al., showed that the presence of risk variants in complement regulatory proteins in patients with systemic lupus erythematosus and/or antiphospholipid syndrome who develop pre-eclampsia, as well as in pre-eclampsia patients lacking autoimmune disease, links complement activation to disease pathogenesis and suggests new targets for treatment of the placental ischemic disease[28].

Thrombophilia and PET

Acquired Thrombophilia

Mothers with antiphospholipid antibodies have a predisposition to PET and IUGR. Indeed, the development of these conditions before 34 weeks in a woman with antiphospholipid antibodies has now become a defining criterion for obstetric antiphospholipid syndrome. This is discussed in more depth in Chapter 16. Other acquired conditions that predispose to thrombosis such as myeloproliferative disease would also be expected to predispose to PET (see Chapter 24).

Genetic Thrombophilias

An association between PET and inherited thrombophilias was first reported by Dekker *et al.* in 1995, who proposed that maternal thrombophilia could act as a genetic constitutional factor for the development of PET[29]. Since then, a large number of retrospective and case-controlled studies have examined the association between different types of thrombophilic mutations and PET. The results of published reports have been inconsistent. Meta-analysis of all case–control studies suggests that only FVL mutation is associated with a minor increased risk of PET (odds ratio, 1.18; 95% confidence interval, 1.14 to 2.87). Overall, studies suggest that women with genetic thrombophilia affected by PET will have more severe PET than those without, but thrombophilia itself does not precipitate the condition.

Prediction of PET

As the exact causative factor that provokes PET is not yet known, at present there is no clear strategy for its prevention and so the clinical and research focus has been on early detection and prediction.

Hyperuricemia is an established marker of severe PET, correlating with the histological severity of renal lesions, and clinically with adverse fetal outcomes, but has a low negative predictive value.

Uterine artery Doppler screening between 20 and 24 weeks identifies mothers at high risk for developing adverse pregnancy outcomes[30]. The correlation between elevated uterine artery resistance and a high risk of PET and/or IUGR was first demonstrated at the end of the second trimester, probably reflecting the ongoing process of trophoblast invasion into the spinal arteries. Bilateral notching at 20–24 weeks identifies the pregnancies that will have IUGR and PET, although

there is a high false-positive rate[30]. Increased levels of soluble fms-like tyrosine kinase 1 (sFlt-1) and reduced levels of soluble placental growth factor (PlGF) have been shown to predict the subsequent development of PET, as early as 5 weeks before the onset of PET[31–33]. Human cancer patients treated with anti-VEGF antibody developed hypertension and proteinuria. In association with increased levels of sFlt-1, symptoms were dramatically worse, and typical of HELLP syndrome, leading the authors to postulate that increased levels of sFlt-1 were responsible for PET, but the combination of increased sFlt-1 and sEng led to HELLP syndrome. In a longitudinal analysis, the rise in soluble endoglin concentrations occurred earlier and was more marked in pregnancies with subsequent pre-eclampsia.

Soluble endoglin (sEng) is a co-receptor for transforming growth factor β1 and β3, expressed on trophoblasts. Its levels are increased in pre-eclampsia[15], and in pregnant rats this has been associated with increased vascular permeability and hypertension. Other serum markers that have been proposed to predict PET as early as the first trimester are placental protein 13 (PP13), placenta-associated plasma protein A (PAPP-A), and long pentraxin 3 (PTX3). All of these markers still need further evaluation in larger multicenter trials.

Management of Pre-eclampsia

At present, the sole effective therapy for pre-eclampsia is delivery and removal of the placenta. Symptoms usually improve within days. Therefore, early diagnosis and timely delivery are imperative for maternal and perinatal survival.

Prevention of PET

Several drugs have been tried for the prevention of PET. Despite the first promising publications, later larger studies showed no evidence for calcium, vitamin C, and vitamin E in PET's prevention. The main drugs that are used for the prevention of PET are antihypertensives and antithrombotics.

Prevention of PET with Antihypertensives

Antihypertensive drugs are used for secondary prevention of PET in women with mild to moderate hypertension developing during or pre-existing the pregnancy. Data from several studies showed that, although there was a reduction in hypertension, it was unlikely that this had a major impact on the progression to PET.

Furthermore, it has been argued that the impact on the fetus of lowering maternal blood pressure could provoke IUGR. Although there is no large randomized trial, beta-blockers have been found to be more likely to have such an impact (eight trials, 810 women; relative risk 1.56, 1.10 to 2.22). The antihypertensive drug methyldopa has often been used in gestational hypertension. Side effects include depression and drowsiness. Other drugs that can be used are labetalol and calcium channel blockers. Atenolol is relatively contraindicated in pregnancy due to possible FGR. Absolutely contraindicated are angiotensin-converting enzyme inhibitors and angiotensin receptor antagonists due to possible teratogenicity. Diuretics should be avoided in general and should be kept only for special indications such as renal or cardiac diseases.

Prevention of PET with Antithrombotics

Antiplatelet Agents

The Collaborative Low-dose Aspirin Study in Pregnancy (CLASP study) was a randomized trial of low-dose aspirin for the prevention and treatment of PET among 9364 pregnant women[34]. The women were randomly assigned 60 mg aspirin daily or matching placebo. To simulate real obstetric practice, the entry criteria were broad and embraced women thought to be at risk of PET and FGR from 12 to 32 weeks' gestation. Primiparous women, women with pre-existing hypertension or a history of IUGR, PET or stillbirth, and women with established PET could all be entered in the study: 74% were entered for prophylaxis of PET, 12% for prophylaxis of IUGR, 12% for treatment of PET, and 3% for treatment of IUGR. Overall, the use of aspirin was associated with a reduction of only 12% in the incidence of proteinuric PET, which was not significant. Nor was there any significant effect on the incidence of IUGR or of stillbirth and neonatal death. Aspirin did, however, significantly reduce the likelihood of preterm delivery (7% aspirin vs 2% control), with an absolute reduction of 5 per 100 women treated. There was a significant trend toward progressively greater reductions in proteinuric pre-eclampsia, the more preterm the delivery. Aspirin was not associated with a significant increase in placental hemorrhage or in bleeding during preparation for epidural anesthesia, but there was a slight increase in use of blood transfusion after delivery. Low-dose aspirin appeared safe for the fetus and newborn infant,

with no evidence of an increased likelihood of bleeding. The rate of stillbirth, neonatal death, or fetal growth retardation occurring before 32 weeks was 5.3% in the aspirin group as compared with 10.6% in the placebo group. These findings do not support routine prophylactic or therapeutic administration of aspirin in pregnancy to all women at increased risk of pre-eclampsia or IUGR. Low-dose aspirin may be justified in women judged to be especially liable to early onset PET severe enough to need very preterm delivery. In such women it seems appropriate to start low-dose aspirin prophylactically early in the second trimester.

The Cochrane Library summarizing data from 37 560 women for 59 trials of aspirin to prevent PET showed that the use of aspirin is associated with a 17% reduction in the risk of pre-eclampsia (46 trials, 32 891 women, relative risk [RR] 0.83, 95% confidence interval [CI] 0.77 to 0.89), an 8% reduction in the relative risk of preterm birth (29 trials, 31 151 women, RR 0.92, 95% CI 0.88 to 0.97; NNT 72 [52, 119]), and a 14% reduction in fetal or neonatal deaths (40 trials, 33 098 women, RR 0.86, 95% CI 0.76 to 0.98; NNT 243 [131, 1666]), and a 10% reduction in small-for-gestational age babies (36 trials, 23 638 women, RR 0.90, 95% CI 0.83 to 0.98) http://www.cochrane.org/CD004659/PREG_antiplatelet-agents-for-preventing-pre-eclampsia-and-its-complications. The authors concluded that antiplatelet agents, largely low-dose aspirin, have moderate benefits when used for prevention of PE and its consequences[34,35].

The Perinatal Antiplatelet Review of International Studies (PARIS) Collaborative Group published a meta-analysis that included 31 randomized trials of PET primary prevention, enrolling a total of 32 217 women and their 32 819 infants[35]. According to their results, antiplatelet agents, particularly aspirin, moderately reduce the relative risk for PET, preterm births before 34 weeks' gestation, and serious adverse pregnancy outcomes. For women randomized to receive antiplatelet agents, the relative risk of developing PET, compared with women in control groups, was 0.90 (95% CI 0.84–0.97). The risk of delivering before 34 weeks' gestation was 0.90 (95% CI 0.83–0.98) and of having a pregnancy with a serious adverse outcome was 0.90 (95% CI 0.85–0.96). Use of antiplatelet agents was not associated with any significant effect on the risk of death of the fetus or newborn, risk of having an infant born small-for-gestational age, or risk for bleeding events for either the women or their babies. No subgroups of women who were substantially more or less likely to benefit from antiplatelet agents than any other were identified[36]. Despite these two large meta-analyses, further studies are required to assess which women are most likely to benefit, when treatment is best started, and at what dose.

The ACCP 2012 guidelines recommend the use of aspirin 80–100 mg/day after 12 weeks' gestation for all women at high risk for pre-eclampsia after the 12th week of gestation[37]; while the Maternal–Fetal Medicine Units High-Risk Aspirin study (MFMU High-Risk Aspirin study) showed that aspirin initiated at <17 weeks' gestation reduced the risk for late-onset pre-eclampsia by 29%, suggesting and supporting the practice of early initiation of aspirin in high-risk women[38]. Interestingly a recent study showed that aspirin inhibits the production of sFLT1 in primary cytotrophoblasts (CTBs) and in HTR-8/SVNeo, suggesting that the aspirin effect may be mediated via inhibition of celecoxib (COX1)[39].

The ASPRE study (ISRCTN13633058) is a multicenter ongoing trial in the European Union to establish whether the prophylactic use of low-dose aspirin from the first trimester of pregnancy in women at increased risk for preterm pre-eclampsia can reduce the incidence of the disease. Results so far show a significant reduction of PET with an aspirin dose of 160 mg.

Heparin and Antithrombin Concentrates

Heparin (subcutaneous low-dose unfractionated heparin or low-molecular-weight heparin) as monotherapy or in combination with aspirin has also been suggested for the prevention of PET in women with high-risk pregnancies, but data are not yet sufficient for a final conclusion. For example, a recent study investigated the effect of low-molecular-weight heparin (LMWH) on pregnancy outcome, on the maternal blood pressure values, and on uteroplacental flow in angiotensin-converting enzyme (ACE) non-thrombophilic women, with insertion/deletion (I/D) polymorphism, with history of PET[40]. The study included 80 women: 41 were treated with dalteparin 5000 IU/day, and 39 did not receive treatment (control group). This study suggests that LMWH may reduce the recurrence of PET, of negative outcomes, and the resistance of uteroplacental flow, and also prevents maternal blood pressure increase in ACE DD homozygote women with a previous history of PET.

Antithrombin (AT) levels are reduced in PET. Previous randomized controlled trials of AT therapy in PET between 24 and 35 weeks' gestation have shown significantly improved maternal symptoms and birth weight[41]. A further trial examined AT therapy in severe PET in women presenting before 32 weeks' gestation: 42 patients were enrolled and each received AT 3000 IU per day for 7 days compared to albumin 582 mg/day for 7 days. An equal number of women discontinued the intervention in the AT and placebo (albumin) groups. AT treatment improved or at least preserved fetal biophysical status. It enabled the pregnancy to reach 34 weeks and fetal growth rate was preserved. However, AT treatment of PET is still largely confined to research settings.

Future Candidates for the Prevention and Treatment of PET

Animal models have shown that pravastatin, a hydrophilic statin that does not cross the placenta, can ameliorate PET in antiphospholipid syndrome, so there is major interest in examining the safety and the efficacy of statins in preventing or treating PET in humans. Currently, a randomized placebo-controlled clinical trial of statins in pre-eclampsia, Statins to Ameliorate early onset Pre-eclampsia (StAMP) trial, is recruiting patients in the UK[42]. In addition, a pilot clinical trial in the United States has started to collect maternal–fetal safety data in high-risk pregnant women receiving pravastatin between the 12th and 17th week of gestation in high-risk women to prevent pre-eclampsia. Epidemiological data collected to date suggest that statins are not major teratogens[43,44].

A recent study is testing in vitro approved drugs to identify candidate compounds with therapeutic potential as pre-eclampsia treatments via their proangiogenic properties; so far, the authors have identified vardenafil as a potential protective agent against pre-eclampsia[45]. The therapeutic mechanism of vardenafil may involve inhibition of the systemic maternal antiangiogenic state that leads to pre-eclampsia, in addition to its vasodilating effect. As concentrations used in this study were high and are unlikely to be useful clinically, further work is needed before testing its safety and effectiveness in humans.

Clinical Management

Planning for the Optimal Timing of Delivery

One can justify PET, of any severity, presenting after 34 weeks as an indication for delivery. If earlier than 34 weeks, the balance of expectant management is set against risk to the mother, but potentially benefits the child in terms of risks of prematurity. Generally, hemodynamic instability, fetal distress, and rapid disease progression are indications for delivery. There is no evidence base to support these decisions, as only small trials of expectant management prior to 34 weeks versus delivery have been carried out.

If an induced preterm delivery is contemplated, it may be necessary to give prostaglandins to ripen the cervix. Steroid therapy to improve fetal lung maturity should also be considered, in discussion with the pediatric team. In general, a vaginal delivery is considered safer than cesarean section for those with complications of PET. For both forms of delivery, a platelet count of greater than 50×10^9/L is recommended, and platelet transfusions may be necessary to achieve this.

Regional anesthesia is also generally preferred, but depends on the platelet count, and guidelines recommend a count of greater than 75×10^9/L, in the setting of normal platelet function. Coagulation parameters should also be checked prior to delivery because of the risk of DIC in PET.

It should be emphasized that the disease may not abate immediately post-delivery and that seizures can occur up to a week later. Hence, seizure prophylaxis, antihypertensive therapy, and frequent monitoring should be continued for an appropriate period, e.g. 12–48 hours for seizure prophylaxis and close monitoring, and up to 12–16 weeks or indefinitely for antihypertensive therapy.

Other Pharmaceutical Management of PET

Antihypertensive Drugs for the Management of PET

The most used antihypertensive drugs in the management of PET are methyldopa, labetalol, and nifedipine. Labetalol is quite safe and effective, decreasing heart rate and having fewer side effects than other drugs (lack of reflex tachycardia, hypotension, or increased intracranial pressure). In general, angiotensin-converting enzyme (ACE) inhibitors, angiotensin receptor-blocking drugs (ARB), and diuretics should be avoided. Nifedipine should be given orally and not sublingually. Concern has been raised about hydralazine as first-line treatment (due to the potential unpredictable hypotension) and the combination of nifedipine and magnesium sulfate.

Magnesium Sulfate

Magnesium sulfate is the drug of choice for the prevention and treatment of pre-eclampsia. The epidemiological and basic science evidence suggesting that magnesium sulfate, when given in early pregnancy to women considered at risk of preterm birth, may be neuroprotective for the fetus has now been confirmed by a recent Cochrane systematic review[46]. It acts by causing cerebral vasodilation, thereby reversing the ischemia produced by cerebral vasospasm during an eclamptic episode. Data suggest that women receiving magnesium sulfate therapy have a 58% lower risk of eclampsia than placebo and that it also reduces the risk for maternal death. A possible side effect is flushing, which occurs in one-quarter of women[47].

Guidelines for the Management of Established PET

The following guidelines are suggested:

- Close inpatient or outpatient monitoring of vital signs, deep tendon reflexes, neurological examination.
- Bed rest and relaxation.
- Fetal monitoring: external fetal monitor, oxcytocin challenge test, biophysical profile.
- Give steroids to accelerate fetal lung maturation when <34 weeks of gestation; betamethasone 12 mg IM/day for two doses, or dexamethasone 6 mg IM/12 hours × four doses.
- Careful fluid restriction to reduce the risk of fluid overload. Total fluid intake should be limited to 80 mL/hour (max 150 mL/hour) or 1 mL/kg/hour; urine output can be tolerated as low as 10 mL/hour.
- Give supplemental oxygen.
- Maintain diastolic blood pressure <110 mmHg and systolic <160 mmHg with antihypertensive drugs.
- Give prophylactic intravenous magnesium sulfate for the prevention of eclampsia during labor and the postpartum.
- Laboratory monitoring: complete blood count, platelet count, coagulation studies in severe PET (PT, PTT, fibrinogen, FDP), urea, serum creatinine, uric acid, serum electrolytes, liver function tests, lactate dehydrogenase.

Guidelines for the Management of Eclampsia

These include:

- Close monitoring.
- Give oxygen.

- Fluid restriction is advisable to reduce the risk of fluid overload. Total fluid should be limited to 80 mL/hour or 1 mL/kg/hour.
- Give magnesium sulfate; alternative drugs include diazepam and phenytoin.
- Give steroids if <34 weeks' gestation.
- Urgent delivery.

Hematological Complications of PET

All the changes taking place during PET due to endothelial cell activation usually produce hematological complications. Thus frequent (at least every 8 hours) full blood count and coagulation screen should be performed in case of severe PET, or where there is suspicion of subsequent development of hematological complications.

Thrombocytopenia

The most common hematological complication of PET is thrombocytopenia, occurring in 18% of pre-eclamptic women. This is probably due to platelet and endothelial activation generating thrombin and causing platelet consumption. In general, the severity of thrombocytopenia is related to the severity of PET. If the platelet count is greater than 40×10^9/L, the risk of bleeding is small. In the majority of cases, thrombocytopenia resolves after delivery, but rarely platelet levels may continue to fall after birth. Severe thrombocytopenia persisting after delivery could be a possible indicator of developing microangiopathic hemolytic anemia and a blood film is required to look for platelet fragmentation.

Management of Thrombocytopenia in PET

Platelet counts of >50×10^9/L in patients with otherwise normal coagulation are regarded as safe for normal vaginal delivery and cesarean section. Concerns over the risk of hematoma formation and neurological damage have led to the use of regional anesthesia not being recommended unless the platelet count is <75×10^9/L with a normal coagulation screen. This recommendation is based on consensus rather than on evidence.

If the platelet count is <50×10^9/L and there is no bleeding, then no treatment is necessary unless there is active bleeding, when it is appropriate to transfuse platelets.

Disseminated Intravascular Coagulation (DIC)

DIC is a clinicopathological syndrome characterized by a systemic activation of coagulation leading to microvascular deposition of fibrin, and thus to consumption of coagulation factors, platelets, and physiological anticoagulants. This produces a reduction in platelet count, a fall in fibrinogen, and a prolongation of the activated partial thromboplastin time (aPTT) and international normalized ratio (INR).

Prolongation of PT and aPTT with severe thrombocytopenia and low fibrinogen levels (<1.0 g/L) are signs of a developing DIC-like state and hence frequent estimation of platelet count, fibrinogen (using Clauss method), prothrombin time (PT), and aPTT is strongly recommended. Laboratory evidence of a consumptive coagulopathy should be sought before microvascular bleeding becomes evident, so that appropriate and aggressive action can be taken to address the underlying cause.

DIC occurs in about 10–12% of all cases of PET and in 7% of severe PET. The etiology of DIC in pre-eclampsia is not well understood, but it is probably a consequence of endothelial cell activation. In only 10–15% of DIC cases in PET, it can become more systemic and even lethal. In PET there is a low-grade fibrin deposition in the renal and placental microcirculation.

DIC in obstetric patients could be a complication of other obstetric conditions or of none related directly with pregnancy. The most common causes of DIC in obstetrics, besides PET, are abruption placentae and amniotic fluid embolism (occurring in more than 50% of obstetric cases), and retained dead fetus, sepsis, and septic abortion.

Management of DIC

Management of DIC involves (1) treating the cause and (2) replacement of missing hemostatic components with blood products. Hematological treatment consists of platelets, FFP, and cryoprecipitate (see Chapter 18C), but avoiding circulatory overload. Novel therapeutic strategies are based on current insights into the pathogenesis of DIC, and include anticoagulant strategies (e.g. directed at switching off coagulation stimulus). Strategies to restore physiological anticoagulant pathways (such as activated protein C concentrate) outside of pregnancy have failed to show any benefit in large RCTs. These have not been evaluated adequately in the management of DIC in pregnancy and postpartum.

HELLP Syndrome

HELLP syndrome (hemolysis, elevated liver enzymes, low platelets) occurs in the second and third trimester of pregnancy and presents occasionally postpartum. There are no clear definition criteria for HELLP. This disorder complicates between 0.5% and 1% of pregnancies and is associated with a maternal morbidity ranging between 1% and 4%. HELLP syndrome is reported in PET with an incidence ranging between 2% and 50% (5% and 15%), depending on the population studied and the diagnostic criteria used: 70% of cases occur antenatally and 30% occur within the first 48 hours to 7 days postpartum. Twenty percent of women who develop HELLP post-labor had no evidence of PET before delivery. The incidence of HELLP is significantly increased among white middle-class and older multiparous women. DIC is found in approximately 20–30% of women with HELLP. Recurrence rates in subsequent pregnancies are 3% for HELLP, 10–14% for IUGR, and 18–20% for PET. The differential diagnosis of HELLP syndrome is shown in Table 22.4

Clinical Presentation of HELLP

The clinical presentation is with fatigue and malaise for a few days, followed by nausea, vomiting, shoulder, neck, epigastric or right upper-quadrant pain, headache, and visual disturbances. Right upper-quadrant or epigastric pain is thought to be due to obstruction of blood flow in the hepatic sinusoids, which are blocked by intravascular fibrin deposits. Usually, the patients present with significant weight gain, due to the associated generalized edema, and with proteinuria greater than 1+ (in 90% of cases). Severe hypertension is not a constant or a

Table 22.4 Differential diagnosis of HELLP syndrome

Acute fatty liver of pregnancy
Gall bladder disease
Gastroenteritis
Appendicitis
Diabetes insipidus
Hemolytic uremic syndrome
Thrombotic thrombocytopenic purpura
Idiopathic thrombocytopenic purpura
Acute renal failure
Pyelonephritis
Glomerulonephritis
Peptic ulcer
Flair of systemic lupus erythematosus
Viral hepatitis

frequent finding in HELLP syndrome. That is why women are often misdiagnosed as having another disease (listed in Table 22.4).

Pathophysiology of HELLP Syndrome

The pathophysiology is not clear, but it is helpful to consider that it represents PET confined to the liver, which may result in necrosis of areas of the liver. According to one theory, pre-eclamptic patients are already prone to spontaneous hemorrhages. The liver is thought to be particularly prone because fibrin split products can deposit in the reticuloendothelial system of the liver. Multiple previous subclinical spontaneous hemorrhages within the small hepatic sinusoids and arterioles may go unnoticed symptomatically and leave the liver in a fragile state. Fibrin thrombi may be left uncleared in the liver. Occasionally, a trigger (such as DIC) may cause extreme hypoperfusion of the liver, leading to infarction.

As the liver is the primary site of plasma protein production and pregnancy is a hypermetabolic condition, it is unsurprising that a specific plasma protein profile was noted in women with HELLP syndrome compared with normal control cases. The primary candidate identified was serum amyloid A (SAA), which differed significantly between the HELLP cases and controls. However, further work is needed to determine if this is truly a predictive marker for the development of HELLP or merely a surrogate of liver impairment.

Complications of HELLP

Possible complications of HELLP syndrome include subcapsular hematoma of the liver, liver infarction, liver rupture, excessive bleeding, DIC, pulmonary edema, acute renal failure, abruptio placentae, perinatal asphyxia, fetal death, and maternal death.

Diagnosis of HELLP Syndrome

The diagnosis is made by the findings of fragmentation on the blood film, low platelets, and abnormal liver function tests, and with abdominal ultrasound. The patient may or may not have signs of PET.

Management of HELLP Syndrome

Stabilization of hypertension, if present, and other manifestations of HELLP, such as seizures or DIC, are required as well as fetal monitoring. The only certain therapeutic measure is prompt delivery, and in the majority of cases women have complete recovery within 24–48 hours after labor, although some women may continue to have symptoms for up to 14 days. In the majority of patients, normalization of platelet count and resolution of HELLP occurs 5 days postpartum. If these signs of disease persist beyond 5 days postpartum (and indeed if they do not begin to improve within 48 hours of delivery), the diagnosis of HELLP should be reconsidered. Ideally, all women with HELLP should be referred to a tertiary hospital. Antihypertensive drugs, steroids, and plasma exchange/plasmapheresis have also been used with variable results.

A Cochrane review summarized the evidence on the effects of corticosteroids on maternal and neonatal mortality and morbidity in women with HELLP syndrome [48]. The 11 randomised controlled studies reviewed, involving 550 women, included use of corticosteroids in the antepartum, intrapartum, and postpartum periods. Although some blood parameters improved, there was no clear benefit on maternal outcome. Dexamethasone improved maternal platelet counts to a greater extent than betamethasone but there was on clear difference in clinical outcomes. The conclusions were that there is insufficient evidence to determine whether steroid use in HELLP decreases the major maternal and perinatal morbidity and the maternal and perinatal mortality. This has been confirmed by a more recent meta-analysis of 15 studies, involving 675 steroid-treated women and 787 controls, showing that steroids significantly improved platelet counts and liver function tests and significantly reduced the need for blood transfusion and duration of hospital stay but had no significant effect on maternal morbidity or mortality[49].

Platelet Transfusions and HELLP Syndrome

A randomized trial of women with class 1 HELLP syndrome received either dexamethasone (n=26) or dexamethasone and platelet transfusions (n=20). Liver function tests were significantly higher in the steroid plus platelets group. Platelet count normalized significantly faster in the dexamethasone only group, and the postpartum stay was more prolonged in the dexamethasone and platelet group. The group that received platelets reported complications such as wound dehiscence, wound infection, and pulmonary edema. A previous report of intrapartum use of platelets when the platelet count was $<40 \times 10^9$/L did not find a significantly lower incidence of hemorrhagic complications. As a result, platelet transfusion is not often used in the management of HELLP unless they are actively bleeding (http://best practice.bmj.com/best-practice/monograph/1000/treat ment/step-by-step.html).

Massive Bleeding Secondary to Placental Abruption

Placental abruption is defined as the premature separation of a normally located placenta. Patients with defective placentation and abnormal placental vasculature, such as in PET, are predisposed to ischemia and rupture of these placental vessels, which is thought to lead to placental abruption. Other risk factors include smoking and cocaine use. Presenting features include mild vaginal bleeding, signs of hypovolemia, fetal compromise, uterine contractions or hypertonicity, DIC, and renal failure. Ultrasonography may be useful to confirm the position of the placenta, or the presence of a large hemorrhage, but is insensitive.

The management of placental abruption, whether expectant or with delivery, depends on the extent of the abruption, the gestational age of the fetus, and the presence of fetal or maternal compromise. A full review is beyond the scope of this chapter and is covered in other sources. In general terms, however, delivery may be vaginal (usually due to the stimulation of rapid labor in response to the abruption) or by cesarean section. The latter scenario may occur in the case of failed progression of labor or in maternal or fetal instability. Expectant management with or without the use of tocolytics may be possible if the presentation of bleeding is less acute and earlier in the pregnancy.

DIC often occurs in association with abruption, particularly with a complete abruption, and may follow within hours. The specific management of DIC has already been mentioned. The hemostatic management of massive bleeding is presented in Chapter 18C.

The maternal complications of placental abruption include massive hemorrhage, DIC, renal failure, and amniotic fluid embolism. Fetal complications relate primarily to premature delivery, i.e. stillbirth (adjusted relative risk of 8.9), growth restriction (adjusted relative risk of 2.0), and complications of prematurity.

Differential Diagnosis of PET and HELLP from Microangiopathic Hemolytic Anemias (MAHA)

The differential diagnosis of thrombotic thrombocytopenic purpura (TTP) and hemolytic uremic syndrome (HUS) from PET and HELLP may be difficult (see Chapter 23). TTP is diagnosed during pregnancy or postpartum, with 75% of episodes occurring around the time of delivery.

Postpartum HUS is a rare syndrome of unknown cause, not related to *E. coli* (D-), but increasingly being recognized as associated with complement abnormalities. The prognosis is poor for both the mother and the fetus. It is recognized that HUS recurs in subsequent pregnancies, although the reason for that is not known. Many pregnant women who survive after HUS develop chronic hypertension and chronic renal failure later in life. Plasma exchange (PE) has low response rates.

Acute Fatty Liver of Pregnancy (AFLP)

HELLP syndrome should be distinguished from AFLP, a rare condition, also associated with thrombocytopenia but without microangiopathic hemolytic anemia. Clinical presentation is similar to that of HELLP, occurring almost always in the third trimester. DIC accompanies AFLP in 90% of cases. Maternal mortality is approximately 15% and fetal mortality <5%.

Summary

- Pre-eclampsia (PET), the new onset of hypertension after 20 weeks of gestation, and proteinuria, resolving after delivery, affects approximately 2–14% of all pregnancies and remains a major cause of maternal and fetal morbidity and mortality worldwide.

- Placental dysfunction is considered to be the central feature in the development of PET.
- The current hypothesis is that PET is a two-stage disease: the first stage is reduced placental perfusion and the second stage is the maternal response to this with endothelial cell activation.
- Proposed placental factors produced from the placenta that affect blood flow, arterial pressure, and maternal endothelial cell activation (ECA) include oxidative stress, cytokines (TNF-α, IL-6), and angiogenic factors (VEGF, sflt-1, sEng).
- Maternal constitutional factors that have been proposed to act as inductors of the maternal syndrome of PET include several dietary factors, metabolic conditions (diabetes, insulin resistance, and uric acid), obesity, metabolic syndrome, folic acid and hyperhomocysteinemia, hyperlipidemia, maternal vitamin D deficiency, and thrombophilia.
- PET is associated with IUGR in one-third of cases.
- Despite PET and IUGR occurring only in pregnancy, they have been shown to have long-term consequences for both mother and fetus. Mothers who have had PET or who have delivered a baby with IUGR experience a two- to eightfold increased risk of atherosclerotic cardiovascular disease in later life.
- The key to good management is early detection and secondary prevention with antihypertensive and antithrombotic drugs (aspirin, heparin).

Case Studies

Case Study 1

A 25-year-old primigravida developed a left popliteal deep vein thrombosis (DVT) in the 9th week of gestation. She received therapeutic low-molecular-weight heparin (enoxaparin 80 mg daily subcutaneously). The uterine artery Doppler scan at 22 weeks of gestation showed bilateral notching and increased mean pulsatility index (PI) (0.6). Three weeks later, in the 25th week, she developed early pre-eclampsia with a BP of 150/100 and proteinurea 3+. Blood tests performed at this week of gestation revealed a positive lupus anticoagulant (she was assumed to have antiphospholipid syndrome although an official diagnosis of APS could not be made at that point, due to the need of a positive blood test at least twice with an interval of 12 weeks between). She was given methyldopa to control her blood pressure; low-dose aspirin was then added at 75 mg/day and enoxaparin was increased to 60 mg twice daily. Her 24-hour protein excretion rate was found to be 650 mg/day. She was hospitalized with close monitoring and required increasing methyldopa to control her blood pressure. At 28 weeks' gestation, due to intrauterine growth restriction and poorly controlled pre-eclampsia (generalized edema and poorly controlled blood pressure) an elective cesarean section was performed. The baby boy weighed only 650 g (<5th centile) and required neonatal intensive care for 10 weeks. The pre-eclampsia settled in the week after delivery. Both mother and infant are well now 6 months later. This case emphasizes the lack of adequate active treatment for early pre-eclampsia, as well as the need for specific diagnostic criteria for obstetric APS.

Case Study 2

A 38-year-old primigravida was well until the 35th week of gestation, when she developed edema and elevated blood pressure. Pre-eclampsia was diagnosed based on a mean blood pressure of 150/95 mmHg and 450 mg of protein in a 24-hour urine test. She was given labetalol in increasing doses and admitted to hospital for rest and monitoring. A week later she experienced visual disturbances and received magnesium sulfate for prevention of eclampsia. Three days later due to increasing proteinuria and blood pressure, and as the baby had normal weight on ultrasound (50th percentile), an elective induction of labor was started. A healthy baby girl was born weighing 2780 g. On the second day after labor, when systemic blood pressure was controlled, liver function tests were abnormal, platelet count fell from 150×10^9/L to 90×10^9/L, and there were a few fragments on the blood film, consistent with a diagnosis of postnatal HELLP syndrome. Management was supportive and it took 6 days for the liver function to return to normal. This case illustrates that late pre-eclamspia usually has a favorable clinical impact for the fetus, and that PET and HELLP syndrome can occur postnatally.

- Hematological complications of PET include thrombocytopenia, disseminated intravascular coagulation (DIC), HELLP syndrome, and massive bleeding after placental abruption.
- Differential diagnosis includes microangiopathic hemolytic anemias (thrombotic thrombocytopenic purpura, TTP, hemolytic uremic syndrome, HUS) and acute fatty liver of pregnancy.

References

1. Kuklina EV, Ayala C, Callaghan WM. Hypertensive disorders and severe obstetric morbidity in the United States. *Obstetrics and Gynecology* 2009; **113**: 1299–1306.

2. World Health Organization. Maternal Mortality in 2005: Estimates Developed by WHO, UNICEF, UNIFPA and the World Bank. Geneva, World Health Organization; 2007.

3. RCOG. *The Investigation and Management of the Small-for-Gestational Age Fetus. Green-Top Guideline No. 31, 2nd Edition*. London: Royal College of Obstetricians and Gynaecologists; 2013, Minor revisions – January 2014.

4. Preeclampsia Foundation. http://www.preeclampsia.org/the-news/1-latest-news/299-new-guidelines-in-pree clampsia-diagnosis-and-care-include-revised-defini tion-of-preeclampsia http://www.preeclampsia.org/the-news/1-latest-news/299-new-guidelines-in-pre-eclamp sia-diagnosis-and-care-include-revised-definition-of-pr e-eclampsia

5. Bhide A, Rana R, Dhavilkar M *et al*. The value of the urinary protein: creatinine ratio for the detection of significant proteinuria in women with suspected preeclampsia. *Acta Obstetricia et Gynecologica Scandinavica* 2015; **94**(5): 542–546.

6. MRACE-UK. https://www.npeu.ox.ac.uk/downloads/fil es/mbrrace-uk/reports/MBRRACE-UK-PMS-Report-2015%20FINAL%20FULL%20REPORT.pdf

7. Roberts JM, Gammill HS. Preeclampsia: recent insights. *Hypertension* 2005; **46**: 1243–1249.

8. Maynard SE, Min JY, Mercham J *et al*. Excess placental soluble fms-like tyrosine kinase 1 (sFlt-1) may contribute to endothelial dysfunction, hypertension, and proteinuria in preeclampsia. *Journal of Clinical Investigations* 2003; **111**: 649–658.

9. Lu F, Longo M, Tamayo E *et al*. The effect of over-expression of sFlt-1 on blood pressure and the occurrence of other manifestations of preeclampsia in unrestrained conscious pregnant mice. *American Journal of Obstetrics and Gynecology* 2007; **196**: 396.

10. Li B, Ogasawara AK, Yang R *et al*. KDR (VEGF receptor 2) is the major mediator for the hypotensive effect of VEGF. *Hypertension* 2002; **39**: 1095–1100.

11. Gilbert JS, Babcock SA, Granger JP. Hypertension produced by reduced uterine perfusion in pregnant rats is associated with increased soluble fms-like tyrosine kinase-1 expression. *Hypertension* 2007; **50**: 1142–1147.

12. Levine RJ, Lam C, Qian C *et al*. Soluble endoglin and other circulating antiangiogenic factors in preeclampsia. *New England Journal of Medicine* 2006; **355**: 992–1005.

13. Venkatesha S, Toporsian M, Lam C *et al*. Soluble endoglin contributes to the pathogenesis of preeclampsia. *Nature Medicine* 2006; **12**: 642–649.

14. Masuyama H, Nakatsukasa H, Takamoto N, Hiramatsu Y. Correlation between soluble endoglin, vascular endothelial growth factor receptor-1 and adipocytokines in preeclampsia. *Journal of Clinical and Endocrinological Metabolism* 2007; **92**: 2672–2679.

15. Redman CW, Sacks GP, Sargent IL. Preeclampsia: an excessive maternal inflammatory response to pregnancy. *American Journal of Obstetrics and Gynecology* 1999; **180**: 499–506.

16. Alijotas-Reig J, Palacio-Garcia C, Llurba E, Vilardell-Tarres M. Cell-derived microparticles and vascular

pregnancy complications: a systematic and comprehensive review. *Fertility and Sterility* 2013; **99** (2): 441–449. doi: 10.1016/j.fertnstert.2012.10.009. Epub 2012 Nov 2.

17. Irgens HU, Reiseter L, Irgens LM, Lie RT. Long-term mortality of mothers and fathers after pre-eclampsia: population based cohort study. *British Medical Journal* 2001; **323**: 1213–1217.

18. Barker DJB (ed.) *Foetal and Infant Origins of Adult Disease*. London: BMJ Publishing Group; 1992.

19. Magnussen EB, Vatlen LJ, Lund-Nilsen *et al.* Pregnancy cardiovascular risk factors as predictors of pre-eclampsia: population based cohort study. *British Medical Journal* 2007; **225**: 978–981.

20. Berends AL, de Groot CJM, Sijbrands EJ *et al.* Shared constitutional risks for maternal vascular-related pregnancy complications and future cardiovascular disease. *Hypertension* 2008; **51**: 1034–1041.

21. Aykas F, Solak Y, Erden A *et al.* Persistence of cardiovascular risk factors in women with previous preeclampsia: a long-term follow-up study. *Journal of Investigative Medicine* 2015; **63**(4): 641–645.

22. Liu X, Olsen J, Agerbo E *et al.* Maternal preeclampsia and childhood asthma in the offspring. *Pediatric Allergy and Immunology* 2015; **26**(2): 181–185. doi: 10.1111/pai.12344.

23. Walker CK, Krakowiak P, Baker A *et al.* Preeclampsia, placental insufficiency, and autism spectrum disorder or developmental delay. *JAMA Pediatrics* 2015; **169**(2): 154–162.

24. Rasmussen S, Irgens LM. History of fetal growth restriction is more strongly associated with severe rather than milder pregnancy-induced hypertension. *Hypertension* 2008; **51**: 1231–1238.

25. Huppetz B. Placental origins of preeclampsia: challenging the current hypothesis. *Hypertension* 2008; **51**: 970–975.

26. Sood R, Kalloway S, Mast AE, Hilard CJ, Weiler H. Fetomaternal cross talk in the placental vascular bed: control of coagulation by trophoblast cells. *Blood* 2006; **107**(8): 3173–3181.

27. Song J, Li Y, An RF. Identification of early-onset preeclampsia-related genes and microRNAs by bioinformatics approaches. *Reproductive Sciences* 2015; **22**(8):954–963.

28. Salmon JE, Heuser C, Triebwasser M *et al.* Mutations in complement regulatory proteins predispose to preeclampsia: a genetic analysis of the PROMISSE cohort. *PLoS Medicine* 2011; **8**(3): e1001013.

29. Dekker GA, de Vries JI, Doelitzsch PM, Huijgens PC, von Blomberg BM, Jakobs C, van Geijn HP. Underlying disorders associated with severe early-onset preeclampsia. *American Journal of Obstetrics and Gynecology* 1995; **173**(4): 1042–1048.

30. Papageorgiou AT, Yu CK, Bindra R, Pandis G, Nicolaides KH. Multicenter screening for pre-eclampsia and fetal growth restriction by transvaginal uterine artery Doppler at 23 weeks' of gestation. *Ultrasound Obstetrics and Gynecology* 2001; **18**: 441–449.

31. Chappell LC, Seed PT, Briley A *et al.* A longitudinal study of biochemical variables in women at risk of preeclampsia. *American Journal of Obstetrics and Gynecology* 2002; **187**: 127–136.

32. Hund M, Allegranza D, Schoedl M *et al.* Multicenter prospective clinical study to evaluate the prediction of short-term outcome in pregnant women with suspected preeclampsia (PROGNOSIS): study protocol. *BMC Pregnancy Childbirth* 2014; **14**: 324. doi: 10.1186/1471-2393-14-324.

33. Palomaki GE, Haddow JE, Haddow HR *et al.* Modeling risk for severe adverse outcomes using angiogenic factor measurements in women with suspected preterm preeclampsia. *Prenatal Diagnosis* 2015; **35**(4): 386–393. doi: 10.1002/pd.4554.

34. CLASP. A randomised trial of low dose aspirin for the prevention and treatment of pre-eclampsia among 9364 pregnant women. CLASP (Collaborative low dose Aspirin Study in Pregnancy) Collaborative Group. *The Lancet* 1994; **343**: 619–629.

35. Askie LM, Duley L, Henderson-Smart DJ, Stewart LA. PARIS Collaborative Group. Antiplatelet agents for prevention of pre-eclampsia: a meta-analysis of individual patient data. *The Lancet* 2007; **369**: 1791–1798.

36. Askie L, Duley L, Henderson-Smart D, Stewart L. Antiplatelet agents for prevention of pre-eclampsia: a meta-analysis of individual patient data. *The Lancet* 2007; **369**: 1791–1798.

37. Bates SM, Greer IA, Middeldorp S, Veenstra DL, Prabulos AM, Vandvik PO. VTE, Thrombophilia, Antithrombotic Therapy, and Pregnancy: Antithrombotic Therapy and Prevention of Thrombosis, 9th ed: American College of Chest Physicians Evidence-Based Clinical Practice Guidelines. *Chest* 2012; **141** (2 Suppl): e691S–e736S.

38. Moore GS, Allshouse AA, Post AL, Galan HL, Heyborne KD. Early initiation of low-dose aspirin for reduction in preeclampsia risk in high-risk women: a secondary analysis of the MFMU High-Risk Aspirin Study. *Journal of Perinatology* 2015; **35**(5): 328–331. doi: 10.1038/jp.2014.214

39. Li C, Raikwar NS, Santillan MK, Santillan DA, Thomas CP. Aspirin inhibits expression of sFLT1 from human cytotrophoblasts induced by hypoxia, via cyclo-oxygenase 1. *Placenta* 2015; **36**(4): 446–453.

40. Mello G, Parretti E, Fatini C *et al.* Low-molecular-weight heparin lowers the recurrence rate of preeclampsia and restores the physiological vascular

changes in angiotensin-converting enzyme DD women. *Hypertension* 2005; **45**: 86–91.

41. Maki M, Kobayashi T, Terao T *et al.* Antithrombin therapy for severe preeclampsia: results of a double-blind, randomized, placebo-controlled trial. BI51.017 Study Group. *Thrombosis and Hemostasis* 2000; **84**: 583–590.

42. International Clinical Trials Registry Platform. Statins to Ameliorate early onset Pre-eclampsia StAMP. 10. ISRCTN Register; 2009. http://www.controlled-trials .com/ISRCTN23410175 (accessed December 2013).

43. Costantine MM, Cleary K; Eunice Kennedy Shriver National Institute of Child Health and Human Development Obstetric–Fetal Pharmacology Research Units Network. Pravastatin for the prevention of preeclampsia in high-risk pregnant women. *Obstetrics and Gynecology* 2013; **121**(2 pt 1): 349–353.

44. Bateman BT, Hernandez-Diaz S, Fischer MA *et al.* Statins and congenital malformations: cohort study. *BMJ* 2015; **350**: h1035.

45. Kakigano A, Tomimatsu T, Mimura K *et al.* Drug repositioning for preeclampsia therapeutics by in vitro screening: phosphodiesterase-5 inhibitor vardenafil restores endothelial dysfunction via induction of placental growth factor. *Reproductive Sciences* 2015; **22** (10): 1272–1280.

46. Doyle LW, Crowther CA, Middleton P *et al.* Magnesium sulphate for women at risk of preterm birth for neuroprotection of the fetus. *Cochrane Database of Systematic Reviews* 2009; **1**: CD004661.

47. McCoy S, Baldwin K. Pharmacotherapeutic options for the treatment of preeclampsia. *American Journal Health-System Pharmacy* 2009; **66**: 337–344.

48. Woudstra DM, Chandra S, Hofmeyr GJ, Dowswell T. Corticosteroids for HELLP syndrome in pregnancy. *Cochrane Database of Systematic Reviews* 2010; (**9**): CD008148.

49. Mao M, Chen C. Corticosteroid therapy for management of hemolysis, elevated liver enzymes, and low platelet count (HELLP) syndrome: A meta-analysis. *Medical Science Monitor: International Medical Journal of Experimental and Clinical Research* 2015; **21**: 3777–3783.

Chapter 23

Thrombotic Thrombocytopenic Purpura and Other Microangiopathies in Pregnancy

Marie Scully and Pat O'Brien

Introduction

The term "thrombotic microangiopathies" (TMAs) describes the clinical and histopathological effects of thrombosis in small vessels seen in this group of conditions. There is usually thrombocytopenia and anemia, and review of the blood film confirms a microangiopathic process, with evidence of red cell fragmentation and often polychromasia. A number of conditions may present with these features, including thrombotic thrombocytopenic purpura (TTP) and atypical hemolytic uremic syndrome (aHUS) (see Figure 23.1). These are acute, potentially life-threatening conditions which carry a significant risk of morbidity and mortality.

However, in pregnancy the differential diagnosis may be very difficult and often a high index of clinical suspicion, together with laboratory investigations, are required to differentiate them from other TMAs which are specific to pregnancy. The diagnostic challenge is the differentiation from acute fatty liver of

pregnancy (AFLP), pre-eclampsia (PET) or eclampsia, HELLP (hemolysis, elevated liver enzymes, low platelets), antiphospholipid syndrome (APS), systemic lupus erythematosus[1], hemolytic uremic syndrome (HUS), and disseminated intravascular coagulation (DIC) (see Table 23.1). Furthermore, features of PET and HELLP, for example, may be part of the presentation of a TMA such as TTP or aHUS.

Moderate-to-Severe Thrombocytopenia Presenting during Pregnancy

Thrombocytopenia is defined by a platelet count $<150 \times 10^9/L$. It results from increased destruction and/or decreased platelet production, and can affect 10% of pregnancies. The most common is *gestational thrombocytopenia*, which represents 75% of all cases. Rarely, the platelet count is below $70 \times 10^9/L$, typically in the

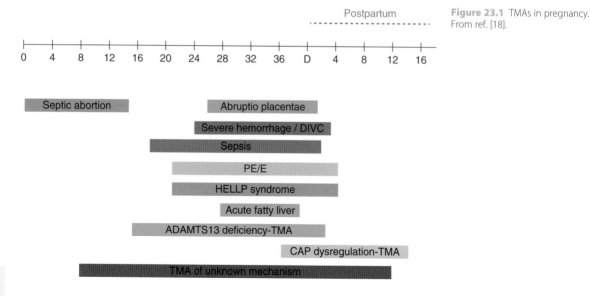

Figure 23.1 TMAs in pregnancy. From ref. [18].

Table 23.1 Typical features in pregnancy-associated microangiopathies

	MAHA	Thrombo-cytopenia	Coagulopathy	HBP	Abdominal symptoms	Renal impairment	Neurological symptoms
PET	+	+	±	+++	±	±	++
HELLP	+	+	±	+	+++	+	±
TTP	++	+++	–	±	+	++	+++
HUS	+	++	±	++	+	+++	±
AFLP	±	+		+	++	+	±
SLE	+	+	±	+	±	++	+
APS	+	++	±	++	–	++	++

MAHA: microangiopathic hemolytic anemia; HBP: high blood pressure; PET: pre-eclampsia; HELLP: hemolysis, elevated liver enzymes and low platelets; TTP: thrombotic thrombocytopenia; HUS: hemolytic uremic syndrome; AFLP: acute fatty liver of pregnancy; SLE: systemic lupus erythematosus; APS: antiphospholipid syndrome.
±: possibly occurs.
+++: definitive feature.

third trimester; it returns to normal within 12 weeks postpartum. It is thought to result from a hemodilutional effect in pregnancy. There is very little risk of hemorrhage to either the mother or the fetus.

Immune thrombocytopenic purpura (ITP) is a result of immunological peripheral platelet destruction. Maternal treatment and precautions during delivery may be required; rarely does it have a severe effect on the fetal platelet count, but it does require checking at birth (see Chapter 5).

PET and HELLP account for 21% of all cases of thrombocytopenia in pregnancy; the platelet count (and other pathological features) usually returns to normal within 3–5 days after delivery (see Chapter 22).

Of those women presenting with thrombocytopenia (platelet count $<75 \times 10^9$/L) during pregnancy, even with normalization after delivery, 5% have been defined as having ADAMTS 13 (a disintegrin and metalloproteinase with a thrombospondin type 1 motif, member 13) of <10%, associated with congenital TTP[2].

Placental Profiles in High-Risk Pregnancies

Abnormal uterine artery blood flow in the second trimester is indicative of an increased risk of placental pathology later in the pregnancy, including intrauterine growth restriction (IUGR) and PET. Uterine artery Doppler examination is often carried out at around 24 weeks' gestation in women considered to

be at increased risk of these disorders. Increased resistance in the uterine arteries (indicated by increased pulsatility index or "notched" waveforms) is associated with a sixfold increase in the risk of thrombotic placental injury, leading to IUGR and/or PET, compared with normal uterine artery Dopplers. However, the sensitivity of this test is poor, so its use is usually restricted to high-risk women. More recently, a meta-analysis suggested that uterine artery Doppler assessment in the first trimester may be useful in predicting early onset PET and other adverse pregnancy outcomes[3]. In early pregnancy, increased levels of biochemical markers such as alpha fetoprotein (AFP), beta-human chorionic gonadotrophin (HCG), and decreased levels of PAPP-A (pregnancy-associated placental protein A) and PP-13 (placental protein 13), in the absence of Down's syndrome and spina bifida, have been associated with an increased risk of PET, IUGR, placental abruption, and intrauterine fetal death (IUFD)[4]. These biochemical markers may improve the identification of the smaller subset of women with a high risk of later developing serious problems related to placental disease.

Thrombotic Thrombocytopenic Purpura

TTP is an acute, potentially life-threatening disorder associated with thrombocytopenia, microangiopathic hemolytic anemia, and symptoms related to microvascular thrombosis. Clinically, in addition to a low platelet count (below 150×10^9/L, but more usually $< 50 \times 10^9/L$), patients are anemic secondary to fragmentation – hemolysis with an associated acute consumption of folate. Corresponding blood film changes include polychromasia, anemia, reduced platelets, and fragmented red blood cells. Bilirubin is often raised, but the direct antiglobulin test is negative and the clotting screen is normal. Lactate dehydrogenase (LDH) is increased, often out of proportion to the degree of hemolysis, due to associated tissue ischemia[5].

von Willebrand factor (VWF), a plasma glycoprotein synthesized by megakaryocytes and endothelial cells, normally circulates as multimers of 500–20 000 kDa. Ultra-large VWF multimers (ULVWFM), which have a molecular weight greater than 20 000 kDa and are not normally detected in plasma, were initially detected in patients with chronic relapsing TTP. Subsequently, in 2001, patients with TTP were found to have a deficiency of VWF-cleaving protease called ADAMTS 13[6]. This enzyme is required to break down ULVWFMs. Failure to do so, due to an inherited deficiency or acquired reduction of ADAMTS 13 (due to autoantibodies to ADAMTS 13), leads to platelet adhesion and aggregation of ULVWFMs and resulting microvascular thrombosis (see Figure 23.2). The thrombi are uniquely composed of platelets and VWF. Platelet transfusions are contraindicated in TTP as they potentiate the effects of platelet aggregation. Pregnancy is a precipitating cause of acute TTP,

accounting for approximately 10% of all cases of TTP in women.

TTP is more common in women (3:2) and 45% of all cases occur in women of childbearing age. There is also a risk of relapse of TTP during subsequent pregnancies in women diagnosed with TTP. More recently it has been identified that late-onset congenital TTP may be associated with pregnancy[7], and other pregnancy-related thrombotic microangiopathies, such as PET and HELLP, may complicate the diagnosis of TTP[8]. Management approaches differ for these conditions, although differentiation may be clinically challenging.

Hemostatic Changes of Normal Pregnancy: Factor VIII, von Willebrand Factor, and ADAMTS 13

Normal pregnancy is associated with marked changes in hemostasis, which are hormonally mediated and protect against severe hemorrhage at the time of delivery, but ultimately result in a hypercoagulable state. Factor VIII and VWF increase in parallel in the first half of pregnancy; thereafter, the increase in VWF is greater throughout the remainder of pregnancy, returning to normal levels over the 6 weeks postpartum. Reciprocal changes of VWF and ADAMTS 13 have been documented. Therefore, with the increased VWF in pregnancy, ADAMTS 13 would be expected to

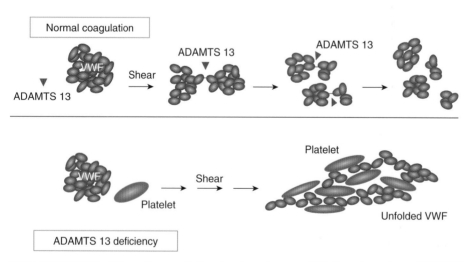

Figure 23.2 Pathophysiology of thrombotic thrombocytopenic purpura (TTP). Normal coagulation: ADAMTS 13 cleaves VWF. VWF multimers bind with platelets and are essential in primary hemostasis. ADAMTS 13 deficiency: lack of ADAMTS 13 results in excessive platelet binding to ultra-large VWF multimers, resulting in microvascular thrombi. From ref. [19].

decrease. A review of ADAMTS 13 in normal women with no history of TTP documented a reduction in ADAMTS 13 activity in the second and third trimesters of pregnancy. A further study in healthy women confirmed a reduction in ADAMTS 13 activity after the first trimester (weeks 12–16) up until the end of the postnatal period when the levels normalized to pre-pregnancy levels. ADAMTS 13 activity was lower in non-pregnant nulliparous women (mean 65%) compared with parous women (mean 83%). In pregnancy and after delivery, mean ADAMTS 13 activity was slightly, but non-significantly, lower in primigravida than in multigravida (68% vs. 74%). ADAMTS 13 was unaffected by platelet count, but was higher in smokers than in non-smokers during pregnancy (mean 79% vs. 70%, respectively). There was a significant correlation between higher VWF:Ag levels and lower ADAMTS 13 activity[9]. The reason for the decrease in ADAMTS 13 during pregnancy may be twofold. Firstly, enzyme levels decrease with excess substrate, VWF. Secondly, a hormonal influence, possibly estrogen, may reduce ADAMTS 13 levels.

Women Presenting with Acute TTP during Pregnancy

Women presenting with TTP during pregnancy appear to fall into two groups: those with often late-onset congenital TTP, frequently first presenting in pregnancy, and those with acquired, antibody-mediated TTP. Congenital TTP may first present during pregnancy and these women are more likely to relapse in subsequent pregnancies. Furthermore, the incidence is probably underestimated and it has been suggested that congenital TTP may constitute 5% of cases of thrombocytopenia in pregnancy. Diagnosis is confirmed with ADAMTS 13 activity <5%, no evidence of an inhibitor, and confirmation by mutational analysis of the ADAMTS 13 gene, revealing a homozygous or compound heterozygous abnormality. In those with acquired TTP, there is evidence of an inhibitor/anti-ADAMTS 13 IgG antibodies[8].

With the availability of ADAMTS 13 activity measurement and detection of inhibitors of ADAMTS 13 (or more specifically IgG antibodies), it may be possible to distinguish TTP from other pregnancy-associated TMAs, specifically if ADAMTS 13 activity is >10% and/or if IgG antibodies are present. In HELLP syndrome, ADAMTS 13 activity is reduced (median 31%,

range 12–43%) but with no inhibitor/antibodies to ADAMTS 13 and higher VWF levels[10].

Clinical presentation of congenital and acquired TTP can be similar. The greatest risk appears to be in the second trimester, when there is an increased risk of IUFD, but in fact a greater proportion present in the third trimester or postpartum. There may be associated features of hypertension, proteinuria, and headaches/migraines that may make differentiation from PET difficult. More "typical" features, such as neurological symptoms, may also occur. Despite the fact that presentation of TTP is more frequent in the third trimester or postpartum, TTP is the most likely diagnosis of a TMA presenting in the first trimester.

Risk Associated with Pregnancy in Women with Previous Acquired Idiopathic (Non-pregnancy-Associated) TTP

A particular concern in women who have had acute TTP unrelated to pregnancy is the risk of relapse from TTP during a subsequent pregnancy. A previous TTP episode is not a contraindication to pregnancy, but close, specialist monitoring is mandatory because of the risk of recurrence.

Treatment of Acute TTP in Pregnancy

Presentation of a TMA requires a review of laboratory parameters as well as clinical features. Platelet count, evidence of red cell hemolysis, and in particular the LDH and blood film, are critical to help aid differential diagnosis. If platelet counts are $<75 \times 10^9$/L, and particularly when $<50 \times 10^9$/L, TTP should be considered. A raised LDH can be a further useful parameter, but ADAMTS 13 activity is definitive. If there is a suggestion of TTP, plasma exchange (PEX) should be started, regardless of whether the disease is felt to be congenital or acquired, in order to ensure remission of the acute scenario.

The primary decision is whether delivery will be associated with remission of the TMA (as in PET or HELLP) or whether PEX should be instigated, as recovery following delivery is unlikely and there is a risk of multiorgan dysfunction/death. A further complicating issue is the more uncommon situation of a woman developing HELLP or PET following delivery.

If TTP develops in the first trimester, PEX may allow continuation of pregnancy with delivery of a live infant. However, TTP can present in the postnatal period or there may be progression of symptoms despite delivery; in this situation PEX is the most appropriate option. Steroids may be useful in HELLP syndrome and in TTP, but for different reasons. They have been used empirically in TTP because of the underlying autoimmune basis of the disorder, and in HELLP may accelerate recovery from delivery (although are rarely used for this indication nowadays because of limited success). However, women presenting with thrombocytopenia, microangiopathic hemolytic anemia[11], neurological features (such as stroke/transient ischemic attacks, seizures, encephalopathy), and renal impairment should be treated with PEX until the diagnosis of TTP is excluded.

Congenital TTP in Subsequent Pregnancies

The risk of relapse in subsequent pregnancies in women with confirmed congenital TTP is such that elective plasma therapy during pregnancy is warranted. Plasma infusions may be satisfactory; however, to deliver sufficient volumes, PEX may be required, particularly later in pregnancy. The optimal frequency of plasma replacement is unknown; the half-life of ADAMTS 13 is 2–3 days and plasma therapy every 1–2 weeks appears satisfactory. It is advisable to consider delivery by 37 weeks' gestation at the latest. Induction of labor and vaginal delivery is encouraged. Low-dose aspirin (LDA) is often also suggested, given the effect of microthrombi formation on the placenta leading to multiple ischemic lesions [8].

Acquired TTP in Subsequent Pregnancies

In women with acquired TTP, it is not as easy to predict those likely to relapse. The previous history of TTP and the ADAMTS 13 activity at the onset of pregnancy may be helpful. A normal ADAMTS 13 at the onset of pregnancy appears to predict women at reduced risk of subsequent relapse. However, if there is low ADAMTS 13 activity (<10%) at the onset of pregnancy, consideration should be given to elective therapy to prevent relapse.

In contrast, women with normal ADAMTS 13 activity at the onset of pregnancy, who maintain normal routine laboratory parameters, ADAMTS 13 activity, and antibody/inhibitor levels throughout pregnancy, do not usually require intervention for TTP. When a reduction in ADAMTS 13 activity (<10%) is identified, therapy to prevent microvascular thrombosis during pregnancy should be started. LDA and/or prophylactic low-molecular-weight heparin (LMWH) should be considered in women with a documented thrombophilia or a past history of venous thromboembolism (VTE) associated with TTP. The aim is to optimize implantation and preserve placental function, as abnormalities of the uteroplacental circulation resulting in later placental insufficiency are often established in the first trimester or early second trimester. However, this therapy has not been formally evaluated in pregnancy-associated TTP. Women with a previous pregnancy loss due to TTP, or those with low ADAMTS 13 activity at the onset of pregnancy, can be assumed to be at increased risk of further episodes of placental disorders in subsequent pregnancies[8,12].

Liver Disease in Pregnancy

Pregnancy normally causes some changes in liver function (see Table 23.2), but clinically abnormal liver function can be detected in 3–5% of all pregnancies. In some cases, pre-existing chronic liver disease may be identified. However, in the majority of cases, pregnancy itself is the precipitant. Hyperemesis gravidarum typically occurs in the first trimester and intrahepatic cholestasis of pregnancy (ICP) in the second or third trimesters. PET, HELLP, and AFLP are also associated with abnormal liver function[13].

Intrahepatic Cholestasis of Pregnancy

ICP has been associated with impaired sulfation and abnormalities of progesterone metabolism. Clinically, initially there is pruritus, which in 10–

Table 23.2 Physiological changes during pregnancy

Test	Change in pregnancy
Bilirubin	Unchanged
Aminotransferases	Unchanged
Alkaline phosphatase	Increase two- to fourfold
Cholesterol	Increase twofold
Prothrombin time	Unchanged
Fibrinogen	50% increase
Hemoglobin	Decrease in later pregnancy
White cells	Increase

25% progresses to jaundice associated with 10- to 20-fold increases in aminotransferase levels, but a less marked rise in bilirubin. The diagnosis is aided by measuring bile acid levels. Treatment is supportive and ursodeoxycholic acid (UDCA) is used. Steroids, although useful for fetal lung maturation pre-delivery, have not been shown to be beneficial compared with UDCA therapy, so should not be used to treat ICP. The main risk of raised bile acid levels is to the fetus; there is an increased risk of placental insufficiency but, more importantly, an association with sudden IUFD, the precise cause of which is not clear. Moreover, there is not a linear relationship between the levels of bile acids in the maternal blood and the risk of IUFD, which makes management more challenging. Resolution of the condition occurs with delivery. However, recurrence occurs in 45–70% of subsequent pregnancies or with the use of the combined oral contraceptive pill; the progesterone-only pill (mini-pill) appears not to increase the risk of recurrence, suggesting that this is an estrogen-related condition[14].

Acute Fatty Liver of Pregnancy

AFLP is a rare disorder (incidence estimated at 1/13 000 births), but is an acute life-threatening illness associated with significant maternal and perinatal mortality[13]. Typically, it presents in the third trimester, between the 30th and 38th weeks of pregnancy, although it has been described in the first and second trimesters on rare occasions. It usually affects primigravid women, although reports of recurrence in subsequent pregnancies have been documented. Clinically, presentation is non-specific with headache, fatigue, nausea, vomiting (70%), and right upper-quadrant or epigastric pain (50%). Progression of the illness is often rapid and, early in the presentation, there may be gastrointestinal hemorrhage, coagulation abnormalities, acute renal failure, infection, pancreatitis, and hypoglycemia. Later in the disease process, liver failure and encephalopathy may occur. Early delivery is imperative for both maternal and fetal reasons. After delivery, improvement in liver function is usually seen within 24–48 hours, and resolution occurs over 1–4 weeks postpartum. Diagnosis of AFLP is suggested by the clinical features and may be confirmed by liver biopsy, although this is rarely necessary as it may be technically difficult in

pregnancy, carries greater risk if clotting is deranged, and the diagnosis is usually made without resort to this invasive procedure. Histologically, there is characteristic microvesicular steatosis with oil red O staining, and cytoplasmic vesiculation as a result of microvesicular fat. Because of the acute presentation and laboratory features including coagulopathy, as mentioned, it is usually not possible to undertake liver biopsy, and the diagnosis is made by a combination of clinical and biochemical features. In routine laboratory tests, the most striking abnormality is that serum aminotransferases are markedly raised and alkaline phosphatase is three to four times the normal level (although this is raised in normal pregnancy because of placental production). There may be a raised white cell count and thrombocytopenia with normoblasts on the blood film. There is DIC (with prolonged PT, aPPT, and reduced fibrinogen). Urea, creatinine, and uric acid levels are raised, and there are elevated ammonia levels and hypoglycemia. The primary differential diagnoses are acute fulminant hepatitis and severe HELLP syndrome, although these are less likely to be associated with hypoglycemia and prolonged PT. The histological features of liver biopsy are described above.

Pathogenesis

With advances in molecular biology, it has become evident that AFLP may, in some cases at least, result from mitochondrial dysfunction. There is a strong association between AFLP and a deficiency of the enzyme long chain 3-hydroxyacyl-CoA dehydrogenase (LCHAD) in the fetus, a disorder of mitochondrial fatty acid β-oxidation. β-oxidation of fatty acids is a major source of energy for skeletal muscle and the heart, while the liver oxidizes fatty acids under conditions of prolonged fasting, during illness, and at periods of increased muscular activity. Mitochondrial β-oxidation of fatty acids is a complex process. LCHAD is part of an enzyme complex, the mitochondrial trifunctional protein (MTP), associated with the inner mitochondrial membrane. MTP contains four α and four β subunits. A hydratase enzyme is located in the amino-terminal domain and LCHAD is located in the carboxy-terminal region of the β subunit. The β subunit contains thiolase enzymatic activity. Defects in the MTP complex are recessively inherited and are due to an isolated LCHAD deficiency, specifically associated with the G1548C mutation, with relatively normal hydratase and thiolase activities. In complete MTP deficiency, there is a marked reduction in all three enzymes. A few hours after birth, children with these disorders, which are primarily LCHAD, present with non-ketotic hypoglycemia and hepatic encephalopathy, progressing to coma or death if untreated. Studies suggest an association between fetal MTP defects and AFLP in the mother. In one study, in every pregnancy in which the fetus had an LCHAD deficiency, the mother developed AFLP or HELLP syndrome. Subsequent work in pregnancies in which the fetus was not LCHAD-deficient found that the pregnancy progressed normally, with no liver dysfunction. In another study of prospectively screened mothers who developed AFLP (27 pregnancies) or HELLP (81 pregnancies), 5 fetuses in the AFLP group, but none in the HELLP group, had an MTP mutation.

The precise mechanism by which an LCHAD-deficient fetus causes AFLP in a heterozygote mother remains unclear. However, there are several hypotheses. The mother who is heterozygote for an MTP defect has reduced capacity to oxidize long chain fatty acids. The stress of pregnancy is associated with altered metabolism, increased lipolysis, and decreased β-oxidation, and the hepatotoxic LCHAD produced by the fetus or placenta may accumulate in the maternal circulation. Therefore, approximately one in five women who develop AFLP may carry an LCHAD-deficient fetus. Screening of newborn infants at birth for this disorder of fatty acid oxidation can be life-saving and allows for genetic counseling in subsequent pregnancies.

Hemolysis, Elevated Liver Enzymes, and Low Platelets

HELLP is a thrombotic microangiopathy, histologically associated with endothelial cell injury, fibrin deposition, platelet activation and consumption, and areas of hepatic hemorrhage and necrosis. The underlying precipitating cause is unknown but it occurs only in pregnancy and the incidence is between 0.17% and 0.85% of all live births. Maternal mortality is 3–4%, with fetal mortality reaching approximately 25%, due mainly to

prematurity. Diagnostically, there is considerable overlap with other TMAs especially PET, and they may represent different points on a single pathological spectrum. There are no obvious precipitating factors associated with development of HELLP and it typically presents between the second and third trimesters, although approximately a quarter of all cases are postpartum. Typical presenting symptoms include upper abdominal pain and tenderness, nausea, vomiting, malaise, headache, and rarely jaundice. There are no clinical or laboratory factors that are diagnostic, but bilirubin is not usually raised. Aminotransferases can be marginally increased or up to 20-fold. HELLP syndrome may be classified according to the degree of thrombocytopenia into HELLP 1 ($\leq 50 \times 10^9$ /L), HELLP 2 (between 50×10^9/L and 100×10^9/L), and HELLP 3 (between 100×10^9/L and 150×10^9/L), although this classification is not commonly used in clinical practice. Serious maternal complications include DIC, placental abruption, acute renal failure, pulmonary edema, and hepatic failure, occasionally requiring liver transplantation. Hepatic rupture is a further rare, acute, life-threatening complication[15] (see Chapter 22).

Pre-eclampsia

PET is classically defined as the triad of hypertension, proteinuria, and edema, but is best thought of as a multisystem disorder resulting from widespread endothelial damage. It is a leading cause of maternal and neonatal morbidity and mortality, affecting 5–10% of all pregnancies. It is more common in primigravid women. It rarely occurs before 24 weeks of gestation and the incidence rises as pregnancy advances, being most common in the third trimester. Liver involvement is common although rarely severe and is the most common cause of hepatic tenderness and liver dysfunction in pregnancy. Severe PET is an indication for delivery because of the increased risk of severe eclampsia, hepatic rupture, DIC, and necrosis, but mild to moderate PET may be managed conservatively for some time when it is desirable to gain fetal maturity before delivery. The high perinatal morbidity and mortality are partly due to the association with placental insufficiency and IUGR, but partly due to premature delivery for maternal indications. Severe PET is complicated in 2–12% of cases by

HELLP syndrome[16], consistent with the idea that these two conditions lie on a spectrum of a single disorder. Renal impairment, eclampsia (convulsions), and abnormalities of the coagulation system are further potential complications (see Chapter 22).

Hemolytic Uremic Syndrome

Shiga-like toxin-producing *E. coli* hemolytic uremic syndrome (STEC HUS) is typically preceded by an illness with a verotoxin-producing bacterium, usually *E. coli* 0157:H7. Atypical HUS (aHUS), is rare and, in the majority of cases associated with pregnancy, occurs postpartum. However, the outcome is often severe, with two-thirds of cases in end stage renal failure (ESRF) within 1 month of diagnosis. aHUS may be familial and has a poorer prognosis than "typical" STEC HUS. Like all TMAs, it is a disease of microvascular endothelial activation, cell injury, and thrombosis, but it is also associated with complement deregulation, leading to an increase in activity in the alternative complement pathway. Mutations within the complement regulatory proteins and activating components are found in 50–60% of cases. Typically, the presentation in HUS is of MAHA, thrombocytopenia, and renal impairment. The primary pathology is in the renal arterioles and interlobular arteries, with widespread endothelial cell swelling, leading to exposure of the underlying basement membrane.

The vessel lumens are occluded by red cells and platelet fibrin thrombi. The pre-glomerular pathology may help in distinguishing from STEC HUS and TTP. There is consequently excess complement activation, particularly along glomeruli, arteriolar endothelium, and basement membranes (see Figure 23.3). Mutations in complement genes controlling the alternative complement pathway affect complement regulatory genes, such as factor H, I, or MCP[17], or complement activating genes, factor B (CBF), or C3 (C3). Single nucleotide polymorphisms and antibodies, such as to factor H, have also been found to play a role. Factor H mutations, mostly heterozygous, account for 15–30% of all cases of aHUS. MCP mutations account for 10–13% of aHUS patients, the majority being heterozygous, with approximately 25% homozygous/compound heterozygous[18].

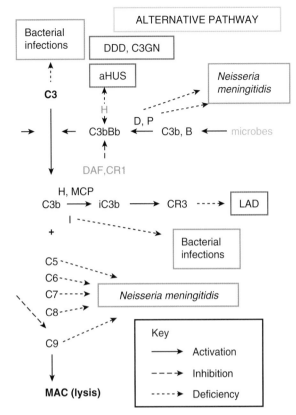

Figure 23.3 Pathophysiology of aHUS: the alternative complement pathway. From ref. [20].

Treatment of Pregnancy-Associated aHUS

Treatment of aHUS is primarily supportive, including red cell transfusion, blood pressure control, and renal dialysis. PEX should be started in the acute setting with identification of a TMA, but with confirmation of ADAMTS 13 levels not in keeping with TTP, complement inhibition with ecluzimab is the therapy of choice. As with TTP, there is an increased risk of fetal loss and PET in patients with aHUS[18]. Patients with a known history of aHUS require counseling pre-pregnancy and specialist management throughout pregnancy.

Exacerbation of Systemic Lupus Erythematosis

SLE is an autoimmune disease, the active phase of which may be associated with thrombocytopenia, hemolytic anemia, pancytopenia, and an increase in

289

double-stranded DNA. The disorder is multisystem and typically there are associated skin and joint symptoms. Serum complement levels may be normal or decreased. An acute exacerbation occurs in 25–30% of women during pregnancy, but it may occur for the first time during pregnancy or in the postpartum period. An acute episode of lupus nephritis, associated with hypertension and proteinuria, may be difficult to differentiate from HELLP or PET. Antiphospholipid antibodies (aPL) may be present in 30–49% of women with lupus and further increase the risk of thrombotic events, tissue ischemia, and TMA. Thrombocytopenia is present in a minority.

Disseminated Intravascular Coagulation

In pregnancy, DIC must not be forgotten as a potential cause of MAHA with an abnormal clotting screen. There is usually an underlying precipitating cause that must be treated, and DIC can be a complication of any of the above TMAs in severe cases. Treatment of DIC requires platelet transfusions to maintain a count $>50 \times 10^9$/L, fresh frozen plasma, and cryoprecipitate or fibrinogen concentrate, depending on the level of abnormality of the coagulation parameters.

Case Studies

Case Study 1

A 39-year-old woman was referred to a tertiary Fetal Medicine Unit. In her previous pregnancy 1 year earlier, she had suffered a fetal loss at 23 weeks' gestation due to severe IUGR. In that pregnancy, ultrasound confirmed fetal growth below the third percentile, with a very high pulsatility index (PI) and reversed end diastolic flow (EDF) in the uterine artery on Doppler scanning. Histological review had confirmed a severely growth restricted fetus with multiple areas of ischemia and infarction in the placenta. In her second pregnancy, she was started on LDA and thromboprophylaxis with LMWH. Fetal growth was on the 50th percentile, but from 33 weeks of gestation, she started to develop severe headaches, despite normal blood pressure. Routine laboratory parameters were essentially normal apart from a reduced platelet count (73×10^9/L), having remained in the normal range until this point. Monitored in hospital, her symptoms remained stable for 3 days, as did her platelet count. On day 4 her platelet count dropped, LDH increased, and the blood film confirmed an MAHA picture. ADAMTS 13 activity was <5%. She received daily PEX and a live infant weighing 3 kg was delivered 2 days later by cesarean section. There was no evidence of an antibody to ADAMTS 13. The diagnosis was late-onset pregnancy-associated congenital TTP.

This case highlights a few features of TTP: second trimester fetal loss is a characteristic feature, the presenting platelet count may not be extremely low, a raised LDH is a useful aid to diagnosis, and prompt therapy with PEX is required.

Case Study 2

A 35-year-old woman, previously fit and well, presented in her first pregnancy at 31 weeks' gestation with rapid-onset edema, hypertension, and blurred vision. She was found to have significant proteinuria (6 g/day). She was admitted to hospital, given IV labetolol and magnesium sulfate, and underwent fetal monitoring. She subsequently had an uncomplicated cesarean section with minimal blood loss.

However, her blood pressure remained raised and she became increasingly unwell over the next 4 days with worsening anemia (despite no obvious blood loss apart from normal lochia), thrombocytopenia, and renal impairment. By this point, her platelets were 26×10^9/L, hemoglobin 80 g/L, she had raised reticulocytes, LDH 3604 IU, CRP 192, and normal coagulation screen. *Pseudomonas aeruginosa* was detected in blood cultures and heavy proteinuria persisted. She was transferred with a presumptive diagnosis of TTP; however, her ADAMTS 13 was in the normal range. She received PEX and antibiotics for sepsis, and her hypertension was treated aggressively (see Figures 23.4 and 23.5). She made a full clinical recovery, with normal hematology and renal parameters and blood pressure, although a raised protein:creatinine ratio and slightly reduced C3 level persisted. Subsequently a mutation was found in the complement factor H gene. A diagnosis of aHUS was confirmed.

This case illustrates the differential diagnosis of TTP, with sepsis/DIC and PET all being possible diagnoses. With the reduced platelet count and very raised LDH, transfer for PEX, and supportive therapy for infection and hypertension, were appropriate. The role of ADAMTS 13 in aiding diagnosis is highlighted and the role of complement inhibitor therapy is important in such cases.

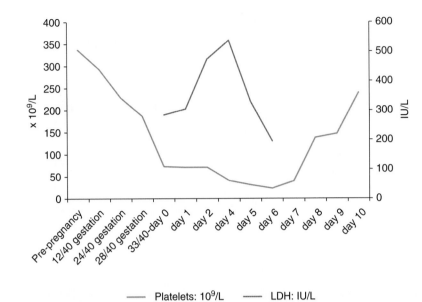

Figure 23.4 Platelet count and LDH before and during presentation of TTP. Normal range for platelets: 150–400 × 10^9/L and LDH: 135–214 IU/L.

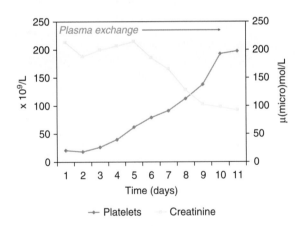

Figure 23.5 Response of platelets and creatinine to PEX. PEX received from day 1 to 9 inclusive.

References

1. Rangarajan S, Kessler C, Aledort L. The clinical implications of ADAMTS13 function: the perspectives of hemostaseologists. *Thrombosis Research* 2013; **132**(4): 403–407.

2. Delmas Y, Helou S, Chabanier P *et al.* Incidence of obstetrical thrombotic thrombocytopenic purpura in a retrospective study within thrombocytopenic pregnant women. A difficult diagnosis and a treatable disease. *BMC Pregnancy Childbirth* 2015; **15**: 137.

3. Velauthar L, Plana MN, Kalidindi M *et al.* First-trimester uterine artery Doppler and adverse pregnancy outcome: a meta-analysis involving 55,974 women. *Ultrasound in Obstetrics and Gynecology* 2014; **43**(5): 500–507.

4. Naljayan MV, Karumanchi SA. New developments in the pathogenesis of preeclampsia. *Advances in Chronic Kidney Disease* 2013; **20**(3): 265–270.

5. Scully M, Hunt BJ, Benjamin S *et al.* Guidelines on the diagnosis and management of thrombotic thrombocytopenic purpura and other thrombotic microangiopathies. *British Journal of Haematology* 2012; **158**(3): 323–335.

6. Sadler JE. Von Willebrand factor, ADAMTS13, and thrombotic thrombocytopenic purpura. *Blood* 2008; **112**(1): 11–18.

7. Moatti-Cohen M, Garrec C, Wolf M *et al.* Unexpected frequency of Upshaw-Schulman syndrome in pregnancy-onset thrombotic thrombocytopenic purpura. *Blood* 2012; **119**(24): 5888–5897.

8. Scully M, Thomas M, Underwood M *et al.* Thrombotic thrombocytopenic purpura and pregnancy: presentation, management, and subsequent pregnancy outcomes. *Blood* 2014; **124**(2): 211–219.

9. Sanchez-Luceros A, Farias CE, Amaral MM *et al.* von Willebrand factor-cleaving protease (ADAMTS13) activity in normal non-pregnant women, pregnant and post-delivery women. *Thrombosis and Hemostasis* 2004; **92**(6): 1320–1326.

10. Lattuada A, Rossi E, Calzarossa C *et al.* Mild to moderate reduction of a von Willebrand factor cleaving protease (ADAMTS-13) in pregnant women with HELLP microangiopathic syndrome. *Hematologica* 2003; **88**(9): 1029–1034.

11. Narayanan P, Jayaraman A, Rustagi RS *et al.* Rituximab in a child with autoimmune thrombotic thrombocytopenic purpura refractory to plasma exchange. *International Journal of Hematology* 2012; **96**(1): 122–124.

12. Shamseddine A, Saliba T, Aoun E *et al.* Thrombotic thrombocytopenic purpura: 24 years of experience at the American University of Beirut Medical Center. *Journal of Clinical Apheresis* 2004; **19**(3): 119–124.

13. Hay JE. Liver disease in pregnancy. *Hepatology* 2008; **47**(3): 1067–1076.

14. Ozkan S, Ceylan Y, Ozkan OV *et al.* Review of a challenging clinical issue: Intrahepatic cholestasis of pregnancy. *World Journal of Gastroenterology* 2015; **21**(23): 7134–7141.

15. Kia L, Rinella ME. Interpretation and management of hepatic abnormalities in pregnancy. *Clinical Gastroenterology and Hepatology* 2013; **11**(11): 1392–1398.

16. Sibai BM. Imitators of severe preeclampsia. *Obstetrics and Gynecology* 2007; **109**(4): 956–966.

17. Caprioli J, Noris M, Brioschi S *et al.* Genetics of HUS: the impact of MCP, CFH, and IF mutations on clinical presentation, response to treatment, and outcome. *Blood* 2006; **108**(4): 1267–1279.

18. Fakhouri F, Vercel C, Fremeaux-Bacchi V. Obstetric nephrology: AKI and thrombotic microangiopathies in pregnancy. *Clinical Journal of the American Society of Nephrology* 2012; **7**(12): 2100–2106.

19. Tsai HM. Autoimmune thrombotic microangiopathy: advances in pathogenesis, diagnosis, and management. *Seminars in Thrombosis and Hemostasis* 2012; **38**: 469–482.

20. Panelius J, Meri S. Complement system in dermatological diseases – fire under the skin. *Frontiers of Medicine* 2015; **2**: 3. https://doi.org/10.3389/fmed.2015.00003.

Chapter 24

Myeloproliferative Neoplasms and Pregnancy

Susan Robinson and Claire Harrison

Introduction

The myeloproliferative neoplasms (MPNs) encompass chronic myelogenous leukemia (CML), polycythemia vera (PV), myelofibrosis (PMF), primary thrombocythemia (also known as essential thrombocythemia or ET), rarer entities such as chronic neutrophilic leukemia, chronic eosinophilic leukemia, chronic myeloproliferative disease unclassifiable, and the mast cell diseases. This chapter will concentrate upon the management of the more common classical Philadelphia negative MPNs: ET, PV, and PMF in pregnancy.

Epidemiology

The incidence of the classical Philadelphia negative MPNs combined is approximately 6/100 000 to 9/100 000, with a peak in frequency between 50 and 70 years of age; they are less frequent in women of reproductive age.

Thrombosis and hemorrhage are a major cause of morbidity in MPN patients; progression to myelofibrosis or an acute leukemia occurs less frequently. Historical case reports of pregnancy in MPNs have suggested significant maternal morbidity and poor fetal outcome. An increase in awareness of MPNs, advanced maternal age, and automation of blood counts to include a platelet count has led to an increase in the diagnoses of MPNs in women of reproductive age. Hence issues concerning the management of these disorders in pregnancy are a real clinical challenge to hematologists and obstetricians. Unfortunately, this challenge is compounded by a lack of clinical data and evidence-based guidance. This chapter provides a summary of the epidemiology, pathogenesis, and diagnosis of the MPNs in pregnancy and a management strategy developed from current experience attained in a tertiary referral center.

Previous Reports of MPN in Pregnancy

A large meta-analysis reported the outcome of 461 pregnancies in women diagnosed with ET[1]. The mean age was 29 years and the mean platelet count

at the beginning of pregnancy was 1000×10^9/L declining to 599×10^9/L in the second trimester. The live birth rate was 50–70%, first trimester loss occurred in 25–40%, and late pregnancy losses in 10%. Rates of placental abruption (3.6%) and intrauterine growth restriction (IUGR) (4.5%) were higher than in the general population. Postpartum thrombotic episodes were reported in 5.2% of pregnancies and pre-/postpartum hemorrhage in 5.2%. In addition, a summary of 208 historical cases of ET collated from case series that included greater than six pregnancies produced comparable data (presented in Table 24.1). The literature for pregnancies affected by PV is sparse; pregnancy outcome in a case series of 18 pregnancies in PV combined with 20 historical reports was concordant with the pregnancy outcomes in ET (and is summarized in Table 24.2)[2]. In PV, first trimester loss was the most frequent complication (21%), followed by late pregnancy loss (18%), IUGR (15%), and premature delivery (13%), which included three neonatal deaths, resulting in a 50% survival rate. Maternal morbidity was also significant including three thromboses, one large postpartum hemorrhage, four cases of pre-eclampsia, and one maternal death associated with evidence of a deep vein thrombosis, pulmonary emboli, sagittal sinus thrombosis, and disseminated intravascular coagulation. Lastly, PMF is the least prevalent MPN in women of childbearing age. Reports to date include a report of four pregnancies in PMF combined with four historical cases and a single case report, which suggest a 50% risk of fetal loss; however, no maternal complications of thrombosis or disease progression were noted but the numbers are probably too small to draw any firm conclusions (summarized in Table 24.3)[3].

Historical reports of pregnancy in MPN are likely to be subject to selection bias, favoring cases associated with a poor outcome. The United Kingdom Obstetric Surveillance Survey (UKOSS) prospective data of MPN in pregnancy are now available and will

Table **24.1** Summary of reported pregnancies affected by ET

Reference	Number of pts	Number of Pregnancies	Previous thrombosis	Previous hemorrhage	Maternal outcome	Live birth total	Pregnancy loss total	Loss <12/40	Loss >12/40	IUGR	Placental abruption	Live birth premature delivery <37/40	Live birth FTD
[16]	3	11	Detail not available	Detail not available	Detail not available	4	7	6	1	Detail not available	1	2	2
[17]	6	9	0	0	1 phlebitis, 1 leg ulcer, 1 PPH	8	1	1	0	0	0	1	7
[18]	8	10	Detail not available	Detail not available	Detail not available	7	3	0	3	Detail not available	0	0	7
[19]	9	15 (1 TOP)	1 VTE, 2 TIA	0	2 VTE, 2 TIA, 1 hemorrhage	9	6	3	2	2	0	4	5
[20]	13	16	1 VTE	0	3 VTE	13	3	3	0	0	0	3	10
[21]	12	30 (1 ectopic)	Detail not available	Detail not available	1 PE	17	13	4	8	2	5	5	12
[22]	9	17	1 CVA, 1 VTE	1 epistaxis	1 TIA, 2 acquired VWD, 3 vaginal bleeds, 2 epistaxis	11	6	6	0	0	0	3	8
[23]	20	43 (2 TOP, 1 ectopic)	Detail not available	Detail not available	Detail not available	22	21	16	2	Detail not available	1	1	21
[24]	12	17	0	0	3 vaginal bleeds	7	10	8	2	0	0	0	7
[25]	16	40	Detail not available	Detail not available	1 eclampsia, 2 pre-eclampsia, 1 vaginal bleed	26 (1 twin)	15	13	2	1	0	2	23
Total	108	208				124 (60%)	85 (41%)	60 (29%)	20 (10%)	5 (2%)	7 (3%)	22 (11%)	102 (49%)

FTD: full-term delivery; IUGR: intrauterine growth restriction; TOP: elective termination of pregnancy.
Adapted from refs. [6] and [7].

Table 24.2 Summary of literature regarding pregnancy in PV

Author	Number of pts	No. of pregnancies	Previous thrombosis	Previous hemorrhage	Treatment during pregnancy	High risk	Maternal outcome	Live birth total	Pregnancy loss total	FTM	Stillbirth (gestation)	IUGR	Placental abruption	Live birth premature delivery <37/40	Live birth FTD
[26]	1	1	No	No	Aspirin + dipyrimadole	No	Death[a]	0	1	1 TOP	0	0	0	0	0
[27]	1	3	No	No	Nil	No	Alive	1	2	2	0	0	0	0	1
	1	2	No	No	Nil	No	Alive PET	2	0	0	0	0	0	0	2 PET
[28]	1	2	Superficial thrombophlebitis	No	None	No	Alive PET	1	1	0	1 (35/40) PET	1	0	0	1
[29]	1	3	No	No	Aspirin, heparin[b] venesection	No	Alive PE postpartum	1	2	0	2 (24/40 and 28/40)[c]	2	0	1 (32/40)	0
[30]	1	4	Yes, CVA	No	Nil	Yes	Alive PET	2	2	0	2(5 + 7 months) PET	0	0	1 (7 months, PET), 1 (8 months)	0
[31]	2	2	No	No	Nil	No	Alive PPH	2	0	0	0	0	0	0	2
[32]	1	2	No	No	Heparin 3/52 postpartum	No	Alive, PE 24/7 postpartum	1	1	1	0	0	0	0	1
[33]	1	1	No	No	Hydroxyurea 9/40 then nil	No	Alive	1	0	0	0	0	0	0	1
[34]	8	18 (1 twin)	Yes (1 patient) No		Varied: venesection, aspirin, interferon, LMWH, vitamin C +E	No	Alive PET in 1	11	7	4	2	3	0	1 (34/40, IUGR), 1 (36/40), 1 (26/40) (NND)	9
Total	18	38	1 CVA 1 thrombophlebitis	None		1 yes	1 death, 4 PET, 2 PE, 1 PPH	22 3 NNDs	16	8	7	6	0	6	17

Adapted from ref. [2].

[a] The patient died with evidence of deep vein thrombosis, pulmonary embolism, sagittal sinus thrombosis, and disseminated intravascular coagulation.

[b] Postpartum heparin after 2nd pregnancy, LMWH throughout third pregnancy, aspirin throughout both pregnancies.

[c] Multiple placental infarcts in first and abnormal uterine artery Doppler waveforms and severe IUGR in third pregnancy.

FTM: first trimester miscarriage; IUGR: intrauterine growth restriction; FTD: full-term delivery; TOP: termination of pregnancy; NND: neonatal death; PE: pulmonary embolism; PET: pre-eclampsia; PPH: postpartum hemorrhage; LMWH: low-molecular-weight heparin.

Table 24.3 Summary of literature regarding PMF in pregnancy

Author	Patients	Number of pregnancies	Previous thrombosis	Previous hemorrhage	Treatment pre-pregnancy	Treatment during pregnancy	Maternal outcome	First trimester miscarriage	Stillbirth (gestation)	IUGR	Placental abruption	Live birth premature delivery <37 wk
[35]	1	1	No	No	Supportive	Supportive	No complications	0	0	0	0	1 elective induction at 36 wk
[36]	1	1	No	No	None	None	No complications	0	30 (placental infarctions)	0	0	0
		2	Placental infarctions	No	None	None	No complications	0	27 (placental infarctions)	0	0	0
		3	Placental infarctions	No	Interferon α	Interferon α	No complications	0	0	1	0	1 elective delivery at 34 wk due to IUGR, birth weight 2000 g
[9]	A	3 (NB. preceding PMF diagnoses)	No	No	Aspirin	Aspirin	Disseminated TB	0	0	0	0	1 FTND
	B	1	Digital ischemia	No	Aspirin	Aspirin, LMWH	Postpartum hemorrhage	0	0	0	0	1 FTND
	B	2	Digital ischemia	No	Aspirin	Aspirin, LMWH	No complications	0	24/40 cardiac malformation	0	0	0
	B	3	Digital ischemia	No	Aspirin	Aspirin, LMWH	No complications	1	0	0	0	0
[37]	1	1	No	No	No	No	Postpartum pneumonia Hematoma	0	0	1	0	emCS 37/40 PET Abnormal cardiotocography
Total	5	9	3	0	3	3		0	3	2	0	4

Adapted from ref. [3].
IUGR: intrauterine growth restriction; FTND: full-term normal delivery; EmCS: emergency cesarean section.

provide clinicians with valuable outcome data according to current UK management of these pregnancies. Data were collected between January 2010 and December 2012 from 58 women, of whom 47 (81%) had ET, 5 (8.6%) PV, 5 (8.6%) MF, and 1 (1.7%) had a MPN-unclassified. There were 58 live births: 56 single and 2 twin deliveries. The incidence of miscarriage was 1.7/100 pregnancies and the perinatal mortality rate was 17/1000 live and stillbirths. Incidences of maternal complications were 8.8% (n=5/57) pre-eclampsia, 8.8% (n=5/57) postpartum hemorrhage, and 3.5% (n=2/57) hematoma postpartum. There were no thrombotic events or admissions to a critical care unit. Delivery was induced in 42% of women and cesarean section was performed in 42% of women. The majority of women (86%, n=49/57) delivered at term (>37 weeks' gestation); however, over 20% (n=11/54) of neonates were low birth weight (<2500 g) and 13% (n=7/54) required admission to a neonatal intensive care unit, although there was no neonatal mortality. These findings confirm a higher rate of stillbirth, pre-eclampsia, cesarean section, and low birth weight in women with MPNs compared to the general population. However, overall, women with MPN appear to have successful pregnancies with better outcomes than previously anticipated.

Pathogenesis

MPNs result from the transformation of a hematopoietic progenitor cell and are characterized by overproduction of mature blood cells. The proliferation of one single cell type predominates, resulting in increased numbers of granulocytes (CML), erythrocytes (PV), platelets (ET), or fibroblasts (PMF). A single, acquired point mutation in the Janus kinase 2 (JAK2) gene occurring in the majority of patients with PV and almost half of those with ET and PMF was discovered in 2005. The mutation is a guanine to thymidine substitution that substitutes phenylalanine for valine at position 617 (V617 F) of the JAK2 protein. This residue is located within the JH2 pseudokinase domain, which negatively regulates the JH1 catalytically active kinase domain. The wild-type JAK2 protein binds to multiple cytokine receptors including the erythropoietin, thrombopoietin, and granulocyte colony-stimulating factor receptors that are essential for hemopoietic stem cell biology and differentiation. The JAK2 protein with the V617 F mutation enables constitutive, cytokine-independent activation of the JAK-STAT, PI3 K, and MAPK signal

transduction pathways at various stages of development and in various lineages of hemopoietic cells (Figure 24.1). A series of further mutations affecting JAK2 exon 12 have also been identified and define a distinctive myeloproliferative neoplasm that affects patients who previously received a diagnosis of PV or idiopathic erythrocytosis. A series of further mutations in the thrombopoietin receptor MPL transmembrane domain also occur; the commonest, W515 L/K, has been described in patients with PMF (5%) and ET (1–3%). The reported mutations have been shown to produce an MPN-like phenotype in various murine models. More recently mutations in exon 9 of the calreticulin gene (CALR) have been described in about a third of ET and PMF patients, almost exclusively those lacking JAK2 mutations[4,5]. Whether or not the JAK2 V617 F mutation is a predictor of poor pregnancy outcome is not as of yet clear. Passamonti *et al.* suggest the presence of the JAK2 V617 F mutation is a predictor of poor pregnancy outcome and that aspirin may be effective in the prevention of pregnancy complications in JAK2 V617 F positive women with ET[6,7]. This association of the JAK2 V617 F mutation and poor pregnancy outcome is supported by Melillo *et al.*[8]; however aspirin did not alter the effects of the JAK2 V617 F mutation. In general interferon appeared to improve outcome (P= 0.034, OR 0.1 [95% CI: 0.013–0.846]), although any potential capability to overcome the unfavorable effect of the JAK2 V617 F mutation remains undefined. In contrast Gangat *et al.*[9] report that aspirin may be associated with a favorable outcome but no association between the presence of the JAK2 V617 F mutation and pregnancy loss. There are limited data concerning outcome of CALR-mutated MPN and pregnancy at the present time, though it appears that patients with this mutation are less likely to have thrombotic events; a recent analysis suggests pregnancies in patients with these mutations may be less eventful[10].

Pathogenesis of Placental Infarction and Thrombosis

Thrombosis is consistently identified as the leading cause of maternal mortality in apparently healthy normal pregnancies. Thrombotic occlusion and subsequent infarction (Figure 24.2) of the placental circulation may be a late manifestation of placental dysfunction or an independent mechanism of

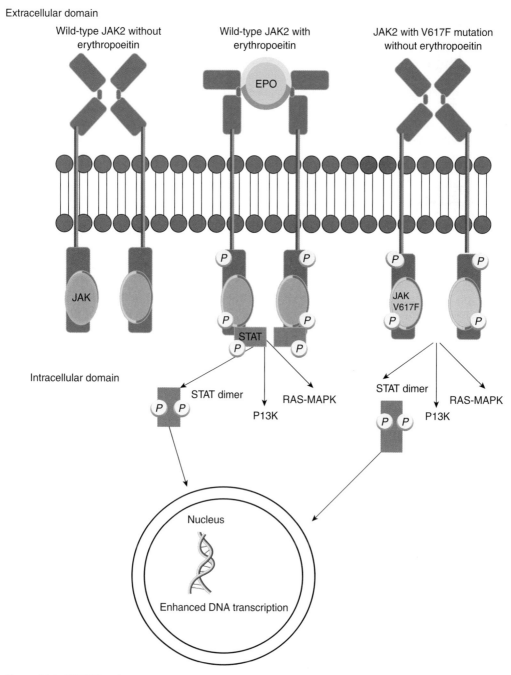

Extracellular domain

Wild-type JAK2 without erythropoeitin

Wild-type JAK2 with erythropoeitin

JAK2 with V617F mutation without erythropoeitin

EPO

JAK

JAK V617F

Intracellular domain

STAT

STAT dimer

P13K

RAS-MAPK

STAT dimer

P13K

RAS-MAPK

Nucleus

Enhanced DNA transcription

Figure 24.1 JAK-STAT pathways.

pregnancy morbidity. In women with ET, placental thrombosis is reported in pregnancies, which results in late fetal loss, preterm delivery, and IUGR. IUGR, which is associated with uteroplacental dysfunction, is known to occur in other acquired and inherited causes of thrombophilia.

Multiple factors are likely to contribute to the pathogenesis of thrombosis in MPNs, including the

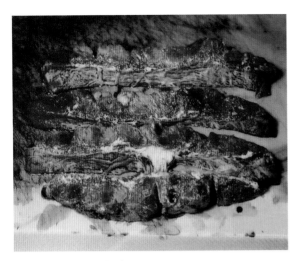

Figure 24.2 Placental infarction.

degree of thrombocytosis, leukocytosis, raised hematocrit, activation of platelets and leukocytes, the formation of platelet–leukocyte aggregates, circulating prothrombotic and endothelial factors, and their interactions[11]. It is of interest to our understanding of how the MPN phenotype contributes to placental dysfunction that, independently, studies of MPNs and pre-eclampsia both report increased platelet activation, platelet–monocyte aggregate formation, and microparticle formation.

Diagnosis

The diagnosis of MPNs in pregnancy requires an increased awareness of these disorders occurring in pregnant women. Suspicion may be secondary to an abnormal full blood count and a thrombotic or hemorrhagic event and should prompt referral to a hematologist. In view of pregnancy morbidities and the likelihood of improved outcome with intervention, these women benefit from a diagnosis being made pre-conceptually or during pregnancy or the postpartum period. The following section details local policy including adaptation for diagnostic investigations in pregnancy.

Primary Thrombocythemia

There is no diagnostic hallmark for this condition. The diagnosis is made by excluding other MPNs and a reactive or secondary cause of a thrombocytosis. Causes of a reactive thrombocytosis include iron deficiency anemia, chronic inflammation (e.g.

rheumatoid arthritis or inflammatory bowel disease), splenectomy, acute hemorrhage, and malignant disease. Where conditions coexist that may cause a reactive thrombocytosis, this may make the diagnosis more difficult. In pregnancy, the platelet count may fall especially during the second and third trimesters, thereby masking the diagnosis.

Historically, the diagnostic criteria for ET were those of the polycythemia vera study group; 40 years on, continual development of the diagnostic criteria for MPNs set the stage for the World Health Organization diagnostic criteria 2001, modified in 2007. The revised WHO criteria require characteristic bone marrow morphology (this is a controversial aspect not universally accepted), a platelet threshold of 450×10^9/L, and molecular analysis for the JAK 2 V617 F mutation and other clonal markers. Investigations should include a blood count, blood film, hematinics, renal and liver profile, CRP, ANA and RhF, genetic screen for the JAK2 V617 F, MPL W515 L/K, CALR and *bcr/abl* mutation, and abdominal ultrasound scan.

Polycythemia Vera

An erythrocytosis requiring investigation is defined as a packed cell volume (PCV) greater than 0.48 in non-pregnant women; in pregnancy this threshold has not formally been defined. To determine whether there is an absolute increase in PCV or an erythrocytosis or an apparent increase due to reduced plasma volume has traditionally required a red cell mass study, which would be contraindicated in pregnancy. Red cell mass scans have been largely superseded by testing for the presence of the JAK2 V617 F mutation, which indicates the presence of the majority of PV cases. The JAK2 V617 F mutation negative erythrocytosis cases may still be PV without a genetic marker or with a JAK2 exon 12 mutation; alternatives include a pseudo/apparent, primary congenital, secondary congenital or acquired, or an idiopathic erythrocytosis, all of which require definition.

The current British Committee for Standards in Hematology guidelines for investigation and management of erythrocytosis[12] suggest a staged approach to investigation as the differential diagnosis is broad and secondary causes must be excluded. This is followed by investigations to confirm or refute a diagnosis of a JAK2 V617 F positive PV. The majority of patients (excluding borderline erythrocytosis) and all ex- and current smokers will require a chest X-ray. This should be avoided in pregnancy unless there is a strong suspicion of a causative lung pathology, in which case appropriate screening should be used. Urinalysis is a simple effective screen for renal disease, which should be performed in all patients at the initial visit. Patients may present with comorbidity, thus regardless of a diagnosis of PV a review of secondary causes is pertinent. Additional investigation of possible secondary causes will vary according to symptoms or signs present.

Myelofibrosis

Myelofibrosis is very rare indeed in women of child-bearing age. To achieve this diagnosis it is necessary to exclude other MPNs (PV, ET, and CML) as well as disorders in which marrow fibrosis can develop as a secondary feature such as metastatic carcinoma, lymphoma, irradiation, TB, and leishmaniasis. The following features are generally necessary to confirm a diagnosis of MF: splenomegaly, increased bone marrow fibrosis (coarse reticulin fibers arranged in parallel in trephine biopsy), a leukoerythroblastic blood film (immature red cells and myeloid precursors with tear-drop-shaped red cells), and the exclusion of secondary causes of myelofibrosis (see above). In all suspected cases of MF a bone marrow aspirate and trephine are required.

Treatment Options

Women of reproductive age with a diagnosis of MPN should receive information and assurance regarding management and outcome of future pregnancies. If fertility issues arise, optimal disease management may need to be re-addressed prior to a timely referral for standard fertility investigation. A risk assessment according to disease status, concomitant illnesses, and prior obstetric history forms the basis for a discussion of the risks and benefits of therapeutic options in pregnancy (Figure 24.3). According to perceived risk, the therapeutic options include aspirin, heparin, venesection, cytoreductive agents, and thromboembolic deterrent stockings. From preconceptual planning to the postpartum period, access to joint care from an obstetrician with experience of high-risk pregnancies and a hematologist in a multidisciplinary setting is paramount.

The preconception to postpartum management plan should include:

- informed multidisciplinary care and education;
- risk assessment and discussion of therapeutic options and implementation of an appropriate management plan;
- additional monitoring during pregnancy;

- further optimization of disease control, if fertility is an issue, prior to timely referral for standard investigation;
- a comprehensive delivery and postpartum plan.

This approach enables optimal disease control with the aim of increasing the possibility of conception, implantation, and maintenance of placental function, thus reducing complications secondary to placental dysfunction, such as IUGR and pregnancy losses. An emphasis on the prevention of thrombosis and hemorrhage and management of events pre- and postpartum is also required.

Two key treatment aims, in high-risk non-pregnant patients with MPNs, are to attain a platelet count less than 400×10^9/L and a PCV less than 0.45 and possibly less than 0.42 in women who remain symptomatic. In pregnancy an increase in the plasma volume reduces both the platelet count and PCV, which is likely to further alter blood cell rheology. Interestingly, it has been suggested that the decrease in platelet count is greater than that expected in a normal pregnancy. One theory is whether the placenta produces an interferon-like substance. An understanding of this physiological dilutional effect and the brisk return to pre-pregnancy levels in the postpartum period in MPN pregnancies is important when considering optimal monitoring intervals and suitable treatment targets. The target PCV and platelet count in pregnant women with MPNs are ongoing debates, but appropriate targets are probably a platelet count of less than 400×10^9/L and a hematocrit of certainly less than 0.45 and probably in the mid-gestation appropriate range.

Aspirin

Low-dose aspirin is considered safe in pregnancy in accordance with the Collaborative Low-dose Aspirin Study in Pregnancy (CLASP), although its use for thromboprophylaxis in MPNs has never been assessed by a controlled trial. The European Collaborative Low-dose Aspirin in Polycythemia Vera (ECLAP) study supports the use of low-dose aspirin in non-pregnant patients with PV. Aspirin has been the most widely used therapy (in at least half of published pregnancies) for pregnancies affected by ET. Although the evidence is both retrospective and based on small numbers, the use of low-dose aspirin in pregnancy in myeloproliferative disorders seems advantageous, and a low risk strategy

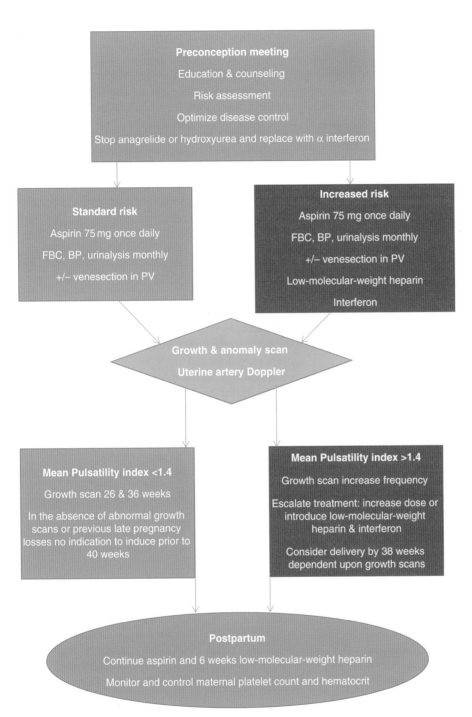

Figure 24.3 Management of MPN in pregnancy.

for the pregnancy. A recent update of the largest case series of pregnant women with ET to date provided analysis of pregnancy outcomes treated with aspirin versus those managed by observation alone. There was no evidence that therapy with aspirin positively influenced pregnancy outcome in women with ET; however, interpretation should be cautious as with all retrospective reports.

301

Low-Molecular-Weight Heparin

The successful use of LMWH in other pregnancies at high risk of thrombosis and in reducing fetal morbidity has drawn attention to the possibility of its use, in addition to aspirin, during pregnancy in women with MPNs with a previous thrombosis or pregnancy-related events.

Our regime for LMWH use, if necessary, in pregnant patients with MPNs is:

- antenatal dose of LMWH, e.g. 40 mg enoxaparin daily or 5000 IU dalteparin daily, increasing to 12 hourly from 16 weeks onwards if the indication is thromboprophylaxis;
- at low body weight (e.g. <50 kg), lower doses of LMWH may be required, e.g. 20 mg enoxaparin daily or 2500 IU dalteparin daily;
- in obese patients (e.g. BMI >30 in early pregnancy), higher doses of LMWH may be required, e.g. 40 mg enoxaparin 12 hourly or 5000 IU dalteparin 12 hourly;
- postpartum dose of LMWH, e.g. 40 mg enoxaparin daily or 5000 IU dalteparin daily for 6 weeks; and
- if the uterine artery Doppler pulsatility index is ≥1.4, increase to a therapeutic dose of LMWH.

In women with previous arterial thrombotic events or in those with recurrent thrombosis on warfarin prior to pregnancy, therapeutic doses of subcutaneous LMWH may be required. Some patients may require monitoring of anti-Xa levels.

Graduated Elastic Compression Stockings (GECS)

GECS may be used antenatally and during the postpartum period. There are no trials to support such practice, but the British Society for Hematology (BSH) guidelines suggest that all women with previous venous thrombosis or a thrombophilia should be encouraged to wear GECS throughout their pregnancy and for 6–12 weeks after delivery.

Cytoreductive Therapy

Cytoreduction is used where necessary to reduce the platelet count or a raised PCV that is resistant to venesection, but these agents should preferably be avoided in pregnancy, particularly in the first trimester. None of the cytoreductive drugs mentioned in this chapter has a product license for use in pregnancy. The expected natural fall of the platelet count and hematocrit during pregnancy may reduce the need for cytoreduction or venesection. However, in high-risk situations where cytoreduction is deemed necessary (see Control of Platelet Count and Hematocrit), interferon α (IFN-α) is the drug of choice. There are no reports of teratogenic effects in animals or adverse effects in the admittedly small numbers of pregnancies exposed to this drug. However, some evidence suggests that IFN-α may decrease fertility and so it is best avoided in women with difficulty conceiving. In relation to hydroxyurea, the outcomes of small numbers of pregnancies have been published and these are mainly without fetal complications, although one stillbirth and one malformed infant have been reported after exposure to hydroxyurea. Teratogenicity in animals has also been reported. Thus the use of hydroxyurea is probably contraindicated at the time of conception and during pregnancy. The use of anagrelide in pregnancy is similarly not recommended because of insufficient documentation of its use in this situation and because of the possibility of thrombocytopenia in the fetus.

Venesection

Although the natural fall in the hematocrit or PCV in pregnancy may obviate the need for venesection, it is an option in resistant cases. If venesection fails to control the PCV, then cytoreduction should be considered. The target PCV for a pregnant woman has yet to be determined. A reasonable target PCV would be the middle of the gestation-appropriate range (Table 24.4). There is currently no evidence for maintaining

Table 24.4 95% ranges for hematological variables during pregnancy

Gestation	First trimester	Second trimester	Third trimester
Hb (g/L)	110–143	100–137	98–137
PCV (L/L)	0.31–0.41	0.30–0.38	0.28–0.39
Platelet count (10^9/L)	174–391	171–409	155–429

Adapted from ref. [13].

Table 24.5 High-risk MPN pregnancy criteria

- Previous venous or arterial thrombosis in mother (whether pregnant or not)
- Previous hemorrhage attributed to MPN (whether pregnant or not)[a]
- Previous pregnancy complication that may have been caused by an MPN:
- *Three or more unexplained consecutive spontaneous miscarriages before 10th week gestation, with maternal anatomic or hormonal abnormalities and paternal and maternal chromosomal abnormalities excluded*
- *One or more unexplained deaths of a morphologically normal fetus at or beyond 10 weeks' gestation*
- *One or more premature births of a morphologically normal fetus before 34 weeks' gestation because of eclampsia, severe pre-eclampsia, or recognized placental insufficiency[b]*
- *A significant ante- or postpartum hemorrhage (requiring red cell transfusion)*
- Platelet count rising to >1500 × 10^9/L prior to pregnancy or during pregnancy[a]
- Diabetes mellitus or hypertension requiring treatment

[a] Indication for cytoreductive treatment but *not* LMWH.
[b] Generally accepted features of placental insufficiency include:

(i) abnormal or non-reassuring fetal surveillance tests;
(ii) abnormal Doppler flow velocity wave forms analysis suggestive of fetal hypoxemia;
(iii) oligohydramnios;
(iv) postnatal birth weight less than the 10th centile for gestational age.

---

it lower than this in pregnancy, although this has been an area of controversy.

Recommendations for Management of MPNs in Pregnancy

An overview of the small groups of MPN patients and individual cases described in the literature does not enable confident management guidelines to be drawn up. The following are recommendations based on current knowledge of this and other thrombophilic states and on personal experience in a tertiary referral unit. Good communication between consultant obstetrician and hematologist is essential.

Preconception Meeting

The patient should ideally have a preconception meeting with both an obstetrician and a hematologist to discuss a plan of management for a future pregnancy, including the necessity for cytoreductive therapy. Ideally, this should be written out and copied to the patient.

Control of Platelet Count and Hematocrit

If a patient is already taking hydroxyurea or anagrelide, this should be gradually withdrawn before conception, followed ideally by a wash-out period of 3 months for hydroxyurea following the last dose. The platelet count and PCV must be closely monitored thereafter. Careful venesection should be commenced if the hematocrit rises above the gestational appropriate range.

Cytoreduction with IFN-α may be necessary in cases with a raised PCV resistant to venesection or persistent thrombocytosis. Most if not all patients with a clear indication for cytoreductive therapy pre-pregnancy will require cytoreduction during pregnancy.

Cytoreduction with IFN-α may also be necessary if any of the factors are present, or if they develop in the index pregnancy, which in our experience defines a high-risk MPN pregnancy (Table 24.5). Treatment should be guided by monitoring the full blood count and by maintaining the platelet count at less than 400 × 10^9/L and the PCV in the appropriate gestational range. IFN-α may also be introduced in patients with abnormal uterine artery Dopplers.

Management of Thrombotic Risk

Assessment of Need for Antithrombotic Medication

The assessment of the need for antithrombotic medication should preferably be done in the preconception meeting, but ongoing individual risk assessment should occur and may warrant commencing or increasing thromboprophylaxis.

Aspirin

In the absence of clear contraindications, i.e. asthma, history of peptic ulceration, or current hemorrhage, all patients should be on aspirin (initially 75 mg once daily) throughout the pregnancy and for at least 6 weeks after delivery. In the event of a platelet count in excess of 1000 × 10^9/L, acquired von Willebrand disease should be excluded prior to commencing aspirin.

Low-Molecular-Weight Heparin

Consider the use of subcutaneous LMWH during pregnancy in addition to cytoreduction in patients with any of the high-risk MPN pregnancy factors listed in Table 24.5 with the exception of hemorrhage and extreme thrombocytosis. LMWH is an option to be introduced in patients with persistently abnormal uterine artery Dopplers. Once adequate hemostasis has been achieved postpartum, all women should be offered 6 weeks of LMWH thromboprophylaxis in the absence of a prior history of a significant hemorrhage. Caution should be applied to cases where women have a previous history of a significant hemorrhage with a platelet count $<1000 \times 10^9$/L and no other obvious cause except for platelet dysfunction secondary to an MPN.

Graduated Elastic Compression Stockings

Consider the use of GECS as a supplementary therapy throughout pregnancy and for 6–12 weeks after delivery in accordance with BCSH and RCOG guidelines.

Maternal and Fetal Monitoring

Maternal Monitoring

Full blood count monitoring, blood pressure, and urine testing should be performed 4 weekly until 24 weeks and thereafter at 2–4-weekly intervals.

Fetal Monitoring

The local protocol for fetal monitoring includes scans at 12 and 20 weeks. If the uterine artery Doppler at 20 weeks is abnormal, consideration should be given to increasing or escalating therapy. Serial growth scans should also be performed.

Uterine artery Dopplers are a predictive test for the development of pregnancy complications such as pre-eclampsia, intrauterine growth restriction, abruption, and fetal death. They are usually performed between 18 and 24 weeks. A systematic review and meta-analysis has shown that an increased pulsatility index is the best predictor of pre-eclampsia (positive likelihood ratio 21.0 among high-risk patients and 7.5 among low-risk patients). It was also the best predictor of overall (positive likelihood ratio 9.1) and severe (positive likelihood ratio 14.6) intrauterine growth restriction among low-risk patients[14]. A mean pulsatility index (mPI) of more than 1.40 is considered a screen positive test[15]. If the mean pulsatility index is less than 1.4, local practice is to perform further growth scans at 20, 26, and 34 weeks. In the presence of a mean pulsatility index of more than 1.4, local practice would be to perform growth scans more frequently and offer escalation of treatment to include heparin and α-interferon.

Delivery

Prior to labor or cesarean section, it is important to discuss the implications of the use of thromboprophylaxis for epidural or spinal anesthesia with the woman and obstetric anesthetist following locally agreed protocols. If a woman develops a hemorrhagic problem while on LMWH, the treatment should be stopped and hematological advice sought; a platelet transfusion may be useful in patients with MPNs. It should be remembered that excess blood loss and blood transfusion are risk factors for VTE, so thromboprophylaxis should be begun or reinstituted as soon as the immediate risk of hemorrhage is reduced. The third stage of labor should be managed actively.

Postpartum Thromboprophylaxis

The time of greatest risk for VTE associated with pregnancy is the immediate puerperium period. The prothrombotic pregnancy phenotype does not revert back to normal until 6 weeks after delivery. All MPN patients should receive 6 weeks of postpartum LMWH thromboprophylaxis unless contraindicated. Aspirin should also be continued for at least 6 weeks. As discussed above, where women have a history of hemorrhage, the addition of postpartum heparin should be cautious and considered on an individual case basis.

Postpartum Assessment

The platelet count and PCV may rise dramatically postpartum, but can usually be controlled with cytoreductive therapy or venesection. Cytoreductive therapy suitable immediately post-delivery if required includes hydroxyurea, IFN-α, and anagrelide, the choice and dose depending on previous experience in that patient. Local practice is to support breast-feeding while maintaining low-dose aspirin. Aspirin is excreted into breast milk at low concentrations. In view of immature metabolism and accumulation in infant's serum this may theoretically result in platelet dysfunction and Reye's syndrome. However, there is only one report of toxicity in a breast-fed infant despite extensive use and the dose used in MPN is low. Heparins are not excreted in breast milk and may be used safely when breast-feeding. Hydroxyurea, IFN-α, and possibly anagrelide are excreted in breast milk, so breast-feeding is contraindicated. Interferon α is variably excreted in breast milk and may be active orally; however, there is an absence of safety data rather than evidence of harm to the neonate. As such in women who wish to breast-feed and in whom cytoreductive therapy remains necessary, local practice would be to continue IFN-α, discuss the theoretical risks alongside the benefits of breast-feeding, and support the mother's decision to breast-feed.

In the current literature, there is no evidence that pregnancy predisposes MPN patients to acceleration of their disease to PMF or acute leukemia, nor would this be anticipated. The most significant risk is of thrombosis in the mother and adverse fetal outcome. A frequent question asked by these patients is what is the chance of their children being affected by MPN. Until recently, it was believed that familial MPN was relatively rare and, while this is true for large kindreds with many affected individuals, it has become apparent that up to 8% of MPN patients may have an affected relative, usually a cousin, aunt, uncle, etc. Parent:child combinations are extremely uncommon and routine testing of children is not recommended.

Case Studies

The following section includes a series of challenging cases, which enable discussion of management options accordingly in these women with complex pregnancies.

Case Study 1

A 37-year-old woman with a diagnosis of ET is referred for a tertiary opinion regarding conception and pregnancy management. The referral to a hematologist and initial diagnosis of ET followed a full blood count screen by her GP. The obstetric history includes one full-term spontaneous vaginal delivery 12 years previously. Following remarriage 3 years ago, she has undergone two spontaneous miscarriages at <10 weeks. The current platelet count is 1700 × 10^9/L; current medication includes aspirin 75 mg daily.

In an attempt to establish when the patient developed ET prior to the official diagnosis, any previous full blood counts could be reviewed. However, this is unlikely to change the management in this case. The diagnosis of ET and obstetric history are suggestive of poor pregnancy outcome secondary to ET. The platelet count enables us to stratify the patient as being at high risk of a vaso-occlusive event and outside of pregnancy would suggest benefit from commencing cytoreductive therapy. With the stated aim to conceive in the near future, the appropriate cytoreductive agent would be interferon α as this could be continued throughout pregnancy. A screen for an acquired von Willebrand disease should be completed prior to continuation of aspirin. The woman should be monitored in her local clinic and the dose of interferon adjusted to maintain a platelet count <400 × 10^9/L. If a pregnancy is confirmed, monitoring according to the treatment algorithm should commence and follow-up could be shared between the local hospital and tertiary referral unit. The patient does not currently meet the criteria to commence LMWH antenatally, although may benefit from heparin and aspirin for 6 weeks postpartum. However, a discussion within the multidisciplinary preconception meeting in view of the patient's age and prior obstetric history may conclude the addition of LMWH from conception as suitable on an individual basis regardless that the history is of two, not three, miscarriages at <10 weeks. Clearly, these complex cases need to be managed upon an individual basis and management plans may need to encompass aspects which are outside of general guidance. Close collaboration between the local hematology and obstetric unit and the tertiary center may enable delivery outside of the tertiary center dependent upon the progress of the individual pregnancy.

Case Study 2

A pregnant 26-year-old woman diagnosed with PV following investigation of menorrhagia and epistaxis 4 years previously is referred for an opinion at 9 weeks' gestation. There is no prior obstetric history, and the current management is low-dose aspirin and venesection. Her current blood count reveals Hb 150 g/L, HCT 0.47, platelets 567 × 10^9/L.

The history of hemorrhage and/or epistaxis may be attributed to MPN in this case and, if so, the woman would meet the criteria to consider interferon in this pregnancy, but this is a relatively soft indication and the authors would not use this treatment in this setting. However, this history should be examined carefully as hemorrhage is rare in these conditions and, even though the platelet count is not markedly abnormal, it would be wise to screen for von Willebrand disease. With no history of thrombotic events or pregnancy complications, there is no indication for antenatal heparin prophylaxis unless uterine artery Dopplers subsequently suggest impaired placental function;

heparin should be given for 6 weeks postpartum. Aspirin should be continued throughout pregnancy. The current PCV is outside the appropriate range for the first trimester and venesection should be considered if tolerated.

Case Study 3

A 32-year-old woman diagnosed with PMF 3 years ago following a recent hepatic vein thrombosis attends clinic to discuss treatment options regarding future pregnancies. She has one healthy daughter of 5 years delivered by cesarean section following a trial of labor which failed to progress. Current medication includes aspirin, warfarin, and hydroxyurea. The question of future cord blood stem cell storage is also raised. Her current blood count shows Hb 110 g/L, PCV 0.35 L/L, platelets 147×10^9/L, WBC 7.6×10^9/L.

In the preconception planning, a management plan regarding anticoagulation, cytoreductive therapy, and review of concomitant liver disease is required. The issues of stem cell storage need to be addressed regarding reasoning and practicalities. Clearly, the woman may have a personal interest in cord stem cell storage and this needs to be addressed pre-conceptually. This complex case would benefit from follow-up and delivery in a tertiary referral center.

The aspirin should be continued throughout pregnancy; testing should be performed in the fortnight following a possible conception in order to stop the warfarin as early as possible and commence LMWH. In view of the history of a hepatic vein thrombosis, a therapeutic dose of LMWH should be used and switched back to warfarin postpartum. Three months prior to conception the hydroxyurea needs to be stopped and interferon commenced. Optimization of any concomitant liver pathology and portal hypertension secondary to the previous hepatic vein thrombosis is important. The obstetric history needs to be reviewed in light of whether portal hypertension and varices are present. The presence of varices may require banding and additional medication, which should be instigated and followed up by the gastroenterology team. The planned mode of delivery according to concomitant pathology needs to be addressed in a multidisciplinary meeting.

Case Study 4

A pregnant 31-year-old female with diabetes is referred at 10/40 with a platelet count of 759×10^9/L from the combined endocrine obstetric clinic and is subsequently diagnosed with PT.

Although there is no previous obstetric history, a diagnosis of diabetes suggests a high-risk pregnancy. Outside of pregnancy, the patient would be in the high risk of vaso-occlusive event group secondary to the diagnosis of diabetes. Low-dose aspirin should be commenced and continued postpartum. A prophylactic dose of LMWH once daily increased to twice daily at 16 weeks followed by 6 weeks' postpartum prophylactic once daily LMWH should be considered. Interferon would also be considered in this case.

Case Study 5

A 29-year-old pregnant woman with a diagnosis of ET with no prior obstetric history or thrombotic events attends clinic at 15/40. Her current blood count is Hb 120 g/L, HCT 0.34, Platelets 580×10^9/L.

Low-dose aspirin throughout pregnancy continued indefinitely postpartum combined with 6 weeks postpartum heparin prophylaxis would be appropriate in this case. Additional treatment will depend upon how the pregnancy progresses.

References

1. Barbui T, Finazzi G. Myeloproliferative disease in pregnancy and other management issues. *Hematology* 2006; **1**: 246–252.

2. Robinson S, Bewley S, Hunt BJ, Radia DH, Harrison CN. The management and outcome of 18 pregnancies in women with polycythemia vera. *Hematologica* 2005; **90**: 1477–1483.

3. Tupule S, Bewley S, Robinson SE *et al.* The management and outcome of 4 pregnancies in women with idiopathic myelofibrosis. *British Journal of Haematology* 2008; **142**: 480–482.

4. Nangalia J, Massie CE, Baxter EJ *et al.* Somatic CALR mutations in myeloproliferative neoplasms with nonmutated JAK2. *New England Journal of Medicine* 2013; **369**: 2391–2405.

5. Klampfl T, Gisslinger H, Harutyunyan AS *et al.* Somatic mutations of calreticulin in myeloproliferative neoplasms. *New England Journal of Medicine* 2013; **369**: 2379–2390.

6. Passamonti F, Randi ML, Rumi E *et al.* Increased risk of pregnancy complications in patients with essential thrombocythemia carrying the JAK2 (617 V>F) mutation. *Blood* 2007; **110**(2); 485–489.

7. Passamonti F, Rumi E, Randi ML. Aspirin in pregnant patients with essential thrombocythemia: a retrospective analysis of 129 patients. *Journal of Thrombosis and Hemostasis* 2010; **8**: 411–413.

8. Melillo L, Tieghi A, Candoni A *et al.* Outcome of 122 pregnancies in essential thrombocythemia patients: a report from the Italian registry. *American Journal Hematology* 2009; **84**: 636–640.

9. Gangat N, Wolanskyj AP, Schwager S *et al.* Predictors of pregnancy outcome in essential thrombocythemia: a single institution study of 63 pregnancies. *European Journal of Haematology* 2009; **82**(5): 350–353.

10. Rumi E, Bertozzi I, Casetti IC *et al.* Impact of mutational status on pregnancy outcome in patients with essential thrombocytemia. *Hematologica* 2015; **100**(11): e443–e445.

11. Harrison CN. Platelets and thrombosis in myeloproliferative diseases. *Hematology* 2005; **1**: 409–415.

12. McMullin MF, Bareford D, Campbell P *et al.* Guidelines for the diagnosis, investigation and management of polycythemia/erythrocytosis. *British Journal of Haematology* 2005; **130**: 174–195.

13. Bain BJ. *Blood Cells*, 3rd edn. Oxford, UK: Blackwell Science; 1995.

14. Cnossen JS, Morris RK, Riet GT *et al.* Use of uterine artery Doppler ultrasonography to predict pre-eclampsia and intrauterine growth restriction: a systematic review and bivariable meta-analysis. *Canadian Medical Association Journal* 2008; **178**(6): 701–711.

15. Llurba E, Carreras E, Gratacos E *et al.* Maternal history and uterine artery doppler in the assessment of risk for development of early- and late-onset pre-eclampsia and intrauterine growth restriction. *Obstetrics and Gynecology International* 2009; Article ID 275613. doi:10.1155/2009/275613.

16. Bellucci S, Janvier M, Tobelem G *et al.* Essential thrombocythemias: Clinical evolutionary and biological data. *Cancer* 1986; **58**: 2440–2447.

17. Beard J, Hillmen P, Anderson CC *et al.* Primary thrombocythemia in pregnancy. *British Journal of Haematology* 1991; **77**: 371–374.

18. Leone G, De Stefano V, D'Addosio A. Essential thrombocythemia pregnancy. *Hematologica* 1991; **76**: 365–367.

19. Pagliaro P, Arrigoni L, Muggiasca ML *et al.* Primary thrombocythemia and pregnancy: treatment and outcome in fifteen cases. *American Journal of Hematology* 1996; **53**: 6–10.

20. Randi ML, Rossi C, Fabris F, Girolami A. Essential thrombocythemia in young adults: treatment and outcome of 16 pregnancies. *Journal of Internal Medicine* 1999; **246**: 517–518.

21. Cincotta R, Higgins JR, Tippett C *et al.* Managament of essential thrombocythemia during pregnancy. *Australia and New Zealand Journal of Obstetrics and Gynecology* 2000; **40**: 33–37.

22. Bangerter M, Guthner C, Beneke H *et al.* Pregnancy in essential thrombocythemia: treatment and outcome of 17 pregnancies. *European Journal of Haematology* 2000; **65**: 165–169.

23. Wright CA, Tefferi A. A single institutional experience with 43 pregnancies in essential thrombocythemia. *European Journal of Haematology* 2001; **66**: 152–159.

24. Candoni A, Fanin R, Michelutti T *et al.* Pregnancy and abortion in women with essential thrombocythemia. *American Journal of Hematology* 2002; **69**: 233–234.

25. Niittyvuopio R, Juvonen E, Kaaja R *et al.* Pregnancy in essential thrombocythemia: experience with 40 pregnancies. *European Journal of Haematology* 2004; **73**: 434–436.

26. Crowley JP, Barcohana Y, Sturner WQ. Disseminated intravascular coagulation following first trimester abortion in polycythemia vera. Increased platelet count apparently contributed to fatal outcome. *Rhode Island Medical Journal* 1987; **70**: 109–112.

27. Centrone AL, Freda RN, McGowan L. Polycythemia rubra vera in pregnancy. *Obstetrics and Gynecology* 1967; **30**: 657–659.

28. Ruch WA, Klein RL. Polycythemia vera and pregnancy: report of a case. *Obstetrics and Gynecology* 1964; **23**: 107–111.

29. Subtil D, Deruelle P, Trillot N, Jude B. Preclinical phase of polycythemia vera in pregnancy. *Obstetrics and Gynecology* 2001; **98**: 945–947.

30. Hochman A, Stein JA. Polycythemia and pregnancy. Report of a case. *Obstetrics and Gynecology* 1961; **18**: 230–235.

31. Harris RE, Conrad FG. Polycythemia vera in the childbearing age. *Archives of Internal Medicine* 1967; **120**: 697–700.

32. Ruggeri M, Tosetto A, Castaman G, Rodeghiero F. Pulmonary embolism after pregnancy in a patient with polycythemia vera. *American Journal of Hematology* 2001; **67**: 216–217.

33. Pata O, Tok CE, Yazici G *et al.* Polycythemia vera and pregnancy: a case report with the use of hydroxyurea in the first trimester. *American Journal of Perinatology* 2004; **21**: 135–137.

34. Robinson S, Bewley S, Hunt BJ *et al.* The management and outcome of 18 pregnancies in women with polycythemia vera. *Hematologica* 2005; **90**: 1477–1483.

35. Taylor UB, Bardeguez AD, Iglesias N, Gascon P. Idiopathic myelofibrosis in pregnancy: a case

report and review of the literature. *American Journal of Obstetrics and Gynecology* 2004; **167**: 38–39.

36. Gotic M, Cvetkovic M, Bozanovic T, Cemerikic V. *[Successful treatment of primary myelofibrosis with thrombocytosis during pregnancy with alfa-interferon.]* *Srp Arh Celok Lek* 2001; **129**: 304–308.

37. Okoli S, Wilkin B, Robinson S, Harrison C. Diagnosis of a myeloproliferative disorder in late pregnancy. *Obstetric Medicine* 2013; **6**(1): 26–27.

Management of Acute Hematological Malignancy in Pregnancy

Sahra Ali and Gill Swallow

Introduction

Diagnosis of malignancy during pregnancy poses a huge challenge to the pregnant patient, her family, and the medical team. The fact that treatment of pregnant women with chemotherapy may pose a risk to the fetus raises therapeutic, ethical, and social dilemmas as well as complicated maternal–fetal conflict.

Patients diagnosed with acute malignancy during pregnancy should be managed jointly by consultant hematologists, obstetricians, anesthetists, and neonatologists. Consideration should be given to the health of both mother and baby and the informed wishes of the mother; the mother's wellbeing should be considered paramount by the managing medical team. The woman should be fully informed about the diagnosis, its treatment, and possible complications during pregnancy.

The general side effects and risks of chemotherapy in a pregnant woman are, in large part, similar to those risks in a non-pregnant individual. These include the risk of sepsis, but of course the potential for teratogenicity is of specific relevance and often at the forefront of the patient's mind. The risk of teratogenesis following cancer treatment appears to be lower than commonly estimated from the available animal data. Therapeutic doses used in humans are often lower than the minimum teratogenic dose applied in animals.

Lymphoma

Lymphoma describes a heterogeneous group of malignancies of the lymphoid system. Although they are broadly divided into two distinct groups, Hodgkin's disease/lymphoma (HL) and non-Hodgkin's lymphoma (NHL), several subtypes exist.

Broadly speaking, lymphoma represents a progressive, clonal expansion of lymphoid cells which may be mature B-cells, T-cells, and/or NK-cells. Disease can occur within the lymph nodes and lymphoid organs, the bone marrow, and peripheral blood as well as extranodal spread. The World Health Organization (WHO) classification of lymphoid malignancies remains the most well-recognized classification system to date[1] (Table 25.1). Each specific subtype of lymphoma has its own distinct pathophysiology, etiology, epidemiology, and prognosis thus treatment is markedly varied. All lymphomas occur rarely during pregnancy and therefore only those more commonly encountered will be discussed in any detail.

Incidence

Overall, HL represents <1% of malignancies in the UK. The incidence is 2.8/100 000 per annum, which equates to approximately 1800 new cases per year. There is a slight male preponderance and a bimodal age distribution: a peak incidence in young adults aged 20–34 years and a further peak in those older than 70 years. In 2011, there were 459 new cases of classical Hodgkin's lymphoma in females aged between 15 and 50 years in the UK[2].

NHL is slightly more common and accounts for 4% of all new malignancies in the UK. Overall incidence is 15.5/100 000 annually or approximately 12 700 new cases per year. Diffuse large B-cell lymphoma represents almost half of these cases with marginal zone lymphoma and follicular lymphoma approximately 20% each. T-cell lymphoma, mantle cell lymphoma, and Burkitt's lymphoma make up the remainder of cases[2].

Lymphoma is the fourth most frequently diagnosed malignancy in pregnancy, complicating up to 1:6000 deliveries[3]. Classical HL occurs more frequently than NHL because the peak incidence of the disease falls within the childbearing years, and it has been estimated that up to 3% of cases occur during concurrent pregnancy[4]. NHL occurs rarely in pregnancy but the incidence is increasing in part due to women delaying pregnancy until later in life as well as the increasing incidence of HIV-associated

Table 25.1 Classification of lymphoid neoplasms

Hodgkin's lymphoma	Mature B cell neoplasms	Mature T-cell and NK-cell neoplasms
Nodular lymphocyte predominant Hodgkin's lymphoma	Chronic lymphocytic leukemia/small lymphocytic lymphoma	T-cell prolymphocytic leukemia
Classical Hodgkin's lymphoma	B-cell prolymphocytic leukemia	T-cell large granular lymphocytic leukemia
	Splenic marginal zone lymphoma	Adult T-cell lymphoma/leukemia
	Hairy cell leukemia	Extranodal NK/T-cell lymphoma, nasal type
	Lymphoplasmacytic lymphoma – Waldenström macroglobulinemia	Enteropathy-associated T-cell lymphoma
	Heavy chain diseases	Mycosis fungoides
	Plasma cell myeloma	Sézary syndrome
	Solitary plasmacytoma	Primary cutaneous T-cell lymphoma
	Extranodal marginal zone lymphoma of mucosa-associated lymphoid tissue (MALT lymphoma)	Peripheral T-cell lymphoma
	Follicular lymphoma	Angioimmunoblastic T-cell lymphoma
	Mantle cell lymphoma	Anaplastic large cell lymphoma, *ALK* positive/*ALK* negative
	Diffuse large B-cell lymphoma	
	Burkitt's lymphoma	

Adapted from the World Health Organization Classification of lymphoid neoplasms[1].

lymphoma in developing countries. Diffuse large B-cell lymphoma (DLBCL) is the subtype of NHL most commonly seen in pregnancy[5,6].

Clinical Presentation

Lymphoma can present in a variety of ways. HL commonly presents with localized painless lymphadenopathy, most often cervical or supraclavicular with mediastinal disease identified in approximately 80% of patients. Initially spread is to adjacent lymph nodes with hematogenous spread to organs occurring later in the disease course. Bone marrow infiltration can occur but is only detectable in 5–18% of patients depending on the staging investigations performed[7].

Different subtypes of NHL present in variable ways; commonly there is widespread painless lymphadenopathy and hepatosplenomegaly is often present at diagnosis. The more aggressive lymphomas such as DLBCL and Burkitt's lymphoma tend to progress rapidly whereas more indolent subtypes such as follicular lymphoma have a more insidious onset. Bone marrow involvement is variable depending on subtype of disease. Several authors have noted a higher than expected incidence of involvement of the reproductive organs and breasts with NHL diagnosed in pregnancy [5,6,8].

Systemic symptoms (also known as "B symptoms") include drenching night sweats, unexplained fever >38°C, and weight loss >10% over 6 months. These are identified in about a quarter of patients with HL at diagnosis[7]. Within the NHL subtypes, B symptoms are more commonly seen in the high-grade lymphomas as opposed to more indolent disease.

Diagnostic and Staging Investigation

The overriding principle in assessing a patient with suspected lymphoma during pregnancy is to obtain sufficient information to make a diagnosis and provide accurate staging to plan treatment while minimizing the impact on and the risk to the fetus.

A diagnosis of lymphoma must firstly be established by the laboratory analysis of affected tissue; an excision or core biopsy of an affected lymph node, extranodal mass or bone marrow biopsy is required. The diagnosis and specific subtype of lymphoma can be confirmed using a combination of histological, immunohistochemical, and cytogenetic analytical methods.

Once the diagnosis is confirmed, further staging investigations are required. Staging provides information regarding the location of disease and extent of any organ involvement, both of which guide the need for immediate intervention as well as having implications for prognosis. Baseline laboratory investigations should include a full blood count, renal and liver function, bone profile, ESR, lactate dehydrogenase (LDH), albumin, serum protein electrophoresis, and testing for human immunodeficiency virus (HIV). Any physiological changes which occur in these parameters during gestation should be borne in mind.

In the non-pregnant population standard staging investigations include computed tomography (CT) and positron emission tomography (PET-CT) scanning; however, both imaging modalities have a risk of fetal toxicity, especially if performed in early gestation. Therefore, alternative imaging with ultrasound scanning, MRI scan (without gadolinium), and chest X-ray with abdominal shielding can be considered in preference. Reassessment should then be performed postnatally. A bone marrow biopsy is required to assess for disease involvement and there is no contraindication to performing this procedure during pregnancy.

Management

There are limited data regarding the optimum management of lymphoma in pregnancy and current clinical practice is based predominantly on case reports, small case series, and expert opinion. The aim of management is to obtain good long-term outcomes for both the mother and fetus, and each woman should be assessed and treated on an individual case basis with multidisciplinary involvement of specialists.

An important decision is the timing of treatment and in particular whether this is necessary pre-delivery. This will depend on the severity and extent of disease at diagnosis, the anatomical sites involved, gestational age of the fetus, and the pace of tumor growth. The embryonic period from the second to eighth weeks after conception represents a time of critical organogenesis and when the embryo is the most sensitive to teratogenic insult. If a diagnosis of lymphoma is made at this very early stage, options for treatment should include a discussion about termination of pregnancy, particularly in the more aggressive lymphomas. As pregnancy progresses, the risk of teratogenicity

becomes lower and the main effect is on fetal growth. Close monitoring with regular growth scans is therefore important.

Hodgkin's Disease

The clinical outcome for Hodgkin's disease (HL) outside of pregnancy is excellent. Therefore, the goal of treatment in pregnancy should remain curative for the mother while minimizing fetal toxicity and optimizing perinatal outcome for the fetus[9]. Outside of pregnancy, the standard of care for management of HL is the use of doxorubicin, bleomycin, vinblastine, and dacarbazine (ABVD) combination chemotherapy[7].

Management of HD in the first trimester is controversial. Options include deferral of treatment until the second trimester, termination of pregnancy with immediate chemotherapy, ABVD chemotherapy while continuing pregnancy, or single agent vinblastine as bridging therapy[9]. Avilés and colleagues collected data over the last 40 years of women exposed to chemotherapy during pregnancy for a variety of hematological malignancies including 54 pregnancies exposed to chemotherapy in the first trimester[10]. Low birthweight for gestational age was the most frequent finding. No congenital abnormalities were detected, subsequent development was normal, and no neoplasm or acute leukemia has been observed in these children. There remains, however, a lack of good-quality data in this regard which has led to inconsistent recommendations among authors; the use of ABVD therefore in the first trimester requires careful consideration and, wherever possible, it should be deferred until the second trimester. Other groups have investigated the use of single agent vinblastine as temporary bridging therapy[4] and shown no teratogenicity and good long-term maternal and fetal outcome. Again, numbers are small and this needs to be borne in mind when planning treatment.

In the second and third trimesters, it may be possible to adopt a watch and wait approach to treatment if the disease stage allows. If treatment is required there is increasing evidence that ABVD in the second and third trimesters can be safely used. Evens and colleagues published the largest case series to date retrospectively, examining treatment, complications, and outcome for 40 patients with HL diagnosed during pregnancy. Seventeen women were treated with ABVD and there was no difference in morbidity and mortality between the groups of women who had received chemotherapy antenatally compared to deferral. All women delivered healthy infants with no malformations or spontaneous pregnancy losses. There was no difference in rates of induction of labor, cesarean section, or low birth weight (infants <10th percentile size for gestational age)[6].

Case reports and small case series report the use of radiotherapy alone for early stage, limited supra-diaphragmatic disease during pregnancy. This would not be standard of care in the non-pregnant patient[7]. Current evidence suggests that although the risk to the fetus appears minimal (provided special attention is paid to the treatment techniques and adequate fetal shielding), in most cases it is feasible to delay radiotherapy until after delivery and to treat with chemotherapy in preference should intervention be required[4,7,9].

Non-Hodgkin's Lymphoma

Management of NHL during pregnancy depends on the histological subtype of disease, gestational age at diagnosis, and the urgency of treatment for the individual patient. More indolent lymphomas often have a protracted course and outside of pregnancy treatment is often delayed until the patient is symptomatic or has other disease-related complications without compromising long-term outcome. Therefore, if the diagnosis is made in pregnancy, initially adopting a "watch and wait" management strategy is appropriate. Treatment in the first trimester is rarely required in these subtypes. If treatment becomes necessary, the regimen chosen will depend on the histological subtype of lymphoma[10].

The most common aggressive lymphoma in pregnancy is diffuse large B-cell lymphoma (DLBCL). Standard of care outside of pregnancy would be immediate treatment with combination chemotherapy cyclophosphamide, doxorubicin, vincristine, and prednisolone along with the monoclonal antibody Rituximab (R-CHOP). Several publications report CHOP chemotherapy alone being used in the second and third trimesters and existing data suggest that this may be administered safely, without adverse fetal outcome[3,5,6,11]. Management of DLBCL with chemotherapy in the first trimester is more difficult as the risks of fetal toxicity with exposure to chemotherapy are higher in earlier gestation. The option of termination of pregnancy, particularly with aggressive disease, should be discussed. In some cases of early disease, it may be possible to delay chemotherapy until the second trimester; however, a careful discussion regarding risks is required[5,11].

Outside of pregnancy, the combination of CHOP chemotherapy and the monoclonal antibody rituximab

(R-CHOP) improves the prognosis of DLBCL; however, data on its use during pregnancy are limited to case reports[12–14]. A more recent review examined pregnancy outcome after the use of maternal rituximab; indications for use were varied and included both hematological malignancy and autoimmune disease. Nintey of 153 pregnancies with known outcomes resulted in live births. There were 22 premature deliveries with one neonatal death at 6 weeks, 11 infants with hematological abnormalities, four neonatal infections, and 2 congenital malformations. It is worth noting, however, that only 20 of these pregnancies were exposed to rituximab antenatally as well as the confounder that many of these women were treated with concurrent medication with teratogenic potential[15].

CNS prophylaxis with high-dose methotrexate should not be given during pregnancy due to the unacceptably high risk to the fetus; treatment should be deferred until after delivery. Methotrexate is able to cross the placenta, even after administration by the intrathecal route, and therefore this should be avoided [11].

Burkitt's lymphoma is a highly aggressive subtype which occurs rarely in pregnancy, hence the literature is limited to case reports[16,17,18]. Owing to its rapidly progressive nature, treatment with combination chemotherapy should begin as soon as possible after diagnosis. Depending on the gestational age at which the diagnosis is made, a discussion regarding termination of pregnancy or (if the pregnancy is sufficiently advanced) early delivery is required. Most chemotherapy regimens for Burkitt's lymphoma include high-dose methotrexate; this carries a high rate of teratogenicity when given in the first trimester and profound fetal myelosuppression if administered in the second and third trimesters. Historically the prognosis for very aggressive lymphomas such as Burkitt's during pregnancy was poor but this may reflect suboptimal treatment administered as a result of pregnancy.

In terms of outcome data, the most recent retrospective study of the management of lymphoma during pregnancy included 50 cases of NHL, 32 of whom required chemotherapy antenatally: 21 women had DLBCL, 7 had T-cell lymphoma, 3 had Burkitt's lymphoma, and 1 had follicular lymphoma. There was no significant difference in maternal or perinatal complications between those women who received antenatal chemotherapy and those women who did not; however, as seen in other publications, there was a trend toward low birth weight in the treated group.

Maternal survival rates in this study were consistent with the expected lymphoma-related outcomes.

Timing of Delivery

A difficult decision when managing patients with malignancy during pregnancy is the timing of delivery. Recent publications examined the long-term cognitive and cardiac outcomes after prenatal exposure to chemotherapy[6,19,20]. The authors concluded that fetal exposure to chemotherapy was not associated with increased CNS, cardiac, growth, or auditory morbidity compared with the general population. The most significant impact on long-term cognitive development was premature delivery, emphasizing the importance of preventing iatrogenic preterm delivery if possible.

Leukemia

Incidence of Acute Leukemia in Pregnancy

Leukemia during pregnancy is uncommon, occurring in approximately 1 in 75 000 to 1 in 100 000 pregnancies. Acute leukemia accounts for the vast majority of these presentations with acute lymphoblastic leukemia (ALL) representing approximately one-third and acute myeloblastic leukemia (AML) two-thirds of cases[21].

Diagnosis

Diagnosis of leukemia in pregnancy is more challenging than in non-pregnant individuals since anemia, which can be multifactorial, is relatively common in pregnancy. Initial suspicion of a more serious cause for anemia is usually triggered by an abnormal blood count and blood film appearances. While both thrombocytopenia and anemia are relatively common findings in pregnancy, neutropenia is rarer and merits further investigation or close monitoring. The presence of circulating blasts on a blood film suggests a diagnosis of hematological malignancy and is an indication for bone marrow biopsy.

Treatment

The published data indicate that pregnancy is not an independent risk factor influencing cancer survival [22]. Chemotherapy can be administered from 14 weeks gestational age onwards. The placental barrier's function is to protect the fetus. Long-term outcome of children antenatally exposed to chemotherapy is comparable to that of children of the same age. Nevertheless, a higher rate of neurodevelopmental problems was encountered after preterm birth[19].

Treatment delays may compromise maternal outcome without improving the outcome for the pregnancy[23]. Without treatment, maternal death can occur within weeks or months[24]. In addition leukemia in a pregnant woman carries an increased risk of miscarriage, fetal growth restriction, and perinatal mortality[24,25,26]. The earlier in gestation the diagnosis of leukemia is made, the higher the incidence of spontaneous miscarriage, premature labor, and fetal growth restriction. Suspected causes of fetal death include maternal anemia, disseminated intravascular coagulation, or leukemic cells affecting blood flow, nutrient exchange, and oxygen delivery in the intervillous spaces of the placenta[24]. Delaying treatment would therefore have an adverse outcome for both mother and baby, and, unless the pregnancy is advanced, treatment should be commenced as early as possible.

When pregnancy is not advanced enough to consider early induction of labor, combination chemotherapy should be offered.

Acute Myeloid Leukemia (AML)

Induction with daunorubicin and cytarabine as per standard AML protocols should be offered (daunorubicin 60 mg/m^2 daily by intravenous infusion on days 1, 3, and 5 and cytosine arabinoside 100 mg/m^2 12 hourly by intravenous push on days 1 to 10 inclusive).

It is still a matter of debate whether in utero exposure to anthracyclines in general is cardiotoxic to the fetus. However, serial prenatal sonographic assessment of fetal cardiac function might have a role in monitoring anthracyclines' cardiotoxicity or cardiac failure[27].

Most fetal malformations observed after anthracycline treatment seem to occur during the first trimester, especially with exposure between 2 to 8 weeks' gestation. In general, daunorubicin or doxorubicin should be used in preference to idarubicin as the latter is more lipophilic, favoring more placental transfer.

Experience of cytarabine administration during pregnancy is limited. The fact that it is an anti-metabolite, however, raises concerns regarding its safety[28]. As with the use of anthracyclines, most fetal malformations seem to occur after exposure during the first trimester. Congenital malformations including limb malformation have been associated with its use in the first trimester, either alone or in combination with other chemotherapies[29,30,31]. Transient cytopenias, intrauterine fetal death, fetal growth restriction, and neonatal death secondary to sepsis have been reported with its use during all trimesters[32,33] though the risk is relatively small.

While there are few data to provide meaningful comment on the effects of hydroxycarbamide in pregnancy, it seems reasonable to avoid the use of this agent except in cases of high white cell count (greater than 100×10^9/L) where the clinician believes early count control with hydroxycarbamide may improve the outcome.

Acute Lymphoblastic Leukemia (ALL)

Single agent chemotherapy might be used such as vinca alkaloid or anthracycline. However, multiagent chemotherapy like conventional ALL induction with standard combinations of drugs, such as vinca alkaloid, corticosteroid, and anthracycline, can be considered. This treatment may induce and maintain remission without remarkable side effects and with mild myelosuppression, until the time at which delivery is safe.

There are no reports on fetal neurotoxicity secondary to vinca alkaloids. It is still a matter of debate whether exposure to anthracycline during pregnancy is cardiotoxic for the fetus. There is no indirect evidence for an increased risk for maternal chemotherapy-related cardiotoxicity. While the fetal effects during the first trimester need to be avoided, the risk of chemotherapy during the second and third trimester is controversial[22]. Hence serial prenatal sonographic assessment of fetal cardiac function might have a role in monitoring anthracyclines' cardiotoxicity or cardiac failure.

Methotrexate should be avoided as well as L-asparginase[24].

Philadelphia Positive Acute Lymphoblastic Leukemia (Ph+ ALL)

The safety of imatinib in pregnancy is still uncertain. However, it can be considered relatively safe in late pregnancy[28].

In most series, pregnant women have been dosed on their actual body weight with dose adjustments for weight gain during pregnancy[24]. This seems reasonable given that the increase in blood volume consequent upon pregnancy and the increased rate of renal drug clearance may act to reduce the area under the curve for drug bioavailability.

Myelodysplastic Syndrome in Pregnancy (MDS)

Incidence

MDS during pregnancy currently appears to be exceptionally rare, but frequency of reporting is increasing perhaps due to a rising incidence of MDS in younger people[34]. While Ikeda et al.[35] outlined that MDS prognosis is not influenced by pregnancy, as no patients in their research developed AML, other authors, such as Siddiqui et al.[36] and Pagliuca et al. [37], referred to some cases of transformation to AML.

Diagnosis

This can be very difficult as the hematological changes during pregnancy can be complex. Other causes of anemia or cytopenia need to be excluded. As with acute leukemias, baseline blood tests, blood film, and bone marrow examination are necessary to confirm the diagnosis and to rule out other causes of cytopenia.

Treatment

Management is mainly supportive. The effect of MDS on the outcome of pregnancy is controversial. While some have reported that pregnancy complicated with MDS has a poor prognosis[36], other investigators have indicated that prognosis is not always poor [38,39]. Probably, the impact of MDS on pregnancy outcome is related to the severity of cytopenias, where more pronounced cytopenias are associated with more frequent adverse events like decreased body weight gain, infections, and hemorrhages.

Anemia and gestational hypertension may be the primary risk factors for poor maternal and fetal outcomes in pregnant patients with MDS. To avoid maternal and neonatal complications, a hemoglobin level above 70 g/L and platelet count above 20×10^9/L during pregnancy should be maintained[40].

Close monitoring and active supportive treatment are recommended. In addition to intermittent blood transfusion, erythropoietin (rhEPO) seems to be an effective treatment for MDS[41].

The outcome of the neonates seems very good but prematurity and small-for-gestational age remain the main problems encountered, probably related to anemia and/or hypertension in the pregnant mother.

Sepsis and Pregnancy

Between 2006 and 2008 cases of sepsis rose to be the leading cause of direct maternal deaths in the UK, with 13 deaths due to group A streptococcal infection (GAS) in this period. Severe sepsis with acute organ dysfunction has a mortality rate of 20 to 40%, which increases to 60% if septic shock develops.

Women receiving chemotherapy for AML during pregnancy are at increased risk of sepsis. Changes in the immune system in pregnancy per se also make a woman more susceptible to infection. In addition, the signs and symptoms of sepsis in pregnant women may be less typical than in the non-pregnant population and are not necessarily present in all cases. Therefore, there should be vigilance for signs of infection and a high index of suspicion is necessary. If there is evidence of sepsis the woman should be managed by a senior team of hematologists, obstetricians, and anesthetists[42].

Women are at particular risk if they have spontaneous preterm premature rupture of membranes (PPROM). If the woman presents with PPROM and has evidence of myelosuppression, delivery should be expedited because of the significant risk of maternal sepsis, regardless of gestation. If the woman presents with PPROM at 28 to 34 weeks' gestation, but is well with no evidence of myelosuppression, delivery is still the preferred option rather than conservative management, but consideration could be given to delaying delivery by 48 hours so that a course of corticosteroids can be administered. Close maternal monitoring in that situation would be paramount. The benefits and risks of delaying delivery and corticosteroids at different gestations should be discussed with the parents. At gestations earlier than 28 weeks, the timing of delivery needs to be decided by the hematologists, obstetricians, and neonatologists in conjunction with the parents, considering the risk of sepsis and the likelihood of fetal survival in order that treatment plans can be individualized.

Supportive Therapies in Pregnancy

Antiemetics

Nausea and vomiting following chemotherapy are expected and may require treatment. According to the UKTIS (UK Teratology Information Service) the first choice antiemetic drugs are the antihistamines cyclizine and promethazine. Prochlorperazine and metoclopramide are considered second-line agents because they may be associated with maternal dystonic reactions. Ondansetron can be used in cases where first- and second-line antiemetic therapies have been unsuccessful[43].

Antibiotics

Patients usually suffer severe neutropenia either at presentation or secondary to chemotherapy. The risk of infection is high especially at induction of delivery and after membrane rupture. Antibiotics might be considered either for prophylactic or therapeutic purposes. Penicillins, erythromycin, metronidazole, and cephalosporins can be safely given. Augmentin should be avoided if possible because of an increased risk of neonatal necrotizing enterocolitis. Clindamycin, piperacillin–tazobactam (Tazocin), carbapenems, and gentamicin can all be used if sepsis is suspected. Relatively limited data exist on the tolerability of aminoglycosides. Quinolones, tetracycline, and sulphonamides should be avoided[44].

Antifungal Agents

Amphotericin B represents the systemic antifungal drug treatment of choice during pregnancy with which there has been the most experience in pregnancy, with no reports of teratogenesis attributed to it. No human data are available regarding the liposomal or lipid-complex preparations, though their lipophilic nature potentially increases transplacental transfer. Animal studies have not, however, revealed evidence of teratogenicity. Ambisome, Abelcet, and amphotericin B share an FDA pregnancy category B rating (http://www.drugs.com/pregnancy-categories.html). Azoles have been demonstrated to have teratogenic effects in animal studies: posaconazole, caspofungin, and itraconazole carry a category C rating and fluconazole category D. Fluconazole is, however, reasonably widely used in pregnancy though at doses of less than 150 mg/day[45]. Given the reduced nephrotoxic effects of lipid-associated drug as compared to standard amphotericin B and the reduced incidence of infusion-related toxicity, liposomal or lipid-complex amphotericin are preferred antifungal agents in the prophylactic and therapeutic setting in pregnancy.

315

Transfusion Requirements

CMV negative blood and blood products should be administered during pregnancy irrespective of serological CMV status, but are not needed during labor. In an emergency if CMV negative products are not available, standard leukodepleted products should be used[46].

Preparation for and Management of Delivery

Planned delivery is preferable to allow timely administration of subsequent chemotherapy. Plans should be made for elective delivery as soon as fetal maturity allows but it should be carefully timed and delivery should be avoided during the maternal nadir period, usually 2 to 3 weeks after treatment. This should allow the mother's blood counts to be improving rather than deteriorating. The delay of delivery for 2 to 3 weeks after chemotherapy also facilitates fetal drug excretion via the placenta thus reducing the risk of neonatal myelosuppression. Chemotherapy administered shortly before delivery might not have been eliminated from the fetus, and drugs might therefore persist in the newborn. This is especially true for preterm babies, who have a limited ability to metabolize or excrete drugs due to the immaturity of the liver and kidneys.

Vaginal delivery is preferable to cesarean section because of the lower risks of infection and quicker recovery and therefore induction of labor is normally recommended, elective cesarean section only being advised for obstetric indications. The woman should be informed of the risks specific to cesarean section and induction of labor. Because of the advantages of a vaginal delivery, if labor has not established after a course of prostin pessaries, consideration may be given to a rest period and then starting the induction process again, although the woman should be informed that the chance of a cesarean section in this situation is higher. The risk of neonatal myelosuppression overall is low and therefore fetal scalp sampling and the use of fetal scalp electrodes, ventouse, and forceps are not contraindicated.

Early involvement of the anesthetic team, to discuss methods of pain control, is recommended. If the mother is moderately to severely neutropenic or is thrombocytopenic, epidural analgesia is not recommended because of the risk of hematoma and infection and alternatives such as pethidine/diamorphine or patient-controlled analgesia should be considered. Intramuscular injections should be avoided if the platelet count is $<50 \times 10^9$/L.

If cesarean section is necessary in a woman who is neutropenic or thrombocytopenic, it should be performed under general anesthesia rather than a regional block (epidural/spinal), again because of the risk of hematoma/infection. If a cesarean section is necessary and the woman has platelets $<50 \times 10^9$/L, consultant hematological involvement is paramount so that platelets are available to cover the operation. IV access should be gained and antibiotic prophylaxis should be used during and after membrane rupture and delivery.

Dexamethasone or betamethasone should be given when preterm delivery is anticipated at 24 to 35 weeks of gestation, to reduce the risks from prematurity including respiratory distress syndrome, intraventricular hemorrhage, necrotizing enterocolitis, and cerebral palsy. Whenever possible these drugs should be given for 48 hours within the week prior to planned preterm delivery[47].

Magnesium sulfate has also been demonstrated to reduce the chance of cerebral palsy and should be considered in the 24 hours before delivery, if delivery is anticipated before 30 weeks[48].

Because of the increased risk of postpartum hemorrhage in women with AML, active management of the third stage is recommended. This includes administration of Syntocinon 5 IU with the delivery of the anterior shoulder and delivery of the placenta by controlled cord traction. Consideration should be given to a prophylactic Syntocinon infusion (20 IU in 500 ml Hartmann's/0.9% sodium chloride) over 4 hours following delivery. Management of postpartum hemorrhage should otherwise be the same as in all pregnant women although consideration should be given to early recourse to carboprost, examination in theater, balloon tamponade, and a B-Lynch suture if there is continuing hemorrhage. In this situation, it is imperative that there is consultant obstetric, anesthetic, and hematological involvement.

For women who are Rh D negative, standard anti-D immunoglobulin prophylaxis should be given[49]. For patients who have a platelet count less than 30×10^9/L, anti-D should be given subcutaneously or intravenously if an appropriate product is available. If Rh D positive platelets need to be given to a woman who is Rh D negative, recent BCSH guidelines should be followed[49].

Case Studies

Case Study 1

A previously well 28-year-old primiparous woman was found to have a 7-cm mass on her routine booking scan. This was initially thought to be a pyosalpinx and a conservative approach was adopted. At detailed scan the mass had increased in size to 14 cm and she underwent an urgent MRI assessment. The patient described episodes of intermittent abdominal pain over previous months with lethargy and minor weight loss. Investigations revealed hemoglobin of 85 g/L, white cell count 12.0×10^9/L, and platelet count 560×10^9/L. She was iron deficient and her lactate dehydrogenase (LDH) was significantly elevated at 1113 U/L.

Biopsy of the mass revealed a diagnosis of diffuse large B-cell lymphoma. Staging investigations with MRI and bone marrow biopsy confirmed that the lymphoma was confined to the pelvic mass: bulky stage 1E disease.

In view of the pelvic bulk and highly proliferative nature of the high-grade lymphoma, treatment with single agent corticosteroid was commenced at 23+2 weeks' gestation and repeat MRI scan 4 weeks later showed stable disease. Following multidisciplinary discussion including the patient and her partner, a decision was made to commence immunochemotherapy using standard dose R-CHOP (rituximab, cyclophosphamide, doxorubicin, vincristine, and prednisolone) with antibiotic and GCSF support. However, at 29 weeks' gestation, immediately prior to commencing chemotherapy, she was admitted in spontaneous labor. There was failure to progress and a pathological CTG leading to emergency cesarean section.

Chemotherapy was commenced 9 days after delivery. Treatment was complicated by recurrent infection at the surgical wound site and small bowel obstruction thought secondary to adhesions 12 weeks postnatally. She went on to receive 6 courses of R-CHOP followed by 2 further courses of rituximab monotherapy and involved field radiotherapy. PET scanning at completion of treatment showed a complete metabolic response and she remains well to date. Her baby spent several weeks on the neonatal unit but remains well with normal development.

A Case Study 2

A 21-year-old G2 P1, with congenital amegakaryocytic thrombocytopenic purpura and psoriasis, and a family history of neonatal amegakaryocytic thrombocytopenic purpura, was found to be pancytopenic by a blood test at 32 weeks' gestation. She was entirely asymptomatic with normal fetal movements. Blood results showed Hb 84 g/L, WBC 2.6×10^9/L, neutrophils 0.43×10^9/L, and platelets 94×10^9/L. There was a prominent population of myeloblasts and bone marrow aspirate and trephine biopsy confirmed hypercellularity and 44% blasts. The karyotype was normal and nucleophosmin1 (NPM1) was the sole abnormality, there was no FMS-like tyrosine kinase-3 (FLT3) mutation.

The risks and benefits of chemotherapy at 32 weeks' gestation were discussed, particularly the risk of fetal pancytopenia and anthracycline cardiotoxicity. The patient opted for induction and a vaginal delivery (without instrumentation, as the history of familial idiopathic amegakaryocytic thrombocytopenia conferred a 50% risk to the fetus of being affected). Single dose intravenous dexamethasone was given and induction took place at 34 weeks' gestation, resulting in the delivery of a healthy child. Antibiotic prophylaxis was given. Norethisterone and bromocriptine were started following delivery to prevent excess vaginal bleeding and lactation, respectively, and contraception was discussed. The patient declined AML17 trial and was treated with standard chemotherapy daunorubicin and cytarabine 3+10, achieving complete morphological remission after the first cycle. She declined a second course of consolidation with high-dose ARA-C, for psychological and family reasons. One year later, she relapsed with 19.7% blasts with the same phenotype as before. FLAG-Ida was given as salvage therapy, achieving complete morphological remission after one cycle. However, she developed *E. coli* and *Streptococcus mitis* neutropenic sepsis with acute heart failure, which was considered to be acute anthracycline-induced cardiotoxicity with multiorgan failure. She recovered after a period of inotropic support on intensive care but has persistent severe dilated cardiomyopathy precluding further chemotherapy and bone marrow transplant. Similarly, heart transplant is contraindicated in the context of AML but with ongoing clinical improvement she may be a candidate for novel or targeted treatments in the context of future relapse. Her child remains healthy, with no hematological issues and normal development.

References

1. Swerdlow SH, Campo E, Pileri SA. The 2016 revision of the World Health Organization classification of lymphoid neoplasms. *Blood* 2016; **127**: 2375–2390.

2. Cancer Research UK. Cancer Research UK Hodgkin Lymphoma Incidence Statistics; 2011. http://www.can cerresearchuk.org/cancer-info/cancerstats/types/hodg kinslymphoma/incidence/uk-hodgkins-lymphoma-in cidence-statistics (accessed May 28 2015).

3. Pereg D, Koren G, Lishner M. The treatment of Hodgkin's and non-Hodgkin's lymphoma in pregnancy. *Hematologica* 2007; **92**: 1230–1237.

4. Bachanova V, Connors JM. Hodgkin lymphoma in pregnancy. *Current Hematologic Malignancy Reports* 2013; **8**: 211–217.

5. Rizack T, Mega A, Legare R, Castillo J. Management of hematological malignancies during pregnancy. *American Journal of Hematology* 2009; **84**: 830–841.

6. Evens A, Advani R, Press OW *et al.* Lymphoma occurring during pregnancy: antenatal therapy, complications, and maternal survival in a multicenter analysis. *Journal of Clinical Oncology* 2013; **32**: 4132–4139.

7. Follows GA, Ardeshna KM, Barrington SF *et al.*; on behalf of the British Committee for Standards in Hematology. Guidelines for the first line management of classical Hodgkin lymphoma. *British Journal of Haematology* 2014; **166**: 34–49.

8. Horowitz NA, Benyamini N, Wohlfart K, Brenner B, Avivi I. Reproductive organ involvement in non-Hodgkin lymphoma during pregnancy: a systematic review. *Lancet Oncology* 2013; **14**: 275–282.

9. Eyre TA, Lau IJ, Mackillop L, Collins GP. Management and controversies of classical Hodgkin lymphoma in pregnancy. *British Journal of Haematology* 2015; **169**: 613–630

10. Avilés A, Natividad N, Maria-Jesus N. Hematological malignancies and pregnancy: Treat or no treat during first trimester? *International Journal of Cancer* 2012; **131**: 2678–2683.

11. Avivi I, Connors JM, Brenner B, Horowitz NA. Non-Hodgkin lymphomas in pregnancy: Tackling therapeutic quandaries. *Blood Reviews* 2014; **28**: 213–220.

12. Guven S, Ozcebe OI, Tuncer ZS. Non-Hodgkin's lymphoma complicating pregnancy: A case report. *European Journal of Gynaecological Oncology* 2005; **26**: 457–458.

13. Decker M, Rothermundt C, Hollander G, *et al.* Rituximab plus CHOP for treatment of diffuse large B-cell lymphoma during second trimester of pregnancy. *Lancet Oncology* 2006; 7: 693–694.

14. Rey J, Coso D, Roger V *et al.* Rituximab combined with chemotherapy for lymphoma during pregnancy. *Leukemia Research* 2009; **33**: 8–9.

15. Chakravarty EF, Murray ER, Kelman A, Farmer P. Pregnancy outcomes after maternal exposure to rituximab. *Blood* 2011; **117** (5): 1499–1506.

16. Antid N, Colovid M, Cemerikid V *et al.* Disseminated Burkitt like lymphoma during pregnancy. *Medical Oncology* 2000; **17**; 233–236.

17. Magloire LK, Pattker CM, Buhimschi CS, Funai EF. Burkitt's lymphoma of the ovary in pregnancy. *American Journal of Obstetrics and Gynecology* 2006; **108**(3): 743–745.

18. Petersen C, Lester DR, Sanger W. Burkitts lymphoma in early pregnancy. *Journal of Clinical Oncology* 2010; **28** (9): 136–138.

19. Amant F, Van Calsteren K, Halaska MJ. Long-term cognitive and cardiac outcomes after prenatal exposure to chemotherapy in children aged 18 months or older: An observational study. *Lancet Oncology* 2012; **13**: 256–264.

20. Amant F, Han SN, Gziri MM, Dekrem J, Van Calsteren K. Chemotherapy during pregnancy. *Current Opinion in Oncology* 2012; **24**(5): 580–586.

21. Hurley TJ, McKinnel JV, Irani MS. Hematologic malignancies in pregnancy. *Obstetric and Gynecology Clinics of North America* 2005; **32**: 595–614.

22. Gziri MM. Effects of chemotherapy during pregnancy on the maternal and fetal heart. *Prenatal Diagnosis* 2012; **32**(7): 614–619.

23. Greenlund LJ, Letendre L, Tefferi A. Acute leukemia during pregnancy: a single institutional experience with 17 cases. *Leukemia and Lymphoma* 2001; **41**: 571–577.

24. Cardonick E, Iacobucci A. Use of chemotherapy during human pregnancy. *Lancet Oncology* 2004; **5**: 283–291.

25. Reynoso EE, Shepherd FA, Messner HA *et al.* Acute leukemia during pregnancy: the Toronto Leukemia Study Group experience with long-term follow-up of children exposed *in utero* to chemotherapeutic agents. *Journal of Clinical Oncology* 1987; **5**: 1098–1106.

26. Cheghoum Y, Vey N, Raffoux E *et al.* Acute leukemia during pregnancy: a report on 37 patients and a review of the literature. *Cancer* 2005; **104**: 110–117.

27. Meyer-Wittkopf M, Barth H, Emons G, Schmidt S. Fetal cardiac effects of doxorubicin therapy for carcinoma of the breast during pregnancy: case report and review of the literature. *Ultrasound in Obstetrics and Gynecology* 2001; **18**: 62–66.

28. Shapira T, Pereg D, Lishner M. How I treat acute and chronic leukemia in pregnancy. *Blood Reviews* 2008; **22**: 247–259.

29. Wagner VM, Hill JS, Weaver D, Behner RL. Congenital abnormalities in baby born to cytarabine treated mother. *Lancet* 1980; **316**: 98–99.

30. Artlich A, Möller J, Kruse K *et al.* Teratogenic effects in a case of maternal treatment for acute myelocytic leukemia – neonatal and infantile course. *European Journal of Pediatrics* 1994; **153**: 488–491.

31. Schafer AI. Teratogenic effects of antileukemic chemotherapy. *Archives of Internal Medicine* 1981; **141**: 514–515.

32. Avilés A, Niz J. Long-term follow-up of children born to mothers with acute leukemia during pregnancy. *Medical and Pediatric Oncology* 1988; **16**: 3–6.

33. Cantini E, Yanes B. Acute myelogenous leukemia in pregnancy. *Southern Medical Journal* 1984; **77**: 1050–1052.

34. Breccia M, Mengarelli A, Mancini M *et al.* Myelodysplastic syndromes in patients under 50 years old: a single institution experience. *Leukemia Research* 2005; **29**: 749–754.

35. Ikeda Y, Masuzaki H, Nakayama D *et al.* Successful management and perinatal outcome of pregnancy complicated with myelodysplastic syndrome. *Leukemia Research* 2002; **26**: 255–260.

36. Siddiqui T, Elfenbein GJ, Noyes WD *et al.* Myelodysplastic syndromes presenting in pregnancy. A report of five cases and the clinical outcome. *Cancer* 1990; **66**: 377–381.

37. Pagliuca A, Mufti GJ, Fenaux P *et al.* Myelodysplastic syndromes during pregnancy. *European Journal of Hematology* 1991; **47**: 310–312.

38. Fadilah SA, Roswati MN. Refractory anemia with excess of blasts in transformation (RAEB-T) during pregnancy with hematological remission following delivery. *British Journal of Haematology* 1999; **104**: 935–936.

39. Essien EM, Sharma U, Upadhaya K, Malik R. Myelodysplastic syndrome and successful pregnancy. *International Journal of Hematology* 1998; **68**: 449–452.

40. Yang Z, Mei-Ying L, Shan-Mi W, Xiao-Hui Z. Pregnancy and myelodysplastic syndrome: an analysis of the clinical characteristics, maternal and fetal outcomes. *Journal of Maternal and Fetal Neonatal Medicine* 2015; **28**(18): 2155–2159.

41. Hellstrom-Lindberg E. Efficacy of erythropoietin in the myelodysplastic syndromes: a meta-analysis of 205 patients from 17 studies. *British Journal of Haematology* 1995; **89**: 67–71.

42. Royal College of Obstetricians and Gynecologists. *Bacterial Sepsis following Pregnancy. Green-Top Clinical Guideline No. 64b.* London: Royal College of Obstetricians and Gynecologists; 2012. http://www.rcog.org.uk/files/rcog-corp/11.6.12GTG64b.pdf (accessed June 1 2014).

43. Einarson A, Maltepe C, Navioz Y *et al.* The safety of ondansetron for nausea and vomiting of pregnancy: a prospective comparative study. *British Journal of Obstetrics and Gynecology* 2004; **111**: 940–943.

44. Lynch CM, Herold AH. Use of antibiotics during pregnancy. Medical News and Events, 1991. http://www.drplace.com/Use_of_antibiotics_during_pregnancy.16.18138.htm (accessed July 11 2017).

45. King CT, Rogers PD, Cleary, JD Chapman, SW. Antifungal therapy during pregnancy. *Clinical Infectious Diseases* 1998; **27**: 1151–1160.

46. The Advisory Committee on the Safety of Blood, Tissues and Organs (SaBTO) position statement. Provision of cytomegalovirus tested blood components position statement; 2012. https://www.gov.uk/government/news/provision-of-cytomegalovirus-tested-blood-components-position-statement-published (accessed July 11 2017).

47. Royal College of Obstetricians and Gynecologists. *Green-Top Clinical Guideline No. 7 Antenatal Corticosteroids to Reduce Neonatal Morbidity and Mortality.* London: Royal College of Obstetricians and Gynecologists; 2010. http://www.rcog.org.uk/files/rcog-corp/GTG%207.pdf (accessed June 1 2014).

48. RCOG. Magnesium Sulphate to Prevent Cerebral Palsy following Preterm Birth. RCOG Scientific Impact Paper No.29. 2011. https://www.rcog.org.uk/globalassets/documents/guidelines/scientific-impact-papers/sip_29.pdf (accessed June 1 2014).

49. Qureshi H, Masse, E, Kirwan D *et al.* BCSH guideline for the use of anti-D immunoglobulin for the prevention of hemolytic disease of the fetus and newborn. *Transfusion Medicine* 2014; **24**: 8–20.

Chapter 26

Late Effects of Chemoradiotherapy on Fertility and Pregnancy

Seonaid Pye and Nina Salooja

Introduction

Advances in treatment for hematological malignancies over the last two decades have led to marked improvements in survival, and for many patients this translates to cure. Consideration of the long-term sequelae of treatments administered is therefore becoming increasingly relevant to the overall management strategies of these disorders and, since many of the potentially treatable hematological cancers occur in children and young adults, this includes concerns about future fertility. The agents used to treat hematological malignancies can affect reproductive potential in a variety of ways. In this chapter we will consider:

- the general effects of chemoradiotherapy on female fertility;
- the incidence of infertility following radiation and chemotherapy;
- the likely outcome of pregnancy in a patient treated for hematological malignancy;
- the strategies available for the preservation of fertility in patients who require potentially sterilizing treatment.

General Effects of Chemoradiotherapy on Fertility

Normal reproduction requires interplay between the gonads and the hypothalamic–pituitary–endocrine axis. In addition, the uterus must be receptive to implantation and capable of effecting appropriate growth in pregnancy. Damage to hormone-producing cells in the hypothalamus, pituitary, or gonads can lead to infertility as well as more direct damage to the germ cells, reproductive tracts, or sexual organs.

In females, the production of germ cells (oocytes) ceases before birth. Thereafter, the number of oocytes decreases throughout life, either by a mechanism of preprogramed cell death (physiological apoptosis) or else post-menarche, in menstruation. When the number of oocytes falls below a critical number, ovulation

and ovarian function cease; a female's fertility potential is therefore related to the number of oocytes present in the ovary.

At the time of birth, surviving oocytes are surrounded by follicular epithelial cells forming primordial follicles. The majority of these are in the ovarian cortex where they remain dormant for years or even decades. During reproductive life cohorts of follicles are sequentially activated for a developmental trajectory which takes 3 months or more to complete and culminates for the minority of growing follicles in the release of a mature egg. Chemotherapy and radiotherapy both lead to an irreversible reduction in the number of oocytes. Several mechanisms have been proposed to account for this including vascular damage to the ovarian stroma[1] and induction of apoptosis in pre-granulosa cells and oocytes[2]. Studies in mice indicate that cyclophosphamide can also disrupt the phosphatidylinositol 3-kinase signaling pathway, leading to excessive recruitment of dormant primordial follicles with subsequent "burnout" of the ovarian reserve[3].

The chance of retaining ovarian function following external insults to germ cell numbers depends on the starting number of follicles and this is related to the age of the patient. Thus, young women who start with high numbers of follicles are more likely to recover menses and fertility following chemoradiotherapy, although they remain at risk of premature ovarian failure. Older women with relatively low numbers of follicles remaining in the ovary pre-treatment frequently experience immediate and irreversible cessation of ovarian function. Biochemically, this is associated with low serum levels of estradiol and significantly elevated levels of gonadotrophic hormones, follicle stimulating hormone (FSH) and luteinizing hormone (LH).

In the last decade, there has been increasing interest in serum levels of anti-mullerian hormone (AMH) as a marker of ovarian reserve[4]. AMH is produced by the granulosa cells of developing follicles and the level does not change significantly with the menstrual cycle. The serum levels do fall, however, after a spontaneous menopause. In patients receiving chemotherapy, serum AMH can fall dramatically within the first few weeks, indicative of damage to the majority of growing follicles. Longitudinal studies which include 6-month follow-up data have shown that recovery of AMH can subsequently occur following some chemotherapeutic agents, although following alkylating agents AMH levels typically remain low. The relationship between AMH and resumption of menses or indeed conception is not clear. Further data are therefore required to demonstrate the clinical utility of AMH measurements in the management of fertility issues in patients with cancer.

Abdomino-pelvic radiation can damage the uterus as well as ovarian tissue. Imaging by ultrasound or MRI scanning indicates that morphological changes occur in the myometrium, endometrium, and vasculature of the uterus. In a study which investigated length and blood flow of the uterus in 10 women aged 15–31 following 20–30 Gy abdominal radiotherapy in childhood, there were significant reductions in uterine length and blood flow compared with women with premature ovarian failure whose treatment had not included abdominal radiation[5].

Cranial irradiation can cause immediate damage to the hypothalamic–pituitary axis, but because these tissues replicate slowly it can also lead to delayed onset of hormone deficiencies. Tissues affected include the neurones, glial cells, and blood vessels.

The Incidence of Infertility Following Radiation

The clinical effects of radiotherapy on fertility depend on the dose and radiation field in addition to patient age as discussed above. Animal studies have shown that increasing doses of ovarian radiation lead to loss of primordial follicles in a dose-dependent manner. The dose at which 50% of human oocytes are lost (LD50) has been estimated to be <2 Gy[6]. Considering the radiation fields, treatment impinging on either the cranium or reproductive tract can lead to impairment of fertility (Table 26.1).

Direct Cranial Irradiation

Irradiation of the hypothalamic–pituitary axis leads to a classical pattern of hormone loss, with growth hormone being the most sensitive and first to be

Table 26.1 Radiation sites relevant to reproductive potential

Site of irradiation	Tissues relevant to fertility potential
Irradiation to the cranium, for example: (a) total body irradiation (b) craniospinal irradiation (c) direct cranial irradiation	Hypothalamic–pituitary axis
Irradiation to the abdomen or pelvis, for example: (a) total body irradiation (b) total lymphoid irradiation (c) craniospinal irradiation (d) direct irradiation to the pelvis or abdomen	Ovaries Uterus Reproductive tract

affected, followed by the gonadotrophins. In adults administered more than 30 Gy for pituitary tumors, the risk of gonadotropin deficiency is 60% at 4 years [7]. Damage from the underlying malignancy may also have contributed to this. Lower doses of cranial radiation are used in patients receiving treatment for acute leukemia. Doses in the range 18–24 Gy may result in isolated growth hormone (GH) deficiency but do not typically lead to central hypogonadism. Nonetheless disturbances in the menstrual hormone cycle have been described with doses in this range, and a report from the Childhood Cancer Survivor Study has shown a reduced likelihood of pregnancy following hypothalamic–pituitary doses greater than 22 Gy compared to a group of sibling controls. In this latter study, patients who had received more than 0.1 Gy radiation to the ovaries were excluded[8].

Direct Abdomino-Pelvic Radiation

Fertility outcome data indicate that doses to the uterus of 25–30 Gy can cause irreversible damage when administered in childhood[9]. Case reports describing successful pregnancy after uterine radiation administered in adult life suggest that the threshold for irreversible damage is likely to be higher in adults[10]. In a study including 84 adult survivors of childhood cancer who had received abdominal and/or pelvic radiation it was concluded that fertility could be preserved in patients who had abdominal radiotherapy that excluded the pelvis[9]. In these patients, the scatter dose to the uterus was estimated to be 4 Gy or less. Of 28 women in this study whose fertility was proven by pregnancy, the mean dose to the uterus was 4.9 +/–9.8 Gy. Of 23 patients who appeared likely to

321

be infertile with amenorrhoea and no recorded pregnancies, the mean dose to the uterus was significantly higher at 18.2 +/–14.6 Gy.

Total Body Irradiation

This affects all of the radiation sites relevant to fertility potential. It is usually given together with chemotherapy as conditioning prior to stem cell transplantation (SCT) and serves two separate functions:

- suppression of the host immune system to allow donor engraftment;
- eradication of hematopoiesis in the host bone marrow.

Doses of 8–15 Gy are administered either as a single dose or in fractions. At these doses, the effects on the hypothalamic–pituitary axis are usually minimal, but both ovarian function and uterine function are compromised. The incidence of ovarian failure is high. In a single-center study, which included 144 women who had received total body irradiation (TBI) as conditioning for SCT, all became amenorrhoeic immediately post-transplant and only 9 of the 144 recovered menses at a median of 4 years following treatment[11]. All who regained ovarian function were aged less than 25 at the time of SCT.

Uterine function following TBI has been less extensively studied, but in a study that included 12 women who had received TBI in childhood, there was a reduction in uterine volume to 40% of adult size despite the use of sex steroid replacement therapy[12]. These patients had received either unfractionated TBI at a midline dose of 8.5–10 Gy (n=4) or a total midline dose of 10.9–11.7 Gy in three fractions (n=8). These data suggest that the adverse effects of radiation may be more marked if given pre-pubertally, before optimum growth of the uterus has been achieved.

The Incidence of Infertility Following Chemotherapy

The likelihood of infertility following chemotherapy depends on:

- the drug(s) administered;
- the doses to which the patient is exposed;
- the underlying disease;
- patient age.

Chemotherapy agents can be divided into classes based upon their mechanism of action (Table 26.2). Meirow[13] provides an elegant analysis of the sterilizing effects of different classes of chemotherapeutic agents (Figure 26.1). Data on 168 patients treated with combination chemotherapy were evaluated and the odds ratio for ovarian failure calculated for exposed versus unexposed patients. Results were then adjusted for age by logistic regression analysis. These data show that alkylating agents and platinum derivatives are associated with the highest risks of ovarian failure with odds ratios of 3.98 and 1.7, respectively.

For many individual drugs, however, the true age-related, dose-related incidence of infertility is unknown because there are insufficient longitudinal data using them as single agents. A notable exception to this is cyclophosphamide for which there are extensive published data. This is because the drug is useful in the treatment of a variety of diseases that affect women of childbearing age: these include breast cancer, autoimmune disorders such as SLE, and hematological malignancies. Cyclophosphamide also plays an important part in conditioning treatment given prior to allogeneic SCT where it can be used as:

- a high-dose single agent (for example, in patients transplanted for severe aplastic anemia, SAA);
- in combination with busulfan (for example, pediatric and adult transplantation for leukemia);
- together with total body irradiation (for example, in adults transplanted for leukemia).

The relationship between ovarian failure and age in women administered cyclophosphamide was clearly demonstrated by a study in which premenopausal women with breast cancer were treated with cyclophosphamide (CY) at a dose of 100 mg/day[14]. The data are illustrated in Table 26.3 and show that a total cumulative dose in excess of 11 g will lead to cessation of menstruation in most women over the age of 30 but not younger women.

Although the cumulative dose administered is important, as illustrated above, data from transplant centers where cyclophosphamide is administered in a single high dose as pre-transplant conditioning suggest that this may be a particularly gonadotoxic approach. Follow-up of 43 women with SAA who received CY in doses of 200 mg/kg as pre-transplant conditioning demonstrated acute cessation of menstruation in all 27 of these patients who were less than 26 years of age at the time of transplant but they subsequently recovered ovarian function, in comparison with only 5 of the 16 women aged >26[15].

More limited data are available on other chemotherapeutic drugs used as single agents. An association of

Table 26.2 Classes of chemotherapeutic agents and their action

Drug class/subclasses	Examples	Mechanism of action
Alkylating agents		
Nitrogen mustards	Cyclophosphamide, chlorambucil, melphalan	DNA damage
Nitrosureas	BCNU (carmustine), lomustine	
Alkyl sulfonates	Busulfan	
Triazines	Dacarbazine	
Ethylenimines	Thiotepa, altretamine	
Platinum drugs[a]	Cisplatin, carboplatin	
Bendamustine		
Antimetabolites	Methotrexate, 5-fluorouracil, 6-mercaptopurine, gemcitabine, cytarabine (Ara-C), fludarabine	Interfere with nucleic acid or nucleotide synthesis
Antibiotics		
Anthracyclines	Daunorubicin, doxorubicin, epirubicin, idarubicin	Various mechanisms, e.g. interference with enzymes involved in DNA synthesis
Other	Bleomycin, mitomycin-C, mitoxantrone[b]	
Topoisomerase inhibitors		
Topoisomerase I	Topotecan	
Topoisomerase II	Etoposide (VP-16), mitoxantrone[b]	
Mitotic inhibitors		
Taxanes	Paclitaxel, docetaxel	
Vinca alkaloids	Vinblastine, vincristine	
Epothilones	Ixabepilone (Ixempra)	
Tyrosine kinase inhibitors	Imatinib, nilotinib, dasatinib, ponatinib	
Immunomodulatory drugs	Thalidomide, lenalidomide, pomalidomide	
Proteasome inhibitors	Bortezomib, carfilzomib	
Miscellaneous	L-asparaginase	

[a] Platinum drugs are grouped here with alkylating agents because they have a similar mechanism of action.
[b] Similar to doxorubicin but also acts as topoisomerase II inhibitor.

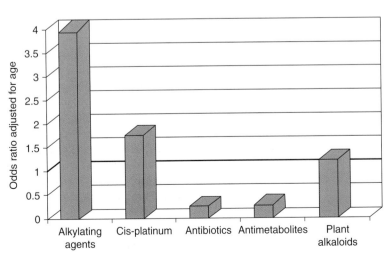

Figure 26.1 In 168 cancer patients treated by combination chemotherapy, the overall ovarian failure rate was 34%, representing an odds ratio of 1.0. Medications were in five drug categories (alkylating agents, platinum derivatives, antibiotics, antimetabolites, and plant alkaloids) and analysis was performed on these groups. The fraction contributed by each of the chemotherapeutic classes was analyzed by the odds ratio of exposed versus non-exposed patients. The results were adjusted for age. Figure reproduced with permission from ref. [45].

Table 26.3 Relationship between dose of cyclophosphamide and age

Age	Number of patients	Number developing amenorrhea	Average cumulative dose at onset of amenorrhea
>40	13	13	5.2 g (range 1.4–8.4 g)
30–40	5	4 (2 subsequently resumed menses)	9.3 g (7–11 g)
20–30[a]	5	3	20.4 g (14–24.5 g)

From Ref. [7].

[a] These patients received other treatment modalities in addition to CY.

busulfan with ovarian failure has been noted as far back as the 1950s with cumulative doses of 150–400 mg associated with acute amenorrhea. More recent data from transplant patients in whom high doses of busulfan (BU) were incorporated into pre-transplant conditioning regimens further highlight the gonadotoxicity of this agent. In a large European multicenter study evaluating pregnancy following SCT, the combination of BU and CY (BUCY) as pre-transplant conditioning appeared more gonadotoxic than CY/TBI as there were no pregnancies in patients with malignant disease who had received BUCY in standard doses for pre-transplant conditioning[16].

There are fewer protocols involving use of chlorambucil as a single agent in young females. In a small study of 10 pre-pubertal girls exposed to cumulative doses of chlorambucil ranging from 9 to 28 mg/kg for autoimmune disease, all had normal pubertal development including normal age at onset of menarche [17]. Larger cumulative doses of 535–750 mg/m^2 administered to women with breast cancer, however, are associated with ovarian failure[18].

Data on drug combinations will now be discussed in the context of the underlying disease.

Acute Leukemias

Conventional treatments for acute myeloid leukemia (AML) and acute lymphocytic leukemia (ALL) are generally less gonadotoxic than those used to treat lymphomas. Typical induction regimens for AML involve drugs such as cytarabine, daunorubicin, and etoposide followed by consolidation treatment, which may incorporate amsacrine or mitoxantrone. The incidence of persistent gonadal damage following treatment with anthracycline-based regimens during childhood or adulthood has been reported as <10%. AML survivors had a 6% incidence of acute ovarian

failure in the Childhood Cancer Survivors Study published in 2006[19].

Acute lymphoblastic leukemia is the commonest childhood cancer, although it also affects adults. In addition to induction and consolidation phases, treatment of ALL also incorporates a maintenance phase and CNS-directed therapy. The latter is generally administered as intrathecal chemotherapy with cranial or craniospinal irradiation reserved for those at high risk (5–20%) of CNS relapse. The drugs commonly used in the treatment of ALL are glucocorticoids, vincristine, anthracycline, and asparaginase. High-dose methotrexate may be administered to those with high-risk disease and a tyrosine kinase inhibitor (imatinib, dasatinib, or ponatinib) is used for patients who have Philadelphia positive ALL. The incidence of persistent gonadal damage in females following treatment of childhood ALL with standard UK ALL protocols is less than 20%. Those who received craniospinal irradiation or cyclophosphamide as part of their treatment are at greatest risk. Data from the Childhood Cancer Survivors Study demonstrated an acute ovarian failure rate in ALL survivors of 14%[19].

Chronic Leukemias

Chronic lymphocytic leukemia is predominantly a disorder of the elderly and so will not be discussed further. Chronic myeloid leukemia (CML) is typically a disorder of middle-aged adults, but a significant number of cases occur in women of childbearing age (15–49). In the past, the mainstay of treatment for chronic myeloid leukemia (CML) has been treatment with hydroxycarbamide (formerly known as hydroxyurea) followed by stem cell transplantation. In the last 15 years, however, there has been considerable success in managing CML with tyrosine kinase inhibitors such as imatinib: the first example of a molecularly targeted therapy. Imatinib was first administered to patients with CML in 1998 and has now been used to treat more than 60 000 patients worldwide. It is given orally and is generally well tolerated. Patients taking imatinib are cautioned against pregnancy because it is teratogenic in animal studies. Nonetheless, 180 pregnancies have been reported in patients who were taking imatinib[20]. Dosage data were not available in every case, but many who conceived were receiving standard doses of 300–400 mg. Animal data also suggest that imatinib at standard dosages is unlikely to impair fertility in either adult male or female animals. However, although human data remain limited, there have been case reports suggesting a detrimental effect on human ovarian function. This is consistent with published data suggesting that higher doses of imatinib can be associated with premature ovarian failure [21].

Lymphomas

Hodgkin's and non-Hodgkin's lymphoma (HL and NHL) together account for approximately 10% of pediatric cancers (4% HL, 6% NHL). With modern treatments for HL, in excess of 90% of children and adolescents can expect to be cured. Alkylating agents have played a major role in many of the combination chemotherapy protocols proposed for the treatment of HL and many of these have therefore been associated with infertility (Table 26.4). In the 1970s, treatment regimens containing nitrogen mustard such as MOPP (nitrogen mustard, vincristine, procarbazine, and prednisolone) and MVPP (nitrogen mustard, vinblastine, procarbazine, and prednisolone) were used and were associated with oligo- or amenorrhea in approximately 20–40% of women. In the mid-1970s, however, it was discovered that a new regimen combining doxorubicin, bleomycin, vinblastine, and dacarbazine (ABVD) was as efficacious a treatment as MOPP or MVPP, but lacked the gonadotoxicity. ABVD remains the gold standard of treatment in many parts of the world and the risk of sterilization in women under the age of 25 is almost zero[22]. Women treated with inverted Y-irradiation, in addition to alkylating agents, have been shown to have a significantly higher risk of premature menopause, however.

Non-Hodgkin's lymphomas (NHL) can be broadly subdivided into low-grade and high-grade lymphomas. One of the mainstays of treatment for all lymphomas expressing the B-cell surface antigen

Table 26.4 Treatment regimens for Hodgkin's disease and likelihood of gonadal failure

Risk of gonadal failure	Combination chemotherapy regimens for Hodgkin's lymphoma
High risk (>80%)	MVPP
	MOPP
	ChlVPP/EVA
	COPP
Intermediate risk	BEAM (BCNU, etoposide, cytarabine and melphalan)
	Dose escalated BEACOPP
	VEBEP
	Alternating ABVD/MOPP or COPP
	CHOP
Low risk (<20%)	VAPEC-B
	BEACOPP
	VEEP
	ABVD

MVPP, mustine, vinblastine, procarbazine, and prednisolone; MOPP, mechlorethamine, vincristine, procarbazine, and prednisone; ChlVPP/EVA, chlorambucil, vinblastine, procarbazine, and prednisone/etoposide, vincristine, and doxorubicin; COPP, cyclophosphamide, vincristine, procarbazine, and prednisone; BEAM, BCNU, etoposide, cytarabine, melphalan; BEACOPP, bleomycin, etoposide, doxorubicin, cyclophosphamide, vincristine, procarbazine, and prednisone; VEBEP, etoposide, epirubicin, bleomycin, cyclophosphamide, and prednisolone; ABVD, doxorubicin (adriamycin), bleomycin, vinblastine, dacarbazine; CHOP, cyclophosphamide, doxorubicin, vincristine, prednisolone; VAPEC-B, vincristine, doxorubicin (adriamycin), prednisone, etoposide, cyclophosphamide, bleomycin; VEEP, vincristine, epirubicin, etoposide, and prednisolone.

CD20 is an anti-CD20 monoclonal antibody. The first of these to be used in clinical practice was rituximab and this, administered with the appropriate chemotherapy regimen, is now standard therapy for such lymphomas whether they are low or high grade. Low-dose oral chemotherapy such as chlorambucil is appropriate for many older patients with low-grade disease as discussed above. Younger patients with an indication for therapy are usually treated with intravenous regimes such as cyclophosphamide, vincristine, and prednisolone or bendamustine, each given with rituximab. There are now significant data on the use of rituximab in pregnancy as it is also approved for the treatment of various autoimmune conditions such as rheumatoid arthritis and idiopathic thrombocytopenic purpura (ITP). Rituximab contains an immunoglobulin G1κ construct and can therefore cross the placenta. Levels in the fetal circulation slowly rise throughout pregnancy, peaking during the last 4 weeks of gestation, thus timing of exposure may be important. Although the drug is classified by the Food and Drug Administration as pregnancy category C based on adverse events in animal reproductive studies, pregnancies have inevitably occurred. A review of 253 pregnancies exposed to the drug was reported in 2011 and of these 153 had known outcomes[23]. Nearly 60% (n=90) resulted in live births and there were 33 reports of first trimester miscarriages (21%). Of the 90 live births, 68 (76%) resulted in full-term deliveries and there were 22 (24%) premature births (<37 weeks' gestation). The women in this series were receiving treatment for a variety of conditions including lymphoma and were thus exposed to other potentially teratogenic agents but regardless the outcomes in the live births were encouraging. It is known that rituximab can cause B-cell depletion in exposed infants but in animal studies these levels returned to normal at 6 months. The data on rituximab are of importance as its use as maintenance therapy as a single agent in many low-grade lymphomas has become common practice in recent years. Patients can receive treatment for a period of up to 2 years post completion of their initial chemotherapy and thus there will be many more years of exposure to the drug. The new anti-CD20 monoclonal antibody Ofatumumab is now also available for specific indications although its use is much less widespread, and thus data relating to use in pregnancy are not available. The advice remains to avoid exposure. Exposure to bendamustine during pregnancy should be avoided as the drug is known to cause significant birth defects in animal studies and it is both teratogenic and mutagenic. The risks of impaired fertility as a result of prior exposure to this drug are not yet clear: amenorrhea is common but rates of infertility are as yet unknown and are likely to be related to a variety of factors such as maternal age.

The gold standard treatment for high grade NHL is a combination of the following drugs: rituximab (375 mg/m^2), cyclophosphamide (750 mg/m^2), doxorubicin, vincristine, and prednisolone (CHOP). Premenopausal women treated using this regimen are likely to develop amenorrhea during chemotherapy, but the majority (95%) will resume menstruation shortly after completion of treatment. The risk of permanent ovarian failure is highest in those aged 40 or more at the time of treatment. Even when higher doses of cyclophosphamide are used, as in "mega-CHOP," in which 2–3 g/m^2 cyclophosphamide are administered, it appears that the risk of persistent ovarian failure may be low, with 92% (12/13) of women regaining ovarian function in one study[24]. Women in this latter study who were aged <40 years were offered gonadotrophin-releasing hormone (GnRH) analogs in parallel with their chemotherapy in an attempt to preserve fertility. A second study which combined data on various chemotherapy regimens for NHL in premenopausal women found a higher incidence of ovarian failure of 44%[25], but the patient characteristics and details of chemotherapy regimens used were not reported, and this is likely to underlie the discrepancy. Childhood NHL is treated with similar protocols to childhood ALL and the risks of infertility and delayed puberty are low. In a recent prospective study of survivors of childhood NHL or ALL, all 40 females treated with chemotherapy alone or chemotherapy plus cranial irradiation underwent spontaneous menarche[26]. Whether these patients will subsequently undergo premature ovarian failure is not known but it seems likely that their reproductive lifespan will be reduced. A Norwegian study which investigated 99 women treated between 1975 and 1992 for lymphoma demonstrated that younger age at treatment delays the development of premature ovarian failure but does not decrease the lifetime risk[27].

Myeloma

Myeloma tends to be a disease of older people with only 4% of cases found in individuals less than 45 years old. There have, however, now been 32 case reports of pregnancies in women with myeloma[28]. This may in part reflect the current trend to delay having a family until later in life. Sixteen of these patients deferred any treatment of their myeloma until after delivery. Most of the live births were delivered by cesarean section and 20 (73%) were premature. Moderate to high-dose steroids were the most commonly used treatment for those women requiring therapy prior to delivery. In some cases this was administered with other agents, e.g. cyclophosphamide. Newer anti-myeloma therapies such as thalidomide or lenalidomide are well known to be contraindicated in pregnancy and hence the manufacturers have a pregnancy prevention program in place. No clinical data for the use of the proteasome inhibitor bortezomib in pregnancy are available and therefore this should be avoided.

The Likely Outcome of Pregnancy in a Patient Treated for Hematological Malignancy

There are several reasons why pregnancy outcome might be adversely affected by prior treatment with chemoradiotherapy. Irradiation to the uterus may affect implantation, potentially predisposing to miscarriage or intrauterine growth retardation. Chemotherapy agents such as cyclophosphamide can cause gene mutations, chromosomal breaks, and rearrangements, raising the possibility of an increased risk of congenital anomaly.

Although the focus of this chapter is on the relationship between chemoradiotherapy and fertility potential, effects on other maternal organs may cause complications for pregnancy and delivery. Cardiac and pulmonary toxicities, for example, are well described following some regimens. Patients at risk of such complications should have a cardio-respiratory review early in pregnancy, including an echocardiogram and pulmonary function tests, and may require assessment by an anesthetist prior to delivery. Similarly, patients with renal impairment will require expert review and monitoring throughout pregnancy.

A report from the Childhood Cancer Survivor Study (CCSS) looked at pregnancy outcome for 4029 pregnancies in 1915 women previously treated for cancers in childhood. The pregnancy outcome of the sibling closest in age to the patient was used for control data. Their results showed that women treated with pelvic irradiation in childhood tended to have smaller babies than the controls and delivered earlier, at an average of 37.23 weeks vs. 38.47 weeks for controls. Use of daunorubicin or doxorubicin was also linked adversely to birth weight but there was no clear dose–response relationship[29].

There are also data to support concerns of an adverse pregnancy outcome resulting from pelvic irradiation in adulthood. Following stem cell transplantation in which total body irradiation is given, there is an increased likelihood of preterm and low birth weight babies[16].

Despite the theoretical concern of congenital anomalies arising in offspring of survivors of cancer treatment, available data do not demonstrate a substantial increase in risk in patients where conventional chemotherapy has been used prior to conception. Studies from the Danish cancer registry[30] and CCSS[31] did not show a statistically significant association between maternal abdomino-pelvic irradiation and congenital anomalies in the offspring. The mean dose of radiation to the ovary in the study from the CCSS was 1.19 Gy; however, larger studies need to be done to investigate whether higher doses of radiation lead to an adverse outcome.

The tyrosine kinase inhibitor imatinib does not appear to damage chromosomes but it is capable of interacting with several target proteins of relevance to embryonic development, such as c-KIT and PDGFR. Female rats administered doses >45 mg/kg (which equates to approximately half the maximum human dose of 800 mg/day, based on body surface area) experienced significant post-implantation loss with increased fetal resorption, stillbirths, non-viable pups, and early pup mortality. Doses higher than 100 mg/kg resulted in fetal loss (Novartis clinical safety statement). In a study which included data on pregnancy outcomes for 125 women exposed to imatinib at conception and during part or all of the first trimester, there were 12 offspring identified with abnormalities, 3 of which were terminated electively. Of the offspring with identifiable anomalies, 3 had strikingly similar complex malformations, which were considered unlikely to have occurred by chance[20].

Effects of Chemotherapy and Radiotherapy During Pregnancy

Diagnosis of a hematological malignancy in pregnancy can create a significant conflict between the wellbeing of the mother versus that of the child. Most chemotherapy agents are potentially teratogenic and the risks to fetus are most marked in the first trimester. Management of hematological malignancy in pregnancy therefore depends on the stage of pregnancy when a diagnosis is made, the drugs required, and the nature of the underlying malignancy, which dictates whether or not treatment can be delayed. The decision about when and how to treat a woman with malignancy in pregnancy requires a multidisciplinary approach with careful counseling of the patient.

In some patients, non-curative treatment can be considered as a holding tactic. In patients with CML, for example, leukapheresis can be used to temporarily control the white cell and platelet counts while the pregnancy continues. In patients with Hodgkin's lymphoma, single agent vinblastine has been used[32].

327

The management of AML in pregnancy has been the subject of a guideline issued by the British Society of Hematology[33]. In keeping with the nature of the topic, 12/19 recommendations are based on Grade C (low) quality data. In general, the authors recommend that for patients with acute leukemia treatment should be commenced with minimal delay using a standard daunorubicin/cytarabine induction regimen. In the first trimester it is reasonable to consider elective termination prior to treatment because the outlook for the fetus is poor and it is safer for the mother to have an elective rather than spontaneous miscarriage in this setting. In the third trimester, if the gestation is greater than 32 weeks then it may be preferable to deliver the baby prior to starting treatment. Between 24 and 36 weeks the risks of premature delivery versus exposure to chemotherapy should be discussed with a neonatologist and hematologist. The timing of delivery in relation to maternal chemotherapy is important because of the risks of fetal neutropenia and ideally delivery should take place at least 3 weeks after administration.

In Hodgkin's lymphoma, there is some experience using the combination ABVD. Data suggest that its use in the second and third trimester of pregnancy can be associated with a good outcome for mother and baby. It has also been used with success in the first trimester but its use at this stage remains more controversial[34].

Fertility Preservation

Management of women who are to receive potentially sterilizing doses of chemoradiotherapy has been the subject of several guidelines including a joint report from three Royal Colleges in the UK[35] and individual reports from the National Institute for Health and Care Excellence (NICE)[36], the American Society for Reproductive Medicine (ASRM)[37], and the American Society of Clinical Oncology (ASCO)[38]. All of these guidelines emphasize the importance of addressing potential infertility with the patient before cancer treatment commences and furthermore discussing all of the available management options.

Some women will have more than one therapeutic option for their cancer in which case women who hope to commence a family after treatment may be able to avoid potentially sterilizing treatment. In women who require pelvic irradiation, it may be possible to laparoscopically transpose the ovaries outside the field of radiation, leaving the ovarian blood supply intact. This is not always successful, however; not only can the ovaries migrate back into the field of radiation, but complications can occur as a result of the procedure such as chronic pain or formation of ovarian cysts. Alternatively, modified field radiation can sometimes be planned to omit/reduce radiation to the ovaries. Scatter radiation can nonetheless contribute to ovarian failure and follow-up remains important.

Embryo cryopreservation is one of the preferred methods of fertility preservation in women who require sterilizing treatment. This technique requires ovarian stimulation over a 2-week period, following which mature oocytes in their second metaphase are collected. These oocytes are fertilized in vitro before freezing. This option is not open to all patients with cancer, however. Ovarian stimulation takes 2 weeks, but conventional protocols time this to the early follicular phase of the menstrual cycle. As a result, it can take 2–6 weeks from presentation to retrieve mature oocytes. Random start stimulation protocols can reduce this time delay to 2–3 weeks[39,40], but even this is prohibitive for many patients with hematological malignancies. Additional complexity arises if the patient lacks a male partner to provide sperm.

In healthy women who attempt pregnancy with transfer of thawed embryos using their own eggs, the pregnancy rate is close to 20% but with decreasing success as age increases. There are several reasons why the outcome of artificial reproductive techniques (ART) may be lower in women with cancer, however. Firstly, women with cancer do not always respond well to stimulation regimens and the quality and number of oocytes may be lower than expected. Secondly, many patients will have compromised endometrial function in addition to ovarian failure as a result of their treatment. This could potentially impede implantation or fetal growth and development. There are some data to support this from a European multicenter study which included nine women who conceived using ART following TBI[16]. Among the pregnancies to these women, the incidence of preterm delivery and low birth weight offspring was high, and median birth weights were lower than expected for gestational age. Although there are a number of case reports of successful pregnancies using cryopreserved embryos following systemic cancer therapy, it is difficult to quote accurate success rates for these patients and some will elect to use a surrogate if available to carry their embryos.

The guideline on fertility preservation from NICE (2013) recommends that embryo or oocyte cryopreservation should be offered to female patients undergoing potentially sterilizing treatment[36]. Furthermore they recommend that vitrification is used in preference to controlled rate freezing if it is available. This is based on data indicating that there have been significantly more clinical pregnancies using oocytes cryopreserved using vitrification compared to controlled rate freezing. The ASRM has also removed the experimental status of oocyte cryopreservation as of 2012 and along with ASCO recommends oocyte or embryo cryopreservation as methods of fertility preservation.

Freezing Ovarian Tissue

This is currently considered experimental and is not available to all patients. Nonetheless it is the only option open to pre-pubertal patients or to those women whose disease will not tolerate a significant delay in treatment. Cortical fragments containing primordial follicles with immature oocytes can be obtained by laparoscopy and frozen. Ideally, ovarian tissue should be obtained before the patient has been exposed to chemotherapy, but this is not always possible and is not an absolute requirement. Attempts to restore ovarian function and fertility have involved reimplanting the ovarian tissue, either orthotopically adjacent to the ovary or heterotopically, for example, into the anterior abdominal wall. Donnez *et al.* summarized data from three centers incorporating 60 cases of reimplanted cryopreserved ovarian tissue [41]. In the majority of cases, ovarian activity was restored; the duration of endocrine activity was variable but the authors suggest that if follicular density is well preserved in the transplanted tissue, 4–5 years may be expected. There were 11 pregnancies some of which involved IVF and at the time of this publication (2013), the total number of reported live births in the literature from this technique was 24.

A major concern when reimplanting cryopreserved ovarian tissue is the possibility of reintroducing cancer cells, particularly as tissue is usually removed before anti-cancer treatment commences [42]. The risk depends on the individual disease but ovarian metastases have been described in leukemia, Hodgkin's, and non-Hodgkin's lymphoma. Testing for malignant cells can take place by histology,

immunohistochemistry, molecular biology, and animal transplantation. Assessment of ovarian tissue taken from patients with leukemia (CML, AML, ALL) by PCR has demonstrated positivity in a number of cases and assessment of tissue in SCID mice confirms the leukemic potential of the tissue[43]. As a result, re-introduction of ovarian tissue from patients with leukemia would not currently be recommended. In the future, maturation in vitro of follicles from cryopreserved tissue may enable production of a viable disease-free alternative. In patients with lymphoma, histologically negative samples of ovarian issue have been transplanted without initiating relapse but in some cases the follow-up time was short[41].

The use of assisted reproductive techniques in cancer patients raises a range of ethical concerns, including several issues relating to consent. Consent takes place when two or more people agree upon a course of action and it implies that:

- agreement occurred without coercion;
- agreement occurred based on the provision of information; and
- the participants have the ability to understand the facts and implications of the action ("competence").

In the UK, consent for long-term cryopreservation of gametes is governed by the Human Fertilization and Embryology Authority (HFEA), and they have constructed guidance and consent forms, which are available at www.hfea.gov.uk. The consent of both partners is required when embryos are cryopreserved and also when embryos are replaced. If either partner withdraws consent, the embryos cannot be used. This point was highlighted by the case of Evans vs. the United Kingdom in the European Court of Human rights when the male partner of Evans withdrew his consent for the use of their embryos when their relationship ended[44]. This may now prompt patients to consider storing both embryos and eggs if the opportunity is available. In the UK, young people aged 16–18 can consent to treatment under the Family Law Reform Act 1969 ("competent minors"). The position in younger patients was established in the case of Gillick vs. West Norfolk Area Health Authority (1985). As a result of this case, children who are of sufficient understanding and capable of expressing their own wishes (Gillick competent) can also make informed decisions. Under HFEA

329

regulations, parents or guardians cannot give consent on behalf of a child for the storage or use of gametes. Immature germ cells obtained from gonadal tissue of pre-pubertal children do not come under this remit, however. The tissue can therefore be recovered with parental consent if it is considered to be in the best interest of the child.

Conclusions

Treatment of hematological cancers is constantly evolving to produce improved survival data and incorporate better tolerated agents. As a result of this, an increasing number of young patients diagnosed with hematological malignancies can now hope to lead relatively normal adult lives and for many this includes the expectation of parenthood. Management of possible infertility should start before cancer treatment is administered and, ideally, should include a full discussion of: (1) treatment options and the likelihood of infertility associated with each option; and (2) strategies for preserving fertility if the chance of sterilization as a result of treatment is high. Full data are not always available, however, particularly where new drugs are used or when experimental methods for preserving fertility are considered. Long-term follow-up studies of patients treated for cancer remain a central priority to provide the core information required for such pretreatment counseling.

Case Studies

Case Study 1

A 24-year-old woman is seen for annual review in a general hematology clinic having had a stem cell transplant conditioned with cyclophosphamide and total body irradiation in adolescence for high-risk acute lymphoblastic leukemia. She is generally well, she has a normal full blood count, and is not experiencing any specific medical problems. To further questioning, she went through puberty at the age of 12 years prior to her diagnosis of leukemia and resumed regular monthly menstrual cycles 6–9 months after treatment. She is not currently planning a family but would like to have children in the future.

You explain to the patient that although she is having normal menstrual cycles at the moment, she is at risk of subfertility and premature ovarian failure as a result of the treatment she has received in the past. You therefore recommend referral to a specialist infertility clinic to consider evaluation of her ovarian reserve and whether she should have eggs frozen at this stage for use in the future.

Following this consultation, she is informed that although she has normal menstrual cycles, parameters indicative of ovarian reserve (including AMH levels and ultrasound data) suggest that she is already subfertile and that her chance of conceiving naturally is low. Furthermore, it is considered that her chance of responding to ovarian stimulation with a view to collecting eggs is poor. She is informed that while spontaneous pregnancy cannot be ruled out completely as a possibility, her best option for parenthood in the future will probably be donor embryos. This will require a healthy uterus and as this may also have been affected by her chemoradiotherapy further tests are arranged to investigate her uterine size and vascularity.

Case Study 2

A 30-year-old woman with a history of previously treated Hodgkin's lymphoma presents with a recurrence in the form of bulky abdominal disease. She has previously been treated with ABVD and so had been anticipating normal future fertility but is informed that she will now require potentially sterilizing treatment. She is determined that all possible steps are taken to preserve her chance of parenthood. She does not have a partner at present so she is unable to consider cryopreserving embryos in advance of treatment. Furthermore, she is informed that her hematology treatment will not tolerate the required minimum delay to collect eggs. The only option therefore is to collect and store ovarian tissue.

She is informed that the procedure is experimental and that few children have been born worldwide to date using this method. She is also warned that her ovarian tissue will be assessed for evidence of lymphoma prior to consideration of reimplantation and that if there is any evidence of lymphoma cells in the tissue it will not be used. She is referred to the closest center that can offer ovarian tissue collection and formal counseling and consent takes place before collecting ovarian cortical strips laparoscopically. These are frozen and stored for possible future use.

References

1. Meirow D, Dor J, Kaufman A *et al.* Cortical fibrosis and blood-vessels damage in human ovaries exposed to chemotherapy. Potential mechanisms of ovarian injury. *Human Reproduction* 2007; **22**: 1626–1633.

2. Tilly JL. Pharmacological protection of female infertility. In Tulandi T, Gosden R (eds) *Preservation of Fertility*. London:Taylor and Francis; 2004: 65–75.

3. Kalich-Philosoph L, Roness H, Carmely A *et al.* Cyclophosphamide triggers follicle activation and 'burnout'; AS101 prevents follicle loss and preserves fertility. *Science Translational Medicine* 2013; **5**: 185ra62

4. Peigne M, Decanter C. Serum AMH level as a marker of acute and long-term effects of chemotherapy on the ovarian follicular content: a systematic review. *Reproductive Biology and Endocrinology* 2014; **12**: 26.

5. Critchley HO, Wallace WH, Shalet SM *et al.* Abdominal irradiation in childhood: the potential for pregnancy. *British Journal of Obstetrics and Gynecology* 1992; **97**: 804–810.

6. Wallace WHB, Thomson AB, Kelsey TW. The radiosensitivity of the human oocyte. *Human Reproduction* 2003; **18**: 117–121.

7. Littley MD, Shalet SM, Beardwell CG *et al.* Hypopituitarism following external radiotherapy for pituitary tumours in adults. *Quaterley Journal of Medicine* 1989; **70**: 145–160.

8. Green DM, Nolan VG, Kawashima MS *et al.* Decreased fertility among female childhood cancer survivors who received 22-27 G hypothalamic/pituitary irradiation: a report from the childhood cancer survivor study. *Fertility and Sterility* 2011; **95**: 1922–1927.

9. Sudour H, Chastagner P, Claude L, *et al.* Fertility and pregnancy outcome after abdominal irradiation that included or excluded the pelvis in childhood tumor survivors. *International Journal of Radiation Oncology Biology Physics* 2010; **76**: 867–873.

10. The T, Stern C, Chander S, Hickey M. The impact of uterine radiation on subsequent fertility and pregnancy outcomes. *BioMed Research International* 2014; Article ID 482968.

11. Sanders JE, Buckner CD, Amos D *et al.* Ovarian function following marrow transplantation for aplastic anemia or leukemia. *Journal of Clinical Oncology* 1988; **6**: 813–818.

12. Holm K, Nysom K, Brocks V *et al.* Ultrasound B-mode changes in the uterus and ovaries and Doppler changes in the uterus after total body irradiation and allogeneic bone marrow transplantation. *Bone Marrow Transplantation* 1999; **23**: 259–263.

13. Meirow D. Reproduction post-chemotherapy in young cancer patients. *Molecular Cell Endocrinology* 2000; **169**: 123–131.

14. Koyama H, Wada T, Nishizawa Y *et al.* Cyclophosphamide-induced ovarian failure and its therapeutic significance in patients with breast cancer. *Cancer* 1977; **39**: 1403–1409.

15. Sanders JE, Hawley J, Levy W *et al.* Pregnancies following high-dose cyclophosphamide with or without high-dose busulfan or total-body irradiation and bone marrow transplantation. *Blood* 1996; **87**: 3045–3052.

16. Salooja N, Szydlo RM, Socie G *et al.* Pregnancy outcomes after peripheral blood or bone marrow transplantation: a retrospective study. *Lancet* 2001; **358**: 271–276.

17. Callis L, Nieto J, Vila A, Rende J. Chlorambucil treatment in minimal lesion nephrotic syndrome: a reappraisal of its gonadal toxicity. *Journal of Pediatrics* 1980; **97**: 653–656.

18. Freckman HA, Fry HL, Mendez FL *et al.* Chlorambucil–prednisolone therapy for disseminated breast carcinoma. *Journal of the American Medical Society* 1964; **189**: 23–26.

19. Chemaitilly W, Mertens AC, Mitby P *et al.* Acute ovarian failure in the Childhood Cancer Survivor Study. *Journal of Clinical Endocrinology and Metabolism* 2006; **91**: 1723–1728.

20. Pye S, Cortes J, Ault P *et al.* The effects of imatinib on pregnancy outcome. *Blood* 2008; **111**: 5505–5508.

21. Christopoulos C, Dimakopoulou V, Rotas E. Primary ovarian insufficiency associated with imatinib therapy. *New England Journal of Medicine* 2008; **358**: 1079–1080.

22. Meirow D, Dor J. Epidemiology and infertility in cancer patients. In Tulandi T, Gosden R (eds) *Preservation of Fertility*. London:Taylor and Francis; 2004: 21–38.

23. Chakravarty E, Murray E, Kelman A *et al.* Pregnancy outcomes after maternal exposure to rituximab. *Blood* 2011; **117**: 1499–1506.

24. Dann EJ, Epelbaum R, Avivi I *et al.* Fertility and ovarian function are preserved in women treated with an intensified regimen of cyclophosphamide, adriamycin, vincristine and prednisone (Mega-CHOP) for non-Hodgkin lymphoma. *Human Reproduction* 2005; **20**; 2247–2249.

25. Meirow D. Reproduction post-chemotherapy in young cancer patients. *Molecular Cell Endocrinology* 2000; **169**: 123–131.

26. Steffens M, Beauloye V, Brichard B *et al.* Endocrine and metabolic disorders in young adult survivors of childhood acute lymphoblastic leukemia (ALL) or

non-Hodgkin lymphoma (NHL). *Clinical Endocrinology* 2008; **69**: 819–827.

27. Huakvik UKH, Dieset I, Bjoro T, Holte H, Fossa SD. Treatment-related premature ovarian failure as a long-term complication after Hodgkin's lymphoma. *Annals of Oncology* 2006; **17**: 1428–1433.

28. Cabañas-Perianes V, Macizo M, Salido E *et al.* Management of multiple myeloma during pregnancy: a case report and review. *Hematological Oncology* 2016; **34**(2): 108–114.

29. Green DM, Whitton JA, Stovall M *et al.* Pregnancy outcomes in female survivors of childhood cancer: a report from the Childhood Cancer Survivor Study. *American Journal of Obstetrics and Gynecology* 2002; **187**: 1070–1080.

30. Winther JW, Olsen JH, Wu H *et al.* Genetic disease in the children of Danish surviors of childhood and adolescent cancer. *Journal of Clinical Oncology* 2012; **30**: 27–33.

31. Signorello LB, Mulvihill JJ, Green DM *et al.* Congenital anomalies in the children of cancer survivors: a report from the childhood cancer survivor study. *Journal of Clinical Oncology* 2012; **30**: 239–245.

32. Bachanova V, Connors JM. Hodgkin lymphoma in pregnancy. *Current Hematologic Malignancy Reports* 2013; **8**: 211–217.

33. Ali S, Jones GL, Culligan DJ *et al.* Guidelines for the management of acute myelod leukemia in pregnancy. *British Journal of Haematology* 2015; **170**: 487–495.

34. Eyre TA, Lau IJ, Mackillop L, Collins GP. Classical Hodgkins lymphoma and pregnancy. *British Journal of Haematology* 2015; **69**: 613–630.

35. Royal College of Physicians, Royal College of Radiologists and RCOG. *The Effects of Cancer Treatment on Reproductive Function. Guidance on Management.* London: RCP; 2007.

36. NICE. NICE Clinical Guideline 156. Fertility: Assessment and Treatment for People with Fertility Problems; 2013. https://www.nice.org.uk

37. The Ethics Committee of the American Society for Reproductive Medicine. Fertility preservation and reproduction in patients facing gonadotoxic therapies: a committee opinion. *Fertility and Sterility* 2013; **100**: 1224–1231.

38. Loren AW, Mangu PB, Beck LN *et al.* Fertility preservation for patients with cancer: American Society of Clinical Oncology Clinical Practice Guideline Update. *Journal of Clinical Oncology* 2013; **31**: 2500–2510.

39. Cakmak H, Katz A, Cedars, MI, Rosen MP. Effective method for emergency fertility preservation: random-start controlled ovarian stimulation. *Fertility and Sterility* 2013; **100**: 1673–1680.

40. Kuang Y, Hong Q, Chen Q *et al.* Luteal-phase ovarian stimulation is feasible for producing competent oocytes in women undergoing in vitro fertilization/intracytoplasmic sperm injection treatment, with optimal pregnancy outcomes in frozen-thawed embryo transfer cycles. *Fertility and Sterility* 2014; **101**: 105–111.

41. Donnez J, Dolmans M, Pellicer A *et al.* Restoration of ovarian activity and pregnancy after transplantation of cryopreserved ovarian tissue: a review of 60 cases of reimplantation. *Fertility and Sterility* 2013; **99**: 1503–1513.

42. Dolmans M, Marinescu C, Saussoy P *et al.* Reimplantation of cryopreserved ovarian tissue from patients with acute lymphoblastic leukemia is potentially unsafe. *Blood* 2010; **116**: 2908–2914.

43. Rosendahl M, Greve T, Anderson CY. The safety of transplanting cryopreserved ovarian tissue in cancer patients: a review of the literature. *Journal of Assisted Reproduction and Genetics* 2012; **30**: 11–24.

44. Lockwood GM. Whose embryos are they anyway? *Clinical Ethics* 2007; **2**: 56–58.

45. Meirow D, Dor J. Epidemiology and infertility in cancer patients. In Tulandi T, Gosden R (eds) *Preservation of Fertility.* London:Taylor and Francis; 2004: 31.

Index

anti-D immunoglobulin prophylaxis,
114–116
first trimester, 115
hematological malignancies, 316
improving safety, 126
ITP, 47
postpartum, 115
recombinant monoclonal antibodies,
126
refusal, 116
routine antenatal (RAADP),
115–116
anti-E antibodies, 125
anti-embolism stockings (AES). *See*
graduated elastic compression
stockings
antiemetics, 315
antifungal agents, 315
antihypertensive agents, 271–272, 274
anti-Kell antibodies, 125, 127
anti-La antibodies, 182–183
anti-mullerian hormone (AMH),
320–321
antiphospholipid antibodies (aPL), 48,
178–179
case study, 186
isolated, without prior problems, 185
laboratory evaluation, 181–182
pathophysiological mechanisms,
178–179
antiphospholipid syndrome (APS),
177–186
case studies, 186
catastrophic (CAPS), 181
classification criteria, 177
clinical features, 179–181, 283
epidemiology, 178
laboratory evaluation, 181–182
management, 182–186
neonatal, 186
pathophysiology and etiology,
178–179
pre-eclampsia, 180, 271
primary (PAPS), 177
secondary (SAPS), 177
seronegative (SNAPS), 185
thromboprophylaxis, 142, 144
antiplatelet agents. *See also* aspirin
peripartum period, 166
pre-eclampsia, 272–273
prosthetic heart valves, 156, 157
anti-Ro antibodies, 182–183, 186
antithrombin, 9–11
concentrates, pre-eclampsia, 273
testing in pregnancy, 132, 194
antithrombin deficiency,
189–190
pregnancy loss, 191
thromboprophylaxis, 132,
142, 144

antithrombotic therapy
inherited thrombophilia, 192–193
myeloproliferative neoplasms,
303–304
pre-eclampsia, 272–273
anti-Xa monitoring
antenatal, 133, 142
peripartum period, 170
prosthetic heart valves, 156–157
apixaban, 134, 145, 151, 173
aplastic anemia, 99
argatroban, 173
ARMS (amplification refractory
mutation system), 85–86
arterial thrombosis
antiphospholipid syndrome, 179
previous, 183
ascites, fetal, 113
L-asparaginase, 314
aspirin
antenatal thromboprophylaxis, 144
antiphospholipid syndrome, 182, 184
inherited thrombophilia, 193, 195
myeloproliferative neoplasms, 297,
300–301, 303, 304
peripartum period, 166
pre-eclampsia, 272–273
prosthetic heart valves, 152, 156, 157
sickle cell disease, 61
thalassemia, 70
assisted reproductive techniques. *See
also* preimplantation genetic
diagnosis
antiphospholipid syndrome,
185, 186
cancer patients, 328–330
asthma, 270
autism spectrum disorder, 270
autoimmune cytopenias, 40–54
autoimmune hemolytic anemia
(AIHA), 40, 51–54
autoimmune neutropenia (AIN), 40,
49–51
azathioprine, 47, 185

balloon tamponade, uterus, 202
Barker hypothesis, 270
basophil count, 3, 4
bendamustine, 326
Bernard–Soulier syndrome (BSS), 44,
242–243
beta 2 glycoprotein 1 antibodies. *See*
anti-beta 2 glycoprotein 1
antibodies
beta-human chorionic gonadotrophin
(hCG), 283
β-thalassemias
antenatal screening, 80
case studies, 74–75
global distribution, 66

prenatal diagnosis, 78, 84, 85, 86
risk of affected offspring, 69
betrixaban, 173
bilirubin
amniotic fluid, 117, 118
hemolytic disease of fetus and
newborn, 112, 113
bisphosphonates, 72
bleeding disorders, heritable. *See*
inherited bleeding disorders
bleeding/hemorrhage
intracranial. *See* intracranial
hemorrhage
maternal von Willebrand disease, 237
neonatal hemophilia, 247, 248–249
neonatal thrombocytopenia, 49, 105
neonatal von Willebrand disease, 239
obstetric. *See* obstetric hemorrhage
blood films
iron deficiency anemia, 20
ITP, 44
vitamin B_{12} deficiency, 33
blood loss estimation, obstetric
hemorrhage, 209, 210
blood transfusion
autoimmune hemolytic anemia, 53
complications of massive, 211–212
fetal, hemolytic disease, 118–119, 122
fixed ratio protocols, severe PPH,
211, 222, 223
hematological malignancies, 316
iron deficiency anemia, 23, 25
neonatal exchange transfusion,
123–124
obstetric hemorrhage, 210–211,
220–223
sickle cell disease, 61–62
thalassemia, 67–68, 70
blood volume, 1, 15
B-Lynch brace suture, 203
bone disease, thalassemia, 72
bone marrow examination
autoimmune neutropenia, 50–51
folate deficiency, 36
idiopathic thrombocytopenic
purpura, 44
iron deficiency, 20–21
vitamin B_{12} deficiency, 33, 34
bone marrow failure syndromes,
inherited, 99
breast-feeding
anticoagulated women, 134, 160, 167
myeloproliferative neoplasms,
304–305
Burkitt lymphoma, 310, 312–313
busulfan, 322–324

C4b-binding protein, 10
calreticulin (*CALR*) gene mutations, 297
carbetocin, 202

339